Professional's Handbook of

DRUG THERAPY
for
PAIN

Professional's Handbook of

DRUG THERAPY
for
PAIN

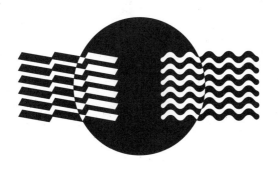

SPRINGHOUSE
Springhouse, Pennsylvania

Staff

Senior Publisher
Donna O. Carpenter

Editorial Director
William J. Kelly

Creative Director
Jake Smith

Art Director
Elaine Kasmer Ezrow

Drug Information Editor
Tracy Roux, RPh, PharmD

Project Editor
Catherine E. Harold

Clinical Project Editor
Christine Damico, RN, MSN, CPNP

Associate Editor
Raphe Cheli

Copy Editor
Beth E. Pitcher

Clinical Editors
Lisa M. Bonsall, RN, MSN, CRNP; Eileen Cassin Gallen, RN, BSN; Theresa P. Fulginiti, RN, BSN, CEN; Nancy LaPlante, RN, BSN; Pamela S. Messer, RN, MSN; Kimberly A. Zalewski, RN, MSN, CEN

Designers
Arlene Putterman (associate design director), Joseph John Clark, Donald G. Knauss, Susan Hopkins Rodzewich

Typographers
Diane Paluba (manager), Joyce Rossi Biletz

Manufacturing
Deborah Meiris (director), Patricia K. Dorshaw (manager), Otto Mezei (book production manager)

Editorial Assistants
Carol A. Caputo, Arlene P. Claffee

Library of Congress Cataloging-in-Publication Data
Professional's handbook of drug therapy for pain.
    p. ; cm.
    Includes bibliographical references and index.
    Analgesics – Handbooks, manuals, etc.
2. Pain – Handbooks, manuals, etc. I. Springhouse Corporation.
    [DNLM: 1. Pain – drug therapy – Handbooks.
WL 39 P964 2001]
RM319 .P76 2001
615'.783—dc21   00-050986
ISBN 1-58255-102-2 (alk. paper)

Contents

Clinical contributors and consultants

Christine Soucy Beason, PharmD
Clinical Pharmacist
The Hospice of the Florida Suncoast
Largo, Fla

Julie Albrecht Bianchi, RN, BSN
Clinical Nurse, Intermediate Intensive
 Care Unit (Surgical)
Thomas Jefferson University Hospital
Philadelphia, Pa

Susan Brown-Wagner, RN, MSN,
AOCN, CRNP
Director, Patient Services/Oncology
 Service Line
Scottsdale Healthcare
Scottsdale, Ariz

Lawrence Carey, PharmD
Clinical Pharmacist Supervisor
Thomas Jefferson Home Infusion
 Service
Philadelphia, Pa

Samyadev Datta, MD, FRCA
Assistant Attending Anesthesiologist
Memorial Sloan-Kettering Cancer
 Center
New York, NY

Christopher A. Fausel, PharmD, BCPS,
BCOP
Clinical Pharmacist, Adult
 Hematology/Oncology
Indiana University Hospital
Indianapolis, Ind

Beverly Sigl Felten, RN, PhD(c), APNP
President
Gero-Psych Nursing, S.C.
Lannon, Wis

David A. Fishbain, MD, MSc, FAPA
Professor, Psychiatry, Neurological
 Surgery, Anesthesiology
University of Miami Pain Center
S. Miami Beach, Fla

Elaine M. Herzog, RN, MS, ANP, CS
Coordinator, Anesthesia Pain
 Management
North Shore University Hospital
Manhasset, NY

Mary L. Heye, RN, PhD, CS
Associate Professor, School of
 Nursing
University of Texas Health Science
 Center at San Antonio
San Antonio, Tex

Lora McGuire, RN, MS
Professor of Nursing
Joliet Junior College
Joliet, Ill

Erin M. McMenamin, RN, MSN, CRNP,
AOCN
Pain Medicine Nurse Practitioner
University of Pennsylvania
Philadelphia, Pa

Roland G. Ottley, PA-C, JD
Director, Healthcare Consulting
Metronome Healthcare Management,
 LLC
Brooklyn, NY

John J. Park, MD
Instructor, Department of
 Anesthesiology
Thomas Jefferson University Hospital
Philadelphia, Pa

John B. Rose, MD
Associate Anesthesiologist
Children's Hospital of Philadelphia
Philadelphia, Pa

Michael L. Schmitz, MD
Associate Professor of Anesthesiology
    and Pediatrics
Arkansas Children's Hospital
Little Rock, Ark

Michele F. Shepherd, RPh, PharmD,
MS, BCPS, FASHP
Clinical Specialist
Abbott Northwestern Hospital
Minneapolis, Minn

Catherine Ultrino, RN, MS, OCN
Assistant Nurse Manager,
    Oncology/Hematology
Boston Medical Center
Boston, Mass

Kathleen M. Woodruff, MS, CRNP
Instructor
Johns Hopkins University School of
    Nursing
Baltimore, Md

Preface

Although health care professionals have known for centuries that pain causes great distress and suffering, only in the last 30 years or so has pain management been considered a distinct discipline in health care. Indeed, some patients still receive inadequate pain control from professionals who lack the knowledge or confidence to treat pain with appropriate assertiveness.

This book will help to remedy that problem. It combines broad coverage of pain management principles with detailed, up-to-date coverage of all the drugs and herbs commonly used in pain management today. It includes not only analgesics, but also important ancillary drugs, such as antidepressants, antiemetics, anticonstipation drugs, and more.

Part 1 starts with an overview of nociception and the more complex response that we call pain. It then provides general principles for assessing pain—which commonly can't be gauged or even detected by standard, objective diagnostic tests. And then it discusses the broad topic of pain management.

Part 2 contains close to 200 drugs commonly prescribed for patients with pain. They're listed in alphabetical order by generic name. Each drug entry includes information essential to the working health care professional: trade names, pharmacologic and therapeutic classifications, pregnancy risk category, controlled substance schedule, indications and dosages, pharmacodynamics, pharmacokinetics, contraindications and precautions, interactions, adverse reactions, overdose and treatment, special considerations, and patient teaching. The special considerations sections highlight important preparation, administration, and warning information, and also issues pertaining to pregnant, breast-feeding, pediatric, and geriatric patients.

Part 3 includes similar detailed coverage for about 25 herbs used for pain management. The herbs are arranged alphabetically by their most common names. Each herb entry includes practical information, such as other common and trade names, how the herb is supplied, reported uses, dosage, actions, cautions, interactions, adverse reactions, special considerations, and patient teaching.

Part 4 includes handy quick-reference appendices. You'll find in-depth coverage of both narcotic and nonnarcotic combination analgesic products, a generous list of pain management resources, and suggestions for further reading about pain management.

Perhaps more than any other disorder, pain combines physical and emotional components that can make pain management a challenging puzzle. Using this book as a key reference will help you solve the puzzle to each patient's benefit.

The *Professional's Handbook of Drug Therapy for Pain* provides an overview of concepts and tools that every clinician should know. It reviews nociception, pain, assessment techniques, and major pain-management principles. It also provides exhaustively reviewed, completely updated drug information on virtually every pain drug in current clinical use—including clinically approved but unlabeled uses. And it provides helpful information on herbs commonly used to manage pain.

Generic drugs

The individual drug entries provide detailed information on virtually all pain drugs in current clinical use, all arranged alphabetically by generic name for easy access. A guide word at the top of each page identifies the generic drug presented on that page. Each generic entry is complete where it falls alphabetically and doesn't require cross-referencing to other sections of the book.

In each drug entry, the generic name precedes an alphabetically arranged list of current trade names. (An open diamond signals products available only in Canada.) Next, the pharmacologic and therapeutic classifications identify the drug's pharmacologic or chemical category and its major clinical uses. Listing both classifications helps explain the multiple, varying, and sometimes overlapping uses of drugs within a single pharmaco-

> ### Defining pregnancy risk categories
>
> ▸ **A:** Adequate studies in pregnant women have failed to show a risk to the fetus.
> ▸ **B:** Animal studies haven't shown an adverse effect on the fetus, but clinical studies in humans are inadequate.
> ▸ **C:** Animal studies have shown an adverse effect on the fetus, but clinical studies in humans are inadequate. The drug may be useful despite its potential risks.
> ▸ **D:** The drug poses a risk to the fetus, but potential benefits may outweigh the risk.
> ▸ **X:** Studies in animals or humans show fetal abnormalities, or adverse reaction reports indicate evidence of fetal risk. The risks involved clearly outweigh potential benefits of using the drug.
> ▸ **NR:** Not rated.

logic class and among different classes. If appropriate, the next line identifies any drug that the Drug Enforcement Agency lists as a controlled substance and specifies the schedule of control as II, III, IV, or V.

Pregnancy risk category identifies the risk of birth defects using one of six categories (A, B, C, D, X, or NR) assigned by the Food and Drug Administration. (See *Defining pregnancy risk categories.*) Drugs in category A usually are considered safe to use in pregnancy; drugs in category X usually are contraindicated.

How supplied lists the preparations available for each drug (for example, tablets, capsules, solution, or injection), specifying available dosage forms and strengths.

Indications and dosages presents all clinically accepted indications with general dosage recommendations for adults and children; dosage adjustments for specific patient groups, such as the elderly and patients with renal or hepatic impairment, are included when appropriate. (Additional information may appear in the *Special considerations* section.) An asterisk signals a clinically accepted but unlabeled use. Dosage instructions reflect current clinical trends in therapeutics and should not be considered as absolute and universal recommendations. For individual application, dosage must be considered according to the patient's condition.

Pharmacodynamics explains the mechanism and effects of the drug's physiologic action.

Pharmacokinetics describes absorption, distribution, metabolism, and excretion of the drug. It includes onset and duration of action, peak levels, and half-life as appropriate.

Contraindications and precautions lists conditions that pose special risks in patients who receive the drug.

Interactions specifies the clinically significant additive, synergistic, or antagonistic effects that result from combined use of the drug with other drugs. Interactions appear in four categories as needed:

drug-drug, drug-herb, drug-food, and drug-lifestyle.

Effects on diagnostic tests lists significant interference with a diagnostic test or its result by direct effects on the test itself or by systemic drug effects that lead to misleading test results.

Adverse reactions lists the undesirable effects that may follow use of the drug; these effects are arranged by body systems (CNS, CV, EENT, GI, GU, Hematologic, Hepatic, Metabolic, Musculoskeletal, Respiratory, Skin, and Other). Local effects that occur at the site of drug administration (by application, infusion, or injection) and adverse reactions not specific to a single body system (for example, the effects of hypersensitivity) are listed under Other. The most common adverse reactions (those experienced by at least 10% of people taking the drug in clinical trials) are in *italic* type; less common reactions are in roman type; life-threatening reactions are in **bold italic** type; and reactions that are both common and life-threatening are in BOLD CAPITAL letters.

Overdose and treatment summarizes the signs and symptoms of drug overdose and recommends specific treatment as appropriate. Usually, this segment recommends emesis or gastric lavage, followed by activated charcoal to reduce the amount of drug absorbed and possibly a cathartic to eliminate the toxin. This section specifies antidotes, drug therapy, and other special care, if known. It also specifies the effects of hemodialysis or peritoneal dialysis for dialyzable drugs.

Special considerations offers detailed recommendations for drug preparation and administration, for care of the patient during therapy, and for use in pregnant, breast-feeding, pediatric, and geriatric patients.

Herbs

Herbs commonly used to manage pain are listed in alphabetical order. In general, the entries for herbs follow the format for drug entries. Alternate names and common trade names, when appropriate, appear below the main herb name. After that, each entry describes how the herb is supplied, reported uses, dosages, actions, cautions, interactions, adverse reactions, and special considerations.

Appendices

The appendices provide a review of narcotic and nonnarcotic analgesic combination products, resources for pain management, and a list of suggested readings.

Guide to abbreviations

ACE	angiotensin-converting enzyme	**GABA**	gamma-aminobutyric acid
ADH	antidiuretic hormone	**GFR**	glomerular filtration rate
AIDS	acquired immunodeficiency syndrome	**GI**	gastrointestinal
		gtt	drops
ALT	alanine aminotransferase	**GU**	genitourinary
aPTT	activated partial thrombo-plastin time	**G6PD**	glucose-6-phosphate dehydrogenase
AST	aspartate aminotransferase	H_1	histamine$_1$
AV	atrioventricular	H_2	histamine$_2$
b.i.d.	twice daily	**HIV**	human immunodeficiency virus
BUN	blood urea nitrogen	**hr**	hour
cAMP	cyclic adenosine monophos-phate	**h.s.**	at bedtime
CBC	complete blood count	**ICU**	intensive care unit
CK	creatine kinase	**I.D.**	intradermal
CMV	cytomegalovirus	**I.M.**	intramuscular
CNS	central nervous system	**IND**	investigational new drug
COPD	chronic obstructive pulmonary disease	**INR**	international normalized ratio
CSF	cerebrospinal fluid	**IPPB**	intermittent positive-pressure breathing
CV	cardiovascular	**IU**	international unit
CVA	cerebrovascular accident	**I.V.**	intravenous
D_5W	dextrose 5% in water	**kg**	kilogram
DNA	deoxyribonucleic acid	**M**	molar
ECG	electrocardiogram	m^2	square meter
EEG	electroencephalogram	**MAO**	monoamine oxidase
EENT	eyes, ears, nose, throat	**mcg**	microgram
FDA	Food and Drug Administration	**mEq**	milliequivalent
		mg	milligram
g	gram	**MI**	myocardial infarction
G	gauge		

ml	milliliter
mm^3	cubic millimeter
NSAID	nonsteroidal anti-inflammatory drug
OTC	over-the-counter
PABA	para-aminobenzoic acid
PCA	patient-controlled analgesia
P.O.	by mouth
P.R.	by rectum
p.r.n.	as needed
PT	prothrombin time
PTT	partial thromboplastin time
PVC	premature ventricular contraction
q	every
q.d.	every day
q.i.d.	four times daily
RBC	red blood cell
RDA	recommended daily allowance
REM	rapid eye movement
RNA	ribonucleic acid
SA	sinoatrial
S.C.	subcutaneous
SIADH	syndrome of inappropriate antidiuretic hormone
S.L.	sublingual
T_3	triiodothyronine
T_4	thyroxine
t.i.d.	three times daily
U	units
USP	United States Pharmacopeia
UTI	urinary tract infection
WBC	white blood cell

PART 1

Principles of pain control

Chapter 1

Understanding pain

Although the experience of pain may seem like a simple one-two punch—you sustain an injury and you feel its effects—the process actually involves complex physiologic and psychological responses that vary from person to person and even from day to day. To understand pain fully, you must consider both its physiologic aspects, called nociception, and its psychological aspects.

▶ NOCICEPTION

Pain-causing events, such as getting a cut or burn, are known as noxious stimuli; they damage or threaten to damage tissue. By doing so, they activate a special category of sensory receptors called nociceptors. Nociceptors connect with the axons of neurons that send information about the pain-causing event to the spinal cord. There, the electrical information activates autonomic and nociceptive reflexes that transmit pain signals supraspinally to the brain.

Functionally, nociception can be divided into four stages: transduction, abstraction, modulation, and plasticity.

Transduction

Transduction is the rapid conversion of stimulus energy (mechanical, chemical, or thermal) into neural activity—specifically into changes in electrical potentials in nerve membranes. (See *Transduction: First step of nociception*, page 4.) When a primary afferent neuron receives a nociceptive stimulus, the axon of this specialized receptor conveys electrical information toward the spinal cord or cranial nuclei. The cell body rests in a dorsal root ganglion or a ganglion of a cranial nerve.

Specialized sensory nerve endings (called somatovisceral receptors) in skin, deep tissue, and viscera convert mechanical, thermal, and chemical energy into action potentials. These sensory receptors are excited only by stimuli applied in the region they innervate, known as their receptive fields. Receptive fields of various primary afferent fibers vary greatly in size. They may be continuous or discontinuous. Adjacent receptive fields overlap extensively.

Although transduction mechanisms differ for thermal, mechanical, and chemical stimuli, they're also similar in that the stimulus interacts with highly specialized transducer molecules embedded in the receptor membrane. The transducer molecule then undergoes a transformation that directly or indirectly opens sodium channels in the receptor membrane. Sodium influx from the extracellular fluid causes the receptor to depolarize, which initiates an action potential.

Transducer molecules vary according to the type of stimulus they transduce. Chemosensitive transducer molecules have binding sites that will accept only one type

Transduction: First step of nociception

In transduction, a mechanical, thermal, or chemical stimulus interacts with receptor molecules at the tips of nociceptive primary afferent neurons (commonly called free nerve endings). As a result, sodium channels open and extracellular sodium flows in, causing the receptor molecule to depolarize, which creates an action potential. Electrical energy then travels to the spinal cord and on to the brain, signaling pain.

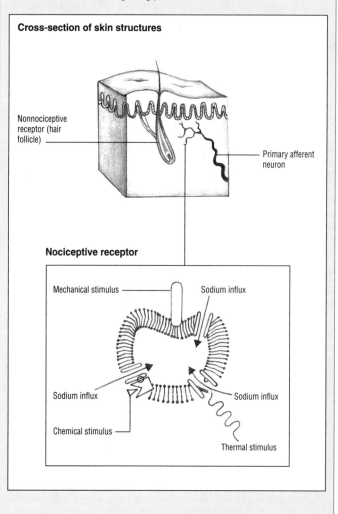

Cross-section of skin structures

Nonnociceptive receptor (hair follicle)

Primary afferent neuron

Nociceptive receptor

Mechanical stimulus

Sodium influx

Sodium influx

Chemical stimulus

Sodium influx

Thermal stimulus

of chemical. Mechanosensitive ionic channels are opened by mechanical distortion of a cell membrane. Thermosensitive transducers have molecular gates that open when heated or cooled.

Different receptors have varying degrees of specificity for different types of stimuli. Receptors that respond to only one type of stimulus energy, heat for example, are termed unimodal receptors. Polymodal receptors respond to two or more types of stimuli. Receptors also differ in their sensitivity, which is the number of action potentials evoked by a given stimulus. Somatovisceral receptors vary greatly in their specificity and sensitivity.

Somatovisceral receptors can be divided into two groups: nonnociceptive, or innocuous, receptors, which can be activated by stimuli that don't cause damage or produce pain, such as touch and hair movement, and nociceptive-specific receptors, or nociceptors, which respond only to stimuli that potentially or actually damage tissue. Although nociceptors are considered specialized pain receptors, nonnociceptive receptors can play a role in pain perception as well.

Nonnociceptive receptors

Although they usually don't signal pain directly, nonnociceptive somatovisceral receptors can affect pain perception in several ways:
▶ In some disorders, innocuous stimuli can become painful, a condition known as hyperalgesia.
▶ Innocuous sensory input can modulate the perception of pain.
▶ In the absence of nociceptive pathways, the nervous system may be able to infer the presence of a noxious stimulus from excessive activity in nonnociceptive primary afferent neurons.

Several types of nonnociceptive sensory receptors exist, each with a distinctive structure, function, depth under the skin, location in the body, response profile, and conduction velocity. They share the features of unimodality, high sensitivity, and low activation threshold. The low activation threshold is what differentiates nonnociceptive receptors from nociceptors; the latter require a higher stimulus energy for activation.

Nociceptive receptors

The most important characteristic of nociceptive somatovisceral receptors is that they respond only to stimuli that damage or threaten to damage tissue. Mechanical, thermal, and chemical stimuli that don't damage tissue don't activate the nociceptors. For example, nociceptors respond when you touch a hot frying pan, but not when you touch a cool one. Commonly called free nerve endings, nociceptors differ from nonnociceptive receptors in several ways:
▶ Nociceptors aren't macroscopically specialized. Under an electron microscope, however, they show a highly complex structure and function that reflects their highly specialized transduction properties.
▶ Some nociceptors are polymodal, whereas all nonnociceptive receptors are unimodal.
▶ The conduction velocity of nociceptors (0.5 to 30 meters/second) is less than that of nonnociceptive primary afferent neurons (30 to 120 meters/second).
▶ Although both nociceptors and nonnociceptive receptors are distributed throughout the body, their

density varies. For example, the fingertips contain many nonnociceptive receptors but relatively fewer nociceptors, presumably because pain sensations might interfere with the sense of touch, for which the fingers are specially adapted. In contrast, the cornea and teeth contain relatively more nociceptors.

▶ Unlike nonnociceptive receptors, nociceptors can be activated by endogenous chemicals, such as inflammatory mediators, or by exogenous compounds.

Stimulating these nociceptors creates the physiologic response that we recognize as pain. Keep in mind, however, that pain doesn't result from a single stimulation of a single nociceptor. For a person to perceive pain, either the action potential must occur repeatedly in a single nociceptor, or the action potential must occur in many nociceptors at once.

Nociceptors occur throughout the skin, deep tissue, and viscera. They include superficial somatic nociceptors, deep somatic nociceptors, and visceral nociceptors.

Superficial somatic nociceptors
Superficial, or cutaneous, somatic nociceptors come in two types: unimodal and polymodal. Unimodal receptors give rise to myelinated afferent nerve fibers with conduction velocities of 2 to 30 meters/second. They're called A-δ fibers. (See *Comparing A-δ and C fibers*.) The receptive field of a typical A-δ fiber ranges from 1 to 8 cm². Activation of these fibers evokes sharp, localized pain. The receptors respond primarily to mechanical and thermal stimuli.

Polymodal nociceptors give rise to unmyelinated afferent nerve fibers with conduction velocities of 0.5 to 2 meters/second. They're called C fibers, and they make up about 75% of all nociceptors. The receptive field of a typical C fiber contains 3 to 20 small areas of less than 1 mm² each. Activation of polymodal nociceptors typically evokes long-lasting, burning pain. These receptors respond to mechanical, thermal, and chemical stimuli—especially to chemicals released during inflammation, exercise, or disease. They also respond strongly to capsaicin, the hot ingredient in chili peppers. Their absolute firing rates are typically lower than unimodal nociceptors.

When both A-δ and C fibers are activated, as from submerging a foot in overly hot bath water, the result is an immediate, sharp, easily localized pain followed by a second, long-lasting, burning pain. That's because the stimulus evoked both the fast and the slow pain fibers.

Deep somatic nociceptors
Deep somatic nociceptors occur in muscle, fascia, connective tissue, and joints. Although similar to cutaneous nociceptors, deep nociceptors respond to somewhat different stimuli. Specifically, they respond most to stimuli that evoke deep pain. For example, they're activated by the excessive force that can occur in traumatic injury and by chemicals (such as lactate and potassium) that can cause muscle pain.

Visceral nociceptors
Years ago, most experts thought that the viscera contained no nociceptors because direct manipulation of an organ produced no pain

Comparing A-δ and C fibers

The brain registers a pain sensation differently based on whether the pain-causing stimulus activated A-δ fibers or C fibers. Both are cutaneous somatic nociceptors, but they differ in several important ways, as described and illustrated below.

A-δ fibers

A-δ fibers are unimodal and give rise to myelinated afferent nerve fibers. They conduct pain signals at 2 to 30 meters/second. They typically have contiguous receptive fields of about 1 to 8 cm² in diameter. These receptors respond mainly to mechanical and thermal stimuli, and they produce sharp, localized pain.

C fibers

C fibers are polymodal and give rise to unmyelinated afferent nerve fibers. They conduct pain signals much more slowly, at 0.5 to 2 meters/second. They typically have punctate receptive fields that contain 3 to 20 areas, each less than 1 mm² in diameter. These receptors respond to mechanical, thermal, and especially chemical stimuli, and they produce long-lasting, burning pain.

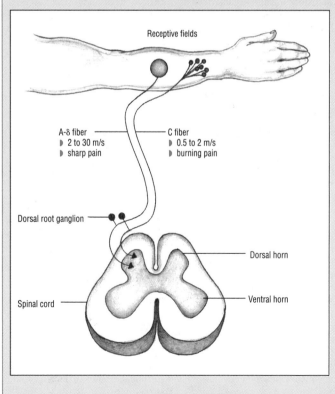

Receptive fields

A-δ fiber
▶ 2 to 30 m/s
▶ sharp pain

C fiber
▶ 0.5 to 2 m/s
▶ burning pain

Dorsal root ganglion

Dorsal horn

Ventral horn

Spinal cord

during light surgical anesthesia. However, disorders such as appendicitis and angina make it clear that pain can indeed arise from internal organs or viscera. It probably does so via slow-conducting, unencapsulated nerve endings of A-δ and C fibers that occur throughout the viscera and somatic structures.

The stimuli that produce pain when applied to the viscera differ from those that produce pain when applied to skin. What's more, stimuli may differ even from organ to organ. For example, in hollow organs, such as the colon and stomach, nociceptors are stimulated by distension. In solid organs, such as the testes, they're stimulated most effectively by compression.

Abstraction

In the second phase of nociception, known as central processing and abstraction, nociceptive neural signals are processed by the central nervous system (CNS) to extract relevant information. To understand this process, imagine the incoming information provided by nociceptors as a "picture" of noxious stimulation.

If you look at a picture that appears in a newspaper, you can see that it's made up of a myriad of tiny dots. Your brain doesn't simply recognize the dots, however; it also recognizes the image conveyed by the picture. The brain does the same thing with the picture of incoming noxious stimuli. In other words, it abstracts the features of the picture that are important—the meaning of the picture. Processing and extraction of relevant features of sensory input is known as abstraction.

Modulation

Modulation, which means control, refers to the exogenous and endogenous ways that pain may be reduced or enhanced. For example, drugs can be used to reduce pain. Cognitive influences can either reduce (distraction, for example) or enhance (anticipation, for example) pain. Many other physical and psychological influences can modulate pain as well.

Indeed, the body itself can modulate nociceptive inputs and the perception of pain. It does so via an anatomically restricted, opioid peptide-related means of pain control located in the midbrain. Here, exogenous opioids and endogenous opioid peptides activate inhibitory influences that descend to the spinal cord.

Neurotransmitters, mainly serotonin and norepinephrine, mediate this descending inhibition. Serotonin is contained in the terminals of neurons descending from the ventral medulla. Norepinephrine is contained in the terminals of neurons descending from the dorsolateral pons. Accordingly, drugs that mimic the actions of serotonin and norepinephrine act as analgesics when delivered directly into the epidural or intrathecal space.

For example, clonidine has been used to treat cancer pain because it acts like norepinephrine in the spinal cord. Opioids given exogenously or released endogenously act at opioid receptors but also in the spinal cord. And certain antidepressants that mimic or facilitate the actions of serotonin or norepinephrine probably provide a helpful adjunct to pain control by allowing a lower opioid dosage and causing tolerance to develop at a slower rate.

Descending pain modulation

This endogenous system of descending modulation can either inhibit or enhance pain. Many influences can activate it. For example, stress, fear, and pain itself can activate inhibitory descending systems. Certain disorders, such as hypertension, can also help activate the descending inhibitory system that reduces pain. Both experimentally-induced increases in blood pressure and pre-existing hypertension lessen a person's sensitivity to noxious stimuli.

Anxiety and apprehension can enhance pain; however, descending facilitation of pain may play a particularly large role in unusual chronic pain states. In fact, it's possible that the pain-facilitating system may be activated but not turned off in these disorders, thus contributing to tonic facilitation, rather than tonic inhibition, of spinal neuron activity.

In certain circumstances, the facilitation of nociceptive information is protective, such as during tissue repair. However, if such a system remains inappropriately activated after tissue repair is complete, typical nonnociceptive stimulation could possibly be perceived as pain. Because the mechanisms of chronic pain are poorly understood, researchers are actively studying the role of endogenous pain-enhancing systems.

Gate control modulation

Some pain modulation systems don't involve descending systems. They include acupuncture, dorsal column stimulation, and transcutaneous electrical nerve stimulation (TENS). These modulation systems are based on a theory of pain transmission known as the gate control theory. It holds that spinal cord cells that transmit nociceptive information to supraspinal sites function as a spinal gate.

According to this model, activity in small-diameter afferent fibers (A-δ and C fibers) opens the gate that allows nociception. In contrast, activity in large-diameter, myelinated, nonnociceptive afferent fibers (A-α and A-β fibers) close the gate that allows nociception. The balance of activity between nociceptive and nonnociceptive afferent fibers can affect the position of the gate. In other words, a relatively open gate means more pain; a relatively closed gate means less pain. The intensity of pain is thereby modulated.

This theory explains at least partially why dorsal column stimulation and TENS work. Electrical stimulation of large-diameter, myelinated fibers in the dorsal column of the spinal cord or in peripheral nerves through the application of a TENS unit closes the gate and reduces pain. Similarly, forms of acupuncture that activate large-diameter peripheral myelinated axons may close the spinal gate. However, various forms of acupuncture probably employ various mechanisms of pain control, all of which can't be explained by the gate control theory.

Plasticity

Perception of sensory stimuli isn't a constant; it changes in response to development, environment, and disease or injury. These changes are collectively called plasticity. Plasticity can be brief (minutes to hours), prolonged (hours to weeks), or even permanent.

Learning and memory are familiar forms of plasticity. The CNS response to nociceptive stimuli also exhibits plasticity. It can result from inflammatory tissue damage, injury to peripheral nerves, or damage to portions of the CNS that mediate pain sensations. It also can result from a person's childhood experience of pain, current attitudes toward pain, and recent traumatic or inflammatory tissue damage.

Allodynia is one example of plasticity. It involves the feeling of pain in response to a stimulus that normally isn't painful. For example, the patient perceives that a bedsheet touching a wounded limb is painful. Another example of plasticity is hyperalgesia. It involves the perception that a normally painful stimulus is more painful than usual. A central pain state can be an example of plasticity as well.

▶ PSYCHOLOGICAL ASPECTS OF PAIN

The concept of pain is distinct from the concept of nociception because the pain experience includes a crucial psychological component. Nociception refers only to the body's physiologic reactions—neural events and reflex responses—to certain stimuli. But the way a person experiences a painful stimulus stems from much more than that physiologic reaction.

The experience of pain is influenced by a person's culture, by anticipation, by previous experience, by various emotional and cognitive contributions, and by the context in which the pain occurs. Accordingly, reactions to stimuli that produce pain vary among people and even for the same person at different times. Nociception is a sensory process. In contrast, the experience of pain is a perceptual process that requires attention to and interpretation of the nociceptive input.

Pain is such a subjective experience that it sometimes may have nothing at all to do with nociception—and vice versa. For example, noxious stimuli applied below the level of a spinal cord injury can cause nociceptive withdrawal reflexes because the peripheral nociceptors and spinal reflex circuitry are intact. However, because the information can't be transmitted past the injury to the brain, the patient perceives no pain.

On the other hand, after having a cerebrovascular accident, certain patients develop deep, aching, or burning pain in the area of sensory loss or neurologic disability contralateral to the cerebral infarct. They experience this pain without any peripheral stimulation. Indeed, various pain syndromes exist without evidence of pathophysiology. Yet the person may experience debilitating pain.

Interpreting the pain experience

When a person touches an unexpectedly hot surface, two things happen: he has a reflex withdrawal from the hot stimulus, and he becomes consciously aware that he just burned himself. The conscious awareness that a peripheral event is painful requires supraspinal integration of the information in several areas of the brain. Most important, it requires interpretation of the event. The combination of supraspinal integration and conscious interpretation make pain a unique experience.

Three ascending tracts

Nociceptive neurons that ascend from the periphery to the brain can be divided into three tracts, all of which travel in the anterolateral quadrant of the spinal cord and each of which performs a slightly different function in the recognition and interpretation of pain.

Neospinothalamic tract

The neospinothalamic tract is, evolutionarily speaking, a relatively young pathway that mediates the sensory-discriminative aspect of pain. It projects to the ventrolateral and ventromedial portions of the thalamus adjacent to but not overlapping the projections of other systems involved in sensory discrimination. From there, the thalamus projects to portions of the parietal lobe of the cerebral cortex that mediate perception and processing of both nonnociceptive and nociceptive information.

Paleospinothalamic tract

An older pathway, the paleospiothalamic tract mediates the motivational-affective aspect of pain. It projects to the intralaminar portions of the thalamus, which are involved with subjective elements of sensory input rather than with discrimination. From there, the intralaminar nuclei project primarily to the limbic system and cortex, which mediate motivational, subjective, and affective sensations and behavior.

Spinobulbar pathway

The spinobulbar pathway actually includes two tracts. The spinoreticular tract ascends to the medulla. The spinomesencephalic tract ascends to the midbrain. There, they activate descending modulation of nociception. Via continued projections from the brainstein or midbrain to the thalamus, they also may influence the motivational-affective component of pain.

Two aspects of pain

The two aspects of the pain experience are sometimes called the sensory-discriminative aspect and the motivational-affective aspect. In the former, neural processes converge to quickly allow a person to pinpoint the location, intensity, and duration of a painful stimulus. For instance, the person who touches a hot surface knows instantly which hand is involved, which finger is affected, and which area of that finger touched the heat. This highly developed ability to quickly characterize and locate the site of pain is best developed in the skin and is relatively poorly developed in deeper tissues such as the viscera.

The motivational-affective aspect of pain involves the emotional responses that make pain personal and unique. The brain sites where these responses take place are different from the sites where sensory-discriminative activities take place. Motivational-affective activities are accomplished by more basic, relatively indirect neural pathways that emotionally color a person's response to nociceptive input. (See *Three ascending tracts*.)

Overlying both the sensory-discriminative and motivational-affective components of pain are cultural and cognitive issues (called the cognitive-evaluative phase) that influence a person's interpretation of and concerns about pain. Cognitive contributions include attention, anxiety, anticipation, and other experiences with pain. For example, if a person had a traumatic previous experience with a painful procedure, then anxiety about the procedure and anticipation of repeated pain will color the person's interpretation of and response to any pain that arises during the procedure. Thus, cognitive contributions can significantly modulate the response and reaction to a painful stimulus.

Evolving view of pain

Over the years, our view of pain has evolved from a completely sensory one to an almost completely psychological one and back to the belief that pain includes both physical and emotional components. Sensory models present pain as entirely caused by physical factors. Psychogenic models claim psychological problems as the primary cause of chronic pain. Indeed, any report of pain that can't be confirmed by observed pathology is viewed even today as pain with a psychological component. The American Psychiatric Association has created three pain-related diagnoses:

⦁ pain disorder associated with psychological factors
⦁ pain disorder associated with a general medical condition
⦁ pain disorder associated with both psychological factors and a general medical condition.

The shortcomings of most of the models described below lie chiefly in their reliance on either physical or psychological factors to explain a pain response—particularly for a person with chronic pain. In reality, the model best able to explain the pain experience is almost certainly the one that best integrates physical and psychological characteristics.

Sensory model

Originally, experts defined pain with a sensory model. In other words, they explained that a painful stimulus caused a pain signal in the person's brain. The amount of pain the person felt linked directly to the amount, degree, or nature of sensory input or physical damage. Clinically, then, you would expect that a person with greater tissue damage would feel and report greater pain.

The sensory model fails for several reasons. For instance, patients with equal degrees and types of tissue damage vary widely in the amount of pain they report. Also, surgical procedures that cut the neurologic pathways on which pain signals travel may fail to alleviate pain. Plus, patients with equal degrees and types of tissue damage respond differently to equal amounts of pain-relieving drugs.

Finally, patients with some painful conditions (such as recurrent headaches) may show no tissue damage at all, despite the use of sophisticated diagnostic procedures, such as computed tomography scans and magnetic resonance imaging.

Pain-prone model

This psychogenic model was proposed to help explain the role of emotions in pain. It posits that a certain type of depression may predispose a person to feel persistent pain. The typical affected person tends to deny emotional and interpersonal problems, to be unable to deal with anger and hostility, to crave affection, to be dependent, and to have a family history of depression, alcoholism, and chronic pain. The theory is that, once the psychological pain creation mechanism has evolved, the person no longer needs peripheral stimulation to feel pain. The problem with this model is that no evidence exists to support it.

Motivational model

This model, suggested by many insurance companies, holds that pain unsubstantiated by observed physical problems must stem from malingering or an exaggeration of symptoms. The assumption here is that patients are motivated primarily by financial gain. However, no studies have shown dramatic improvement in pain reports after a person receives a disability award. The official position of the Institute of Medicine is that malingering is extremely rare in patients who complain of chronic pain.

Operant conditioning model

In the operant conditioning model, behavioral manifestations of acute pain—such as withdrawal, avoidance of activities believed to worsen pain, and attempts to escape from noxious sensations—are thought to be subject to the principles of operant conditioning. These principles include positive reinforcement, negative reinforcement, and avoidance learning. (See *Principles of operant conditioning.*)

The operant view proposes that acute pain behaviors such as avoidance of painful activities may be controlled by external reinforce-

> ## Principles of operant conditioning
>
> Operant conditioning includes three major concepts: positive reinforcement, negative reinforcement, and avoidance learning.
>
> *Positive reinforcement* occurs when a behavior elicits positive consequences or a reward of some type. As a result, the person is motivated to repeat the behavior. Pain behaviors may be positively reinforced, for example, when a person receives attention from others for limping or grimacing.
>
> *Negative reinforcement* occurs when stopping a behavior elicits positive consequences or a reward. Pain behaviors may be negatively reinforced, for example, when a person receives attention from others when he stops complaining about his minor aches and pains.
>
> *Avoidance learning* occurs when performing a behavior helps to avoid a negative consequence or a loss of reward. For example, a person with a back injury may undergo avoidance learning when he understands that exercise, although it may be painful, will ultimately help to avoid increased disability through loss of muscle strength, flexibility, and endurance.

ments. This concept has also been called secondary gain. For example, when back pain flares up, a woman may lie down on the floor and hold her back. Her husband may unknowingly reinforce his wife's pain behaviors by spending extra time with her, rubbing her back, or bringing her something to eat. Another powerful way he may reinforce her pain behaviors is by permitting her to avoid undesirable activities when her back is painful.

It's important to recognize that this model doesn't suggest conscious deception or malingering (in which the person consciously fakes symptoms for some gain, usually financial). The pain sufferer doesn't communicate pain as a conscious way to elicit attention or avoid undesirable activities. Rather, reinforcement of pain behaviors is more likely the result of a gradual, unintended process that neither person recognizes.

The operant conditioning model may provide the basis for effective treatment of selected patients with chronic pain. Treatment aims to eliminate pain behaviors by withdrawing attention from them and positively reinforcing well behaviors. However, like other pain models, this one has flaws. For instance, it uses overt behaviors as the sole basis for understanding pain, distress, and suffering. In reality, we have no way of deciding whether an observed behavior results from pain, from a structural abnormality, or from a coping response.

Respondent conditioning model

Some people think of chronic or recurrent acute pain as fitting in the classical or respondent conditioning model. Thus, if a nociceptive stimulus is frequently paired with a neutral stimulus, the neutral stimulus will eventually come to elicit a pain response. For example, patients who receive painful treatments from a physical therapist may become conditioned to having a negative emotional response to the physical therapist, to the treatment room, or to any other stimulus linked to the original nociceptive stimulus. The negative emotional reaction may cause muscle tensing, worsening of pain, and a reinforcement of the association between the physical therapist and the pain.

Over time, the patient may associate a growing number of stimuli with pain production—a process called stimulus generalization. Sitting, walking, engaging in cognitively demanding work or social interaction, having sex, or even thinking about these activities may increase anticipatory anxiety and cause physiologic and biochemical changes.

Subsequently, patients may display maladaptive responses to many activities other than those that initially induced pain. Physical abnormalities thought to result from chronic pain, such as a distorted gait, decreased range of motion, and muscle fatigue, may actually be secondary to maladaptive behavior changes adopted through learning. As pain becomes associated with a growing list of situations and activities, the patient will avoid them, resulting in greater physical deconditioning, isolation, physical and emotional disability, and ultimately more pain.

Social learning model

From a social learning perspective, the acquisition of pain behaviors can occur via observation and modeling. People, especially children, acquire new behaviors by observing others. They acquire attitudes about health, health care, symptoms, and physiologic processes—as well as appropriate responses to injury and disease—from their parents and social environment. They may ignore or overreact to symptoms, depending upon their social learning experiences.

Ample experimental evidence points to the role of social learning in pain. Physiologic responses to pain stimuli may be conditioned by observing others in pain. For example, patients on a burn unit have much opportunity to observe the responses of other burn patients. In another example, the children of people with chronic pain tend to display more illness behaviors, make more visits to the school nurse, and choose more pain-related responses to defined scenarios than children of healthy parents. Differences in social learning may be one reason why people with similar physical problems have highly variable behavioral responses.

Gate control model
The gate control model, now more than three decades old, is an integrative model that includes both physiologic and psychological factors in its definition of pain. It proposes that the dorsal horn substantia gelatinosa of the spinal cord contains a spinal gating mechanism that inhibits or facilitates transmission of peripheral nerve impulses to the brain, depending on the diameters of the active peripheral fibers and the influence of certain brain processes. In short, it postulates that the spinal gate is influenced by the relative amount of activity in afferent, large-diameter (myelinated) and small-diameter (unmyelinated) nociceptive fibers that converge in the dorsal horns.

The gate control model contradicts the notion that pain is either somatic or psychogenic and instead says that both concepts potentiate or moderate pain percep-

tion. In this model, for example, pain isn't understood to result from depression or vice versa. The two are seen as evolving simultaneously. The gate control theory's emphasis on ascending and descending modulation of dorsal horn input, and the dynamic role of the brain in pain processes and perception, fosters inclusion of psychological variables, such as past experience, attention, mood, and other cognitive activities, into current research and therapy.

Cognitive-behavioral model
This most recent pain model incorporates many of the psychological variables of operant and respondent learning, namely anticipation, avoidance, and reinforcement. However, it suggests that cognitive factors (particularly expectations) rather than conditioning should take central importance. The model suggests that so-called conditioned reactions, such as feeling anxiety and pain when thinking about exercise, are largely self-activated based on learned expectations rather than being automatically evoked based on conditioned stimuli. The critical factor for the cognitive-behavioral model, therefore, isn't that events occur together in time, but that people learn to predict them and to engage in anticipatory anxiety and avoidance behaviors.

The cognitive-behavioral perspective suggests that behavior and emotions are influenced by personal interpretations rather than solely by the objective characteristics of an event. This model emphasizes that the experience of pain is influenced by the ongoing reciprocal relationships among physical, cognitive, affective, social, and behavioral influences. Thus, the experience of pain is shaped by personal attitudes and beliefs that filter and interact reciprocally with sensory experience. emotions, social influences, and behavioral responses. Moreover, these behaviors may elicit responses from significant others that reinforce both adaptive and maladaptive modes of thinking, feeling, and behaving.

Thus, this model is reciprocal and synergistic. Pain management strategies based on this model stem from certain central assumptions about people and the conditions that influence pain perception. (See *Tenets of the cognitive-perceptual model.*)

In the cognitive-behavioral model, people with pain are viewed as having negative expectations about their own ability to control the pain experience or to engage in certain activities without pain. These negative judgments and expectations may reduce the person's coping efforts and activity, which may in turn contribute to psychological distress (helplessness) and subsequent physical limitations.

Over time, the physical factors that contributed to the original pain experience may play a less important role in the reason for the patient's disability. Meanwhile, secondary problems caused by deconditioning may worsen and maintain the pain.

Beliefs about pain

Patients' attitudes, beliefs, expectations of themselves, coping resources, and thoughts about the health care system affect the entire spectrum of their pain behaviors. Because behavior and emotions are influenced by the interpretation of events, not simply by the facts

of those events, patients may differ greatly in their beliefs about pain. For instance, patients who believe their pain results from ongoing tissue damage or a progressive disease are likely to experience more suffering and behavioral dysfunction than those who view their pain as the result of a stable, manageable problem. A person who awakens with a headache believing that it results from excessive alcohol consumption responds very differently from someone who believes his headache suggests a brain tumor.

The beliefs that these scenarios represent have a direct relationship with a patient's coping ability, focus of attention, and outlook for rehabilitation. In other words, certain beliefs may lead to maladaptive coping, increased suffering, and greater disability.

Coping

A person's beliefs, judgments, and expectations about the consequences of an event—and the person's belief in his ability to influence the outcome—can affect his ability to function in two ways: by directly influencing his mood and by altering his coping ability.

For example, patients with low back pain typically fail to comply with prescribed exercise tasks independent of the physical exertion they require or the actual pain they cause. Instead, the previous experience of pain may tend to foster a negative view of their abilities and an expectation of increased pain when they exercise. Together, these beliefs form a rationale for avoiding exercise.

The expectation of exercise-related pain reinforces patients' beliefs about the pervasiveness of their disability. Patients who believe that disability is a necessary reaction to pain, and that activity is dangerous, are most likely to experience continued disability. Their failure to perform prescribed activities robs them of the corrective feedback that could help to counteract their beliefs, and it reinforces the perception of helplessness and incapacity.

In contrast, developing positive coping strategies may alter the perception of pain intensity and promote the patient's ability to manage or tolerate pain and to continue everyday activities. Coping consists of spontaneously employed, purposeful acts and includes both overt and covert behaviors. Overt coping strategies include rest, drug therapy, and the use of relaxation and other such techniques. Covert coping strategies include distraction, reassuring oneself that the pain will diminish, seeking information, and solving problems.

Active coping strategies (efforts to function in spite of pain or to distract oneself from pain) lead to adaptive functioning. Passive coping strategies (depending on others for help in pain control and restricting one's activities) lead to greater pain and depression. Although the overall benefits of active coping strategies are clear, little evidence exists to support one active coping strategy over another. A strategy may be helpful in one situation or for one person and not helpful in a different situation or for another person. Likewise, certain strategies may be helpful at one time and maladaptive or ineffective at another.

The larger issue is that patients who know how to use adaptive coping strategies experience less

> ### Tenets of the cognitive-perceptual model
>
> The cognitive-perceptual model of pain perception stems from five basic beliefs:
>
> - People actively process information rather than simply reacting to the environment. To make sense of stimuli, a person filters and organizes information based on prior learning, information-processing strategies, and more.
> - Thinking influences a person's affect and physiologic arousal, both of which may influence behavior. Conversely, affect, physiology, and behavior can influence thinking.
> - Successful interventions to alter maladaptive behavior focus on maladaptive thoughts and feelings as well as on behaviors. Changing only thoughts, only feelings, or only behaviors doesn't necessarily change the other two.
> - Behavior is reciprocally determined by both the environment and the person. Because people don't simply respond passively to their environment, they in essence create their own environment. A patient who seeks medical attention for symptoms creates an environment different from that created by the person who self-medicates.
> - Because people develop and maintain maladaptive thoughts, feelings, and behaviors, they can also change those maladaptive modes of responding.

pain and increased pain tolerance. The most important feature of poor coping seems to be "catastrophizing" (extremely negative thoughts about one's plight) rather than choosing poorly among adaptive coping strategies.

Attention

Pain can change the way a person processes pain-related and other information by focusing attention on bodily signals. As these signals change, the patient may ascribe the changes to a worsening of the underlying disease—a tendency that typically results in increased reports of pain. Patients who don't attribute their symptoms to worsening of the disease tend to report less pain, even when their disease is actually progressing in a similar manner.

Keep in mind that a person's beliefs and expectations about a disease are difficult to change once they're formed. Patients tend to avoid experiences that could invalidate their beliefs, and they guide their behavior in keeping with these beliefs. Consequently, they may receive little or no corrective feedback.

Rehabilitation

Beliefs about pain are also important in influencing a patient's level of disability, response to treatment, and compliance with prescribed activities. Successful rehabilitation seems to be accompanied by an important cognitive shift; the patient must change from believing that he's helpless and passive to believing in his ability to function regardless of pain.

Clearly, patients who have chronic pain or recurrent acute pain must learn to minimize the role of pain in determining their level of function. People who find a number of successful methods for coping with pain tend to suffer less than those who feel helpless.

In fact, results from numerous treatment outcome studies have shown that changes in pain level don't need to parallel changes in activity level, drug use, a return to work, the ability to cope with pain, or the pursuit of further treatment.

This ability to minimize the role of pain may stem in part from a personal conviction that one can successfully execute a course of action to produce a desired outcome. This concept, known as self-efficacy, is crucial to coping and successful rehabilitation. Patients can build a sense of self-efficacy by performing increasingly difficult subtasks or tasks similar to those prescribed for rehabilitation. A belief in self-efficacy grows from the patient's conviction that the demands of his situation won't exceed his ability to cope.

The problem, of course, is that some types of pain are difficult to control. People with chronic pain and limited success in controlling it perceive the pain to be outside of their personal control and are unlikely to try new pain-management strategies. Instead, they grow frustrated and demoralized by pain that interferes with rewarding recreational, occupational, and social activities. Such people commonly resort to passive coping strategies, such as inactivity, self-medication, or alcohol to reduce emotional distress and pain.

People who feel little personal control over their pain are also more likely to "catastrophize" the impact of a pain episode and any situations that tend to worsen pain. Depression and anxiety, which are common among people with chronic pain, can influence pain perception. Indeed, anxiety about pain can change pain thresholds and tolerance levels. Depression-related symptoms can reduce the person's capacity for successful coping techniques.

Physical links

Clearly, physical factors can affect a patient's psychological condition. Likewise, psychological factors may affect not only a person's mood and coping ability, but also the physiologic characteristics of nociception. Cognitive interpretations and affective arousal may influence physiology by increasing autonomic sympathetic nervous system arousal and by promoting endogenous opioid (endorphin) production.

Autonomic arousal

Thinking about pain and stress can raise muscle tension levels, especially in already painful areas. Chronic and excessive sympathetic nervous system arousal is the immediate precursor of increased skeletal muscle tone (hypertonicity) and may set the stage for hyperactive muscle contraction and muscle contraction persistence, all of which can cause muscle spasm and pain.

Patients who exaggerate the significance of their problems or focus too closely on them, whether consciously or unconsciously, may influence sympathetic arousal and thereby predispose themselves to further injury or otherwise complicate the process of recovery.

Opioid production

Researchers have clearly shown that a person's thoughts can influence the role played by endogenous CNS opioids in controlling pain. In one study, they provided cognitive training in which patients received instructions and then practiced using different coping strategies for alleviating pain. The study had several interesting findings:

▶ Patients' expectations about their ability to control pain and disability increased with cognitive training.
▶ Patients' feelings of self-efficacy predicted their pain tolerance.
▶ Naloxone, an opioid antagonist, blocked the pain-relieving effects of cognitive coping.

Naturally, the third finding implicates the direct effect of thoughts on endogenous opioids—endorphins. Thus, it's reasonable to conclude that self-efficacy may influence pain perception at least partially via the endogenous opioid system.

In another study, the researcher provided stress management treatment to patients with rheumatoid arthritis. This autoimmune disorder, which may result from impaired functioning of suppressor T-cells, causes inflammation of various serous membranes, especially the synovial membranes. Thus, it results in joint pain and stiffness, among other symptoms.

The study findings were remarkable: patients with higher (or increased) feelings of self-efficacy displayed greater numbers of suppressor T-cells. Levels of self-efficacy also related directly to the degree of pain and joint impairment patients experienced. The researchers concluded that feelings of self-efficacy can have a direct effect on physiology.

▶ SUCCESSFUL TREATMENT

Naturally, the goal of any health care professional is to minimize the effect of pain on the patient's life and to maximize the positive influence of a person's feelings of self-efficacy and control on the management and resolution of pain. Doing so requires attention both to the nociceptive and to the emotional aspects of the pain experience.

Clearly, people respond to painful physical conditions in part based on their subjective interpretation of illness and symptoms. Their beliefs about the meaning of pain and about their own ability to function despite discomfort are important aspects of the ability to cope with pain. For example, a person who believes he has a very serious debilitating condition, that disability is a necessary aspect of pain, that activity is dangerous, and that pain is an acceptable reason to reduce one's responsibilities, will likely result in maladaptive responses.

Many factors can facilitate or disrupt a patient's sense of control, such as personal beliefs and expectations about pain, coping ability, social supports, the disorder involved, the health care system, legal implications, and the response of employers. These factors also influence a patient's investment in treatment, acceptance of responsibility, perceptions of disability, adherence to treatment recommendations, and support from significant others.

From the cognitive-behavioral perspective, assessment and treatment of patients with persistent pain requires a broad strategy that addresses all relevant psychosocial and behavioral factors in addition to biomedical ones. This pain management perspective provides patients with techniques to regain personal control over the life-changing effects of pain as well as the skills to modify the affective, behavioral, cognitive, and sensory facets of the pain experience.

During treatment, patients discover that they're more capable than they thought, thus increasing their sense of personal competence. Cognitive techniques help to place affective, behavioral, cognitive, and sensory responses under the patient's control.

Treatment that increases perceived control over pain and decreases "catastrophizing" is known to reduce pain severity ratings and functional disability. Maintaining this sense of control—and the behavioral changes it fosters—depends on the patient's belief that successful pain control stems from his own efforts. An integrative model of pain that incorporates physical, psychosocial, and behavioral factors and the changes that occur in these relationships over time can help set patients on the road to successful management of many painful conditions.

Chapter 2

Assessing pain

Most people are more afraid of pain than just about anything else. When pain develops, patients naturally want you to determine its cause and do something to relieve it as quickly as possible. The problem is, however, that pain is a subjective experience that varies widely from person to person. That makes pain tough to assess.

Sometimes, pain warns of an obviously life-threatening physical problem. Sometimes, it seems to have no physical cause at all. Somehow, you need to assess each patient's unique experience of pain and then quantify the results so you can communicate accurately with the patient, her loved ones, and other members of the health care team.

This chapter reviews the types of pain you'll be assessing, and it outlines proven techniques for getting to the bottom of your patients' pain problems.

▶ TYPES OF PAIN

Pain is usually classified by its duration or its source. Classifying pain by duration is important because pain caused by tissue injury can lead to permanently altered sensations over time. Classifying pain by source is important because pain mechanisms involving superficial structures differ from pain mechanisms involving the viscera.

Duration

Pain classified by duration may be acute or chronic.

Acute pain

Acute pain is a warning signal that results from a specific, identifiable source. The source may be minor, such as a venipuncture or a paper cut. Or it may represent a serious or life-threatening problem, such as a fractured femur. Acute pain causes a withdrawal reflex and, if it results from a significant physical threat, it causes certain autonomic reflexes. (See *Autonomic reflexes: How acute and chronic pain differ*, page 22.)

Activation of the sympathetic nervous system is the major difference between acute and chronic pain. This stimulation causes the release of epinephrine and other catecholamines, which produce physiologic reactions similar to those of a "fight or flight" reaction.

Sympathetic activation directs immediate attention to the site of injury, promotes reflexive withdrawal, and fosters other actions that prevent further damage and enhance healing. For example, if a child places her hand on a hot stove, her autonomic response system immediately generates a reflex withdrawal that jerks the hand away and minimizes the tissue damage.

All in all, acute pain serves an important protective function, announcing the need to take care of

Autonomic reflexes: How acute and chronic pain differ

Acute pain may cause certain physiologic and behaviorial changes that you won't observe in a patient with chronic pain.

TYPE OF PAIN	PHYSIOLOGIC EVIDENCE	BEHAVIORAL EVIDENCE
Acute	▶ Increased respirations ▶ Increased pulse ▶ Increased blood pressure ▶ Dilated pupils ▶ Diaphoresis	▶ Restlessness ▶ Distraction ▶ Worry ▶ Distress
Chronic	▶ Normal respirations, pulse, blood pressure, and pupil size ▶ No diaphoresis	▶ Reduced or absent physical activity ▶ Despair, depression ▶ Hopelessness

an injured area and, if necessary, to seek medical attention for it. All sources of acute pain activate both the sensory-discriminative and the motivational-affective aspects of pain interpretation. These two forces join to help the affected person make judgments about the seriousness of the pain-causing event.

Prolonged pain
Prolonged pain lasts days to weeks. It may be the most common type of acute pain, and it always results from tissue injury and inflammation. Examples include sunburn, a sprain, and surgery. One consequence of this type of tissue injury and inflammation is the release or synthesis of chemicals at the site of injury that can greatly increase the sensitivity of nearby tissues. This increased sensitivity, called hyperalgesia, is normal in prolonged acute pain and typically declines over time.

Like shorter versions of acute pain, prolonged pain serves an important protective function. The tenderness and increased sensitivity of tissue surrounding the site of an injury help to protect the site and prevent further damage.

Recurrent pain
Several pain-causing problems can't be categorized neatly into the acute pain model because they're recurrent, such as migraine headaches and temporomandibular disorders. Each painful episode may be relatively brief, but the episodes recur after variable lengths of time, often without identifiable provocation.

For example, a migraine headache may last for several hours and then resolve spontaneously. The affected person may be headache-free for days, weeks, or months, only to have another migraine episode at an unpredictable time. After that headache runs its course, the person faces another headache-free period followed by another headache.

Some recurrent pain syndromes do have identifiable causes. For example, sickle cell disease causes painful episodes caused by vaso-occlusive crises.

In the case of some recurrent conditions, such as migraine headache, the pain seems to serve no useful purpose because no protective action can be taken and no tissue damage can be prevented. In the case of sickle cell disease, however, acute pain episodes may serve a useful function by encouraging the affected person to seek medical treatment.

Chronic pain

Chronic pain isn't protective and doesn't warn of significant tissue damage. It typically results from nerve damage, such as brain injury, tumor growth, or inexplicable, abnormal responses by the central nervous system to tissue injury. It typically is defined as pain that lasts longer than 6 months.

Chronic pain commonly has no obvious pathology and continues long after an initial injury has apparently been repaired or surgery has corrected the damage. The average duration of treatment for patients who visit chronic pain clinics exceeds 7 years. Treatment lasting 20 to 30 years is common.

Obviously, the motivational-affective and cognitive aspects of chronic pain are highly significant. Chronic pain can produce a wide range of challenging emotions, such as fear, anger, anxiety, and hopelessness.

Besides the personal suffering and debilitation caused by chronic pain, tremendous economic and societal consequences result as well. Millions of Americans have chronic pain severe enough to limit or bar their participation in careers, family life, and even activities of daily living. Severe, intractable, chronic pain raises the risk of decreased function, pain behaviors, depression, doctor shopping, opioid dependence, and suicide.

Despite advances in our understanding of anatomy and physiology, and despite new and sophisticated drugs and medical-surgical treatments, chronic pain continues to present a perplexing puzzle to health care providers and significant distress to patients. No treatment currently available can consistently and permanently relieve chronic pain in all people.

Source

Pain can be categorized as either somatic or visceral depending on its origin. If somatic pain arises from skin, it's called superficial pain. If it arises from muscle, joints, or connective tissue, it's called deep pain. Visceral pain arises from internal organs and differs in significant ways from somatic pain.

Somatic pain

The skin is continuously exposed to the environment and thus to a wide variety of stimuli. Skin is densely innervated by specialized sensory receptors, including nociceptors, which enable a person to distinguish light touch from a noxious pinch and to easily localize the movement of even a single hair on the back of the hand. Various skin sensations, such as itching, touch, temperature, and pain are relatively easy for a person to distinguish and to localize.

Superficial pain is thus best characterized by a person's ability to easily and accurately localize it. Because the skin forms a protective barrier against the environment, noxious stimuli applied to skin typically evoke protective withdrawal reflexes.

In the case of deep somatic tissues (such as muscles, joints, and connective tissues), most sensory nerve activity doesn't reach the level of consciousness. People aren't aware of it. As a result, the main sensation that can reach a person's consciousness about these tissues is pain. Joint sprains and deep muscle bruises can be very painful.

Damage to a joint or muscle typically doesn't evoke the kind of withdrawal reflex caused by noxious stimulation of the skin. However, pain in joints and muscles serves a similar protective function. Joints and muscles are innervated by nociceptors and, as is true for skin, pain from these deeper structures tends to be well localized. A person rarely attributes the source of muscle or joint pain to the wrong muscle or joint.

Because pain in joints and muscles commonly results from tissue injury and inflammation, the sensitivity of nociceptors innervating the injured tissue increases, and the sensory channel for pain undergoes a reversible plastic change. One consequence of such plasticity is referral of pain to the overlying skin. Careful sensory examination of the overlying skin will reveal that its sensitivity to stimulation has increased and it has become hyperalgesic. In this example of an injured joint or muscle, referred pain and hyperalgesia help to pro-

tect the deeper structures from further damage.

Visceral pain

Visceral pain is a separate type of pain with a quality that is, in most ways, unlike the quality of pain in skin, muscles, or joints. Visceral pain is diffuse and difficult to localize. It typically is referred to other deep visceral or nonvisceral structures and to the skin. On the skin, it occupies different locations than the dermatomes, whose locations coordinate with specific spinal cord segments. (See *Somatotopic organization of sensory input.*)

The complexity of visceral pain is illustrated well by angina pectoris, the pain caused by an insufficient myocardial oxygen supply. Angina typically is referred to the skin and muscles of the upper left chest, shoulder, and arm. But a similar pattern of referred pain may stem from gallbladder obstruction or esophageal problems. Consequently, esophageal and gallbladder pain can be confused with angina. In this and other situations, the source of visceral pain can be difficult to identify.

Indeed, the source of visceral pain can be difficult even for the affected person to localize. What's more, because most people have little experience with visceral pain and little knowledge about what could be causing it, they tend to feel quite disturbed by it—especially if it's recurrent or deep and aching. Indeed, the most intense chronic visceral pain stems from tumor growth that distends and distorts a large organ.

Somatotopic organization of sensory input

Sensory input is organized somatotopically by the central nervous system (CNS). In other words, nonnociceptive and nociceptive receptors are organized into adjacent areas that form a sort of map projected by the CNS onto the skin.

Dermatomes are one example of somatotopy. A dermatome represents the area for which a single posterior spinal root supplies afferent nerve fibers. When you consider all such areas of innervation, you get a map of dermatomes that correspond to all of the originating nerve sources, as shown on the left. Presumably, accurate mapping by the CNS aids in the spatial perception of somatic stimuli.

In contrast, the viscera don't seem to be somatotopically organized. As a result, it's more difficult to localize stimuli that originate in the viscera. Instead, sensations from the viscera may be referred to certain general areas, as shown on the right.

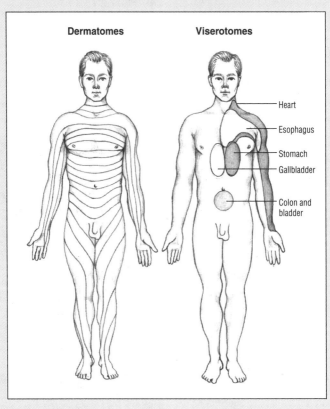

Dermatomes   **Viscerotomes**

Heart
Esophagus
Stomach
Gallbladder
Colon and bladder

▶ ASSESSMENT STEPS

If your patient has acute pain, you may be able to consider certain physical attributes when gathering assessment data. These data include heart rate, blood pressure, respiratory rate, and pupil size. For most types of pain, however, your most important—often your only—source of information will be the patient's description of what she feels. If she has chronic or recurrent pain, consider giving her a self-monitoring record to help her accurately describe the occurrence and severity of symptoms. (See *Self-monitoring record for patients with pain.*) And make sure your assessment includes a detailed interview and pertinent physical examination.

Patient interview

To obtain a full picture of your patient's pain, you'll need to perform a patient interview. If your patient has acute pain from a traumatic injury, your interview may last no more than a few seconds. If, on the other hand, she has a chronic condition with no apparent cause, your interview may be lengthy and repeated.

When interviewing a patient who has chronic pain, focus not only on factual information but also on thoughts and feelings—not just the patient's but also those of the family and loved ones. During the interview, do your best to adopt the patient's perspective. Focus your attention on the patient's reports of specific thoughts, behaviors, emotions, and physiologic responses that precede, accompany, and follow pain episodes or exacerbations, as well as on the environmental conditions and conse-quences of the patient's typical responses to these situations.

As you talk, note the relationships between cognitive, affective, and behavioral components of the patient's pain experience. Doing so will help you later, when you and the patient work together to develop appropriate goals, alternative responses to pain episodes, and possible reinforcements for these alternatives. Also, try to determine what influence the patient's pain has had on her mental state, relationships, and occupation.

Specialist evaluation

Throughout your interview, stay alert for red flags that could indicate the need for a more thorough evaluation by a pain specialist. To help determine that need, consider the answers to questions like these:

▶ Has the patient's pain lasted 3 months or more despite appropriate interventions and a lack of progressive disease?

▶ Does the patient report nonanatomical changes in sensation, such as glove anesthesia?

▶ Does the patient seem to have unrealistic expectations of you or of treatment?

▶ Does the patient complain vigorously about treatments received from previous health care providers?

▶ Does the patient have a history of previous painful or disabling medical problems?

▶ Does the patient have a history of substance abuse?

▶ Does the patient display obvious pain behaviors, such as grimacing or moving in a rigid and guarded fashion?

▶ Is any litigation pending related to the patient's pain?

Self-monitoring record for patients with pain

A self-monitoring record, sometimes called a pain diary, helps you better understand your patient's symptoms, their timing and severity, and the patient's methods of responding to them. It also helps patients understand the active role they must play in managing their pain. Consider asking your patient to keep such a diary before your first interview or the patient's first interview with a pain specialist.

Name: _____

Date/time	Symptoms (How bad, 0 to 10?) Situation (What were you doing or thinking?)	How did you feel? (How bad, 0 to 10?)	What were you thinking?	What did you do? With what result?

▶ Is the patient receiving disability compensation?
▶ Was the patient employed before the pain began?
▶ Was the patient injured on the job?
▶ Does the patient have a job to which she can return?
▶ Does the patient have a history of frequently changing jobs?
▶ Did a major stressful life event occur just before the pain started or worsened?

▶ Does the patient have an inappropriately or excessively depressed or elevated mood?
▶ Has the patient given up many activities (social, recreational, sexual, occupational, physical) because of pain?
▶ Does the patient report a high level of marital or family conflict?
▶ Do the patient's significant others reinforce pain behaviors, such as doing the patient's chores or rubbing the patient's back?

▶ Does anyone else in the patient's family have chronic pain?

▶ Does the patient resist the process of planning to resume activities if the pain subsides?

If the patient has positive responses to only a few of these questions, she probably doesn't need a referral to a pain specialist. However, if she has positive responses to many of these questions, carefully consider a referral.

Assessment tools

Standardized assessment tools offer several advantages over semistructured and unstructured interviews. They're easy to administer, they take less time, and they can uncover important issues that warrant a more thorough investigation. The self-monitoring instrument mentioned earlier in the chapter is one such tool that's particularly helpful for patients with chronic pain.

Other self-reporting methods are available as well, particularly for pain intensity. For instance, you can ask the patient to quantify her pain by giving it a general rating, such as mild, moderate, or severe. Or you can ask her to give it a number between 0 and 10, where 0 equals no pain and 10 equals the most severe pain imaginable. Other intensity rating scales are available as well. (See *Using pain intensity rating scales.*)

Keep in mind that you can use these scales not just for the sensory aspect of pain but also for the motivation-affective aspect. Simply modify the scale by using a different descriptive term, such as distress.

Other pain assessment instruments of various lengths and complexities are available. (See *Pain assessment guide*, pages 30 and 31.) Especially for patients with chronic pain, you may well need more information than a simple rating scale can offer.

Physical examination

For most health problems, the physical examination serves to measure function and detect physical problems. For a patient whose main complaint is pain, however, the physical examination serves a less specific purpose. That's largely because the physical examination commonly can't directly confirm a patient's report of pain or reduced function.

For significant numbers of patients with pain, no physical pathology can be identified. Even with sophisticated advances in imaging technology, a less than perfect correlation exists between identifiable pathology and reported pain. For example, on magnetic resonance images, up to 30% of healthy, asymptomatic people have the structural abnormalities commonly associated with back pain.

The fact is that tests commonly used in physical examinations, such as muscle strength, range of motion, and even X-rays, have little value in predicting long-term functional capacity. What's more, a patient's functional ability can be significantly influenced by her motivation to communicate pain, distress, and suffering to you and other health care providers.

When it comes to pain assessment, even the functional portion of your examination will probably rely primarily on self-reporting by the patient. Ask about her ability to perform a range of functional activities, such as climbing stairs, sitting for specific periods of time,

Using pain intensity rating scales

These scales are examples of the rating systems you can use to help a patient quantify her current pain level. To obtain information for a longer period of time, have the patient keep a pain diary that includes repeated use of one of these scales.

Visual analog scale
Place a line across the scale that indicates your current level of pain.

No pain |_____| Pain as bad as it can be

Descriptive scale
Place a line across the scale that indicates your current level of pain.

No pain   Mild   Moderate   Severe

Numeric scale
Circle the number below that indicates your current level of pain.

No pain | 0   1   2   3   4   5   6   7   8   9   10 | Pain as bad as it can be

Box scale
Place an X through the number that indicates your current level of pain.

0	1	2	3	4	5	6	7	8	9	10

No pain   Most severe pain

Pediatric scale

1   2   3   4   5   6

lifting specific weights, and performing activities of daily living. Also, ask about the level of pain the patient experiences while performing these activities.

Several instruments are available to help you assess your patient's physical function. They include the Roland-Morris Disability Scale, the Sickness Impact Profile, and the Oswestry Disability Scale. Each includes questions designed to elicit specific information that you can use to quantify your patient's condition.

Despite the obvious limitations of self-report instruments, they have several advantages: economy,

Pain assessment guide

Patient name: _____

Patient goal: _____

Past medical conditions: _____

Past surgeries and hospitalizations: _____

Recent tests and results: _____

Drug allergies and reactions: _____

Do you drink alcohol? (Specify substance and amount.) _____

Do you smoke? (Specify substance and amount.) _____

Do you use drugs? (Specify substance and amount.) _____

When did your pain begin? _____

Are you aware of something that started it? _____

Where is your pain?

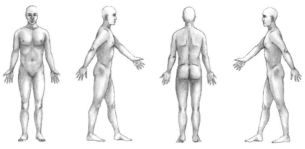

How severe is your pain right now? (Circle the number.)

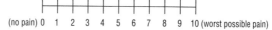

(no pain) 0   1   2   3   4   5   6   7   8   9   10 (worst possible pain)

How would you describe your pain? (Circle all that apply.)

Shooting	Stabbing	Gnawing	Sharp
Dull	Aching	Numb	Throbbing
Radiating	Burning	Unbearable	

Pain assessment guide *(continued)*

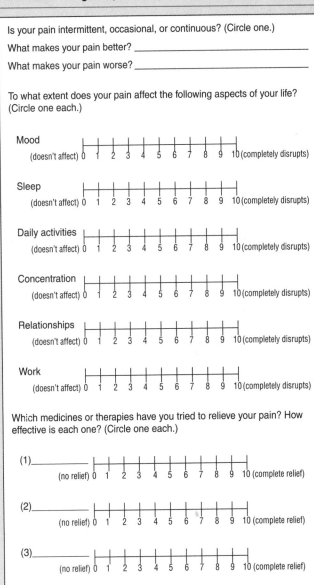

Is your pain intermittent, occasional, or continuous? (Circle one.)

What makes your pain better? _____

What makes your pain worse? _____

To what extent does your pain affect the following aspects of your life? (Circle one each.)

Mood
(doesn't affect) 0 1 2 3 4 5 6 7 8 9 10 (completely disrupts)

Sleep
(doesn't affect) 0 1 2 3 4 5 6 7 8 9 10 (completely disrupts)

Daily activities
(doesn't affect) 0 1 2 3 4 5 6 7 8 9 10 (completely disrupts)

Concentration
(doesn't affect) 0 1 2 3 4 5 6 7 8 9 10 (completely disrupts)

Relationships
(doesn't affect) 0 1 2 3 4 5 6 7 8 9 10 (completely disrupts)

Work
(doesn't affect) 0 1 2 3 4 5 6 7 8 9 10 (completely disrupts)

Which medicines or therapies have you tried to relieve your pain? How effective is each one? (Circle one each.)

(1)_____
(no relief) 0 1 2 3 4 5 6 7 8 9 10 (complete relief)

(2)_____
(no relief) 0 1 2 3 4 5 6 7 8 9 10 (complete relief)

(3)_____
(no relief) 0 1 2 3 4 5 6 7 8 9 10 (complete relief)

Pain behavior checklist

A pain behavior is something a person uses to communicate pain, distress, or suffering to others. Place a check in the box next to each behavior you observe or infer while talking with your patient.

☐ Grimacing

☐ Moaning

☐ Sighing

☐ Clenching teeth

☐ Holding or supporting the painful body area

☐ Sitting rigidly

☐ Frequently shifting posture or position

☐ Moving in a guarded or protective manner

☐ Moving very slowly

☐ Limping

☐ Taking medication

☐ Using a cane, cervical collar, or other prosthetic device

☐ Walking with an abnormal gait

☐ Requesting help with walking

☐ Stopping frequently while walking

☐ Lying down during the day

☐ Avoiding physical activity

☐ Being irritable

☐ Asking such questions as, "Why did this happen to me?"

☐ Asking to be relieved from tasks or activities

efficiency, and utility for assessment of a wide range of patient behaviors, some of which may be private (such as sexual relations) or unobservable (such as thoughts and emotional arousal). Although the validity of self-reporting is often questioned, studies have revealed fairly close relationships between self-reports, disease characteristics, health care providers' ratings of functional abilities, and objective functional performance.

Observation

Especially for patients with pain, observation may form a key aspect of your assessment. Patients display a broad range of responses that communicate to others their pain, distress, and suffering. Some are controllable; others, such as perspiring, are not. As you observe a patient in the waiting room, during your interview, or during a structured series of physical tasks, record the pain behaviors you observe. (See *Pain behavior checklist*.) Then use your observations to help quantify your patient's pain.

Keep in mind that the uncontrollable autonomic activity characteristic of acute pain dissipates over time. If your patient has chronic pain, don't take the absence of autonomic activity as an indication that her pain has declined or resolved.

Many overt behaviors can be considered pain behaviors:
▶ verbal reports
▶ vocalizations, such as sighs and moans
▶ altered motor activities
▶ facial expressions
▶ body postures and gesturing, such as limping or grimacing
▶ functional limitations, including reclining for extended periods

▶ actions taken to reduce pain, such as taking medication.

Keep in mind that personal attention and escape from unpleasant activities (such as work) may reinforce these behaviors even after the initial cause of pain has resolved.

One way to "observe" pain behaviors when you can't be personally present is through a diary that the patient keeps. In it, she can record the amount of time she spends or the number of times she performs specific pain behaviors, such as reclining, sitting, or taking medication. It also allows her to describe the circumstances surrounding the behavior.

For example, a patient might note that she took pain medication after arguing with her husband, and that the husband apologized for upsetting her when he saw her take the drug. This case illustrates the point that recognizing the consequences of pain behavior can help to identify a pattern of behavior that may relate to more than simply the patient's pain. For this patient, the husband may be providing positive reinforcement that unwittingly encourages increased drug use.

Even using the best interview, examination, and observation techniques will leave you with a clinical assessment of chronic pain that's subjective and possibly unreliable. Consequently, a precise diagnosis and even a clear identification of the anatomical origin of pain may be impossible. Despite these limitations, the patient's history and physical examination remain the basis of medical diagnosis and may be the best guide for interpreting the results of sophisticated imaging procedures and other traditional diagnostic tests.

▶ PSYCHOLOGICAL CHARACTERISTICS

Don't forget that your assessment of a patient's pain must include psychological as well as physical characteristics. This is especially true for patients with chronic pain. The effect of pain on a person's life becomes especially complex when the pain persists long enough to be considered chronic. A range of psychological, social, and economic factors can influence the person's perception and reports of pain, and vice versa.

If your patient has chronic pain, you should assess not only the physical sources of the pain but also the patient's moods, fears, expectations, coping efforts, and resources. Also, investigate the responses of the patient's significant others and the impact of pain on the patient's life. In short, your assessment must focus on the whole patient, not just on the cause of the patient's pain.

As the basis of your psychological assessment, start with these questions:

▶ How extensive is the patient's physical impairment?
▶ How much is the patient suffering, disabled, and unable to enjoy her usual activities?
▶ How appropriate is the patient's behavior in light of her condition?
▶ Does the patient show evidence of symptom amplification, such as depression or anxiety?

Psychogenic pain

The failure to find a physical basis for a patient's complaints of pain may lead some clinicians to think the pain is psychogenic. Make this conclusion with great caution. Naturally, it would be naïve to assume that psychogenic pain doesn't exist. However, it's equally important to acknowledge that pain—sometimes pain from unknown pathology—induces emotional distress. If you see a patient in distress and with chronic pain, don't assume that the distress lies at the root of the pain.

What's more, the use of traditional psychological measures, such as the Minnesota Multiphasic Personality Inventory, to identify specific individual differences in reports of pain must be approached cautiously because most of these tools weren't developed for or standardized on this population.

Recently, a number of psychological assessment instruments have been developed for use specifically with pain patients. One of these, which assesses both psychosocial and behavioral aspects of chronic pain, is the West Haven-Yale Multidimensional Pain Inventory, a 60-item, three-part questionnaire. The first part assesses patients' perceptions of pain severity, the impact of pain on various areas of life, affective distress, feelings of control, and support from significant others. The second section assesses the patients' perceptions of significant others' responses to their pain complaints. The third section examines changes in patients' functional activities, such as household chores and socializing.

When objective physical findings fail to substantiate complaints of pain, or when descriptions of its severity seem excessive in light of physical findings, you'll face difficulty in making a comprehensive evaluation. Nonetheless, you'll need to use what evidence you can to decide when it's appropriate to refer a patient for psychological or psychiatric assessment by a specialist in evaluating chronic pain. (See *Psychological assessment of patients with pain*.)

Emotional results of pain

Because pain is subjective, suffering and disability are difficult to prove, disprove, or quantify. Plus, the experience of pain is influenced by cultural conditioning, expectations, social contingencies, mood, and perceptions of control as well as physical pathology. The central point is this: The patient who reports the pain is the subject of evaluation, not the pain itself.

Never lose sight of the fact that patients with chronic pain, especially those with no known pathology, may become enmeshed in and battered by the quest for relief. They go from doctor to doctor, laboratory test to laboratory test, and imaging procedure to imaging procedure in a continuing search for a fitting diagnosis and successful treatment.

For many such patients, pain becomes the central focus of their lives. They withdraw from society, lose their jobs, and alienate family and friends. Thus, it's hardly surprising that many pain patients feel anxious, demoralized, helpless, hopeless, frustrated, angry, and isolated. A significant portion of these patients (study results say 30% to 90%) develop depression. Other common problems caused by chronic pain include anxiety, drug abuse and dependence, anger, violence, and suicide.

The fact is that patients with chronic pain unrelated to a known disease—even those with recurrent acute pain—commonly feel rejected by the very elements of society they need for support. They may

Psychological assessment of patients with pain

If you refer your patient to a pain specialist for a psychological assessment, the initial interview probably will cover topics such as these:

▶ What the patient thinks is wrong
▶ The patient's thoughts about the causes, treatments, and future impact of the pain
▶ What the patient worries about, such as disease progression or increased pain
▶ Problems that have resulted from pain, including work, relationship, and financial problems
▶ Situations, activities, and people that change the intensity, duration, or frequency of pain
▶ Ways the patient expresses pain
▶ How others know when the patient's pain is intense or present
▶ What effect the patient believes the pain is having on others
▶ What the patient's family, friends, coworkers, and employers think about the patient's pain
▶ How others respond to the patient's pain complaints, pain behaviors, and functional limitations

▶ Secondary gains, such as attention and freedom from unpleasant activities
▶ Pattern of drug use
▶ Current and previous substance abuse
▶ Current mood, sleep pattern, and appetite
▶ What the patient tries or has tried to do to reduce pain
▶ Work history, including job changes, satisfaction, and interactions with coworkers and supervisors
▶ Patient's expectations of health care providers and treatments
▶ Views of previous health care providers and treatments
▶ History of pain in patient or family members
▶ Previous and current stressful events
▶ Current and past family and marital relationships
▶ Motivation for rehabilitation and self-management

become frustrated with and lose faith in a medical system that initially promises a cure and then becomes indifferent or skeptical when treatments prove ineffective. As the likelihood of returning to work and earning a full income becomes more elusive, the pile of medical bills for unsuccessful treatments continues to grow.

In time, people with chronic pain may begin to feel that they're being blamed by their health care providers, employers, and even family members when their pain fails to respond to treatment. Third-party payers may even sug-

gest that the person is faking pain for financial gain. In this battle-ground environment, the patient must find a way to overcome such difficulties as constant fear, disturbed sleep, disruption of her usual activities, treatment-induced complications, inadequate or maladaptive support systems, the risk of dependence on potent drugs, the inability to work, financial difficulties, and possible prolonged litigation.

Thus, the emotional distress that you observe in a patient with chronic pain may stem from a variety of sources. Moreover, the presence of an undiagnosed, possibly life-threatening, painful condition that many people consider psychogenic or malingering is itself a source of stress and can initiate psychological distress or aggravate a premorbid psychiatric condition.

Although the assessment and treatment of pain—especially chronic pain—can be a frustrating and ultimately unsuccessful venture, you must resist the urge to lose heart or blame the patient. A great variety of nondrug pain management techniques are available, along with a generous selection of analgesic drugs. By assessing your patient carefully and fully, you can increase the likelihood that she'll find relief from her pain.

Chapter 3

Managing pain

Besides causing profound psychological suffering, pain also produces a host of negative physiologic effects, including the release of stress hormones, impaired immune responses, altered respiratory patterns, and suppressed coughing. These physiologic responses can, in turn, delay recovery from an illness by encouraging pneumonia, discouraging ambulation, and preventing effective participation in physical therapy.

In short, uncontrolled or poorly controlled pain decreases physical and mental health. In contrast, the aggressive prevention and treatment of pain yields significant benefits for patients, including faster recovery rates and shorter hospital stays. Perhaps because pain can be so difficult to treat, a wide variety of drug and nondrug treatments have been developed for patients with all types of pain. This chapter reviews drugs commonly used to manage pain, methods for using these drugs wisely, major types of nondrug therapies for pain, and cognitive-behavioral elements of pain management.

Naturally, the pain management methods outlined here must go hand-in-hand with appropriate management of underlying diseases. For example, an attack of acute cholecystitis, although painful, needs more than simply pain control. Indeed, removal of the diseased gallbladder is what ultimately resolves the patient's pain. In the meantime, however, the methods outlined here can help you control the patient's pain before and after surgery. They also can help you control pain caused by cancer.

▶ DRUGS
Many types of drugs can be used to control pain. Best known among them are nonsteroidal anti-inflammatory drugs (NSAIDs), acetaminophen, opioids, and local anesthetics. Psychotropic drugs, such as antidepressants and anticonvulsants, are sometimes used to control certain types of pain or the emotional problems that can result. Other types of drugs used to manage certain types of pain or pain-related problems include anticholinergics, antihistamines, barbiturates, corticosteroids, histamine$_2$-receptor (H_2-receptor) antagonists, and hydantoin derivatives.

Nonsteroidal anti-inflammatory drugs
NSAIDs are used mainly to provide temporary relief of mild to moderate pain and inflammation. They're commonly used to treat headache, dysmenorrhea, arthralgia, myalgia, neuralgia, and mild to moderate pain caused by certain dental or surgical procedures. These drugs are widely used because they can be taken orally, because they don't cause central nervous system (CNS) or respiratory depression at therapeutic doses,

Signs and symptoms of aspirin toxicity

Mild
Nausea and vomiting
Tinnitus
Vertigo

Moderate
Acneform eruption
Confusion
Diarrhea
Drowsiness
Electrolyte imbalances
Hyperthermia
Hyperventilation

Severe
Cardiovascular collapse
Coma
Hallucinations
Seizures

and because many of them are available without a prescription.

Oral NSAIDs are also used for long-term treatment of rheumatoid arthritis, juvenile arthritis, and osteoarthritis. In osteoarthritis, NSAIDs are used primarily for analgesia. In rheumatoid conditions, they reduce pain, stiffness, swelling, and tenderness. However, they don't stop or reverse the disease process. NSAIDs are also used as adjunctive treatment for pain caused by cancer, particularly in patients with bone metastasis.

Although the drugs that make up the NSAID group have several different chemical structures, all are weak organic acids with similar analgesic and fever-reducing effects. The antipyretic, anti-inflammatory, and analgesic properties of NSAIDs stem from their ability to reduce prostaglandin synthesis by inhibiting the enzyme cyclooxygenase. Besides preventing the activation of primary afferents that convey pain information from the periphery to the CNS, NSAIDs also may produce analgesia by influencing enzymes and neurotransmitter systems in the brain and spinal cord.

Although no NSAID has been proven clearly superior to aspirin with regard to efficacy or toxicity, newer NSAIDs do offer some advantages:
▶ They may cause fewer adverse effects.
▶ Some can be given once daily.
▶ Because some newer NSAIDs require a prescription, some patients may consider them to be more powerful and more acceptable than aspirin.

Commonly used NSAIDs include aspirin, phenylpropionic acid derivatives, indomethacin, piroxicam, nabumetone, ketorolac, and COX-2 inhibitors.

Aspirin

Aspirin has a long history of effectiveness, relative safety, and low cost. Those characteristics, combined with the fact that it's available without a prescription, make it the standard against which all other NSAIDs are measured. Aspirin is effective against pain, inflammation, and fever. A single 650-mg dose achieves maximum analgesic and antipyretic effects, although doses up to 5 g daily are needed to achieve maximum anti-inflammatory effects.

Aspirin is effective when taken orally and is rapidly absorbed from the stomach and small intestine. Toxicity usually isn't life-threatening, and symptoms are mild. (See *Signs and symptoms of aspirin toxicity*.) Tinnitus is a common warning sign of toxic plasma levels. If it occurs, the dosage should be decreased.

Phenylpropionic acid derivatives

These drugs—the largest group of aspirin alternatives—were developed largely in an effort to reduce the adverse gastrointestinal (GI) effects of aspirin. This group includes fenoprofen, flurbiprofen, ibuprofen, ketoprofen, naproxen, and oxaprozin. Oxaprozin has a very long half-life, which means that it can be taken once daily.

These drugs typically cause fewer GI effects than aspirin, and taking them with milk, food, or an antacid can reduce the GI effects still further. Some evidence suggests that these drugs also may be more effective than aspirin. Consequently, they're becoming increasingly common—especially the over-the-counter versions of ibuprofen and naproxen. Keep in mind that people who have hypersensitivity reactions to aspirin may have similar reactions to these drugs.

Indomethacin

Indomethacin is a derivative of indoleacetic acid. It inhibits cyclo-oxygenase and prostaglandin synthesis and has potent antipyretic, anti-inflammatory, and analgesic properties. However, its adverse effects limit its use; indeed, indomethacin isn't recommended for general use. Instead, it's recommended for several specific conditions, including acute gouty arthritis and ankylosing spondylitis. Indomethacin also is used to accelerate closure of the ductus arteriosus in premature infants.

About 20% of people who start taking indomethacin stop taking it because of the adverse effects. Adverse GI effects include abdominal pain, diarrhea, ulcerations, and hemorrhage. Acute pancreatitis has been reported. CNS effects occur in 20% to 25% of people who take the drug long-term; they include severe frontal headaches, dizziness, and mental confusion. Hematologic effects, including neutropenia, thrombocytopenia, and aplastic anemia, and hypersensitivity reactions, such as rashes, pruritus, urticaria, and acute attacks of asthma have also been reported.

Piroxicam

Piroxicam is equivalent to indomethacin as an inhibitor of prostaglandin synthesis and is effective against fever, inflammation, and pain. It's well absorbed orally, and plasma levels peak in 3 to 5 hours. The 50-hour half-life allows a single daily dose.

Although about 20% of people who take piroxicam report having adverse effects, only about 5% of them stop taking the drug as a result. As with other NSAIDs, piroxicam causes GI irritation, inhibits platelet aggregation, and can cause hypersensitivity reactions in people sensitive to aspirin.

Nabumetone

Nabutemone is a nonactive prodrug, structurally similar to naproxen, whose major metabolite is an NSAID when metabolized by the liver. The average half-life of the active metabolite is 24 hours in adults. The drug relieves pain and inflammation from rheumatoid arthritis and osteoarthritis. It has efficacy similar to other NSAIDs but has fewer adverse effects.

Ketorolac

Ketorolac was the first injectable NSAID. It has antipyretic, anti-inflammatory, and analgesic properties. It's used for short-term pain management, particularly in emergency departments. That's because it doesn't cause CNS and respiratory depression, as opioids do, and because it has no risk of dependence.

Ketorolac is also available in an oral form. However, because it has a high risk of adverse effects, it's currently used only for short-term management of moderate to severe pain.

COX-2 inhibitors

Researchers discovered in the early 1990s that cyclooxygenase had two isoforms; they called these compounds COX-1 and COX-2. COX-1 seems to be responsible for protecting the gastric mucosa, among other functions, and COX-2 seems to be responsible for moderating inflammation. Because traditional NSAIDs affect both COX forms, these drugs tend to have certain adverse GI effects. Theoretically at least, the selective COX-2 inhibitors provide anti-inflammatory therapy without the adverse effects.

The drugs celecoxib (Celebrex) and rofecoxib (Vioxx) are members of this recently developed drug class, now used in adults for rheumatoid arthritis and osteoarthritis. They tend to cause less gastric irritation than other NSAIDs, and they have no effect on platelet aggregation or bleeding times. However, because COX-2 may have several functions, the efficacy and adverse effects of these selective inhibitors are still under investigation.

Acetaminophen

Acetaminophen is similar to the NSAIDs because it weakly inhibits prostaglandin synthesis; however, acetaminophen is unlike NSAIDs in several ways:
▶ It doesn't have significant anti-inflammatory properties.
▶ It doesn't interfere with platelet aggregation.
▶ It doesn't affect uric acid levels.
These differences may be because acetaminophen inhibits CNS cyclooxygenase more effectively than it inhibits peripheral cyclooxygenase.

Acetaminophen has analgesic and antipyretic effects similar to those of aspirin. It's the drug of choice for people who need a mild analgesic or antipyretic and for whom aspirin is contraindicated:
▶ patients hypersensitive to aspirin
▶ patients with a history of ulcers
▶ patients with gout
▶ children with viral infections
▶ patients who take anticoagulants.

Acetaminophen is metabolized in the liver, and its most serious adverse effect is hepatotoxicity. The amount of liver damage is related directly to the amount of drug ingested; patients who already have liver disease are particularly susceptible. Hepatotoxicity occurs when metabolic systems in the liver are overwhelmed and a highly active, toxic metabolite accumulates.

Opioids

Opium has been used for centuries to relieve severe pain, diarrhea, cough, anxiety, and insomnia. Obtained from exudate of the poppy seed pod, opium contains about 20 alkaloids, including morphine, codeine, papaverine, and thebaine.

Opioids are usually understood to include natural and semisynthetic alkaloid derivatives from opium and their synthetic surrogates. Their actions mimic those of morphine. Most of these drugs are classified as Controlled Substance Schedule II by the Federal Drug Enforcement Agency because they have a high risk for addiction and abuse. Opioids continue to be the most effective analgesics available for moderate to severe pain. They're especially effective for visceral pain. Opioids relieve severe, dull, constant pain better than they relieve sharp, stabbing pain.

Drug effects

In contrast to NSAIDs, which are commonly called peripheral analgesics, opioids are called central analgesics. That's because opioids produce their primary effects in the CNS. The main general effect of opioids in the CNS is inhibition.

For example, opioids modulate pain information relayed supraspinally on ascending pathways, as by the spinothalamic tract. They do so by presynaptically inhibiting neurotransmitter release from A-δ and C fibers and by postsynaptically inhibiting dorsal horn neuronal activity.

Opioids also inhibit transmission of pain information in the spinal cord via several descending inhibitory systems. Opioid receptors have been localized in regions of the brain stem that support descending inhibition. At the spinal level, neurotransmitters, such as norepinephrine and serotonin, mediate the inhibition that originates in the brain stem.

Central perception of pain occurs in the thalamus and cortex. Opioids modulate pain perception by inhibiting neurons in these regions as well. That's why patients report that their reactions to painful stimuli are very much affected by opioids. In addition, opioids cause analgesia, respiratory depression, sedation, other central effects, and peripheral effects.

Analgesia

Opioids are effective analgesics and produce significant analgesia without the loss of other sensory abilities, such as vision, hearing, and touch. Opioids suppress both the perception of and the reaction to pain. Patients report that they're still aware of pain, but that it no longer causes discomfort.

Respiratory depression

Brain stem respiratory centers contain high concentrations of opioid receptors. When a patient receives an opioid, chemoreceptors in the brain stem become less responsive to carbon dioxide. As a result, all opioids produce dose-dependent respiratory depression. In opioid overdose, respiratory arrest is the usual cause of death.

The respiratory depression produced by opioids is a major disadvantage of their use. Administer these drugs carefully to patients with such respiratory conditions as asthma, chronic obstructive pulmonary disease, and emphysema. Tolerance does develop to the respiratory depressant effects produced by opioids, but even in opioid-tolerant patients, fatal respiratory depression can be produced by very high doses.

Sedation

Opioids commonly cause sedation and mental clouding. Significant CNS depression can occur if opioids are combined with other depressant drugs, such as barbiturates or antipsychotics. The sedative effects produced by opioids can limit their use by some people, but tolerance to sedation does develop. Don't use opioids for their sedative-hypnotic effects unless the patient's insomnia results from pain.

Other central effects
Other effects of opioids may include euphoria, cough suppression, miosis, nausea and vomiting, and truncal rigidity (increased tone of the large trunk muscles). Euphoria, a sense of well-being, is the affective response experienced by most people who take opioids for pain relief. In contrast, 25% of people who take opioids but aren't in pain experience dysphoria, a sense of restlessness and malaise.

Opioids have long been recognized as effective cough suppressants, an effect that results from suppression of the cough reflex center in the brain stem.

Miosis, or constriction of the pupils, is a CNS effect produced by most opioid agonists. Because little tolerance develops to this effect, miosis can be used as an indicator of opioid use or abuse, although you should keep in mind that other drugs and disorders can also alter pupil diameter.

Early in therapy, opioids can stimulate the chemoreceptor trigger zone in the medulla and cause nausea and vomiting in some patients. This effect is transient and more common among ambulatory patients than bedridden patients, suggesting a secondary effect on the vestibular apparatus. Larger or continued doses suppress the chemoreceptor trigger zone.

Some patients develop truncal rigidity after rapid administration of large doses of opioids given for anesthesia. This effect may be mediated at both the supraspinal and spinal levels. It can interfere with respiratory function, particularly in compromised patients.

Peripheral effects
Although most opioid receptors are in the brain or spinal cord, some opioid receptor sites are in the periphery. Consequently, opioids can lead to certain peripheral effects, including constipation, certain cardiovascular (CV) effects, and other effects.

Constipation is a common adverse effect of opioids. Stimulation of opioid receptors in the GI tract increases the resting tone and decreases propulsion. Minimal tolerance develops to this effect, and constipation can be significant and limiting, particularly in patients who need opioids for chronic pain.

Most opioids have no significant direct effects on the CV system at analgesic doses. However, intravenous (I.V.) administration of opioids can cause histamine release that, in turn, can cause hypotension as well as flushing and itching at the injection site. Opioids also can worsen hypovolemic shock; use them cautiously in patients who have decreased blood volume.

Opioids can increase urethral sphincter tone and lead to urine retention, especially after surgery. Also, therapeutic doses of opioids may prolong labor and alter the degree to which a woman can cooperate in childbirth. Opioids also constrict the smooth muscles of the biliary tract and the sphincter of Oddi, which may produce symptoms of biliary colic and epigastric

Opioid receptors and their effects

Opioid receptors are located in the central nervous system (CNS) and in other tissues, such as the nerves of the gastrointestinal tract. Opioids relieve pain by binding at receptor sites in the CNS. A drug that binds at two or more receptor sites may have more benefits than a drug that binds at only one type of receptor. For example, a drug that acts as an agonist at kappa sites and an antagonist at mu sites may provide analgesia without the risk of respiratory depression. Although drugs may exhibit higher affinities for certain receptors than others, none is selective for only one receptor type.

RECEPTOR	EFFECT
Mu (μ)	analgesia, sedation, miosis, euphoria, constipation, respiratory depression, physical dependence
Kappa (κ)	analgesia, sedation, miosis, dysphoria
Sigma (σ)	affective behavior

distress. They can also precipitate biliary colic in patients with bile duct or gallbladder disease.

Classification

Usually, opioids are classified by their function—as agonists, mixed agonist-antagonists, or antagonists. Opioid agonists bind to receptors to produce an effect. (See *Opioid receptors and their effects*.) For example, morphine, the prototypical opioid, binds to mu (μ) receptors.

Opioids with mixed agonist-antagonist properties function as agonists in opioid-naive patients; in opioid-tolerant patients they can precipitate withdrawal symptoms.

Opioid antagonists bind to receptors, but they don't produce an effect. For example, naloxone competes with opioids for receptors, thus blocking opioid effects. Mixed agonist-antagonist opioids may act as agonists at one type of receptor and antagonists at another type. For example, pentazocine acts as an agonist at kappa (κ) receptors and as an antagonist at μ receptors.

Opioid agonists

Many opioids are available for treating moderate to severe pain. (See *Common uses for opioids*, page 44.) Most have pharmacologic properties similar to those of morphine—the standard against which other analgesics are measured. To date, no other opioid has proven clearly superior to morphine as an analgesic. Other opioid agonists include meperidine, methadone, and tramadol.

Morphine and related compounds

Morphine is available for oral use and for injection. However, oral administration results in significant first-pass metabolism, and oral doses are only one-sixth to one-third as potent as parenteral doses.

Codeine, hydromorphone, oxycodone, and oxymorphone, are structurally related to morphine and can be used in its place. Hydromorphone is now considered a second-line choice after morphine. Heroin also is a morphine-

Common uses for opioids

Opioids may be administered for a wide variety of reasons and conditions, such as these:
▶ postoperative pain
▶ severe, chronic pain from terminal cancer
▶ anxiety in patients with dyspnea caused by acute pulmonary edema and acute left ventricular failure
▶ induction of anesthesia
▶ adjunctive therapy to maintain general or regional anesthesia
▶ primary anesthesia during surgery
▶ dry, nonproductive cough
▶ diarrhea.

related compound with significant analgesic properties. Although the use of heroin is prohibited in the United States because of the potential for drug abuse, it's used to treat cancer pain in some countries.

Meperidine and related compounds

Meperidine is a synthetic μ receptor agonist with effects similar to those of morphine. Meperidine is available for oral use and for injection. Like morphine, it's less bioavailable when given orally. Meperidine has a significantly shorter half-life than morphine, and frequent dosing is needed to maintain pain relief. As a result, meperidine isn't routinely recommended. What's more, if its metabolite, normeperidine, accumulates, the patient may develop CNS excitation, which may include seizures, tremors, and muscle twitches.

Fentanyl, sufentanil, and alfentanil are synthetic opioids structurally related to meperidine. They're μ receptor agonists and are about 80 times more potent than morphine. Currently, no oral forms of these drugs are available. High doses can be used as primary anesthetics when you need to minimize CV effects. They also can be used intrathecally and epidurally for postoperative analgesia. Fentanyl is available in a transdermal form for treating chronic intractable pain.

Methadone

Methadone is used for pain relief and for treating opioid abstinence syndromes. It too has pharmacologic properties similar to morphine, but it offers several advantages over morphine:
▶ extended suppression of withdrawal symptoms in opioid-dependent patients
▶ slower development of tolerance and physical dependence
▶ milder withdrawal symptoms after abrupt termination of the drug.

Tramadol

Tramadol is a unique central-acting analgesic with a dual mechanism of action. A synthetic analogue of codeine, tramadol binds weakly to opioid receptors and inhibits the reuptake of both norepinephrine and serotonin. It has a half-life of 6 to 7 hours and is available as tablets. It's currently used to treat moderate to severe pain.

Opioid agonist-antagonists

This class of drugs has varying degrees of agonist and antagonist activity with poorly understood pharmacology. Each drug is believed to act on different opiate receptors in the CNS, to a greater or lesser degree, thus producing slightly different effects. These drugs are potent analgesics with somewhat less addiction potential than the pure narcotic agonists.

Opioid agonist-antagonists are used mainly as analgesics, particularly in patients at high risk for drug dependence or abuse. Some are used as preoperative or preanesthetic medication, to supplement balanced anesthesia, or to relieve prepartum pain.

However, these drugs aren't recommended as first-line choices for pain relief because they can produce morphine-like psychic and physiologic dependence. Plus, drug tolerance can develop with repeated administration. And administration to patients previously treated with opioid agonists can cause withdrawal symptoms.

Common agonist-antagonists include pentazocine, nalbuphine, butorphanol, and buprenorphine.

Pentazocine

Pentazocine is an agonist at κ receptors and a weak antagonist at μ receptors. It has effects similar to those of morphine, including respiratory depression, tolerance, and physical dependence. Currently, pentazocine is the only mixed agonist-antagonist given orally.

Nalbuphine

Nalbuphine, a κ agonist and μ antagonist, is structurally related to both naloxone and oxymorphone. It has a spectrum of effects similar to those of pentazocine. In contrast to morphine, the respiratory depression produced by nalbuphine hits a ceiling; increasing doses beyond 30 mg produces no further respiratory depression. Nalbuphine isn't classified as a controlled substance, and few cases of abuse have been reported. Nalbuphine is available as an injectable for parenteral administration.

Butorphanol

Butorphanol, thought to be a κ agonist, has a pharmacologic profile similar to that of pentazocine. Butorphanol isn't classified as a controlled substance, and addicts actually express a dislike for it. It's available for injection and for intranasal use.

Buprenorphine

Buprenorphine is a semisynthetic opioid derived from thebaine, an alkaloid found in opium. It's a partial agonist at μ receptors and is 25 to 50 times more potent than morphine. The analgesic effects produced by buprenorphine are similar to those of morphine, but the respiratory depressant and sedative effects are much less significant. Buprenorphine is currently available only for parenteral administration in the United States.

Opioid antagonists

Opioid antagonists, such as naloxone and naltrexone, produce little analgesia. Indeed, they produce few effects at all when given to a patient who hasn't received an opioid agonist. Clinically, opioid antagonists are used as diagnostic agents for opioid abuse, to reverse opioid-induced respiratory depression, and as pharmacologic deterrents to opioid addicts. When endogenous opioid systems are activated, as in hypovolemic shock, endotoxic shock, or spinal cord injury, for example, opioid antagonists may be useful in treating them.

Naloxone

Naloxone is a competitive antagonist at μ, κ, and σ opioid receptors. Low subcutaneous (S.C.) doses produce no discernable subjective effects: higher doses produce only slight drowsiness. The drug is absorbed readily from the GI tract, but it's metabolized rapidly by the liver and, as a result, must be given parenterally. Naloxone has a half-life that's significantly shorter than that of morphine, so multiple doses may be needed to reverse the depressant effects of opioids.

Naltrexone

Naltrexone has a longer duration of action than naloxone (10 hours) and is more effective in oral doses. It has a high affinity for μ receptors and is a competitive antagonist. The drug is used as part of long-term treatment for opioid and alcohol addiction. By preventing the euphoria that normally results from the use of opioids, naltrexone helps to discourage their illicit use.

Local anesthetics

Local anesthetics block the sensation of pain by interfering with the propagation of peripheral nerve impulses along nerve axons. When applied to a localized area, they can produce analgesia and muscle relaxation without hypnosis or sedation. As a class, local anesthetics can be identified by the suffix, "-caine." Examples include benzocaine, lidocaine, and procaine.

Local anesthetics block the conduction of action potentials along nerve axons by blocking the influence of stimulation on sodium channels. Local anesthetics must cross the cell membrane to be effective because they produce their effects by binding at specific sites near the intracellular end of sodium channels. As the local anesthetic block develops, the threshold for excitation increases, the conduction rate of action potentials slows and, if sodium conductance is blocked along a critical length of axon, the ability to conduct action potentials fails.

Local anesthetics affect different types of nerve fibers to varying degrees, based mainly on fiber size, length, and firing frequency. Large-diameter, myelinated A fibers, which convey information about motor function, pressure, proprioception, and touch, are relatively insensitive to local anesthetics. In contrast, small-diameter sensory fibers, which convey information about temperature and pain, are very sensitive to local anesthetics. Sensory traits listed in increasing order of resistance to conduction block include pain, cold, warmth, touch, and deep pressure.

Routes of administration

Depending on the extent and duration of anesthesia needed, local anesthetics can be administered by several different routes. Anesthesia of mucous membranes—such as the nose, mouth, throat, and trachea—and of injured skin can be achieved by applying a topical anesthetic directly to surface membranes. Aqueous solutions can be used to cover large surfaces. Ointments or viscous gels can be used for restricted areas. Some local anesthetics, such as benzocaine, may be effective when applied topically but ineffective when administered parenterally.

Injecting a local anesthetic into the S.C. or submucosal tissues rapidly anesthetizes nerve endings in specified regions of the peripheral nervous system. The anesthetic also can be used in nerve block fashion by injecting it close to a nerve trunk but proximal to the intended area of anesthesia. Following diffusion of the drug, tissues normally innervated by the distal portion of the affected nerve are anesthetized.

Finally, giving a local anesthetic solution in the subarachnoid space of the spinal cord can produce CNS anesthesia in all structures of the body below the diaphragm. The local anesthetic is usually administered in the lumbar subarachnoid space to avoid damage to the spinal cord. Cerebrospinal fluid distributes the anesthetic to the spinal cord; the dose and volume of anesthetic administered determine the extent of distribution.

The epidural space can be used as an alternative to the subarachnoid space, but epidural anesthesia usually is slower in onset, typically requires more drug, and may be more difficult to control than spinal anesthesia.

Adverse effects
Local anesthetics can provide reversible analgesia within well-defined, localized regions of the body, but they don't selectively depress peripheral nerve conduction, and they can interfere with nerve conduction in any excitable tissue, particularly CNS tissue and cardiac tissue. Systemic effects can occur if large amounts of drug are absorbed into the blood from the site of injection. However, adverse effects can be minimized if these drugs are administered properly and in combination with a vasoconstrictor. (See *How to avoid the adverse effects of local anesthetics.*) Also, keep in mind that

> ### How to avoid the adverse effects of local anesthetics
>
> ▌ Take a careful history.
> ▌ Use the smallest dose possible that will provide effective anesthesia.
> ▌ Use proper injection techniques, and aspirate before giving the local anesthetic to avoid intravascular injection.
> ▌ Inject slowly.
> ▌ Avoid repeated injections into the same site over a prolonged period of time.
> ▌ Use a vasoconstrictor with the local anesthetic (except in fingers, toes, ears, or penis) because many local anesthetics inhibit myogenic activity and autonomic tone and produce vasodilation at the administration site. The vasoconstrictor localizes the anesthetic, decreases systemic absorption, and prolongs the duration of action. Epinephrine is considered the most effective vasoconstrictor for use with local anesthetics.

the risk of contact dermatitis increases among staff who frequently handle local anesthetics, particularly those of the ester type.

Central effects
Because local anesthetics are lipid-soluble, they can cross the blood-brain barrier and pass from the peripheral circulation into the CNS. These neurons are very sensitive to local anesthetics, and initial signs and symptoms of CNS effects include light-headedness, dizziness, numbness, visual and auditory disturbances, and feelings of disorientation. If blood levels are high enough, seizures may oc-

cur, followed by respiratory and CV depression and a loss of consciousness.

Cardiovascular effects

Local anesthetics can directly affect cardiac tissue. Some of these effects can be beneficial and have been used to advantage. For example, local anesthetics can be used to treat cardiac arrhythmias. At nontoxic levels, they increase the effective refractory period of cardiac tissue and decrease cardiac automaticity. At toxic levels, membrane excitability and conduction velocity are depressed throughout the heart, which leads to decreased cardiac output, hypoxia and, ultimately, circulatory collapse.

Psychotropic drugs

The human pain response is a complex phenomenon with both physiologic and affective components. The affective component can be influenced by many factors, including past experiences with pain, both personal and cultural, the reactions of others to pain, and the emotional context in which pain is experienced. Psychotropic drugs influence multiple neurotransmitter systems in the brain, and changes in CNS neurotransmission could account for their analgesic effects. These changes aren't always comparable, however, and additional studies will be needed to understand the specific mechanisms that account for their analgesic effects.

Drugs that may be used to treat various aspects of the pain experience and its aftermath include antidepressants, antipsychotics, and anxiolytics.

Antidepressants

Certain antidepressants have proven effective at relieving some chronic pain states, such as diabetic neuropathy, rheumatoid arthritis, and migraine headaches. The mechanisms by which these drugs reduce pain are unclear. However, many patients with chronic pain also have evidence of depression; perhaps these drugs' analgesic effects are related in part to their physiologic effects, such as sedation, muscle relaxation, and decreased anxiety.

This isn't the whole explanation, however, for several reasons. For one thing, the analgesic effects of antidepressants occur more quickly than their antidepressant effects. Also, relief of chronic pain has been reported by patients who have no evidence of clinical depression. Plus, not all antidepressants are effective analgesics. A more likely explanation for the analgesic effects of some antidepressants may involve their actions on the CNS catecholamine system and their ability to increase synaptic levels of dopamine, norepinephrine, and serotonin.

Antidepressants known to relieve some kinds of pain in some patients include tricyclic antidepressants and selective serotonin reuptake inhibitors.

Tricyclic antidepressants (especially amitriptyline, desipramine, doxepin, imipramine, and nortriptyline) can be helpful for treating severe, burning, neuropathic pain, especially when combined with anticonvulsants, although it may take 2 to 4 weeks for therapeutic effects to occur. Tricyclic antidepressants also may help to reduce pain in patients with cancer, low back pain, and headache.

Doses for analgesia are lower than for depression. Amitriptyline at low doses is the first choice for chronic pain in most patients. However, doxepin is the drug of choice for elderly patients because of their increased risk of orthostatic hypotension.

Selective serotonin reuptake inhibitors aren't as effective as tricyclic antidepressants in treating chronic pain, but they have fewer adverse effects. They may be used if tricyclic antidepressants fail to relieve a patient's pain or if the adverse effects are intolerable. It may take 3 to 5 weeks for pain-relieving effects to occur.

Antipsychotics
Antipsychotics that may help in treating chronic pain—especially neuropathic pain—include phenothiazines, thioxanthenes, and butyrophenones. Because most patients with chronic pain don't experience delusions, the analgesic effects of these drugs are probably distinct from their antipsychotic effects. Antipsychotics influence multiple neurotransmitter systems in the CNS. Unlike antidepressants, antipsychotics inhibit dopamine, norepinephrine, serotonin, and histamine neurotransmission.

Anxiolytics
Benzodiazepines are the most important class of anxiolytics; they affect transmission of norepinephrine, serotonin, dopamine, and gamma-aminobutyric acid (GABA). In general, these drugs don't produce significant analgesic effects. However, they may still serve several purposes for patients with pain. For one, they can help to relieve the anxiety, excessive muscle tension, and insomnia that can accompany chronic pain.

For another, their sedative-hypnotic and amnestic properties may make them useful before surgery. And because oral forms of diazepam can relax skeletal muscles, this drug can be used to treat neurologic conditions that cause muscle spasms and tetanus. The mechanism of such action is unknown, but the drug probably inhibits spinal polysynaptic and monosynaptic afferent pathways.

Anticholinergics
Anticholinergics are used to treat various spastic conditions, including acute dystonic reactions, muscle rigidity, parkinsonism, and extrapyramidal disorders. They also are used to reverse neuromuscular blockade, to prevent nausea and vomiting from motion sickness, to help treat peptic ulcer disease and other GI disorders, and preoperatively to decrease secretions and block cardiac reflexes. They may be useful as an adjunct for malignant bowel obstruction, reducing peristalsis and secretions. The transdermal scopalamine patch is the drug of choice for this purpose.

Anticholinergics competitively antagonize the actions of acetylcholine and other cholinergic agonists in the parasympathetic nervous system. Lack of specificity for site of action increases the risk of adverse effects along with the therapeutic effects.

Belladonna alkaloids are natural anticholinergics that have been used for centuries. Many semisynthetic alkaloids and synthetic anticholinergics are available; however, most offer few advantages over naturally occurring alkaloids.

Antihistamines

Antihistamines, which are synthetic H_1-receptor antagonists, have many applications related specifically to chemical structure. Some antihistamines are used primarily to treat allergy symptoms, such as rhinitis or pruritus, whereas others are used more often for their antiemetic and antivertigo effects. Still others are used as sedative-hypnotics, local anesthetics, and antitussives. Some evidence suggests a role in analgesia.

For patients with pain, you're most likely to use an antihistamine to counter opioid-induced pruritus, nausea, and vomiting. Use caution when administering an antihistamine to a patient who also receives as opioid because of the additive CNS depressant effects.

Barbiturates

Before the advent of benzodiazepines, barbiturates were used extensively as sedative-hypnotics and antianxiety drugs. They're structurally related compounds that act throughout the CNS, particularly in the mesencephalic reticular activating system, which controls the CNS arousal mechanism. Barbiturates decrease both presynaptic and postsynaptic membrane excitability. The exact mechanism of action at these sites isn't known, nor is it clear which cellular and synaptic actions result in sedative-hypnotic effects.

Barbiturates can produce all levels of CNS depression, from mild sedation to coma to death. They facilitate the actions of GABA. They also exert a central effect, which depresses respiration and GI motility. The principal anticonvulsant mechanism of action is reduction of nerve transmission and decreased excitability of the nerve cell. Barbiturates also raise the seizure threshold.

Most currently available barbiturates are used as sedative-hypnotics for short-term (up to 2 weeks) treatment of insomnia because of their nonspecific CNS effects. Barbiturates aren't used routinely as sedatives, although they may be used as preanesthetic sedatives. Barbiturate-induced sleep differs from physiologic sleep by decreasing rapid eye movement sleep cycles. A few short-acting barbiturates are used as general anesthetics. Phenobarbital is an effective anticonvulsant.

Corticosteroids

Corticosteroids are classified according to their activity into two groups: mineralocorticoids and glucocorticoids. The mineralocorticoids regulate electrolyte homeostasis. The glucocorticoids regulate carbohydrate, lipid, and protein metabolism; inflammation; and the body's immune responses to diverse stimuli. Many corticosteroids exert both kinds of activity. These drugs can be used both systemically and topically. (See *Using topical corticosteroids*.)

Systemic corticosteroids dramatically affect almost all body systems. They're thought to act by controlling the rate of protein synthesis; they react with receptor proteins in the cytoplasm of sensitive cells in many tissues to form a steroid-receptor complex. The steroid-receptor complex migrates into the nucleus of the cell, where it binds to chromatin. Information carried by the steroid of the receptor protein directs the genetic apparatus to transcribe ribonucleic acid, resulting in the synthesis of specif-

Using topical corticosteroids

Topical corticosteroids relieve inflammatory and pruritic skin disorders, including localized neurodermatitis, psoriasis, atopic or seborrheic dermatitis, the inflammatory phase of xerosis, anogenital pruritus, discoid lupus erythematosus, lichen planus, granuloma annulare, and lupus erythematosus.

These drugs also may relieve irritant or allergic contact dermatitis. Rectal disorders responsive to this class of drugs include ulcerative colitis, cryptitis, inflamed hemorrhoids, post-irradiation or factitial proctitis, and pruritus ani.

Oral lesions, such as nonherpetic oral inflammatory and ulcerative lesions and routine gingivitis, may respond to treatment with topical corticosteroids as well.

Over-the-counter topical corticosteroids can be used for minor skin irritations, such as itching; rash from eczema, dermatitis, insect bites, poison ivy, poison oak, or poison sumac; and dermatitis from exposure to soaps, detergents, cosmetics, and jewelry.

Drug action

The exact mechanism by which topical corticosteroids exert anti-inflammatory effects is unclear; however, many researchers believe they stimulate transcription of messenger ribonucleic acid in individual cell nuclei to synthesize enzymes that stimulate biochemical pathways that decrease the inflammatory response.

Topical corticosteroids are minimally absorbed and cause fewer adverse effects than systemic corticosteroids. Fluorinated derivatives are absorbed more than other topical corticosteroids. The degree of absorption depends on the application site, the amount applied, the relative potency, the presence of an occlusive dressing (which may increase penetration by 10%), the condition of the skin, and the vehicle carrying the drug.

Ointments are best for dry, scaly areas. Solutions, gels, aerosols, and lotions are best for hairy areas. Creams can be used for most areas except those in which dampness may cause maceration. Gels and lotions can be used for moist lesions; however, gels may contain alcohol, which can dry and irritate the skin. Topical preparations are classified by potency into six groups: group I is the most potent, group VI the least potent.

Special considerations

When applying a topical corticosteroid, remember to wash your hands thoroughly before and afterwards. Gently clean the area to be treated; to increase drug penetration, consider washing or soaking the area before applying the drug.

Apply the drug sparingly in a light film; rub it in lightly. Avoid the patient's eyes unless you're using an ophthalmic product. Also, avoid prolonged application in areas near the eyes, genitals, rectum, on the face, and in skin folds. High-potency topical corticosteroids are more likely to cause striae and atrophy in these areas because of their higher absorption rates.

---

ic proteins that serve as enzymes in various biochemical pathways. Because the maximum pharmacologic activity lags behind peak blood levels, corticosteroid effects may result from modification of enzyme activity rather than from direct action by the drugs.

Drug uses

Among other actions, these drugs can be used to treat inflammation, to produce immunosuppression, to ease rheumatic and collagen disorders, and to reduce some types of cancer pain.

Inflammation

A major use of systemic glucocorticoids is treatment of inflammation. The anti-inflammatory effects depend on the direct local action of the steroids. Glucocorticoids decrease the inflammatory response via several actions:

▶ stabilizing leukocyte lysosomal membranes, which prevents the release of destructive acid hydrolases from leukocytes
▶ inhibiting macrophage accumulation in inflamed areas
▶ reducing leukocyte adhesion to the capillary endothelium
▶ reducing capillary wall permeability and edema formation
▶ decreasing complement activation
▶ antagonizing histamine activity and release of kinin from substrates
▶ reducing fibroblast proliferation, collagen deposition, and subsequent scar tissue formation.

Immunosuppression

The full mechanism by which these drugs exert immunosuppressive action is unknown. Glucocorticoids reduce activity and volume in the lymphatic system, producing lymphocytopenia, decreasing immunoglobulin and complement concentrations, decreasing passage of immune complexes through basement membranes, and possibly depressing the reactivity of tissues to antigen-antibody interaction.

Other uses

Systemic glucocorticoids are also used to treat many other painful disorders, such as these:

▶ rheumatic and collagen diseases, such as arthritis, polyarteritis nodosa, and systemic lupus erythematosus
▶ thyroiditis
▶ severe dermatologic diseases, such as pemphigus, exfoliative dermatitis, graft versus host disease, lichen planus, and psoriasis
▶ allergic reactions
▶ inflammatory ocular disorders
▶ respiratory diseases, such as asthma, sarcoidosis, and lipid pneumonitis
▶ hematologic diseases, such as autoimmune hemolytic anemia and idiopathic thrombocytopenia
▶ cancers, including leukemias and lymphomas
▶ cancer pain, especially in bone metastasis, headache from increased intracranial pressure, or nerve compression
▶ neuropathic pain
▶ GI diseases, such as ulcerative colitis, regional enteritis, and celiac disease.

Other indications include myasthenia gravis, organ transplants, nephrotic syndrome, and septic shock. Glucocorticoids may help maintain motor and sensory function when given in large I.V. doses shortly after an acute spinal cord injury or compression. In palliative care, corticosteroids help reduce pain, increase appetite, and improve mood and quality of life.

Histamine$_2$-receptor antagonists

The introduction of H$_2$-receptor antagonists has revolutionized the treatment of peptic ulcer disease. These drugs structurally resemble histamine and competitively inhibit the action of histamine on H_2 receptors in gastric parietal cells. As a result, they reduce gastric acid output and concentration regardless of the stimulatory compound (histamine, food, insulin, caffeine) or basal conditions.

Specifically, these drugs are indicated for duodenal ulcer, gastric ulcer, hypersecretory states, and reflux esophagitis. They've also been used off-label to prevent stress ulcers in critically ill patients, to treat short-bowel syndrome, to prevent allergic reactions to I.V. contrast medium, and to eradicate *Helicobacter pylori* in the treatment of peptic ulcers.

Hydantoin derivatives

Hydantoins, of which phenytoin is the prototype, are used mainly to control tonic-clonic and partial seizures. Parenteral phenytoin and fosphenytoin are used to treat status epilepticus, to prevent and treat seizures during neurosurgery, and to provide a short-term substitute for oral phenytoin therapy. The hydantoins work by inhibiting the spread of seizure activity in the motor cortex; they stabilize the seizure threshold against hyperexcitability produced by excessive stimulation and decrease posttetanic potentiation that accompanies abnormal focal discharge.

Certain anticonvulsants (notably carbamazapine and gabapentin) may help to relieve neuropathic pain in adults. Carbamazepine is a dibenzazepine derivative with anticonvulsant and psychotropic properties. It's the drug of choice for treating the pain of trigeminal neuralgia and may be helpful in other neurologic disorders that cause severe pain.

Gabapentin is an analogue of the inhibitory neurotransmitter GABA and is used mainly as an anticonvulsant to treat partial seizures. Although its mechanism of action isn't fully understood, the drug has proven effective in a growing number of patients with intractable neurogenic pain. It's gaining in popularity.

▶ COMMON THERAPIES

Pain management is most successful when tailored to the type of pain the patient has: acute pain, chronic pain, or cancer pain.

Acute pain

Acute pain from trauma, surgery, or acute disease is expected to last for a fairly well-defined period of time, during which medical management will treat the problem and stop the pain. It's possible, therefore, to use drugs and invasive treatments that are effective for short time periods but perhaps not reasonable for extended periods.

Acute pain may be constant (as in a burn), intermittent (as in a muscle strain that hurts only with activity), or both (as in an abdominal incision that hurts a little at rest and a lot with movement or coughing). Accordingly, management of acute pain requires that you consider these varying levels of pain.

First choices

Consider the range of drugs available for treating acute pain as a ladder based on the severity of the patient's pain, on preexisting illnesses, and on the likelihood of complications. At the bottom of the ladder, for minor pain problems, acetaminophen, NSAIDs, and COX-2 inhibitors are common choices. The anti-inflammatory effects of these drugs may actually be helpful in rapid healing and restoration of normal function.

Oral opioids

The next step up the ladder is to oral opioids. Opioids are the most effective analgesics available; they continue to be the cornerstone of pain management. Some give long-lasting relief; others last only 2 to 4 hours. Most familiar opioids have a short duration and make reasonable choices for moderate pain, especially if activity-related. More severe activity-related pain should be controlled by reducing activity along with opioid use.

For fairly severe pain that's expected to last several days or more, consider a long-acting opioid, either a slow-release form or a drug with a long half-life. Slow-release morphine and methadone are commonly used, as is oxycodone. With the increasing focus of medicine on the cost-benefit ratio, the use of oral drugs, even for a patient in the hospital, should be the first choice if the patient is allowed oral intake.

Patients vary greatly in their analgesic requirements, so opioid dosing schedules should be individualized for each patient to maximize analgesic effects and minimize adverse effects. For example, because opioid metabolism and elimination decrease with age, pain relief provided by opioids may increase with age. Thus, opioid doses that provide effective analgesia for older patients may not be appropriate for younger patients and vice versa.

A number of nonanalgesic drugs can be used as adjuncts to pain management with oral opioids. They include sleeping aids, muscle relaxants to decrease muscle spasm, and antihistamines to reduce adverse effects (such as itching) and provide mild sedation.

Parenteral opoids

The next step up the ladder for managing acute pain is to parenteral opioids. The pharmacokinetic properties of many opioids make them most effective when administered parenterally. For acute pain, you'll most likely deliver parenteral opioids by injection. Patient-controlled analgesia (PCA) offers another option for managing acute pain. (See *Benefits of patient-controlled analgesia.*) You also may deliver them via regional analgesia. Other routes may be helpful as well, such as the intranasal route.

Injection

The standard for parenteral opioid administration is I.M. injection on an intermittent basis, usually every 4 to 6 hours. However, because pain relief may last only 2 hours in some patients, they may face a substantial amount of pain—besides the pain of the injection and the 15- to 30-minute wait for pain relief to begin.

Regional analgesia

Opioids can be administered by other routes as well, such as the epidural and intrathecal routes. These usually are used in conjunction with a local anesthetic to produce CNS anesthesia below the level of insertion in the spine. Because the patient retains motor ability and nonnociceptive sensation below the level of the epidural catheter, this is also a popular method of controlling acute postoperative or traumatic pain.

In the United States the pain of childbirth is commonly relieved via an epidural catheter. By placing the catheter at various levels in the epidural space, it's possible to relieve not only labor pain but also pain from abdominal or thoracic incisions and even pain caused by broken ribs.

When local anesthetics are infused through catheters, they reduce all sensation in the nerves near the tip of the catheter. The number of nerves affected is influenced by flow rate. Because opioid receptors are in the spinal cord, opioids given through an epidural catheter are regionally effective in a manner similar to local anesthetics. However, morphine may diffuse through cerebrospinal fluid and affect brain receptors as well.

Although this epidural technique sounds like a panacea for pain, it does have some drawbacks. Head and neck pain commonly can't be treated in this fashion because nerves supplying pain sensitivity to those areas don't travel through the epidural space. Plus, local anesthetics change more than sensation; they can also cause the blood vessels to dilate significantly, sometimes causing blood pressure to fall below acceptable levels. Adequate hydration can help prevent or lower the risk of this adverse event. Higher concentrations of local anesthetics also block the motor nerve fibers, causing muscle weakness. If this change affects the patient's legs, it stops ambulation and can slow the patient's recovery if allowed to continue.

Epidural administration of opioids allows a relatively high opioid level at the spinal pain receptors without the usual nausea, vomiting, sedation, or constipation.

Benefits of patient-controlled analgesia

Patient-controlled analgesia (PCA) is a popular method of controlling acute postoperative pain using an electronic injection device controlled in part by the patient. The computerized device holds a syringe of medication that's attached directly to the patient's intravenous (I.V.) line. By pushing a button, the patient can give himself a small dose of opioid through the I.V. line. The PCA device won't allow administration of an overdose, and most devices can deliver a constant infusion along with on-demand boluses.

Small, on-demand boluses of opioid allow the patient to adjust the drug to his own needs. Also, by providing small but frequent doses, PCA reduces the adverse effects caused by high systemic opioid levels.

Another important benefit of PCA is that it provides patients with a greater sense of personal control, which may reduce anxiety and improve analgesia. It also is particularly useful for patients who are reluctant to ask for pain medication. Patient-controlled epidural devices have become available for pain management as well.

However, the risk of these problems still exists. Another possible adverse effect, if the patient demands absolutely no pain, is itching. Although it can be severe enough for the patient to refuse further epidural administration, it usually is merely a nuisance.

Nerve blocks
Peripheral nerve blocks by single injection or placement of a catheter near the nerve can be performed

for pain after surgery or injury. Anesthesiologists are trained to perform nerve blocks to anesthetize various regions of the body so that surgery can be performed without a general anesthetic. In fact, these same techniques can be used after surgery to relieve pain, and a single injection can last as long as 8 to 12 hours. If pain relief is needed for a longer period of time, a catheter may be inserted to allow repeat administration or a continuous infusion. In general, only local anesthetics are used through these catheters. Delivering opioids by this method hasn't proven consistently helpful.

Chronic pain

Chronic pain is poorly defined because the shift from an acute pain problem to a chronic pain problem develops gradually. Many experts choose a point at 3 to 6 months when they consider that acute pain has become chronic pain.

Unlike acute pain, chronic pain may not have an expected end point. Even with medical management, it may last for the rest of the patient's life in some cases. Under these circumstances, treatments that have significant risks or a reduced likelihood of long-term effectiveness may not be reasonable choices. Indeed, drug treatment alone is almost never effective for long-term chronic pain. Treatment for chronic pain typically includes drug therapy, nondrug therapies, temporary or permanent invasive therapies (such as nerve blocks or surgery), cognitive-behavioral treatments, and self-management techniques. It must focus on rehabilitation rather than cure.

The rehabilitation approach has several clear goals:

▶ to maximize the patient's functional abilities, both physical and psychological
▶ to minimize the pain the patient experiences during rehabilitation and for the rest of his life
▶ to teach the patient how to manage whatever pain remains as well as how to handle pain exacerbations that arise because of increased activity or for unexplained reasons.

Medical treatment for chronic pain should always be determined in the context of the patient's long-term benefit rather than on the narrow basis of today's pain complaint. Naturally, the choice of drug therapy for a patient with chronic pain must consider this wider goal first and foremost.

First choices

Drugs most commonly used for chronic pain are the NSAIDs. These drugs are typically more effective for inflammation-related pain, but they are direct analgesics and, consequently, can also reduce noninflammatory pain.

The other group of drugs commonly used to treat chronic pain on a long-term basis is antidepressants. Many antidepressants are available, each with different adverse effects profiles. However, in general, they all increase the activity of one or more CNS pathways that inhibit pain perception. Unfortunately, the response rate to antidepressants, alone or with other drugs, is significantly less than 100%. Many patients receive no benefit from them at all.

Opioids

The use of opioids for chronic pain has been a source of great controversy because they can lead to tol-

Understanding tolerance, dependence, and addiction

Successful administration of opioids requires that you understand three concepts: tolerance, dependence, and addiction.

Tolerance
Tolerance occurs when a specified amount of drug becomes less effective when taken over a prolonged period of time. This change is common to the opioids. Consequently, a patient's need for larger opioid doses over time doesn't necessarily imply dependence or addiction.

Dependence
Dependence may be physical, psychological, or both. Physical dependence means that if a drug is abruptly discontinued, the patient will develop withdrawal symptoms. For opioids, these symptoms represent increased activity in the sympathetic and central nervous systems. They may include a flulike syndrome, malaise, achiness, marked diarrhea, nausea, vomiting, increased heart rate and blood pressure, profuse sweating, and perhaps confusion, seizures, or even death. Gradual opioid withdrawal greatly reduces or eliminates these symptoms.

Psychological dependence involves the patient's belief that he must take a drug to cause or to stop a particular effect. The desired effect of opioids is to reduce pain, although many patients state that taking an opioid allows them to function. Psychological dependence has some similarities to addiction.

Addiction
Addiction is a complex of behaviors associated with drug-seeking or manipulative behavior and involves taking a drug for effects other than pain relief. With opioids, the effect usually is euphoria or sedation.

When describing a patient's relationship to an opioid, be careful. Avoid using the word *addiction*, with its social, medical, and legal implications, when you really mean physical dependence or tolerance.

---

erance, dependence, and addiction. (See *Understanding tolerance, dependence, and addiction.*) When considering opioids for chronic pain, follow these guidelines. First, try to attain satisfactory pain management without opioids. Second, make sure the patient takes part in a rehabilitation program that includes a behavioral approach to pain management before starting long-term opioid use. And third, assess the behavioral issues that determine whether long-term opioid use is appropriate.

Opioids are delivered most commonly by the oral route. However, other routes are available as well, such as the sublingual (S.L.) route and the transdermal route.

Sublingual administration
Buprenorphine, a synthetic opioid with reduced sedative and respiratory depressant effects, has been proven effective with S.L. administration and is being used outside the United States. A lipophilic compound, it's easily absorbed through the oral mucosa. Other oral morphine preparations have been effective with S.L. administration as well.

An oral transmucosal form of fentanyl can be used as a preoperative sedative, anxiolytic, and analgesic. Fentanyl doesn't produce effective analgesia with a single S.L. dose, but it does provide analgesia when incorporated into a candy base that the patient can suck until pain relief occurs. This noninvasive route of administration may be particularly effective for children.

Transdermal administration

Fentanyl is currently available in transdermal form. Its main advantage is that it converts a short-acting drug into one that produces up to 72 hours of analgesia once plasma levels reach steady state. Because an S.C. depot of the drug must develop after initial application of the product, several days may to need to pass before steady state plasma levels and effective analgesia occur. Conversely, it may take a few days for plasma levels to decrease in cases of toxicity or adverse affects. Thus, alternative means of analgesia are needed during the initial period of the transdermal application. Obviously, transdermal routes of administration aren't appropriate for acute pain because of the slow onset of analgesia.

Subcutaneous and intravenous administration

S.C. and I.V. infusions can also provide a consistent plasma level of opioid and thus a consistent level of relief of relatively constant pain. I.V. boluses with or without the I.V. infusion can deliver rapid increases in the opioid level and, therefore, rapid relief of breakthrough pain. The capacity to deliver an I.V. bolus of opioid is very important for relieving intermittent increases in pain. Relief typically takes 3 to 10 minutes, much less time than an I.M. injection takes.

When a patient isn't an appropriate candidate for long-term opioid therapy, the pain management team must establish a humane weaning program to reduce opioids already in use while avoiding withdrawal symptoms and minimizing pain. There's usually significant iatrogenic cause for opioid dependence under these circumstances, and labeling the patient as a medication abuser or addict is inappropriate. Other drugs prescribed for pain, such as benzodiazepines, barbiturates, and similar drugs, should also be humanely reduced and eliminated if possible.

Nerve blocks

Nerve blocks, or injection therapy, for chronic pain management typically fit one of three basic categories: diagnostic blocks, short-term therapeutic blocks, and destructive, or neurolytic blocks. Diagnostic blocks consist of a local anesthetic injected into an area thought to be a pain source or around the nerves supplying an area thought to be a pain source. This process reveals the relative significance of that source in the patient's complaints. Keep in mind that a placebo response occurs in about 30% of the normal population, giving many false-positive responses. Diagnostic blocks may be performed two or three times to rule out this placebo effect.

Short-term therapeutic blocks can be injected at the site of a pain source or along the path of the nerves to the spinal cord. Nerve blocks can be remarkably effective for some patients by helping them to complete a rehabilitation program faster and with reduced pain.

However, keep in mind that the ability to temporarily block chronic pain isn't a sufficient reason to perform a therapeutic block. In fact, for some patients, it's harmful to create dramatic pain relief, only to have pain return in a short time.

For a patient who does receive a short-term therapeutic block, use objective measures when determining improvement in the patient's condition (physical activity, ability to focus on behavioral techniques, and so forth).

Occasionally a patient will have long-term or apparently permanent pain relief from a short-term block. This response can't be explained medically except by invoking the patient's return to normal activity or the rather unscientific principle of "breaking the pain cycle" as the probable cause of relief. These long-term positive responses are fairly rare and shouldn't be presented to patients as any reasonable expectation.

A remarkable phenomenon can occur with patients who have had permanent neurolysis. After a while, typically 6 to 12 months, the perception of pain in the treated area often recurs. A number of theories explain this phenomenon, including regeneration of nerves and changes in afferent processing mechanisms in the CNS. The recurring pain is frequently somewhat different from the initial pain but, unfortunately, often far more severe. The new pain is usually neuralgic and very difficult to treat or even to reduce. The problem of recurring pain also appears when a neurosurgical procedure interrupts a nerve; therefore, neurosurgical nerve-interruption procedures should also be viewed skeptically for most chronic pain problems.

Spinal cord stimulator

Spinal cord stimulators are most useful for neuralgic pain in an area on one side of the body that isn't adequately controlled by less invasive treatment. For a select group of patients with these complaints, insertion of a spinal cord stimulator can produce remarkable pain relief that allows those patients to return to more normal function. The cord stimulation system involves very specific placement of stimulating electrodes in the epidural space close to the spinal cord. Spinal cord stimulators are intended for lifelong implantation with only occasional battery changes.

This procedure is not a panacea, however, and like any other treatment option, it has its problems and failures. The electrodes can move or break, making them nonfunctional. Even with continued appropriate stimulation, some patients lose pain relief over time. Some patients get no relief from the procedure and, indeed, may experience increased pain with the stimulation. Obviously, in those patients who get no relief, the system would not be permanently placed.

Spinal catheter

Analgesia via spinal catheters involves an infusion or sometimes a bolus injection, usually of an opioid or local anesthetic, into the epidural space in a manner similar to the epidural infusion used to control acute pain. Controversy exists over the use of such catheters for patients with chronic pain, largely because the same tolerance and dependence issues arise with this technologically advanced system as with simple oral administration of opioids. Plus, the cost of placing the catheter and refilling the pump is relatively high. And complications may include infection of the spinal cord or brain.

For these reasons, spinal catheters are usually reserved for cancer pain. As the safety record of these devices improves, and as data on long-term use accumulates, they may begin to play a greater role in managing chronic pain.

Cancer pain

Cancer pain is managed in the context of the assumption that the patient has an undefined but probably shortened life expectancy. Consequently, treatment commonly focuses on pain relief at any cost. As in acute pain, treatments inappropriate for long-term use may be appropriate for treating cancer pain, although quality of life and the patient's functional abilities are extremely important as well.

Undertreated cancer pain diminishes the patient's activity, appetite, and sleep. It may prevent the patient from working productively, enjoying recreation, or taking pleasure in the usual family and society roles. The psychological effect of cancer pain can also be devastating. Whether the pain results from cancer or its treatment, it may cause the patient to lose hope, believing that the terminal disease is progressing. The result may be worsening helplessness, anxiety, and depression. Both physical and mental suffering can be diminished by adequate pain control.

Keep in mind, however, that cancer pain is a complex problem. It may originate from several sources, including bone, muscle, nerves, or visceral structures. And it may have several etiologies, including these:

‣ tumor progression and related pathology
‣ invasive diagnostic or therapeutic procedures
‣ toxicity of chemotherapy and radiation therapy
‣ infection
‣ muscle aches from limitations in physical activity.

First choices

Drug therapy adjusted to the progress of the patient's disease effectively relieves cancer pain in a large number of patients. Opioids provide the cornerstone of treatment for cancer pain. The World Health Organization has developed a simple, effective method (called the analgesic ladder) for choosing the appropriate therapy for cancer pain.

NSAIDs or acetaminophen are used alone for mild pain and combined with opioids and adjuvant analgesics if pain intensity increases. (See *Adjuvant therapy for cancer pain*.) A combination of NSAIDs and opioids can provide better analgesia than either can provide alone. NSAIDs also exhibit a "dose-sparing" effect on opioids. In other words, giving acetaminophen or another NSAID together with an opioid provides effective analgesia at a lower-than-usual opioid dose. NSAIDs don't produce tolerance or physical or psychological dependence, but there is a ceiling on their analgesic potential.

Opioids

The next step on the analgesic ladder employs opioids. The oral route is preferred because it's the most convenient and cost-effective. Full agonists are typically used for cancer pain because they offer analge-

Adjuvant therapy for cancer pain

Opioids are rightfully recognized for their analgesic value in treating cancer pain. However, other drugs may help as well.

▸ NSAIDs can help to manage osseous metastases.
▸ Antidepressants, anticonvulsants, sodium channel blockers, amphetamines, and corticosteroids can help to control neuropathic and other pain syndromes while limiting adverse opioid effects.
▸ Tricyclic antidepressants can be especially useful for patients with neuropathic pain, such as dysesthetic or burning pain. These drugs may also help to restore a normal nighttime sleep pattern and improve the patient's mood.
▸ Corticosteroids have been shown to decrease pain and increase appetite and activity, although some evidence suggests that they may do so for only 2 to 4 weeks. These drugs also raise some risks, such as immunosuppression, infection, proximal myopathy, psychiatric symptoms, and possibly a higher risk of adverse gastrointestinal and cardiovascular effects. Thus, the relative risk versus the benefit of using these drugs should be considered on an individual basis.

▸ Phenothiazines (antipsychotics sometimes used as sedatives or antiemetics) and benzodiazepines (sedatives often used as anxiolytics) probably don't help with analgesia. However, they may have beneficial effects on anxiety, sleep disturbance, and muscle spasms. Their use is appropriate as long as they don't take the place of appropriate opioid therapy or psychosocial interventions.
▸ Amphetamines can significantly increase the analgesic effect of morphine while decreasing sleepiness and increasing activity, appetite, and intellectual performance. However, certain patients (especially elderly patients) may experience decreased appetite, increased anxiety, increased delirium, or a paranoid reaction. These reactions may be less common with methylphenidate, which has a shorter half-life than dextroamphetamine. When opioid-related sedation becomes a limiting factor and the patient still has pain, an amphetamine may significantly decrease the pain and increase function.

sia without a ceiling effect. Don't give an agonist-antagonist to a patient who regularly takes an agonist because withdrawal symptoms may result.

Opioid tolerance and physical dependence are expected with long-term opioid treatment and shouldn't be confused with psychological dependence or addiction. For most cancer patients, the first indication of tolerance is a decrease in the duration of analgesia for a given dose.

Effective pain relief is best accomplished by anticipating and preventing pain. For a patient with persistent or daily pain, give an opioid on a regular schedule rather than as needed. As the drug is being adjusted to effect, the patient can take additional doses as needed to cover breakthrough pain. The optimal dose is one that controls pain with the fewest adverse effects, such as sedation, mental clouding, nausea, and constipation. If a particular adverse effect is poorly tolerated, try switching to another opioid to help manage it.

Usually, opioid analgesics with longer durations of action (such as controlled-release morphine, methadone, levorphanol, and the fentanyl patch) are preferred because they provide sustained analgesia and demand less frequent administration. Mild and incident pain can be relieved by codeine, hydromorphone, oxycodone, or immediate-release morphine, depending on the severity of the pain and the adverse drug effects.

Intramuscular, intravenous, and subcutaneous routes

Alternate routes of administration may be needed at times. I.M. and I.V. routes are commonly used, and the S.C. route can be considered as well. Studies have shown that S.C. dosing produces stable blood levels that correlate closely with continuous I.V. infusion. S.C. PCA has proven as effective as I.V. PCA. A weekly change of infusion site reduces the risk of local toxicity and infection, and can easily be performed by home health services.

Other routes to consider for administering opioids include rectal, nasal, S.L., buccal, and transdermal routes. Rectal administration is common in hospice settings. Variable absorption rates represent the main disadvantage of rectal administration. Absorption rates depend on the placement site, rectal contents, and individual differences in venous drainage from the rectum.

Intraspinal administration

Intraspinal opioid therapy probably represents the most significant advancement in contemporary cancer pain management. It provides reversible analgesia that's more likely to be effective for multiple pains, bilateral pain, or pain that crosses the midline. Intraspinal opioid therapy works best for somatic and visceral pain, both of which are common in cancer. A trial application using the less invasive percutaneous catheters can easily help to predict the patient's response to this therapy.

By means of a catheter, the opioid is introduced into either the epidural (peridural) space or the subarachnoid (intrathecal) space. Intraspinal analgesia classically refers to the administration of opioids only, which leaves the motor, sensory, and sympathetic systems unaffected. However, combinations of opioids and dilute concentrations of local anesthetics, which potentially can cause motor weakness, sensory anesthesia, and interference with sympathetic function at higher doses, are becoming more common. Studies have confirmed the synergism between local anesthetics and opioids.

Morphine is the most commonly used opioid and the most hydrophilic (water-soluble), reaching peak effect in 30 to 60 minutes and having a duration of analgesia of 6 to 24 hours with intrathecal administration. Epidural administration provides an even more delayed onset. The lipophilic (fat-soluble) drugs such as sufentanil and fentanyl peak in about 10 minutes and last 2 to 5 hours. They don't spread as readily in the epidural space; therefore, when delivered by epidural catheter, these drugs must be placed near the site of pain.

Adverse effects of intraspinal opioids include respiratory depression and loss of normal GI motility. The risk of respiratory depression generates the most clinical concern and can occur early (less than 2 hours after a dose) or late (4 to 24 hours after a dose). Lipophilic drugs are more likely to cause early respiratory depression; morphine may cause late respiratory depression. Fortunately, such depression occurs relatively rarely, if at all, in opioid-tolerant cancer patients. Pruritus is also uncommon in cancer patients, although it's very common in opioid-naïve patients. It typically responds to antihistamines or an opioid antagonist given systemically.

As with neurolysis and neurosurgery, the most widely accepted indication for chronic therapy with intraspinal opioids is intractable pain unresponsive to aggressive drug treatment. Some would argue for earlier administration of intraspinal opioids because of their reversibility and low risk, but the cost of the equipment and follow-up care may be a limiting factor.

Palliative radiation and chemotherapy

Radiation therapy and chemotherapy may be used to complement drug therapy and may enhance its effectiveness. That's because these therapies can eradicate or substantially depopulate tumor cells; therefore, they directly target the cause of pain. A balance is needed between the killing of tumor cells and the adverse effects of radiation or chemotherapy on normal tissue.

Local anesthetic nerve blockade

Anesthetic nerve blockade is a procedure in which a local anesthetic is injected around nerves or ganglia or into the epidural or intrathecal spaces of the spinal cord. For cancer pain, local anesthetic nerve blocks may fulfill diagnostic, prognostic, and therapeutic roles. Although this technique doesn't typically provide long-term relief, it does provide immediate relief of regional pain and can be invaluable in guiding future treatment.

Diagnostic nerve blocks can identify the source of pain and determine whether it's visceral or sympathetic, as opposed to somatic. Local anesthetic blocks may also be used to predict the efficacy of permanent ablative procedures, such as celiac plexus neurolysis (permanent destruction of the celiac ganglion), rhizotomy (permanent interruption of the dorsal root of a spinal nerve), or sympathectomy (permanent interruption of some portion of the sympathetic nerve pathways). They also allow the patient to experience the changes that are likely to accompany a more definitive procedure, such as neurolysis.

Even if the patient experiences temporary relief from a local anesthetic nerve block, however, that doesn't guarantee the long-term success of a surgical or neurolytic block. The pain-relieving effects of any neurodestructive procedure can be thwarted by postsurgical nerve regeneration, chronic deafferentation syndrome, and dysesthesias, among other complications. However, because a lack of response to local anesthetic blocks reliably predicts failure of permanent procedures, it remains helpful to perform these predictive blocks when a more permanent procedure is being considered.

Neurolysis: When is it warranted?

Neurolytic blockade may be considered if a patient meets all of these criteria:
- limited life expectancy
- localized or regional pain
- adequate response to local anesthetic block
- pain unrelieved by less invasive treatments.

Neurolysis

The term *neurolysis* means destruction of nerves. Thus, neurolysis is the permanent destruction of nerve tissue using various ablative techniques, including the injection of a neurolytic substance, such as phenol or ethyl alcohol. Although a fair amount of research has been devoted to finding drugs that destroy nerves safely, predictably, and consistently, we've thus far found no substance that consistently destroy nerves without destroying other tissue.

Phenol has some local anesthetic properties, so the injection isn't especially painful. The appropriate concentration of phenol depends largely on the carrier solution used. It may be glycerin, water, saline, or radiopaque dye.

Alcohol injection is commonly painful; however, it relieves pain almost immediately and may improve in effectiveness over 1 to 2 weeks. Alcohol tends to destroy tissue more completely than phenol and therefore may offer a more permanent block in areas where nerves can regenerate. Ethyl alcohol is used in concentrations of 50% to 100%, with 100% being extremely damaging to any tissue near the injection site.

Although newer nondestructive analgesic infusion techniques may have decreased the need for neurolysis, it may still be appropriate. Neurolysis should be performed by an experienced clinician and only after more conservative options have failed. (See *Neurolysis: When is it warranted?*)

Keep in mind that the sympathetic nervous system is extremely good at regenerating, peripheral nerves are fairly good at regenerating, and the spinal cord and brain are essentially incapable of regenerating.

Orthopedic procedures

Tumor involvement in bone can cause such complications as muscle weakness, decreased ambulation, joint stiffness or contractures, spinal deformities, osteopenia from inactivity, thromboembolism, and hypercalcemia. Performing surgical fixation of impending or completed pathologic fractures, maintaining the patient's ambulatory status, and encouraging rehabilitation programs (such as physical and occupational therapy) can reduce or avoid these problems that can lead to reduced functional ability.

Bone pain that isn't likely to result in fracture can be treated with local radiation therapy, which is the mainstay of pain control with metastatic lesions and multiple myeloma (malignant neoplasm of plasma cells, usually arising in the bone marrow). However, surgical stabilization followed by radiation therapy to permit healing is indicated if the patient has an impending fracture in a weight-bearing limb. Radiation therapy alone may be sufficient for lesions in the axial skeleton, which heal more readily.

Lesions of the spine are often detected early because patients usually present with back pain before there is significant bone destruction; however, following radiation therapy, if pain recurs, if the spine is unstable, or if a neurologic deficit progresses, surgery may be necessary.

Neurosurgical procedures

More conservative methods of pain management must be exhausted before neurosurgery is considered, and an experienced clinician must evaluate the patient. Procedures to ablate nervous tissue are typically avoided unless the patient has a life-shortening cancer. If the patient's life expectancy is less than 90 days, pain is usually managed with opioids or a percutaneous procedure, such as neurolytic injection or nonincisional neurosurgery. Neurodestructive surgery would be more appropriate in a cancer patient whose life expectancy is 6 months or greater.

The more common of these neurosurgical procedures include percutaneous radiofrequency coagulation, peripheral neurectomy, dorsal rhizotomy, cordotomy, and myelotomy.

Stereotaxy

Stereotaxy is a precise method of using three-dimensional coordinates to target certain brain structures and create lesions there. Using stereotaxy, radiofrequency and chemical removal of the pituitary gland offer the possibility of pain relief in all areas of the body. This procedure works best for hormone-dependent tumors, such as prostate and breast cancers; however, it's almost as successful with hormone-independent tumors.

It also works for bilateral or diffuse bone pain from metastatic disease that hasn't responded to other hormone, radiation, or medical therapies.

Complications of stereotaxy include anterior hypopituitarism, visual and oculomotor disturbances, and the recurrence of pain in 3 to 4 months. Transient confusion or other cognitive disorders may occur as well. Hormone replacement therapy may be needed to replace pituitary secretions. As with other destructive procedures, the long-term failure rate limits its usefulness.

▶ NONDRUG THERAPIES

Many nondrug and nonsurgical therapies can be used to help relieve pain. They include thermotherapy, cryotherapy, hydrotherapy, electrical therapy, manipulation, acupuncture, immobilization, exercise, and complementary therapies. (See *Selected nondrug therapies: Precautions and contraindications*, pages 66 and 67.)

Thermotherapy

Thermotherapy includes hot packs, paraffin baths, ultrasound, and microwave or shortwave diathermy.

A hot pack is a cloth-covered pouch with a silica gel core. It's externally heated and provides superficial regional conduction heating to the patient's trunk, spine, or limbs. It's used for muscle spasm, tendinitis, and bursitis.

A paraffin bath uses paraffin mixed with mineral oil to create a soak. This therapy provides regional conduction heating to arthritic limbs and hands.

Ultrasound uses energy generated by a quartz crystal and passed from an applicator through trans-

Selected nondrug therapies: Precautions and contraindications

THERAPY	PRECAUTIONS AND CONTRAINDICATIONS
Hot pack	▶ May increase core body temperature, increase blood flow, cause burns, and aggravate inflammatory response. ▶ Contraindicated by active bleeding, active infection, neoplasm, skin desensitization, vascular insufficiency.
Paraffin bath	▶ May cause burns, skin intolerance. ▶ Contraindicated by active bleeding, active infection, neoplasm, skin desensitization, vascular insufficiency.
Ultrasound	▶ May cause cavitation (gas bubble formation in tissue), periosteal superheating over bony surfaces. ▶ Contraindicated by previous spinal surgery or use over eye, fluid-filled sac, neoplasm.
Cryotherapy	▶ May produce mild or relative hypothermia, vascular constriction. ▶ Contraindicated by cryoglobulinemia, paroxysmal cold hemoglobinuria, Raynaud's syndrome, vascular insufficiency.
Pool therapy	▶ Water temperature may produce unwanted systemic effects and must be chosen appropriately. Patient unable to swim must wear life vest. ▶ Contraindicated by bowel or bladder incontinence, chemical sensitivity, open wound.
Hubbard tank, whirlpool	▶ Water temperature may produce unwanted systemic effects and must be chosen appropriately.
Iontophoresis	▶ Contraindicated by implanted cardiac pacemaker or defibrillator, insulin or baclofen pump.
Transcutaneous electrical nerve stimulation	▶ May produce variable effects. ▶ Contraindicated by implanted cardiac pacemaker or defibrillator, insulin or baclofen pump.
Traction	▶ Use caution to avoid injury or excessive pressure to area being treated, skin breakdown, vascular congestion when using inversion or suspension. ▶ Contraindicated by acutely herniated disk or artificial joint, spinal instability, underlying metastatic disease or multiple myeloma.
Massage	▶ Passive massage must be combined with active exercise for full recovery. ▶ Contraindicated for use over active phlebitis, arterial structures, bony prominences, compromised tissue, exposed nerves.

THERAPY	PRECAUTIONS AND CONTRAINDICATIONS
Selected nondrug therapies: Precautions and contraindications *(continued)*	
Manual manipulation	▶ Proper clinical assessment, evaluation, and testing are essential before therapy to minimize risks. Slight discomfort may be felt immediately after treatment. ▶ Contraindicated by active infection or bleeding, disk herniation, fractures, metastases, neoplasm, spinal instability.
Acupuncture	▶ Needles must be sterile to avoid risk of human immunodeficiency virus, hepatitis B transmission. Procedure causes some risk of hemothorax, pneumothorax.
Bed rest	▶ Can't be used indefinitely. Possible complications include bone loss, muscle atrophy, phlebitis, pulmonary embolism, skin breakdown, venous stasis. Early mobilization is essential to recovery.
Braces and orthotics	▶ Watch for dependence on brace, muscle atrophy, and dysfunction. Early selective or isometric exercise is important.

mission gel applied to the skin over targeted areas of body. The procedure provides deep heating to soft tissue and bone. It increases blood flow, raises the pain threshold, and increases tissue metabolism.

In diathermy, microwaves or shortwaves are selectively absorbed by tissues with high water content. This procedure provides electromagnetic conversion heating in soft tissue. Microwaves are especially effective for sprains, strains, herniated disks, rotator cuff tears, and arthritis. Shortwaves are used for low back pain and tenosynovitis.

Cryotherapy

Cryotherapy uses either a waterproof pack of ice and water or a soft plastic pouch of cold-retaining gel. It provides superficial regional cooling to decrease edema and the inflammatory response. It also in-

duces a mild nerve block. Cryotherapy is used mainly for rheumatoid arthritis.

Hydrotherapy

Hydrotherapy may be performed in a pool, a Hubbard tank, or a whirlpool. Pool therapy allows immersion of the patient's whole body in water. Convection heating or cooling can be used, if desired. The water removes the effects of gravity while allowing for nonimpact exercise. It also allows systemic heating or cooling to relieve joint pain, low back pain, arthritis, osteoporosis, and spasticity after spinal cord injuries.

A Hubbard tank is an individual tank that also allows immersion of the patient's whole body in water. Convection heating or cooling can be used, if desired. This therapy is particularly useful for burn patients. It allows you to closely regulate temperature and to add electrolytes.

A whirlpool gently agitates water to ease muscle sprains, chronic spinal conditions, and wound debridement.

Electrical therapy

Electrical therapy may use iontophoresis or transcutanous electrical nerve stimulation (TENS). Iontophoresis uses a direct, continuous unidirectional (galvanic) flow of current to contract denervated muscle, reduce pain, retard muscle atrophy, and increase tissue metabolism, blood flow, and lymph flow. It's used to relieve low back pain, sprains, bursitis, sciatica, and shoulder muscle spasms.

TENS uses an alternating current delivered from a small battery through lead wires attached to the body. It produces muscle relaxation for mild to moderate musculoskeletal or neuropathic pain. It also alleviates muscle spasticity and localized pain problems. And it may be useful in spinal cord injuries where the cord isn't severed.

Manipulation

Manipulation refers to traction, massage, and manual manipulation. Traction uses a weight-and-pulley system to apply a distracting force to a patient's spine or limb, thus separating normally contingent bony surfaces or enlarging the space in a joint without displacing associated ligaments. It's used for limb fracture, vertebral fracture, and dislocation related to spinal cord injury. Applying less force produces soft tissue stretching and relief of muscle spasm.

Massage uses rubbing, kneading, and manipulation of soft tissues. Light or deep techniques can be used. Also, mechanical devices are available. Massage can be used to help relieve muscle spasms, loosen soft tissue adhesions, enhance muscle flexibility, deactivate trigger points, and improve blood and lymph flow.

Manual manipulation employs forceful movements to articulate a joint in a manner not possible for patients to achieve on their own. It also can restore range of motion and provide passive stretching of adhesions in periarticular or intraarticular areas. These techniques are used commonly by osteopaths and chiropractors.

Acupuncture

In acupuncture, sterile, stainless steel needles are inserted into the body at precisely mapped trigger points. Skin penetration is minimal. Bleeding usually doesn't occur, and no chemicals are used. Acupuncture can be used to relieve arthritis pain, neuralgia, and neck, back and myofascial pain, although the amount of pain relief produced can vary. It can be quite effective in relieving musculoskeletal pain.

Immobilization

Immobilization can be accomplished through bed rest and through braces or orthotics. In bed rest, the anti-gravity effect helps to ease pain exacerbated by weight-bearing or repetitive motion. It also reduces edema.

Braces and orthotics range from soft fabric garments to complex metal and plastic implements used to immobilize or improve the function of a specific body part. These devices are used for fractures and for joint and soft-tissue injuries.

Exercise

Exercises to help relieve pain may include active or passive range-of-motion exercise and isotonic, isometric, and isokinetic exercise. Passive range of motion is applied to paralyzed extremities to mobilize the limb and prevent contractures; active or active-assistive range of motion is applied to partially paralyzed or arthritic limbs, and to patients recovering from fracture, ligament sprain, and muscle tendon strain.

Isotonic exercise, which involves active muscle contraction, may be performed with or without resistance to increase strength and muscle size and bulk. Isometric exercise, which involves active muscle contraction while the joint remains still, can be used for patients with restricted joint mobility or septic or inflammatory arthritis. It increases muscle strength but not bulk. And isokinetic exercise, which is active exercise performed against variable resistance, forces maximal muscle exertion throughout the range of motion. It increases muscle strength and bulk.

Complementary therapies

Other nondrug therapies that help to relieve pain, many by promoting relaxation and serenity, include guided imagery, distraction, deep breathing, biofeedback, pet therapy, horticulture therapy, music therapy, and storytelling. Some patients with rheumatoid arthritis, osteoarthritis, neuropathic pain, and refractory pain report receiving benefits from magnet therapy.

▶ COGNITIVE-BEHAVIORAL THERAPY

Especially for patients with chronic pain, cognitive-behavioral therapy guided by a mental health professional can do much to help manage the condition. Cognitive-behavioral therapy helps patients to identify, evaluate, and correct maladaptive conceptualizations and dysfunctional beliefs about themselves and their predicaments. Additionally, patients are taught to recognize the connections between and the consequences of cognition, affect, and behavior.

The strategy of cognitive-behavioral intervention is to help patients relinquish the belief that illness or disability is exclusively a medical problem that precludes personal control. (See *Goals of the cognitive-behavioral approach to pain management,* page 70). Cognitive-behavioral intervention approaches the patient optimistically, emphasizing both the effectiveness of the intervention and the patient's ability to alleviate much personal suffering, even if he can't completely control the disease and physical limitations. It proceeds in four steps: reconceptualization, skills acquisition, skills consolidation, and generalization and maintenance.

Reconceptualization

People's thoughts can greatly influence their moods, behaviors, and even some physiologic processes. Conversely, moods, behaviors, and physiologic activity can influence thoughts. Thus, it's important that people who are in pain notice the thoughts and feelings that are linked to pain episodes. Cognitive reconceptualization, also called cognitive restructuring, is a means of encouraging people to identify and change the stress-inducing thoughts and feelings associated with their pain.

Goals of the cognitive-behavioral approach to pain management

▸ Educate patients about the nature of pain and the relationships among pain, suffering, and disability.

▸ Modify maladaptive thoughts and feelings associated with emotional distress, such as exaggerated perception of danger or loss, poor self-esteem, and anger. Combat demoralization.

▸ Teach patients how and when to use coping techniques for specific challenges, for example, coping skills, practical problem solving skills, and self-control and self-management skills to diminish emotional distress.

▸ Foster a sense of self-control and power to counteract feelings and perceptions of helplessness and hopelessness.

▸ Teach patients to anticipate problems and deal with them as they arise, thus preventing relapse.

Pain diary

Many people with persistent pain find it hard to accept the idea that their thoughts and emotions can actually affect their bodies. To convince patients of this fact, it's useful to have them use a pain diary to self-monitor the thoughts and feelings that precede, accompany, and follow an episode or flare-up of pain.

Once specific, pain-related thoughts and emotions are identified, patients can consider alternative thoughts and strategies that might be used in similar circumstances. They can try these alternative thoughts and record the effects.

Changing thoughts

The crucial element in successful treatment is effecting a shift from habitual and ineffective responses to systematic problem-solving and planning, control of affect, behavioral persistence, and disengagement when appropriate. Reconceptualization continues throughout treatment to continually challenge patients' beliefs about their helplessness in the face of their symptoms. Patients learn to view symptoms and impairments as experiences they can differentiate, modify systematically, and control personally. Reconceptualization of the maladaptive view of physical symptoms provides incentive for patients to develop coping skills to control those symptoms.

Keep in mind that maladaptive thoughts commonly fall within a common set of cognitive errors that affect pain perception and disability. A cognitive error may be defined as a negatively distorted belief about oneself, one's situation, or the future. (See *Thinking about pain: Common errors*.) Cognitive errors commonly observed in those with chronic pain can be related to emotional difficulties that stem from living with pain. Some have suggested that the cognitive error of "catastrophizing" is the most important factor in poor coping, rather than differences in specific adaptive coping strategies.

Once cognitive errors contributing to pain perception, emotional distress, and disability are identified they become the target of intervention. Patients are usually asked to generate alternative, adaptive ways of thinking and responding. For example, they might choose to say, "I'll just take one day at a time," or "I'll try to

Thinking about pain: Common errors

COGNITIVE ERROR	DEFINITION
Overgeneralizing	Extrapolation from the occurrence of a specific event or situation to a large range of possible situations. For example, "The failure of this coping strategy means that none of them will work for me."
Catastrophizing	Focusing exclusively on the worst possibility, regardless of its likelihood. For example, "This pain in my back means my condition is degenerating, and my whole body is falling apart."
All-or-none thinking	Considering only the extreme "best" or "worst" interpretation of a situation without regard to the full range of alternatives. For example, "If I'm not feeling perfectly well, I can't enjoy anything."
Jumping to conclusions	Accepting an arbitrary interpretation without a rational evaluation of its likelihood. For example, "The doctor is avoiding me because he thinks I'm a hopeless case."
Selective attention	Selectively attending to negative aspects of a situation while ignoring positive aspects. For example, "Physical exercises only make me feel worse than I already do."
Negative prediction	Assuming the worst. For example, "I know this coping technique won't work," or "If I lose my hair from the chemotherapy, then I know my husband won't find me attractive anymore."
Mind reading	Making assumptions about the thoughts behind another person's words or actions. For example, "My family members don't talk to me about my pain because they don't care about me."

relax and calm myself down," or "Getting angry doesn't accomplish anything; I'll try to explain how I feel."

Patients will usually be asked to practice these adaptive thoughts at home and to review them during therapy sessions. Therapists should applaud their patients for learning to change. Because changing habitual thought patterns takes time, therapists should also encourage patients to reinforce themselves simply for making the effort to change, not just for attaining results.

Skills acquisition
In all rehabilitation, whether physical or psychological, patients must understand the rationale for learning specific skills and performing specific tasks. Patients who don't understand these rationales or who haven't addressed personal issues or sources of confusion are less likely to persevere in the face of obstacles. Thus, they're less likely to benefit from therapy.

Effective coping strategies are thought to alter both the perceived intensity of pain and the ability to tolerate pain while continuing daily activities. Studies have suggested that there is no one best coping skill to manage pain and disability. Rather than teach only a specific coping strategy, it may be more helpful to introduce patients to many different coping skills, which they may combine as needed.

Perhaps more important than the specific tactics chosen are the strategic goals of enhancing self-control and intrinsic motivation. The manner in which the various skills are described, taught, and practiced may be more important than the skills themselves.

It's essential for therapists to focus on patients' perspectives and perceptions of each skill and assignment. Skills that may be most helpful in managing chronic pain include problem solving, relaxation, and assertive communication skills.

Skills consolidation

During the skills-consolidation phase of cognitive-behavioral therapy, patients practice and rehearse the skills gained during the skills acquisition phase, and they apply those skills outside the clinic. This treatment phase employs mental rehearsal (in which the patient imagines using the skills in different situations), role playing, and role reversal.

An important goal of rehabilitation is development of the patient's ability to use newly learned skills in his own environment. Thus, home practice of all skills learned during the skills acquisition phase is critical.

Generalization and maintenance

This final phase of cognitive-behavioral therapy focuses on possible ways of predicting and either avoiding or coping with symptoms and symptom-related problems that arise after therapy ends. During this phase of treatment, patients are helped to identify high-risk situations—such as an unsupportive spouse or conflict with a child—and to note the types of responses that may be needed to cope successfully.

During this treatment stage, therapists encourage patients to anticipate specific, symptom-worsening events (such as stress, exercise, and conflicts) and to plan ways to cope with them. Naturally, no patient can anticipate all possible problems. Rather, the goal is to give the patient the belief that he has the skills needed to respond appropriately to problems.

More specifically, relapse prevention helps patients understand that minor setbacks are inevitable and that they don't signal total failure. Rather, these setbacks should be viewed as cues to use the coping skills mastered during treatment. Most important, patients must accept ongoing personal responsibility for their adherence to the treatment plan.

PART 2

Drugs

▶ acetaminophen
**Acephen, Anacin-3, Atasol◇,
Bromo-Seltzer, Feverall, Panadol,
Robigesic◇, Tempra, Tylenol**

Pharmacologic classification:
para-aminophenol derivative

Therapeutic classification:
antipyretic, nonnarcotic analgesic

Pregnancy risk category B

How supplied
Available without a prescription
Caplets: 160 mg, 500 mg, 650 mg
Capsules: 325 mg, 500 mg
Solution: 48 mg/ml, 80 mg/ml◇,
100 mg/ml, 80 mg/5 ml, 120 mg/
5 ml, 160 mg/5 ml, 167 mg/5 ml,
500 mg/15 ml
Sprinkle capsules: 80 mg, 160 mg
Suppositories: 80 mg, 120 mg,
125 mg, 300 mg, 325 mg, 650 mg
Suspension: 48 mg/ml, 80 mg/
ml◇, 100 mg/ml, 80 mg/5 ml◇,
160 mg/5 ml
Syrup: 16 mg/ml
Tablets: 160 mg, 325 mg, 500 mg,
650 mg
Tablets (chewable): 80 mg, 120 mg,
160 mg

Indications and dosages
Mild pain
Adults and children over age 12:
325 to 650 mg P.O. or P.R. q 4 to 6
hours p.r.n. Maximum, 4 g daily
(2.6 g daily for long-term therapy).
Children ages 11 to 12: 480 mg q
4 to 6 hours.
Children ages 9 to 10: 400 mg q 4
to 6 hours.
Children ages 6 to 8: 320 mg q 4
to 6 hours.
Children ages 4 to 5: 240 mg q 4
to 6 hours.

Children ages 2 to 3: 160 mg q 4
to 6 hours.
Children ages 12 to 23 months:
120 mg q 4 to 6 hours.
Children ages 4 to 11 months: 80
mg q 4 to 6 hours.
Children age 3 months or less: 40
mg q 4 to 6 hours.

Pharmacodynamics
Analgesic action: May result from
increased pain threshold.
Antipyretic action: Drug probably
acts directly on the hypothalamic
heat-regulating center to block the
effects of an endogenous pyrogen.
Sweating and vasodilation dissipate heat.

Pharmacokinetics
Absorption: Drug is absorbed
rapidly and completely in the GI
tract. Plasma levels peak in 10
minutes to 2 hours, slightly faster
for liquid forms.
Distribution: Drug is 25% protein-
bound. Plasma levels don't correlate well with analgesic effect, but
they do correlate with toxicity.
Metabolism: About 90% to 95% of
drug is metabolized in the liver.
Excretion: Acetaminophen is excreted in urine. Elimination half-
life ranges from 1 to 4 hours. In
acute overdose, prolonged half-life
correlates with toxic effects. Half-
life over 4 hours may result in hepatic necrosis; half-life over 12
hours may result in coma.

Contraindications and precautions
No known contraindications. Use
cautiously in patients with history
of chronic alcohol abuse because
hepatotoxicity has occurred after
therapeutic doses. Also, use cautiously in patients with hepatic or

CV disease, impaired renal function, or viral infection.

Interactions
Drug-drug
Antacids: may delay and decrease acetaminophen absorption. Assess patient's response.
Anticoagulants, thrombolytics: may potentiate effects of these drugs. Monitor patient's coagulation tests.
Anticonvulsants, isoniazid, rifampin: increased risk of hepatotoxicity. Monitor patient's hepatic function.
Lamotrigine: possible decrease in serum lamotrigine levels. Assess drug effects.
Phenothiazines: increased risk of hypothermia with large acetaminophen doses. Monitor patient's response.

Drug-herb
Watercress: may inhibit oxidative metabolism of acetaminophen. Avoid use together.

Drug-food
Caffeine: increased acetaminophen effects. Monitor patient's response.
Food: delays and decreases acetaminophen absorption. Give drug on an empty stomach.

Drug-lifestyle
Alcohol use: increased risk of liver toxicity. Discourage concomitant use.

Effects on diagnostic tests
May cause false-positive results on urine 5-hydroxyindoleacetic acid test.

Adverse reactions
Hematologic: hemolytic anemia, *leukopenia, neutropenia, pancytopenia.*
Hepatic: jaundice, *severe liver damage at toxic doses*.
Metabolic: hypoglycemia.
Skin: rash, urticaria.

Overdose and treatment
Overdose may cause anemia, CNS stimulation, coma, cyanosis, delirium, emesis, fever, hepatotoxicity, jaundice, methemoglobinemia progressing to CNS depression, seizures, skin eruptions, vascular collapse, and death. Acetaminophen poisoning develops in stages:
▶ Stage 1 (12 to 24 hours after ingestion): anorexia, diaphoresis, nausea, vomiting.
▶ Stage 2 (24 to 48 hours after ingestion): clinically improved; liver function test results are elevated.
▶ Stage 3 (72 to 96 hours after ingestion): peak hepatotoxicity.
▶ Stage 4 (7 to 8 days after ingestion): recovery.

To treat overdose, immediately induce emesis with ipecac syrup (if patient is conscious) or perform gastric lavage. Give activated charcoal via nasogastric tube. Oral acetylcysteine (Mucomyst) can minimize hepatic injury from acetaminophen poisoning by supplying sulfhydryl groups that bind with acetaminophen metabolites. It's most effective if started within 12 hours after ingestion; however, it may be helpful even after 24 hours. Remove charcoal before giving acetylcysteine because charcoal may interfere with absorption. Then give 140 mg/kg, followed by 70 mg/kg every 4 hours for 17 more doses. Doses

---

Reactions may be *common*, uncommon, *life-threatening*, or COMMON AND LIFE-THREATENING.

vomited within 1 hour after administration must be repeated.

Hemodialysis may help remove drug from the body. Monitor laboratory values and vital signs closely. Provide symptomatic and supportive measures, including respiratory support and correction of fluid and electrolyte imbalances. Determine plasma drug levels at least 4 hours after overdose. If they indicate hepatotoxicity, perform liver function tests every 24 hours for at least 96 hours.

Special considerations
▶ Acetaminophen has little anti-inflammatory effect. Even so, it may have substantial benefits for patients with osteoarthritis, probably from its analgesic effects.
▶ Many OTC products and combination analgesics contain acetaminophen. Consider them when calculating patient's total daily dose, and limit patient to 4 g/day of acetaminophen.
▶ If patient is on sodium-restricted diet, consider the sodium content when prescribing effervescent buffered acetaminophen granules.
▶ Assess patient's level of pain before and after giving drug.
▶ Because acetaminophen increases the risk of renal toxicity and hepatotoxicity, monitor patient's BUN, serum creatinine level, liver function tests, and CBC as needed.
▶ Patients who can't tolerate aspirin may be able to tolerate acetaminophen.
▶ Refrigerate acetaminophen suppositories.
▶ Besides analgesic use, acetaminophen is also used for fever.
▶ Monitor patient's vital signs, especially temperature, to evaluate antipyretic effectiveness.

Breast-feeding patients
▶ Low levels of drug appear in breast milk, but no adverse effects have been reported.

Pediatric patients
▶ If possible, avoid giving children more than five doses daily for more than 5 days.

Geriatric patients
▶ Elderly patients are more sensitive to drug. Use with caution.

Patient teaching
▶ Teach patient how to administer prescribed form of drug.
▶ Urge patient not to routinely combine drug with NSAIDs.
▶ Tell adult patient not to take drug for more than 10 days without consulting prescriber. Warn him that high doses or unsupervised long-term use can cause liver damage.
▶ Explain that even moderate amounts of alcohol increase the risk of liver damage, especially on an empty stomach.
▶ Caution patient not to take acetaminophen for a fever above 103° F (39° C), a fever that lasts longer than 3 days, or a recurrent fever.
▶ If patient receives high-dose or long-term therapy, emphasize the need for regular follow-up visits.
▶ Warn patient to avoid taking tetracycline antibiotics within 1 hour after taking buffered acetaminophen effervescent granules.
▶ Tell patient not to use acetaminophen for arthritic or rheumatic conditions without consulting prescriber. Drug may relieve pain but not other symptoms.
▶ If patient has had rectal bleeding, warn against suppository form.
▶ Tell patient not to take other prescribed drugs, OTC medications,

or herbal remedies without consulting prescriber.

▶ activated charcoal
Actidose-Aqua, CharcoAid, CharcoCaps, Insta-Char

Pharmacologic classification:
adsorbent

Therapeutic classification:
antidiarrheal, antidote, antiflatulent

Pregnancy risk category NR

How supplied
Available without a prescription
Capsules: 260 mg
Powder: 30 g, 50 g
Suspension: 0.625 g/5 ml, 0.7 g/5 ml (50 g), 1 g/5 ml, 1.25 g/5 ml
Tablets: 325 mg, 650 mg
Tablets with 40 mg simethicone: 200 mg
Tablets (delayed-release) with 80 mg simethicone: 250 mg

Indications and dosages
Poisoning or overdose with acetaminophen, amphetamines, antimony, aspirin, atropine, arsenic, barbiturates, camphor, cocaine, cardiac glycosides, glutethimide, ipecac, malathion, morphine, opium, oxalic acid, parathion, phenol, phenothiazines, phenytoin, poisonous mushrooms, potassium permanganate, propantheline, propoxyphene, quinine, strychnine, sulfonamides, or tricyclic antidepressants (adjunct)
Adults and children: 5 to 10 times the estimated weight of drug or chemical ingested (or 1 g/kg). Mix 30 to 100 g in 250 ml water to make a slurry. Give orally, preferably within 30 minutes of inges-

tion. Give larger doses if stomach contains food. Activated charcoal 20 to 60 g may be given q 4 to 12 hours (gastric dialysis) to enhance removal of some drugs from blood. Monitor serum drug level.
Dyspepsia, flatulence
Adults: 600 mg to 5 g P.O. as a single dose or 975 mg to 3.9 g t.i.d. after meals.

Pharmacodynamics
Antidote and antidiarrheal actions: Adsorbs ingested toxins and nontoxic irrtants, inhibiting GI absorption, diarrhea, GI discomfort.
Antiflatulent action: Charcoal adsorbs intestinal gas.

Pharmacokinetics
Absorption: None.
Distribution: None.
Metabolism: None.
Excretion: Activated charcoal is excreted in feces.

Contraindications and precautions
No known contraindications.

Interactions
Drug-drug
Acetylcysteine, oral drugs: inactivated by charcoal. Remove charcoal by gastric lavage before giving these drugs.

Drug-food
Milk products: decrease the effectiveness of activated charcoal. Avoid use together.

Effects on diagnostic tests
None reported.

Adverse reactions
GI: black stools, constipation, nausea.

Overdose and treatment
No information available.

Special considerations
▶ Don't give oral dose to a semiconscious or unconscious patient; instead, use a nasogastric tube.
▶ Activated charcoal is most effective when given within 30 minutes after toxin ingestion; a cathartic is commonly given with or after activated charcoal to speed removal of the toxin-charcoal complex.
▶ Powder form is most effective. Mix it with tap water to form a thick syrup. A small amount of fruit juice or flavoring may be added to make it more palatable.
▶ Because activated charcoal adsorbs and inactivates syrup of ipecac, give charcoal only after emesis is complete.
▶ If patient vomits shortly after a dose, repeat dose as needed.
▶ If giving charcoal for other than poisoning, give other oral drugs 1 hour before or 2 hours afterward.
▶ Giving activated charcoal for more than 72 hours may impair patient's nutritional status. Monitor patient's response to treatment.
▶ When giving activated charcoal as an antidote for opioid poisoning, monitor blood pressure, heart rate, and respiratory rate.
▶ Activated charcoal may be given orally to decrease colostomy odor.
▶ Drug may also be used for GI disturbances, such as halitosis, anorexia, nausea, and vomiting, in uremic patients.

Patient teaching
▶ Tell patient to call poison information center or hospital emergency department before taking activated charcoal as an antidote.
▶ Instruct patient to mix activated charcoal with 8 ounces of water or juice to form a thick syrup.
▶ Caution patient that milk products may lessen the effectiveness of charcoal mixture.
▶ If patient uses activated charcoal to reduce diarrhea or flatulence, instruct him to take other oral drugs 1 hour before or 2 hours after activated charcoal. Urge patient to notify prescriber if diarrhea persists after 2 days of therapy or if fever or flatulence persist after 7 days.
▶ Warn patient that activated charcoal blackens stool.

▶ alfentanil hydrochloride
Alfenta

Pharmacologic classification:
opioid

Therapeutic classification:
adjunct to anesthesia, analgesic, anesthetic

Controlled substance schedule II

Pregnancy risk category C

How supplied
Available by prescription only
Injection: 500 mcg/ml in 2-, 5-, 10-, and 20-ml ampules

Indications and dosages
Analgesic adjunct in the maintenance of general anesthesia with barbiturate, nitrous oxide, and oxygen
Adults: initially, 8 to 20 mcg/kg I.V., increased by 3 to 5 mcg/kg I.V. Or give a continuous infusion of 0.5 to 1 mcg/kg/minute.

---

*Unlabeled use

Pharmacodynamics

Analgesic and anesthetic actions:
Alfentanil is a potent opiate receptor agonist with a quick onset and short duration of action.

Pharmacokinetics

Absorption: Administered I.V., alfentanil has an immediate onset.
Distribution: Redistributed quickly after absorption; drug is more than 90% protein-bound.
Metabolism: Drug is metabolized in the liver; half-life is about 1½ hours.
Excretion: Drug is excreted in urine.

Contraindications and precautions

Contraindicated in patients hypersensitive to drug. Use cautiously in patients with decreased respiratory reserve, head injury, hepatic impairment, pulmonary disease, or renal impairment.

Interactions

Drug-drug

Anticholinergics: risk of paralytic ileus. Monitor patient closely.
Cimetidine: possible increased respiratory and CNS depression, causing apnea, confusion, disorientation, or seizures. Avoid concurrent use.
CNS depressants, such as antihistamines, barbiturates, benzodiazepines, general anesthetics, muscle relaxants, opioid analgesics, phenothiazines, sedative-hypnotics, and tricyclic antidepressants: potentiated CNS depression, hypotensive effects, respiratory depression, and sedation. Monitor patient closely during concurrent use.
Diazepam: vasodilation, decreased blood pressure, and possible CV depression if given close to high doses of alfentanil. Monitor patient closely.
Drugs extensively metabolized in the liver, such as digitoxin, erythromycin, phenytoin, rifampin: possible accumulation and enhanced effects of these drugs. Monitor patient's hepatic function and response to treatment.

Drug-lifestyle

Alcohol use: potentiates respiratory and CNS depression, sedation, and hypotensive effects of alfentanil. Discourage concomitant use.

Effects on diagnostic tests

None reported.

Adverse reactions

CNS: anxiety, confusion, headache, sedation, sleepiness.
CV: *arrhythmias, asystole, bradycardia,* hypertension, hypotension, tachycardia.
EENT: blurred vision.
GI: increased plasma amylase and lipase levels, *nausea, vomiting.*
Respiratory: *bronchospasm,* chest wall rigidity, hypercapnia, *laryngospasm, respiratory arrest, respiratory depression.*
Skin: pruritus, urticaria.

Overdose and treatment

Overdose commonly causes CNS depression, miosis, and respiratory depression. It may cause apnea, bradycardia, cardiopulmonary arrest, circulatory collapse, hypotension, hypothermia, pulmonary edema, seizures, and shock.

To treat acute overdose, ensure adequate respiratory exchange. If patient has significant respiratory or CV depression, give naloxone. Repeated doses may be needed be-

---

Reactions may be *common,* uncommon, *life-threatening,* or COMMON AND LIFE-THREATENING.

cause alfentanil has a longer duration of action than naloxone. Provide symptomatic and supportive treatment, including continued respiratory support and correction of fluid or electrolyte imbalance. Closely monitor vital signs, laboratory values and neurologic status.

Special considerations
▶ Drug may be given I.V. or by epidural route, and only by staff specially trained to give it. Keep naloxone and resuscitation equipment available during I.V. use.
▶ Assisted or controlled ventilation is needed. Monitor patient closely.
▶ Drug is compatible with D_5W, D_5W in lactated Ringer's solution, and normal saline solution. Most clinicians use infusions that contain 25 to 80 mcg/ml.
▶ Use a tuberculin syringe or its equivalent to give a small volume. Or use an infusion pump.
▶ Monitor patient for skeletal muscle rigidity because drug can cause it, especially at higher doses.
▶ Alfentanil has less sedative effect then fentanyl.
▶ Alfentanil also can be used as an anesthetic for general anesthesia or monitored anesthesia care.

Breast-feeding patients
▶ Drug appears in breast milk. Give cautiously to breast-feeding women.

Pediatric patients
▶ Safe use in children under age 12 hasn't been established.

Geriatric patients
▶ Elderly patient typically need lower doses because they may be more sensitive to therapeutic and adverse effects, especially apnea.

Patient teaching
▶ Explain the anesthetic effect of alfentanil as well as preoperative and postoperative care measures.

▶ amitriptyline hydrochloride
Amitriptyline, Elavil, Levate◇, Novotriptyn◇

Pharmacologic classification: *tricyclic antidepressant*

Therapeutic classification: *antidepressant*

Pregnancy risk category NR

How supplied
Available by prescription only
Injection: 10 mg/ml
Tablets: 10 mg, 25 mg, 50 mg, 75 mg, 100 mg, 150 mg

Indications and dosages
Neuropathic pain (adjunct)*
Adults: 25 mg/day P.O. h.s. Increase by 25 mg/day every 72 hours until desired therapeutic effect occurs or you reach maximum of 200 mg/day.
◫ DOSAGE ADJUSTMENT. Give 10 mg P.O. t.i.d. and 20 mg h.s. to elderly or adolescent patients.

Pharmacodynamics
Analgesic action: Unknown.
Antidepressant action: Amitriptyline inhibits reuptake of norepinephrine and serotonin in CNS nerve terminals (presynaptic neurons), resulting in increased levels and enhanced activity of these neurotransmitters in the synaptic cleft. It inhibits serotonin reuptake more actively than norepinephrine.

◇ Available in Canada only   *Unlabeled use

Pharmacokinetics
Absorption: Drug is absorbed rapidly from the GI tract after oral administration and from muscle tissue after I.M. administration.
Distribution: Drug is distributed widely into the body, including the CNS and breast milk; it's 96% protein-bound. Levels peak in 2 to 12 hours, reach steady state in 4 to 10 days, and achieve full therapeutic effect in 2 to 4 weeks.
Metabolism: Drug is metabolized by the liver to the active metabolite nortriptyline. Significant first-pass effect may account for variability of serum levels in different patients taking the same dosage.
Excretion: Mostly in urine.

Contraindications and precautions
Contraindicated in patients hypersensitive to drug, within 14 days of taking an MAO inhibitor, and during the acute recovery phase after MI. Also contraindicated in patients with a history of seizures because tricyclic antidepressants lower the seizure threshold.

Use cautiously in patients with recent history of MI and in those with unstable heart disease or renal or hepatic impairment.

Interactions
Drug-drug
Antiarrhythmics (disopyramide, procainamide, quinidine), pimozide, thyroid hormones: increased risk of arrhythmias and conduction defects. Monitor cardiac function.
Anticholinergics, such as antihistamines, antiparkinsonians, atropine, meperidine, phenothiazines: risk of oversedation, paralytic ileus, visual changes, and severe constipation. Monitor patient closely.

Barbiturates, haloperidol, phenothiazines: possible altered amitriptyline metabolism and decreased efficacy. Monitor patient's response to treatment.
Beta blockers, cimetidine, methylphenidate, oral contraceptives, propoxyphene, selective serotonin reuptake inhibitors: may inhibit amitriptyline metabolism, increasing plasma levels and toxicity. Assess patient for adverse effects.
Central-acting antihypertensives, such as clonidine, guanabenz, guanadrel, guanethidine, methyldopa, reserpine: decreased hypotensive effects. Monitor patient's response to treatment.
CNS depressants, including analgesics, anesthetics, barbiturates, narcotics, tranquilizers: possible oversedation. Monitor patient closely.
Disulfiram, ethchlorvynol: increased risk of delirium and tachycardia. Monitor patient closely.
Metrizamide: increased risk of seizures. Monitor patient closely.
Sympathomimetics commonly found in nasal sprays, including ephedrine, epinephrine, phenylephrine, and phenylpropanolamine: may increase blood pressure. Monitor patient's blood pressure.
Warfarin: may increase PT, INR, and the risk of bleeding. Monitor patient's coagulation studies.

Drug-lifestyle
Alcohol use: additive effects. Avoid concurrent use.
Heavy smoking: induces amitriptyline metabolism and decreases efficacy. Discourage smoking.
Sun exposure: risk of photosensitivity. Urge precautions.

Effects on diagnostic tests
None reported.

Reactions may be *common*, uncommon, ***life-threatening***, or COMMON AND LIFE-THREATENING.

Adverse reactions

CNS: anxiety, ataxia, *coma,* delusions, disorientation, dizziness, drowsiness, extrapyramidal symptoms, fatigue, hallucinations, headache, insomnia, peripheral neuropathy, restlessness, *seizures,* tremor, weakness.
CV: *arrhythmias, CVA, ECG changes,* edema, *heart block,* hypertension, *orthostatic hypotension, MI, tachycardia.*
EENT: *blurred vision,* increased intraocular pressure, mydriasis, tinnitus.
GI: anorexia, constipation, diarrhea, *dry mouth,* epigastric distress, nausea, paralytic ileus, vomiting.
GU: urine retention.
Hematologic: *agranulocytosis,* eosinophilia*, leukopenia, thrombocytopenia.*
Hepatic: elevated liver function test results.
Metabolic: hyperglycemia, hypoglycemia.
Skin: *diaphoresis,* photosensitivity, rash, urticaria.
Other: *hypersensitivity reaction.*

Overdose and treatment

The first 12 hours after acute ingestion are a stimulatory phase characterized by excessive anticholinergic activity that includes agitation, confusion, constipation, dilated pupils, dry mucous membranes, hallucinations, hyperthermia, ileus, irritation, parkinsonian symptoms, seizures, and urine retention. CNS depression follows and may include decreased or absent reflexes, cardiac irregularities, conduction disturbances, cyanosis, hypotension, hypothermia, quinidine-like effects on the ECG, sedation, and tachycardia. Metabolic acidosis may follow hypotension, hypoventilation, and seizures. Delayed cardiac anomalies and death may occur.

Treatment is symptomatic and supportive. Maintain patient's airway, body temperature, and fluid and electrolyte balance. Induce emesis with ipecac if gag reflex is intact; follow with gastric lavage and activated charcoal to prevent further absorption. Dialysis is of little use. Physostigmine may be cautiously used to reverse the symptoms of tricyclic antidepressant poisoning in life-threatening situations. Give parenteral diazepam or phenytoin for seizures, parenteral phenytoin or lidocaine for arrhythmias, and sodium bicarbonate for acidosis. Don't give barbiturates; they may worsen CNS and respiratory depressant effects.

Special considerations

▶ Although amitriptyline is the best documented tricyclic antidepressant for analgesia, it's the least tolerated because of its anticholinergic effects.
▶ Parenteral form is for I.M. use only. Don't give drug by I.V. route.
▶ Switch to oral route as soon as possible.
▶ I.M. administration may yield a shorter onset of action than oral administration.
▶ Drug commonly causes sedation; tolerance may develop over several weeks.
▶ Full dose may be given at bedtime to help offset daytime sedation.
▶ Discontinue drug at least 48 hours before surgical procedures.
▶ Abrupt withdrawal of long-term therapy may cause nausea, headache, and malaise (which don't indicate addiction).
▶ Drug may promote a shift to mania or hypomania in depressed pa-

tients, particularly those with bipolar disorder.
▶ Monitor patient for response to treatment and for adverse effects Therapeutic effects may not occur 7 to 10 days after treatment starts.
▶ Drug also may be used for depression, for anorexia or bulimia with depression, for intractable hiccups, and to prevent migraine and cluster headaches.
▶ Drug may be helpful for chronic pain.

Breast-feeding patients
▶ Drug appears in breast milk in concentrations equal to or greater than those in maternal serum. About 1% of the ingested dose appears in the breast-fed infant's serum. The potential benefit to the mother should outweigh the possible adverse reactions in the infant.

Pediatric patients
▶ Drug isn't recommended for children under age 12.

Geriatric patients
▶ Elderly patients may have an increased risk of adverse cardiac effects and severe orthostatic hypotension.

Patient teaching
▶ Tell patient to take drug exactly as prescribed and not to double the dose if he misses one.
▶ Explain that full effects of drug may not become apparent for up to 4 weeks after therapy starts.
▶ Advise patient that full dose may be taken at bedtime to alleviate daytime sedation or in early evening to avoid morning hangover.
▶ Suggest taking drug with food or milk if it causes stomach upset.

▶ Urge patient to lie down for about 30 minutes after initial doses and to rise slowly from lying or sitting positions to prevent dizziness or fainting.
▶ Caution patient not to drink alcoholic beverages during therapy.
▶ Warn patient to avoid hazardous activities until full CNS effects of drug are known.
▶ Suggest ice or sugarless chewing gum or hard candy to ease dry mouth. Stress the importance of dental hygiene because a dry mouth can encourage dental caries.
▶ Tell patient to avoid excessive exposure to sunlight because photosensitivity may occur.
▶ Warn patient not to stop taking drug suddenly.
▶ Encourage patient to report troublesome or unusual effects, especially confusion, movement disorders, rapid heartbeat, dizziness, fainting, or difficulty urinating.

▶ **amobarbital**

▶ **amobarbital sodium**
Amytal

Pharmacologic classification:
barbiturate

Therapeutic classification:
anticonvulsant, sedative-hypnotic

Controlled substance schedule II

Pregnancy risk category D

How supplied
Available by prescription only
Capsules: 200 mg
Powder for injection: 250-mg, 500-mg vials
Tablets: 30 mg

Indications and dosages
Sedation
Adults: usually 30 to 50 mg P.O. b.i.d. or t.i.d. but may range from 15 to 120 mg b.i.d. to q.i.d.
Children: 2 mg/kg/day P.O. in four equal doses.

Pharmacodynamics
Anticonvulsant action: The exact site and mechanism of action are unknown. Parenteral amobarbital suppresses the spread of seizure activity produced by epileptogenic foci in the cortex, thalamus, and limbic systems by enhancing the effect of GABA. Both presynaptic and postsynaptic excitability are decreased.
Sedative-hypnotic action: Drug acts throughout the CNS as a non-selective depressant with an intermediate onset and duration of action. Particularly sensitive to this drug is the mesencephalic reticular activating system, which controls CNS arousal. Amobarbital decreases both presynaptic and postsynaptic membrane excitability by facilitating the action of GABA.

Pharmacokinetics
Absorption: Amobarbital is absorbed well after oral administration and 100% after I.M. administration. Action begins in 45 to 60 minutes.
Distribution: Drug is distributed well throughout body tissues and fluids.
Metabolism: Amobarbital is metabolized in the liver by oxidation to a tertiary alcohol.
Excretion: Less than 1% of a dose is excreted unchanged in the urine; the rest is excreted as metabolites. The half-life is biphasic, with a first phase of about 40 minutes and a second phase of about 20 hours. Duration of action is 6 to 8 hours.

Contraindications and precautions
Contraindicated in patients hypersensitive to barbiturates and patients with bronchopneumonia, other severe pulmonary insufficiency, or porphyria.

Use cautiously in patients with suicidal tendencies, acute or chronic pain, history of drug abuse, hepatic or renal impairment, or pulmonary or CV disease.

Interactions
Drug-drug
Antidepressants, antihistamines, MAO inhibitors, opioids, sedative-hypnotics, tranquilizers: additive or potentiated CNS and respiratory depressant effects. Avoid concurrent use.
Beta blockers, carbamazepine, corticosteroids, digitoxin (not digoxin), doxycycline, estrogens (including oral contraceptives), xanthines (including theophylline): enhanced hepatic amobarbital metabolism. Monitor patient's response to treatment.
Disulfiram, MAO inhibitors, valproic acid: decreased amobarbital metabolism and increased risk of toxicity. Monitor patient closely.
Griseofulvin: decreased GI absorption of griseofulvin and possible impaired effectiveness. Monitor patient's response to treatment.
Phenytoin: unpredictable fluctuations in serum phenytoin levels. Monitor closely.
Rifampin: increased amobarbital metabolism and possible decreased drug levels. Monitor patient's response to treatment.

◇ Available in Canada only   *Unlabeled use

Warfarin and other oral anticoagulants: enhanced enzymatic degradation of anticoagulants. Monitor coagulation studies because patient may need increased anticoagulant dosage.

Drug-food
Food: decreases drug absorption. Give drug before meals or on an empty stomach to enhance absorption rate.

Drug-lifestyle
Alcohol use: additive or potentiated CNS and respiratory depressant effects. Don't use together.

Effects on diagnostic tests
Amobarbital may cause false-positive results on the phentolamine test, and it may impair absorption of cyanocobalamin. It also may decrease serum bilirubin levels in neonates, epileptic patients, and patients with congenital nonhemolytic unconjugated hyperbilirubinemia. It alters EEG patterns (low-voltage, fast-activity) for some time after therapy stops.

Adverse reactions
CNS: *drowsiness, hangover, lethargy,* paradoxical excitement, physical and psychological dependence, somnolence, syncope.
CV: *bradycardia,* hypotension.
GI: nausea, vomiting.
Hematologic: exacerbation of porphyria.
Respiratory: *apnea, respiratory depression.*
Skin: *Stevens-Johnson syndrome,* rash, reactions at injection site (pain, irritation, sterile abscess), urticaria.
Other: *angioedema.*

Overdose and treatment
Overdose may cause areflexia, coma, confusion, fever, hypothermia, jaundice, oliguria, pulmonary edema, respiratory depression, shock with tachycardia and hypotension, slurred speech, somnolence, sustained nystagmus, and an unsteady gait.

Treatment aims to maintain and support ventilation and pulmonary function and support cardiac function and circulation with vasopressors and I.V. fluids as needed. If patient is conscious with a functioning gag reflex and ingestion was recent, then induce emesis with ipecac syrup. If emesis isn't appropriate and patient has a cuffed endotracheal tube in place, consider gastric lavage. Follow with activated charcoal or a sodium chloride cathartic. Measure fluid intake and output, vital signs, and laboratory values. Maintain body temperature.

Alkalinization of urine may be helpful in removing amobarbital from the body; hemodialysis may be useful in severe overdose.

Special considerations
▶ For I.M. use, prepare 20% solution by using 1.25 or 2.5 ml of sterile water for injection with 250 or 500 mg of amobarbital. For I.V. use, reconstitute powder for injection with sterile water for injection. Use 2.5 or 5 ml (for 250 or 500 mg of amobarbital) to make 10% solution. Roll vial in hands rather than shaking it.
▶ Give reconstituted parenteral solution within 30 minutes after opening the vial.
▶ Don't give solution that's cloudy or precipitated 5 minutes after reconstitution.

Reactions may be *common*, uncommon, *life-threatening*, or COMMON AND LIFE-THREATENING.

Give I.M. dose deep into large muscle mass. Don't exceed 5 ml in any one injection site. Sterile abscess or tissue damage may result from inadvertent superficial I.M. or S.C. injection.

Drug usually isn't used as a sedative or sleeping aid; barbiturates have been replaced by safer benzodiazepines for these uses.

Give oral form before meals or on an empty stomach to enhance absorption rate.

Restrict I.V. use to conditions in which other routes aren't feasible (unconscious or resistant patient, need for prompt action).

Don't exceed 50 mg/minute; final dosage is based on patient response.

Keep emergency resuscitative equipment available.

Giving full loading doses over short periods of time to treat status epilepticus may require ventilatory support in adults.

Monitor patient's cardiopulmonary status frequently for possible changes. Monitor CBC for possible adverse reactions.

Monitor renal and hepatic studies to ensure adequate drug removal.

Monitor PT and INR carefully when patient receiving amobarbital starts or ends anticoagulant therapy. Anticoagulant dosage may need to be adjusted.

Amobarbital is also indicated as a preanesthetic drug, an anticonvulsant, and a treatment for insomnia.

Breast-feeding patients

Amobarbital passes into breast milk and may cause drowsiness in the infant. If so, discontinue drug or change dosage as needed. Use with caution.

Pediatric patients

Safe use in children under age 6 hasn't been established.

Use of amobarbital may cause paradoxical excitement in some children.

Geriatric patients

Elderly patients usually require lower doses.

Confusion, disorientation, and excitability may occur in elderly patients. Use with caution.

Patient teaching

Warn patient about possible hangover effects.

Tell patient to avoid alcohol while taking drug.

Warn patient about possible physical or psychological dependence with prolonged use.

amoxapine
Asendin

Pharmacologic classification:
dibenzoxazepine, tricyclic antidepressant

Therapeutic classification:
antidepressant

Pregnancy risk category C

How supplied
Available by prescription only
Tablets: 25 mg, 50 mg, 100 mg, 150 mg

Indications and dosages
Analgesic adjunct for phantom limb pain, chronic pain, migraine, chronic tension headache, diabetic neuropathy, tic douloureux, cancer pain, peripheral neuropa-

thy with pain, post-herpetic neu-
ralgia, arthritic pain*
Adults: 100 to 300 mg/day P.O.
☒ DOSAGE ADJUSTMENT. For elderly
patients, recommended starting
dose is 25 mg P.O. b.i.d. to t.i.d.

Pharmacodynamics
Analgesic action: Unknown.
Antidepressant action: Drug probably inhibits reuptake of norepinephrine and serotonin in CNS
nerve terminals (presynaptic neurons), which results in increased
levels and enhanced activity of
these neurotransmitters in the
synaptic cleft. Amoxapine has a
greater inhibitory effect on norepinephrine reuptake than on serotonin. Drug also blocks CNS
dopamine receptors, which may
account for the higher occurrence
of movement disorders with this
drug.

Pharmacokinetics
Absorption: Amoxapine is absorbed rapidly and completely
from the GI tract after oral administration.
Distribution: Drug is distributed
widely into the body, including the
CNS and breast milk. It's 92%
protein-bound. Levels peak in 8 to
10 hours and reach steady state in
2 to 7 days. Proposed therapeutic
plasma levels (parent drug and
metabolite) range from 200 to
500 ng/ml.
Metabolism: Drug is metabolized
by the liver to the active metabolite
8-hydroxyamoxapine; a significant
first-pass effect may explain variable serum levels in different patients taking the same dosage.
Excretion: Amoxapine is excreted
in urine and feces (7% to 18%);
about 60% of a dose is excreted as

the conjugated form within 6 days.
Plasma half-life is about 8 hours.

Contraindications and precautions
Contraindicated during the acute
recovery phase after MI, in patients
hypersensitive to drug, and in patients who took an MAO inhibitor
within 14 days or who take a drug
that prolongs the QT interval.
   Use cautiously in patients with
angle-closure glaucoma, CV disease, a history of seizures, a history of urine retention, or increased
intraocular pressure.

Interactions
Drug-drug
Antiarrhythmics (disopyramide,
procainamide, quinidine), pimo-
zide, thyroid hormones: increased
risk of arrhythmias and conduction
defects. Monitor patient's cardiac
function.
Anticholinergics, such as antihista-
mines, antiparkinsonians, atropine,
meperidine, phenothiazines: risk
of oversedation, paralytic ileus, visual changes, and severe constipation. Monitor patient closely.
Antivirals, protease inhibitors: altered metabolism of these drugs.
Monitor response to treatment.
Barbiturates, haloperidol, phe-
nothiazines: possible altered
amoxapine metabolism and decreased efficacy. Monitor patient's
response to treatment.
Beta blockers, cimetidine,
methylphenidate, oral contracep-
tives, propoxyphene: may inhibit
amoxapine metabolism, increasing
plasma levels and toxicity. Assess
patient for adverse effects.
Central-acting antihypertensives,
such as clonidine, guanabenz, gua-
nadrel, guanethidine, methyldopa,

Reactions may be *common*, uncommon, *life-threatening*, or COMMON AND LIFE-THREATENING.

reserpine: decreased hypotensive effects. Monitor patient's response to treatment.
CNS depressants, including analgesics, anesthetics, barbiturates, narcotics, tranquilizers: possible oversedation. Monitor patient closely.
Disulfiram, ethchlorvynol: increased risk of delirium and tachycardia. Monitor patient closely.
Metrizamide: increased risk of seizures. Monitor patient closely.
Sympathomimetics commonly found in nasal sprays, including ephedrine, epinephrine, phenylephrine, and phenylpropanolamine: may increase blood pressure. Monitor patient's blood pressure.
Warfarin: may increase PT, INR, and the risk of bleeding. Monitor patient's coagulation studies during concurrent use.

Drug-lifestyle
Alcohol use: additive effects. Don't use together.
Heavy smoking: induces amoxapine metabolism and decreases efficacy. Discourage smoking during therapy.
Sun exposure: risk of photosensitivity. Urge precautions.

Effects on diagnostic tests
Drug may prolong conduction time (elongation of QT and PR intervals, flattened T waves on ECG).

Adverse reactions
CNS: anxiety, ataxia, confusion, *dizziness, drowsiness, EEG changes,* excitation, fatigue, headache, insomnia, nervousness, nightmares, restlessness, **seizures,** *tardive dyskinesia,* tremor, weakness.

CV: edema, hypertension, *orthostatic hypotension,* palpitations, *tachycardia.*
EENT: *blurred vision.*
GI: *constipation, dry mouth,* excessive appetite, nausea.
GU: **acute renal failure** (with overdose), *urine retention.*
Hematologic: *leukopenia.*
Hepatic: elevated liver function test results.
Metabolic: hyperglycemia, hypoglycemia.
Skin: *diaphoresis,* rash.
Other: **neuroleptic malignant syndrome** (high fever, tachycardia, tachypnea, profuse diaphoresis).

Overdose and treatment
The first 12 hours after acute ingestion are a stimulatory phase with excessive anticholinergic activity that includes agitation, confusion, constipation, dilated pupils, dry mucous membranes, hallucinations, hyperthermia, ileus, irritation, parkinsonian symptoms, seizures, and urine retention. CNS depression follows and may include decreased or absent reflexes, cardiac irregularities, conduction disturbances, cyanosis, hypotension, hypothermia, quinidine-like effects on the ECG, sedation, and tachycardia.

Overdose with amoxapine produces a much higher incidence of CNS toxicity than do other antidepressants. Acute deterioration of renal function (evidenced by myoglobin in urine) occurs in 5% of overdosed patients; this is most likely to occur in patients with repeated seizures after the overdose. Seizures may progress to status epilepticus within 12 hours. Metabolic acidosis may follow hypotension, hypoventilation, and seizures.

Treatment is symptomatic and supportive. Maintain patient's airway, body temperature, and fluid and electrolyte balance. Monitor patient's renal function because of the heightened risk of renal failure. Induce emesis with ipecac if gag reflex is intact; follow with gastric lavage and activated charcoal to prevent further absorption. Dialysis is of little use. Give parenteral diazepam or phenytoin for seizures, parenteral phenytoin or lidocaine for arrhythmias, and sodium bicarbonate for acidosis. Don't give barbiturates; they may worsen CNS and respiratory depressant effects.

Special considerations
▶ Drug is also used for depression.
▶ Doses for chronic pain typically are lower than those for depression.
▶ Amoxapine may be useful for treating neuropathic pain.
▶ To reduce daytime sedation, give drug on a fixed schedule at h.s.
▶ Tolerance to sedative effects usually develops over the first few weeks of therapy.
▶ Discontinue drug at least 48 hours before surgical procedures.
▶ Monitor patient for tardive dyskinesia and other extrapyramidal symptoms that may result from dopamine-blocking activity.
▶ Assess male and female patients for gynecomastia because drug may increase cell division in breast tissue.
▶ Abrupt withdrawal of long-term therapy may cause nausea, headache, malaise (which don't indicate addiction).
▶ Amoxapine creates a high risk of seizures.
▶ Drug may promote a shift to mania or hypomania in a depressed patient with bipolar disorder.

Breast-feeding patients
▶ Amoxapine is excreted in breast milk at a fraction of maternal serum levels: 20% as parent drug and 30% as metabolites. Make sure that potential benefits to mother outweigh possible adverse reactions in infant.

Pediatric patients
▶ Drug isn't recommended for patients under age 16.

Geriatric patients
▶ Elderly patients typically receive lower dosages because they're more sensitive to therapeutic and adverse effects.
▶ Elderly patients are much more susceptible to tardive dyskinesia and extrapyramidal symptoms than younger patients.

Patient teaching
▶ Tell patient to take drug exactly as prescribed; to reduce daytime sedation, recommend full dose at bedtime.
▶ Urge patient to lie down for about 30 minutes after initial doses and to rise slowly to prevent dizziness.
▶ Explain that full effects of drug may not become apparent for at least 2 weeks or more after therapy begins, perhaps not for 4 to 6 weeks.
▶ Suggest that patient takes drug with food or milk if it causes stomach upset.
▶ Caution against doubling the dose to compensate for a missed one.
▶ Warn patient to avoid hazardous activities until full CNS effects of drug are known.
▶ Suggest ice or sugarless chewing gum or hard candy to ease a dry mouth.
▶ Tell patient not to drink alcoholic beverages during therapy.

▸ Inform patient that exposure to sunlight, sunlamps, or tanning beds may cause burning of the skin or abnormal pigment changes.

▸ Warn patient not to stop drug abruptly.

▸ Encourage patient to report unusual or troublesome reactions immediately, especially confusion, movement disorders, rapid heartbeat, dizziness, fainting, or difficulty urinating.

▸ amphetamine sulfate

Pharmacologic classification:
amphetamine

Therapeutic classification:
CNS stimulant, short-term adjunctive anorexigenic, sympathomimetic amine

Controlled substance schedule II

Pregnancy risk category C

How supplied
Available by prescription only
Tablets: 5 mg, 10 mg

Indications and dosages
Attention deficit disorder with hyperactivity
Children age 6 and older: 5 mg/day P.O. Increase by 5 mg weekly until desired response occurs. Dosage rarely exceeds 40 mg/day. Give first dose upon awakening and additional doses at 4- to 6-hour intervals.
Children ages 3 to 5: 2.5 mg/day P.O. Increase by 2.5 mg weekly until desired response occurs.
Narcolepsy
Adults: 5 to 60 mg/day P.O. in divided doses or a single dose.

Children over age 12: 10 mg/day P.O. Increase by 10 mg weekly, p.r.n.
Children ages 6 to 12: 5 mg/day P.O. Increase by 5 mg weekly, p.r.n.

Pharmacodynamics
Anorexigenic action: Anorexigenic effects probably occur in the hypothalamus, where decreased smell and taste acuity decreases the appetite.
CNS stimulant action: The cerebral cortex and reticular activating system appear to be the primary sites of amphetamine activity; they release nerve terminal stores of norepinephrine, promoting nerve impulse transmission. At high dosages, effects are mediated by dopamine.

Pharmacokinetics
Absorption: Drug is absorbed completely within 3 hours after oral administration; therapeutic effects persist for 4 to 24 hours.
Distribution: Drug is distributed widely throughout the body, with high concentrations in the brain. Therapeutic plasma levels are 5 to 10 mcg/dl.
Metabolism: Drug is metabolized by hydroxylation and deamination in the liver.
Excretion: Drug is excreted in urine.

Contraindications and precautions
Contraindicated in patients with hypersensitivity or unusual reactions to sympathomimetic amines, in patients who took an MAO inhibitor with 14 days, in agitated patients, and in patients with advanced arteriosclerosis, glaucoma, a history of drug abuse, hyperthyroidism, moderate to severe hypertension, or symptomatic CV disease.

Use cautiously in elderly, debilitated, hyperexcitable, suicidal, or homicidal patients.

Interactions
Drug-drug
Acetazolamide, antacids, sodium bicarbonate: enhanced amphetamine reabsorption and prolonged duration of action. Monitor patient closely.

Ammonium chloride, ascorbic acid: enhanced amphetamine excretion and shortened duration of action. Monitor patient's response to treatment.

Antihypertensives: antagonized hypertensive effects. Monitor patient's blood pressure closely.

Barbiturates: counteract amphetamine effects by CNS depression. Avoid concurrent use.

CNS stimulants: additive effects. Avoid concurrent use.

Guanethidine: decreased guanethidine effectiveness. Avoid concurrent use.

Haloperidol, phenothiazines: decreased amphetamine effects. Avoid concurrent use.

Insulin: altered insulin requirements. Monitor blood glucose levels closely.

MAO inhibitors or drugs with MAO-inhibiting effects, such as furazolidone: possible hypertensive crisis. Monitor patient's blood pressure closely.

Drug-food
Caffeine: additive effects. Avoid concurrent use.

Effects on diagnostic tests
Amphetamines may interfere with urinary steroid determinations.

Adverse reactions
CNS: chills, dizziness, dysphoria, euphoria, headache, *hyperactivity, insomnia,* irritability, *restlessness, talkativeness,* tremor.
CV: *arrhythmias,* cardiac valve damage, hypertension, *palpitations,* pulmonary hypertension, *tachycardia.*
GI: anorexia, constipation, diarrhea, dry mouth, metallic taste.
GU: altered libido, impotence.
Metabolic: elevated plasma corticosteroid levels, weight loss.
Skin: urticaria.

Overdose and treatment
Acute overdose may cause arrhythmias, circulatory collapse, coma, confusion, delirium, diaphoresis, fever, flushing, hyperreflexia, hypertension, increasing restlessness, insomnia, irritability, mydriasis, seizures, self-injury, tachypnea, tremor, and death.

Provide symptomatic, supportive treatment. If ingestion was within 4 hours, induce emesis or perform gastric lavage. Activated charcoal, a sodium chloride cathartic, and urine acidification may enhance excretion. Forced fluid diuresis may help. In massive ingestion, hemodialysis or peritoneal dialysis may be needed. Keep patient in a cool room, monitor his temperature, and minimize external stimulation. Give haloperidol for psychotic symptoms and diazepam for hyperactivity.

Special considerations
▶ Drug may enhance analgesic effects and counteract the sedative effects of opioids.
▶ Amphetamines may be useful for managing CNS effects in terminally ill patients.

▶ Avoid administration after 4 p.m. to prevent insomnia.
▶ Don't give amphetamine capsules for initial dose or when adjusting dosage. Once dosage has been established, capsules can be substituted if once-daily dosing is needed.
▶ Monitor patient for desired effects.

Pediatric patients
▶ Use of amphetamines for hyperactivity is contraindicated in children under age 3.
▶ Amphetamines aren't recommended for weight reduction in children under age 12.

Patient teaching
▶ Warn patient about possible drowsiness, and instruct him to avoid hazardous activities until full CNS effects of drug are known.

▶ aspirin
ASA, Ascriptin, Aspergum, Bufferin, Ecotrin, Empirin, Halfprin, Novasen◇, ZORprin

Pharmacologic classification: *salicylate*

Therapeutic classification: *anti-inflammatory, antiplatelet, antipyretic, nonnarcotic analgesic*

Pregnancy risk category D

How supplied
Available by prescription only
Tablets (enteric-coated): 975 mg
Tablets (extended-release): 800 mg
Available without a prescription
Chewing gum: 227.5 mg
Suppositories: 60 mg, 120 mg, 125 mg, 200 mg, 300 mg, 600 mg
Tablets: 81 mg, 325 mg (5 grains), 500 mg, 650 mg
Tablets (enteric-coated): 81 mg, 162 mg, 165 mg, 325 mg, 500 mg, 650 mg
Tablets (extended-release): 650 mg

Indications and dosages
Arthritis
Adults: 3.6 to 5.4 g/day P.O. in divided doses.
Children: 80 to 130 mg/kg/day P.O. in divided doses.
Mild pain or fever
Adults: 325 to 650 mg P.O. or P.R. q 4 hours, p.r.n.
Mild pain
Children: 65 mg/kg/day P.O. or P.R. divided q 4 to 6 hours, p.r.n.
Kawasaki (mucocutaneous lymph node) syndrome
Adults: 80 to 100 mg/kg/day P.O. in four divided doses. Some patients may require up to 180 mg/kg/day to maintain serum salicylate levels above 200 mcg/ml during the febrile phase. After the fever subsides, reduce dosage to 3 to 5 mg/kg once daily. Therapy usually continues for 6 to 8 weeks.

Pharmacodynamics
Analgesic action: Aspirin produces analgesia by an ill-defined effect on the hypothalamus (central action) and by blocking generation of pain impulses (peripheral action). The peripheral action may involve blocking of prostaglandin synthesis via nonspecific inhibition of cyclooxygenase enzyme isoforms 1 and 2.
Anti-inflammatory action: Exact mechanism is unknown, but aspirin probably inhibits prostaglandin synthesis. It also may inhibit the synthesis or action of other mediators of inflammation.

◇ Available in Canada only   *Unlabeled use

Antipyretic action: Aspirin relieves fever by acting on the hypothalamic heat-regulating center to produce peripheral vasodilation. This action increases peripheral blood supply and promotes sweating, which promotes heat loss and cooling by evaporation.

Anticoagulant action: At low doses, aspirin appears to impede clotting by blocking prostaglandin synthetase action, which prevents formation of the platelet-aggregating substance thromboxane A. This interference with platelet activity is irreversible and can prolong bleeding time. However, at high doses, aspirin interferes with prostacyclin production, a potent vasoconstrictor and inhibitor of platelet aggregation, possibly negating its anticlotting properties.

Pharmacokinetics

Absorption: Aspirin is absorbed rapidly and completely from the GI tract. Therapeutic blood salicylate levels for analgesia and anti-inflammatory effect are 150 to 300 mcg/ml. Responses vary.

Distribution: Aspirin is distributed widely into most body tissues and fluids. Protein-binding to albumin is concentration-dependent and ranges from 75% to 90%. It decreases as serum level increases. Severe toxic effects may occur at serum levels above 400 mcg/ml.

Metabolism: Aspirin is hydrolyzed partially in the GI tract to salicylic acid with almost complete metabolism in the liver.

Excretion: Aspirin is excreted in urine as salicylate and its metabolites. Elimination half-life ranges from 15 to 20 minutes.

Contraindications and precautions

Contraindicated in patients hypersensitive to drug or other NSAIDs, in children with chickenpox or flu-like symptoms, and in patients with bleeding disorders (such as hemophilia), G6PD deficiency, telangiectasia, or von Willebrand disease.

Use cautiously in patients with GI lesions, hepatic impairment, hypoprothrombinemia, renal impairment, thrombotic thrombocytopenic purpura, or vitamin K deficiency.

Interactions
Drug-drug

Antacids, urine alkalizers: at high doses of these drugs, blood aspirin levels decrease. Monitor patient for decreased salicylate effect.

Anticoagulants, thrombolytics: may potentiate platelet-inhibiting effects of aspirin. Monitor patient's CBC and coagulation studies closely.

Corticosteroids: enhance aspirin elimination. Monitor patient's response to treatment.

Drugs that are highly protein-bound, such as phenytoin, sulfonylureas, warfarin: may lead to displacement of these drugs or aspirin, causing adverse effects. Monitor patient's response closely.

GI-irritant drugs (such as antibiotics, other NSAIDs, steroids): may potentiate adverse GI effects of aspirin. Use together cautiously.

Lithium carbonate: possible decreased renal lithium clearance, thus increasing serum lithium levels and the risk of adverse effects. Monitor patient closely.

Ototoxic drugs (such as aminoglycosides, bumetanide, capreomycin, cisplatin, erythromycin, ethacrynic acid, furosemide, vancomycin): may potentiate ototoxic effects. Monitor patient for altered hearing. *Phenylbutazone, probenecid, and sulfinpyrazone:* uricosuric effects antagonized by aspirin. Monitor patient's response to treatment. *Urine acidifiers, such as ammonium chloride:* increased blood aspirin levels. Monitor for aspirin toxicity.

Drug-herb
Horse chestnut, kelpware, prickly ash, red clover: may increase risk of bleeding. Monitor patient closely.

Drug-food
Food: may delay and decrease aspirin absorption. Monitor patient for effect.

Drug-lifestyle
Alcohol: may potentiate adverse GI effects of aspirin. Discourage concurrent use.

Effects on diagnostic tests
Aspirin interferes with urine glucose analysis using Diastix, Chemstrip uG, glucose enzymatic test strip, Clinitest, and Benedict's solution. It also interferes with urinary 5-hydroxyindoleacetic acid and vanillylmandelic acid tests. Serum uric acid levels may be falsely increased. Aspirin may interfere with Gerhardt's test for urine acetoacetic acid.

Adverse reactions
EENT: *hearing loss, tinnitus.*
GI: *dyspepsia, **GI bleeding**, GI distress, nausea, occult bleeding.*
Hematologic: *leukopenia, prolonged bleeding time, **thrombocytopenia.***

Hepatic: abnormal liver function studies, ***hepatitis.***
Skin: bruising, *rash,* urticaria.
Other: ***angioedema, hypersensitivity reactions (anaphylaxis,*** asthma), ***Reye's syndrome.***

Overdose and treatment
Overdose may cause acute renal failure, EEG abnormalities, GI discomfort, hyperthermia, oliguria, restlessness, tinnitus, and metabolic acidosis with respiratory alkalosis, hyperpnea, and tachypnea because of increased CO_2 production and direct stimulation of the respiratory center.

To treat aspirin overdose, empty the patient's stomach immediately. If patient is conscious, induce emesis with ipecac syrup. If not, perform gastric lavage. Give activated charcoal via nasogastric tube. Provide symptomatic and supportive measures, including respiratory support and correction of fluid and electrolyte imbalances. Closely monitor patient's laboratory parameters and vital signs. Enhance renal excretion by giving sodium bicarbonate to alkalinize urine. Use cooling blanket or sponge bath if patient's rectal temperature is above 104° F (40° C). Hemodialysis is effective in removing aspirin, but is only used in severe poisoning or in patients at risk for pulmonary edema.

Special considerations
▶ There's a ceiling to the analgesic effects of aspirin.
▶ 650 mg of aspirin equals 50 mg of oral meperidine.
▶ Enteric-coated products are absorbed slowly and aren't suitable for acute therapy. They're ideal for long-term therapy, as for arthritis.

▶ For patients unable to take anything by mouth, rectal aspirin suppositories are effective.

▶ Monitor patient's CBC and coagulation studies during therapy.

▶ Tinnitus is a common warning sign of toxic plasma levels; if it occurs, decrease dosage.

▶ Stop aspirin therapy 1 week before elective surgery, if possible.

▶ No evidence exists that aspirin reduces the risk of transient ischemic attacks in women.

▶ Moisture may cause aspirin to lose potency. Store in a cool, dry place, and avoid using tablets that smell like vinegar.

▶ Aspirin is also indicated as an antipyretic, anti-inflammatory, and antiplatelet drug.

Breast-feeding patients
▶ Salicylates are distributed into breast milk; avoid use during breast-feeding.

Pediatric patients
▶ Because of their connection to Reye's syndrome, aspirin and other salicylates shouldn't be given to children who have chickenpox or flulike symptoms.

▶ Don't use long-term salicylate therapy in children under age 14; safety hasn't been established.

Geriatric patients
▶ Patients older than age 60 may be more susceptible to the toxic effects of aspirin. Use with caution.

▶ Effects of aspirin on renal prostaglandins may cause fluid retention and edema, a significant drawback for elderly patients and those with heart failure.

Patient teaching
▶ Tell patient to take drug with food or after meals to avoid GI upset.

▶ Instruct patient to avoid aspirin if he's allergic to tartrazine dye.

▶ If patient receives high-dose, long-term aspirin therapy, instruct him to watch for petechiae, bleeding gums, and signs of GI bleeding.

▶ Because aspirin is a leading cause of poisoning, warn parents to keep aspirin out of children's reach, and encourage use of child-resistant cap.

▶ atenolol
Tenormin

Pharmacologic classification:
beta blocker

Therapeutic classification:
antianginal, antihypertensive

Pregnancy risk category C

How supplied
Available by prescription only
Injection: 5 mg/10 ml
Tablets: 25 mg, 50 mg, 100 mg

Indications and dosages
Prevention of migraine headaches
Adults: 25-100 mg P.O. b.i.d.
Chronic stable angina pectoris
Adults: 50 mg P.O. once daily; may increase to 100 mg/day after 7 days for optimal effect. Maximum, 200 mg/day.

☒ DOSAGE ADJUSTMENT. If patient's creatinine clearance is 15 to 35 ml/minute/1.73 m^2, give 50 mg/day. If creatinine clearance is below 15 ml/minute/1.73 m^2, give 25 mg/day. If patient receives hemodialysis, give

25 to 50 mg after each treatment under close supervision.

Pharmacodynamics

Antianginal action: Drug decreases myocardial contractility and heart rate (negative inotropic and chronotropic effect), thus reducing myocardial oxygen consumption.
Antihypertensive action: Atenolol may reduce blood pressure by adrenergic receptor blockade, thereby decreasing cardiac output by decreasing the sympathetic outflow from the CNS and by suppressing renin release. At low doses, atenolol, like metoprolol, selectively inhibits cardiac beta$_1$-receptors; it has little effect on beta$_2$-receptors in bronchial and vascular smooth muscle.
Antimigraine action: Unknown.
Cardioprotective action: Atenolol reduces PVCs, chest pain, and enzyme elevation by an unknown mechanism, thus improving survival after MI.

Pharmacokinetics

Absorption: About 50% to 60% of dose is absorbed. Effects begin within 60 minutes and peak at 2 to 4 hours. Antihypertensive effect persists for about 24 hours.
Distribution: Drug is distributed into most tissues and fluids except the brain and CSF; about 5% to 15% is protein-bound.
Metabolism: Minimal.
Excretion: About 40% to 50% of a dose is excreted unchanged in urine; the rest in feces as unchanged drug and metabolites. Plasma half-life is 6 to 7 hours; longer as renal function decreases.

Contraindications and precautions

Contraindicated in patients with sinus bradycardia, greater than first-degree heart block, overt cardiac failure, or cardiogenic shock.

Use cautiously in patients at risk for heart failure and in those with bronchospastic disease, diabetes, hyperthyroidism, and Raynaud's disease.

Interactions
Drug-drug

Alpha-adrenergic drugs (such as those found in OTC cold remedies), indomethacin, NSAIDs: may antagonize hypertensive effects. Monitor blood pressure.
Antihypertensives: may potentiate antihypertensive effects. Monitor patient's blood pressure closely.

Effects on diagnostic tests

Atenolol may alter exercise tolerance and ECG results.

Adverse reactions

CNS: *dizziness,* drowsiness, *fatigue,* lethargy, vertigo.
CV: ***bradycardia, heart failure,*** hypotension, intermittent claudication.
GI: diarrhea, nausea.
GU: elevated BUN and creatinine.
Metabolic: hyperglycemia, hyperkalemia, hypoglycemia.
Musculoskeletal: leg pain.
Hepatic: elevated transaminase, alkaline phosphatase.
Metabolic: fever.
Respiratory: ***bronchospasm,*** dyspnea.
Skin: rash.

Overdose and treatment

Overdose may cause bradycardia, bronchospasm, heart failure, and severe hypotension. After acute ingestion, induce emesis or perform gastric lavage. Follow with activated charcoal to reduce absorption. Thereafter, treat symptomatically and supportively.

Special considerations
▶ Atenolol I.V. has a rapid onset of protection against reinfarction.
▶ Patients who can't tolerate atenolol I.V. after an MI may receive some benefit from atenolol P.O. However, gastric absorption may be delayed in the early phase of MI, possibly from physiologic changes from MI or possibly from the effects of morphine.
▶ Give single daily dose P.O. at same time each day.
▶ Drug may be taken without food.
▶ Don't stop drug abruptly.
▶ Monitor serum glucose levels in patients with diabetes because drug may cause hypoglycemia. Dosages of insulin or oral antidiabetic drugs may need adjustment.

Breast-feeding patients
▶ Safety hasn't been established. An alternative feeding method is recommended during therapy.

Pediatric patients
▶ Safety and efficacy in children haven't been established; make sure potential benefits outweigh risk.

Geriatric patients
▶ Elderly patients may need lower maintenance dosages because of increased bioavailability or delayed metabolism.
▶ They also may experience enhanced adverse effects.

Patient teaching
▶ Stress the importance of not missing doses.
▶ Warn patient not to double the dose if he misses one, especially if he takes the drug once daily.
▶ Advise patient to consult prescriber before taking OTC cold medications.

▶ **auranofin**
Ridaura

Pharmacologic classification:
gold salt

Therapeutic classification:
antiarthritic

Pregnancy risk category C

How supplied
Available by prescription only
Capsules: 3 mg

Indications and dosages
Rheumatoid arthritis
Active systemic lupus erythematosus*, Felty's syndrome*, psoriatic arthritis*
Adults: 6 mg/day P.O., either as 3 mg b.i.d. or 6 mg once daily. After 4 to 6 months, may increase to 9 mg/day. If response inadequate after 3 months at 9 mg/day, discontinue drug.

Pharmacodynamics
Antiarthritic action: Auranofin suppresses or prevents, but doesn't cure, adult or juvenile arthritis and synovitis. It has an anti-inflammatory effect in active arthritis, probably by altering the immune system. Drug decreases high serum levels of immunoglobulins and rheumatoid factors in pa-

tients with arthritis. However, the exact mechanism of action remains unknown.

Pharmacokinetics
Absorption: When given P.O., 25% of the gold in auranofin is absorbed through the GI tract. Plasma level peaks in 1 to 2 hours.

Distribution: Drug is 60% protein-bound and is distributed widely in body tissues. Oral gold from auranofin is bound to a higher degree than gold from the injectable form. Synovial fluid levels are about 50% of blood levels. No correlation between blood-gold levels and safety or efficacy has been determined.

Metabolism: The metabolic fate of auranofin is not known, but drug probably isn't broken down into elemental gold.

Excretion: 60% of absorbed auranofin (15% of the administered dose) is excreted in urine, the remainder in feces. Average plasma half-life is 26 days, compared with about 6 days for gold sodium thiomalate.

Contraindications and precautions
Contraindicated in patients with history of severe gold toxicity, necrotizing enterocolitis, pulmonary fibrosis, exfoliative dermatitis, bone marrow aplasia, severe hematologic disorders or history of severe toxicity caused by previous exposure to other heavy metals.

Use cautiously with other drugs that cause blood dyscrasia or in patients with renal, hepatic, or inflammatory bowel disease; rash; or bone marrow depression. Use of

drug in pregnant women is not recommended.

Interactions
Drug-drug
Drugs that increase the risk of blood dyscrasia: possible additive hematologic toxicity. Monitor patient closely.

Effects on diagnostic tests
Serum protein-bound iodine test, especially when done by the chloric acid digestion method, gives false readings during and for several weeks after gold therapy.

Adverse reactions
CNS: confusion, hallucinations, *seizures.*
EENT: conjunctivitis.
GI: anorexia, *abdominal pain,* constipation, *diarrhea,* dysgeusia, dyspepsia, flatulence, glossitis, metallic taste, *nausea, stomatitis, ulcerative colitis.*
GU: *acute renal failure,* glomerulonephritis, hematuria, *nephrotic syndrome,* proteinuria.
Hematologic: *agranulocytosis,* anemia, *aplastic anemia,* eosinophilia, *leukopenia, thrombocytopenia* with or without purpura.
Hepatic: jaundice, elevated liver enzymes.
Respiratory: interstitial pneumonitis.
Skin: alopecia, *dermatitis,* erythema, exfoliative dermatitis, *pruritus, rash,* urticaria.

Overdose and treatment
Overdose may cause encephalopathy and peripheral neuropathy from neurotoxicity.

In acute overdose, empty gastric contents by induced emesis or gastric lavage. When severe reactions to gold occur, corticosteroids, dimercaprol (a chelating agent), or penicillamine may be given to aid recovery. Prednisone 40 to 100 mg daily in divided doses is recommended to manage severe renal, hematologic, pulmonary, or enterocolitic reactions to gold.

Dimercaprol may be used concurrently with steroids to facilitate the removal of the gold when steroid treatment alone is ineffective. Use of chelating agents is controversial, and caution is recommended. Appropriate supportive therapy is indicated as necessary.

Special considerations
▶ Indicated only for inflammatory pain from rheumatoid arthritis.
▶ May take 3 to 4 months before full effect is seen.
▶ Stop drug if platelet count decreases below 100,000/mm^3.
▶ When switching from injectable gold, start auranofin at 6 mg/day P.O.
▶ Monitor CBC and liver enzymes.

Breast-feeding patients
▶ Drug isn't recommended for use during breast-feeding.

Pediatric patients
▶ Safe dosage hasn't been established; use in children currently isn't recommended.

Geriatric patients
▶ Give usual adult dose.
▶ Use cautiously in elderly patients with decreased renal function.

Patient teaching
▶ Reassure patient that beneficial drug effect may take 3 months. However, if response is inadequate

after 6 to 9 months, auranofin will probably be discontinued.
▶ Encourage patient to take drug as prescribed and not to alter the dosage schedule.
▶ Tell patient to continue taking other prescribed drugs, such as NSAIDs, because auranofin has no intrinsic analgesic properties.
▶ Diarrhea is the most common adverse reaction. Tell patient to continue taking drug if mild diarrhea develops; however, tell him to call immediately about bloody stool.
▶ Dermatitis is a common adverse reaction. Tell patient to report rash or other skin problems right away.
▶ Stomatitis is another common adverse reaction. Tell patient that stomatitis is often preceded by a metallic taste; advise him to call immediately if it occurs.

▶ aurothioglucose
Solganal

▶ gold sodium thiomalate
Aurolate

Pharmacologic classification:
gold salt

Therapeutic classification:
antiarthritic

Pregnancy risk category C

How supplied
Available by prescription only
aurothioglucose
Injection (suspension): 50 mg/ml in sesame oil in 10-ml vial
gold sodium thiomalate
Injection: 50 mg/ml with benzyl alcohol

Indications and dosages
Rheumatoid arthritis
aurothioglucose
Adults: initially, 10 mg I.M., followed by 25 mg for second and third doses at weekly intervals. Then, 50 mg weekly until 800 mg to 1 g has been given. If improvement occurs without toxicity, 25 to 50 mg is continued at 3- to 4-week intervals indefinitely.
Children ages 6 to 12: one-quarter usual adult dose. Don't exceed 25 mg per dose.
gold sodium thiomalate
Adults: initially, 10 mg I.M., followed by 25 mg in 1 week. Then, 25 to 50 mg weekly to total dose of 1 g. If improvement occurs without toxicity, give 25 to 50 mg q 2 weeks for 2 to 20 weeks; then, give 25 to 50 mg q 3 to 4 weeks as maintenance therapy. If relapse occurs, resume weekly injections.
Children: initially, 10 mg I.M. Then, 1 mg/kg I.M. weekly, not to exceed 50 mg for a single injection. Follow adult spacing of doses.

Pharmacodynamics
Anti-inflammatory action: Drug probably inhibits sulfhydryl systems, which alters cellular metabolism. May also alter enzyme function and immune response and suppress phagocytic activity.

Pharmacokinetics
Absorption: Rapidly absorbed after I.M. administration. Levels peak in 3 to 6 hours.
Distribution: Absorbed gold concentrates in the lymph nodes, bone marrow, liver, kidneys, spleen, and synovial fluid, especially in arthritic joints. It's widely distributed in other body tissues and highly protein-bound.

Metabolism: Unknown.
Excretion: Excreted in urine and feces.

Contraindications and precautions
Contraindicated in patients with hypersensitivity to drug and in those with history of severe toxicity from previous exposure to gold or other heavy metals. Also contraindicated in those with hepatitis, exfoliative dermatitis, severe uncontrollable diabetes, renal disease, hepatic dysfunction, uncontrolled heart failure, systemic lupus erythematosus, colitis, Sjögren's syndrome, urticaria, eczema, hemorrhagic conditions, or severe hematologic disorders and in those who have recently received radiation therapy.

Use with extreme caution, if at all, in patients with rash, marked hypertension, compromised cerebral or CV circulation, or history of renal or hepatic disease, drug allergies, or blood dyscrasias.

Interactions
Drug-drug
Azathioprine, cyclophosphamide, hydroxychloroquine, methotrexate, penicillamine, phenylbutazone: increased risk of adverse effects. Avoid concomitant use.

Drug-lifestyle
Sun or ultraviolet light exposure: photosensitivity reactions may occur. Urge precautions.

Effects on diagnostic tests
Serum protein-bound iodine test, especially when done by chloric acid digestion method, gives false readings during and for several weeks after therapy.

Adverse reactions

CNS: confusion, hallucinations, *seizures.*
CV: *bradycardia,* hypotension.
EENT: corneal gold deposition, corneal ulcers.
GI: abdominal cramps, anorexia, *diarrhea, metallic taste,* nausea, *stomatitis,* ulcerative enterocolitis, vomiting.
GU: *acute renal failure,* acute tubular necrosis, albuminuria, hematuria, nephritis, nephrotic syndrome, proteinuria.
Hematologic: *agranulocytosis,* anemia, *aplastic anemia,* eosinophilia, *leukopenia, thrombocytopenia.*
Hepatic: elevated liver function test results, *hepatitis,* jaundice.
Skin: *dermatitis,* diaphoresis, erythema, exfoliative dermatitis, photosensitivity, *rash.*
Other: *anaphylaxis, angioedema.*

Overdose and treatment

Overdose may result from increasing dosage too rapidly and may cause rapid appearance of toxic reactions, such as hematuria, proteinuria, thrombocytopenia, and granulocytopenia. Fever, nausea, vomiting, diarrhea, rash, urticaria, exfoliative dermatitis and severe pruritus may also occur.

Treatment includes discontinuing drug, giving dimercaprol, and providing supportive measures.

Special considerations

▶ Drug should only be given I.M. and only under constant supervision by staff thoroughly familiar with drug toxicities and benefits.
▶ Give gold salts I.M., as ordered, preferably intragluteally. Drug is pale yellow; don't use if it darkens.

▶ Immerse aurothioglucose vial in warm water; shake vigorously before injecting.
▶ When injecting gold sodium thiomalate, keep patient supine for 10 to 20 minutes to minimize hypotension.
▶ Watch for anaphylactoid reaction for 30 minutes after giving drug.
▶ Keep dimercaprol available to treat acute toxicity.
▶ If adverse reactions are mild, some rheumatologists resume gold therapy after 2 to 3 weeks' rest.
▶ Analyze patient's urine for protein and sediment changes before each injection.
▶ Monitor CBC, including platelet count, before every other injection.
▶ Monitor platelet counts if patient develops purpura or ecchymosis.
▶ Check liver function test results.

Breast-feeding patients

▶ Small amounts of gold are distributed into breast milk and may cause adverse reactions in the nursing infant. Not recommended for use in nursing mothers.

Pediatric patients

▶ Safety and effectiveness in patients less than age 6 years have not been established.

Patient teaching

▶ Inform patient that joint pain may increase for 1 to 2 days after injection but usually subsides.
▶ Tell patient that benefits may not appear for 3 to 4 months.
▶ Urge patient to avoid sunlight and artificial ultraviolet light.
▶ Urge medical follow-up.
▶ Advise patient to report rash or skin problems immediately and to stop drug until reaction subsides. Pruritus may precede dermatitis;

pruritic skin eruptions during gold therapy should be considered a reaction until proven otherwise.
❱ Advise patient to report unusual bleeding or bruising.
❱ Instruct patient to report a metallic taste. Promote oral hygiene.
❱ Warn women of childbearing age about the risks of gold therapy during pregnancy.

❱ baclofen
Lioresal

Pharmacologic classification:
chlorophenyl derivative

Therapeutic classification:
skeletal muscle relaxant

Pregnancy risk category C

How supplied
Available by prescription only
Tablets: 10 mg, 20 mg
Intrathecal kit: 500 mcg/ml, 2,000 mcg/ml

Indications and dosage
Spasticity in multiple sclerosis and other spinal cord lesions
Adults: initially, 5 mg P.O. t.i.d. for 3 days. Dosage may be increased (based on response) at 3-day intervals by 15 mg (5 mg/dose) daily up to maximum of 80 mg daily.
Intrathecal administration in adults: Dilute with sterile preservative-free normal saline injection and give intrathecal bolus of 50 mcg in 1 ml over at least 1 minute. Watch for response for 4 to 8 hours. A positive response consists of a significant decrease in muscle tone or frequency or severity of spasm. If initial response is inadequate, repeat dose with 75 mcg in 1.5 ml 24

hours after last injection. Repeat observation of patient over 4 to 8 hours. If the response is still inadequate, repeat dosing at 100 mcg in 2 ml 24 hours later. If still no response, patient should not be considered for an implantable pump for chronic baclofen administration. Ranges for chronic doses are 12 to 2,003 mcg/day.
Post-implant dose adjustment in adults: If the screening dose produced the desired effect for over 8 hours, the initial intrathecal dose is the same as the test dose; this dose is infused intrathecally for 24 hours. If the screening dose produced the desired effect for less than 8 hours, the initial intrathecal dose is twice the test dose, followed slowly by 10% to 30% increments at 24-hour intervals.

Pharmacodynamics
Skeletal muscle relaxant action: Precise mechanism of action is unknown, but drug appears to act at the spinal cord level to inhibit transmission of monosynaptic and polysynaptic reflexes, possibly through hyperpolarization of afferent fiber terminals. It may also act at supraspinal sites because baclofen at high doses produces generalized CNS depression. Baclofen decreases the number and severity of spasms and relieves associated pain, clonus, and muscle rigidity and therefore improves mobility.

Pharmacokinetics
Absorption: Drug is rapidly and extensively absorbed from the GI tract, but is subject to individual variation. Peak plasma levels occur at 2 to 3 hours. Also, as dose increases, rate and extent of absorption decreases. Onset of therapeu-

---

tic effect may not be immediately evident; varies from hours to weeks. Peak effect is seen at 2 to 3 hours.

Distribution: Studies indicate that baclofen is widely distributed throughout body, with small amounts crossing the blood-brain barrier. About 30% is plasma protein-bound.

Metabolism: About 15% is metabolized in the liver via deamination.

Excretion: 70% to 80% is excreted in urine unchanged or as its metabolites; remainder, in feces.

Contraindications and precautions

Contraindicated in patients with hypersensitivity to drug. Use cautiously in patients with renal impairment or seizure disorders or when spasticity is used to maintain motor function.

Interactions
Drug-drug

Antidiabetic drugs, insulin: increased blood glucose levels. Monitor patient's glucose levels, and adjust dosages as needed.

CNS depressants, antipsychotics, anxiolytics, general anesthetics, and narcotics: additive CNS effects. Monitor patient closely.

MAO inhibitors, tricyclic antidepressants: possible CNS depression, respiratory depression, and hypotension. Avoid using together; if necessary, monitor patient closely.

Drug-lifestyle

Alcohol use: additive CNS effects. Discourage concomitant use.

Effects on diagnostic tests

None reported.

Adverse reactions

CNS: CNS depression *(potentially life-threatening with intrathecal administration),* confusion, dizziness, drowsiness, dysarthria, *fatigue,* headache, *hypotonia,* insomnia, *seizures, weakness.*

CV: *CV collapse* (secondary to CNS depression), hypertension, hypotension.

EENT: blurred vision, nasal congestion, slurred speech.

GI: constipation, *nausea, vomiting.*

GU: urinary frequency.

Hepatic: increased AST and alkaline phosphatase levels.

Metabolic: hyperglycemia, weight gain.

Respiratory: dyspnea, *respiratory failure* (secondary to CNS depression).

Skin: diaphoresis, pruritus, rash.

Overdose and treatment

Overdose may cause absence of reflexes, coma, drowsiness, marked salivation, muscular hypotonia, respiratory depression, seizures, visual disorders, and vomiting.

Treatment requires supportive measures, including endotracheal intubation and positive-pressure ventilation. If patient is conscious, remove drug by inducing emesis. If patient is comatose, perform gastric lavage after endotracheal tube is in place with cuff inflated. Don't use respiratory stimulants. Monitor patient's vital signs closely.

Special considerations

▶ Baclofen is used to reduce choreiform movements in Huntington's chorea; to reduce rigidity in Parkinson's disease; to reduce spasticity in CVA, cerebral lesions, cerebral palsy, and rheumatic disorders; for analgesia in trigeminal neuralgia; and for treatment of unstable bladder.

▶ Intrathecal administration should be performed only by qualified persons familiar with administration techniques and patient management problems.

▶ Adverse reactions may be reduced by slowly decreasing dosage. Abrupt withdrawal can result in hallucinations, seizures, or acute worsening of spasticity.

▶ In some patients, smoother response may be obtained by giving daily amount in four divided doses.

▶ Patient with epilepsy may have increased risk of seizures. Use EEG, observation, and interview to detect possible loss of seizure control.

▶ If patient is diabetic, assess for increased blood glucose levels.

▶ Initial loss of spasticity caused by drug may affect patient's ability to stand or walk; provide assistance as needed. In some patients, spasticity helps maintain upright posture and balance.

▶ Observe patient's response to drug. Signs of effective therapy may appear in a few hours to 1 week and may include diminished frequency of spasms, reduced severity of foot and ankle clonus, increased ease and range of joint motion, and enhanced performance of daily activities.

▶ During prolonged intrathecal baclofen therapy for spasticity, about 10% of patients become refractory to baclofen therapy and need a break from therapy to regain sensitivity to its effects.

▶ Stop drug if signs of improvement don't occur in 1 or 2 months.

▶ Failure of implantable pump or catheter can result in sudden loss of intrathecal drug effectiveness.

Pediatric patients
▶ Use of oral form isn't recommended for children under age 12.

▶ Safety of intrathecal administration in children under age 4 hasn't been established.

Geriatric patients
▶ Elderly patients are especially sensitive to drug. Observe carefully for adverse reactions, such as confusion, depression, and hallucinations. Lower doses are usually indicated.

Patient teaching
▶ Tell patient to report adverse reactions promptly. Most can be reduced by decreasing dosage. Drowsiness, dizziness, and ataxia are more common over age 40.

▶ Warn patient not to use other CNS depressants, including alcohol, during therapy.

▶ Caution patient to avoid hazardous activities.

▶ Tell diabetic patient that baclofen may raise blood glucose levels and may require adjustment of insulin dosage during therapy. Urge patient to promptly report changes in urine or blood glucose tests.

▶ Caution patient against taking OTC drugs without consulting prescriber. Explain that hazardous drug interactions are possible.

▶ Warn patient not to stop drug abruptly, but rather to withdraw it gradually over 1 to 2 weeks according to prescriber's plan. Abrupt withdrawal after prolonged use may cause acute spasticity, agitation, anxiety, auditory and visual hallucinations, and severe tachycardia.

▶ benzocaine
Americaine, Americaine-Otic Dermoplast, Hurricane, Lanacane, Maximum Strength Anbesol, Orabase Gel, Orajel Mouth-Aid, Otocain, Solarcaine

Pharmacologic classification:
local anesthetic (ester)

Therapeutic classification:
anesthetic

Pregnancy risk category C

How supplied
Available without a prescription
Gel: 20%
Lotion: 0.5% to 8%
Ointment, cream, and dental paste: 1% to 20%
Otic solution: 20%
Topical solution: 20%
Topical spray: 20%

Indications and dosages
Local anesthetic for dental pain or dental procedures
Adults and children: Apply topical gel (20%) or dental paste to area, p.r.n.
Local anesthetic for pruritic dermatoses, pruritus, or other irritations
Adults: Apply topical preparation (1% to 20%) to affected area, p.r.n.
Relief of pain and pruritus in acute congestive and serous otitis media, acute swimmer's ear, and other forms of otitis externa
Adults: 4 to 5 drops (otic) in external auditory canal; insert cotton into meatus; repeat q 1 to 2 hours.

Pharmacodynamics
Analgesic action: Acts at sensory neurons to produce a local anesthetic effect by altering membrane permeability to nerve conduction ions.

Pharmacokinetics
Absorption: Effects peak in 5 minutes.
Distribution: Unknown.
Metabolism: Unknown.
Excretion: Effects last 15 to 45 minutes. Mechanism of excretion is unknown.

Contraindications and precautions
Contraindicated for use in eyes and in patients hypersensitive to any component of the drug or related substances, serious burns, secondary infection in the area, or perforated tympanic membrane or discharge.
Use cautiously in patients with severely traumatized mucosa or local sepsis.

Interactions
None significant.

Effects on diagnostic tests
None reported.

Adverse reactions
CV: edema.
Skin: burning, erythema, irritation, itching, rash, stinging, tenderness, urticaria.

Overdose and treatment
Overdose is unlikely; however, methemoglobinemia has been reported after topical application for teething pain. CNS or CV depression may occur as well.

Treat symptomatically; if needed, give methylene blue 1% 0.1 ml/kg I.V. over at least 10 minutes. Maximum dose is 5 g/day.

Special considerations
▶ Drug may be useful as a lubricant to facilitate passage of laryngoscopes or gastroscopes. It also may be helpful before painful debridement of leg ulcers.
▶ Use with antibiotic to treat underlying cause of pain because drug alone may mask more serious condition.
▶ Keep container tightly closed and protected from moisture.
▶ Monitor patient for response to treatment.
▶ Discontinue drug if hypersensitivity develops.

Pediatric patients
▶ Excessive use may cause methemoglobinemia in infants. Don't use drug in children under age 1.

Patient teaching
▶ Tell patient to report pain that lasts longer than 48 hours, burning, itching, or lack of response.
▶ Instruct patient to keep container tightly closed and protected from moisture.
▶ To reduce the risk of bite trauma after oral application, tell patient not to eat or chew gum until local anesthetic effect has worn off.

▶ bisacodyl
Bisco-Lax, Dulcolax, Fleet Laxative

Pharmacologic classification: *diphenylmethane derivative*

Therapeutic classification: *stimulant laxative*

Pregnancy risk category B

How supplied
Available without a prescription
Rectal suspension: 10 mg/30 ml
Suppositories: 10 mg
Tablets: 5 mg

Indications and dosages
Constipation; preparation for delivery, surgery, or rectal or bowel examination
Adults: 10 to 15 mg/day P.O. Up to 30 mg may be used for thorough evacuation needed for examinations or surgery. Alternatively, give one suppository (10 mg) or 30 ml of rectal suspension P.R. daily.
Children ages 6 to 12: 5 mg/day P.O. Alternatively, give half of suppository (5 mg) or 15 ml of rectal suspension P.R. daily.

Pharmacodynamics
Laxative action: Bisacodyl has a direct stimulant effect on the colon, increasing peristalsis and enhancing bowel evacuation.

Pharmacokinetics
Absorption: Absorption is minimal; action begins 6 to 8 hours after oral administration and 15 to 60 minutes after P.R. administration.
Distribution: Bisacodyl is distributed locally.

Metabolism: Drug is absorbed minimally; bisacodyl is metabolized in the liver.
Excretion: Drug is excreted primarily in feces; some in urine.

Contraindications and precautions

Contraindicated in patients hypersensitive to drug and in patients with abdominal pain, gastroenteritis, intestinal obstruction, nausea, rectal bleeding, symptoms of appendicitis or acute surgical abdomen, vomiting.

Interactions
Drug-drug
Antacids and drugs that increase gastric pH levels: may cause premature dissolution of enteric coating, resulting in intestinal or gastric irritation or cramping. Avoid concurrent use.

Drug-food
Milk: may cause premature dissolution of enteric coating, resulting in intestinal or gastric irritation or cramping. Avoid concurrent use.

Effects on diagnostic tests
None reported.

Adverse reactions
CNS: dizziness, faintness, muscle weakness with excessive use.
GI: *abdominal cramps, burning sensation in rectum* (suppositories), diarrhea (high doses), laxative dependence with long-term or excessive use, *nausea, vomiting.*
Metabolic: alkalosis, fluid and electrolyte imbalance, hypokalemia, protein-losing enteropathy with excessive use, tetany.

Overdose and treatment
No cases have been reported.

Special considerations
▶ Drug may be helpful in preventing opioid-induced constipation.
▶ Monitor patient's response.

Breast-feeding patients
▶ Drug may be used during breast-feeding.

Patient teaching
▶ Tell patient to take drug as directed to avoid laxative dependence.
▶ To avoid GI irritation, instruct patient to swallow tablets whole (rather than crushing or chewing them) with 8 oz (240 ml) of fluid.
▶ Urge patient not to take drug within 1 hour of milk or antacid.

▶ bupivacaine hydrochloride
Marcaine, Sensorcaine, Sensorcaine MPF, Sensorcaine MPF Spinal

Pharmacologic classification: *amide local anesthetic*

Therapeutic classification: *local anesthetic*

Pregnancy risk category C

How supplied
Available by prescription only
Injection: 0.25%, 0.5%, 0.75%

Indications and dosages
Dosages given are for the drug without epinephrine.
Epidural block
Adults: 25 to 50 mg (10 to 20 ml) of 0.25% solution; 50 to 100 mg (10 to 20 ml) of 0.5% solution; 75

---

to 100 mg (15 to 30 ml) of 0.75% solution, single-dose only.

Caudal block
Adults: 37.5 to 75 mg (15 to 30 ml) of 0.25% solution; 75 to 150 mg (15 to 30 ml) of 0.5% solution.

Spinal block
Adults: 7.5 to 12 mg (1 to 1.6 ml) of 0.75% solution (in dextrose 8.25%).

Peripheral nerve block
Adults: 12.5 mg (5 ml) of 0.25% solution; 25 mg (5 ml) of 0.5% solution.

Retrobulbar block
Adults: 15 to 30 mg (2 to 4 ml) of 0.75% solution.

⧄ DOSAGE ADJUSTMENT. Dosage differs with anesthetic procedure, area to be anesthetized, vascularity of area, number of neuronal segments to be blocked, degree of block, duration of anesthesia desired, and individual patient conditions and tolerance. Always use incremental doses.

Pharmacodynamics
Local anesthetic action: Drug blocks the generation and conduction of nerve impulses by increasing the threshold for electrical excitation in the nerve, by slowing propagation of the nerve impulse, and by reducing the rate of the action potential.

Pharmacokinetics
Absorption: Depends on dose, concentration, and route of administration because absorption from the site of administration is affected by vascularity of tissue. After injection for caudal, epidural, or peripheral nerve block, levels peak in 30 to 45 minutes.

Distribution: Bupivacaine is 95% protein-bound. Drug is distributed to some extent to all tissues.
Metabolism: Metabolized primarily in the liver.
Excretion: Bupivacaine is mostly excreted in urine, only 5% as unchanged drug.

Contraindications and precautions
Contraindicated in patients hypersensitive to bupivacaine or any local anesthetic of the amide type. Avoid 0.75% bupivacaine in obstetric patients and don't use solutions of bupivacaine for the production of obstetric paracervical block anesthesia. Also contraindicated for I.V. regional anesthesia (Bier Block). Don't use preserved solutions for caudal or epidural anesthesia.

Use cautiously when administering to patients with hypotension, heart block, hepatic disease, or impaired CV function.

Interactions
Drug-drug
Beta blockers: enhanced sympathomimetic effects when used with bupivacaine and epinephrine. Use with caution.
Butyrophenones, phenothiazines: may reduce or reverse pressor effect of epinephrine. Monitor patient.
Chloroprocaine: may lessen bupivacaine's action. Don't use together.
CNS depressants: may cause additive CNS effects. Reduce dosage of CNS depressants.
Enflurane, halothane, isoflurane, related drugs: increased risk of arrhythmias when used with bupivacaine and epinephrine. Use with extreme caution.

MAO inhibitors, tricyclic antide-pressants: severe, sustained hypertension when used with bupivacaine and epinephrine. Concurrent use should be avoided.

Effects on diagnostic tests
None reported.

Adverse reactions
CNS: anxiety, nervousness, *seizures* (followed by drowsiness, dizziness, tremors).
CV: *arrhythmias*, *bradycardia*, *cardiac arrest*, edema, *heart block*, hypotension, myocardial depression.
EENT: blurred vision, tinnitus.
GI: nausea, vomiting.
Respiratory: *respiratory arrest*, *status asthmaticus.*
Skin: erythema, pruritus, urticaria.
Other: *anaphylaxis*, angioneurotic edema.

Overdose and treatment
Acute emergencies are generally related to high plasma levels. Toxic reactions usually involve the CNS and CV systems.

To treat toxic reactions, immediately establish and maintain a patent airway or administer controlled ventilation with 100% oxygen. If necessary, use drugs to control seizures. Treatment of circulatory depression may require I.V. fluids, vasopressors, or both. If you have trouble maintaining a patent airway or patient needs prolonged ventilatory support, endotracheal intubation may be indicated. If a pregnant patient develops maternal hypotension or fetal bradycardia, keep patient in left lateral decubitus position, if possible, or manually displace the uterus off the great vessels.

Special considerations
▶ Local anesthetics should be administered only by persons experienced in diagnosing and managing drug-related toxicity and other emergencies.
▶ Keep resuscitative equipment, drugs, and oxygen immediately available.
▶ Check solution before giving it. Discard if it contains particulate matter or it's pinkish or slightly darker than yellow.
▶ Don't use disinfectants that contain heavy metals for skin or mucous membrane disinfection because they may cause swelling and edema.
▶ Use epinephrine solutions cautiously in patients with CV disorders and in body areas that have limited blood supply (such as ears, nose, fingers, and toes).
▶ Give a test dose of a local anesthetic with a fast onset (preferably one that contains epinephrine) before giving bupivacaine as epidural anesthesia. Monitor patient for increased heart rate and for CNS and CV toxicity.
▶ Aspirate for blood or CSF before injecting bupivacaine to avoid intravascular or intrathecal injection. (Intravascular injection is still possible even if no blood is aspirated.)
▶ Give the smallest dose and lowest concentration needed to produce the desired result. Reduce dosages for young, elderly, and debilitated patients and patients with cardiac or liver disease.
▶ Give epidural doses in incremental volumes of 3 to 5 ml, with enough time between doses to detect toxicity.
▶ Small doses of local anesthetics injected into the head and neck area may produce adverse reac-

---

Reactions may be *common*, uncommon, *life-threatening*, or COMMON AND LIFE-THREATENING.

tions similar to the systemic toxicity seen with unintentional intravascular injections of larger doses. Monitor patient's circulatory and respiratory status.
▶ The 0.75% concentration is indicated for nonobstetrical surgery patients who need a long duration of profound muscle relaxation.
▶ Continuously monitor CV and respiratory status and patient's state of consciousness after each injection. Restlessness, anxiety, incoherent speech, lightheadedness, numbness and tingling of mouth and lips, metallic taste, tinnitus, dizziness, blurred vision, tremors, twitching, depression or drowsiness may be early signs of CNS toxicity.
▶ Discard partially used bottles that don't contain preservatives.

Pregnant patients
▶ Local anesthetics rapidly cross the placenta and can cause maternal, fetal, and neonatal toxicity. Adverse reactions may involve alterations in the CNS, peripheral vascular tone, and cardiac function.

Breast-feeding patients
▶ No data are available to demonstrate whether drug appears in breast milk. Use cautiously in breast-feeding women.

Pediatric patients
▶ Administration to children under age 12 isn't recommended.

Geriatric patients
▶ Dosage reductions are recommended.

Patient teaching
▶ Advise patient that anesthetized part of the body may have temporary loss of sensation and motor activity.

▶ buprenorphine hydrochloride
Buprenex

Pharmacologic classification: *narcotic agonist-antagonist, opioid partial agonist*

Therapeutic classification: *analgesic*

Controlled substance schedule V

Pregnancy risk category C

How supplied
Available by prescription only
Injection: 0.3 mg/ml in 1-ml ampules

Indications and dosages
Moderate to severe pain
Adults and children over age 13: 0.3 mg I.M. or slow I.V. q 6 hours, p.r.n. May repeat 0.3 mg 30 to 60 minutes after initial dose, or increase to 0.6 mg per dose if necessary. S.C. administration isn't recommended.
Adults*: 25 to 250 mcg/hour via I.V. infusion (over 48 hours for postoperative pain), 60 to 180 mcg via epidural injection.
Pain from circumcision*
Children ages 9 months to 9 years: 3 mcg/kg I.M. along with surgical anesthesia.

Pharmacodynamics
Analgesic action: Exact mechanism of action is unknown, although drug may be a competitive antagonist at some opiate receptors

---

and an agonist at others, thus relieving moderate to severe pain.

Pharmacokinetics

Absorption: Drug is absorbed rapidly after I.M. administration. Onset of action occurs in 15 minutes. Effects peak 1 hour after dosing.

Distribution: About 96% of drug is protein-bound.

Metabolism: Drug is metabolized in the liver.

Excretion: Duration of action is 6 hours. Drug is excreted mainly in feces as unchanged drug with about 30% excreted in urine.

Contraindications and precautions

Contraindicated in patients hypersensitive to drug.

Use cautiously in elderly or debilitated patients and in patients with acute alcoholism, adrenal insufficiency, CNS depression, coma, delirium tremens, head injuries, hepatic impairment, increased intracranial pressure, intracranial lesions, kidney impairment, kyphoscoliosis, prostatic hyperplasia, respiratory impairment, thyroid irregularities, and urethral stricture.

Interactions
Drug-drug

Barbiturate anesthetics (such as thiopental): administration within a few hours of each other may produce additive CNS and respiratory depressant effects and apnea. Separate doses, and monitor patient closely.

CNS depressants (antihistamines, barbiturates, benzodiazepines, opioid analgesics, phenothiazines, sedative-hypnotics), tricyclic antidepressants, muscle relaxants: additive effects. Reduce buprenorphine dosage as needed.

Diazepam: may increase the risk of respiratory and CV collapse (rare). Monitor patient closely.

General anesthetics: concomitant administration may also cause severe CV depression. Monitor patient closely if using together.

MAO inhibitors: concomitant use may produce adverse effects. Use with caution.

Drug-lifestyle

Alcohol use: may potentiate respiratory and CNS depression, sedation, and hypotensive effects. Discourage use.

Effects on diagnostic tests

None reported.

Adverse reactions

CNS: confusion, *dizziness,* euphoria, *headache,* **increased intracranial pressure,** nervousness, *sedation, vertigo.*

CV: **bradycardia,** hypertension, *hypotension,* tachycardia.

EENT: blurred vision, *miosis.*

GI: constipation, dry mouth, *nausea,* vomiting.

GU: urine retention.

Respiratory: dyspnea, hypoventilation, **respiratory depression.**

Skin: *diaphoresis,* pruritus.

Overdose and treatment

To date, there has been limited experience with overdose. Safety of buprenorphine in acute overdose is expected to be better than that of other opioid analgesics because of its antagonist properties at high doses. Overdose may cause CNS depression, respiratory depression, and miosis (pinpoint pupils). Other

---

Reactions may be *common,* uncommon, **life-threatening,** or COMMON AND LIFE-THREATENING.

acute toxic effects may include apnea, bradycardia, cardiopulmonary arrest, circulatory collapse, hypotension, hypothermia, pulmonary edema, seizures, and shock.

To treat acute overdose, establish adequate respiratory exchange. If patient has significant respiratory or CV depression, give a narcotic antagonist (naloxone) to reverse respiratory depression. Give repeated doses if needed because the duration of buprenorphine is longer than that of naloxone. Monitor patient's vital signs closely. If naloxone doesn't completely reverse buprenorphine-induced respiratory depression, mechanical ventilation and higher-than-usual doses of naloxone and doxapram may be needed.

Provide symptomatic and supportive treatment (continued respiratory support, correction of fluid or electrolyte imbalance). Closely monitor patient's laboratory parameters, vital signs, and neurologic status.

Special considerations
▶ Buprenorphine 0.3 mg is equal to 10 mg morphine or 75 to 100 mg meperidine in analgesic potency; duration of analgesia is longer than either.
▶ Adverse effects may not be as readily reversed by naloxone as those of a pure agonist, and naloxone doses may need to be higher than usual.
▶ Drug may cause acute opioid withdrawal if given to patients taking opioid agonists on a long-term basis.
▶ Drug isn't recommended for chronic pain.
▶ Give by direct I.V. injection into a vein or the tubing of a free-flowing, compatible I.V. solution over at least 2 minutes.
▶ Monitor patient's response to treatment.
▶ Drug may also be used to reverse fentanyl-induced anesthesia.

Breast-feeding patients
▶ It isn't known whether drug is excreted in breast milk; use with caution.

Geriatric patients
▶ Administer with caution. Elderly patients typically need lower doses because they may be more sensitive to therapeutic and adverse effects.

Patient teaching
▶ Caution patient to avoid hazardous activities during therapy.
▶ Instruct patient to avoid alcohol and other CNS depressants.

▶ butabarbital sodium
Butisol

Pharmacologic classification:
barbiturate

Therapeutic classification:
sedative-hypnotic

Controlled substance schedule III

Pregnancy risk category D

How supplied
Available by prescription only
Elixir: 30 mg/5 ml
Tablets: 15 mg, 30 mg, 50 mg, 100 mg

Indications and dosages
Sedation
Adults: 15 to 30 mg P.O. t.i.d. or q.i.d.

Preoperative sedation
Adults: 50 to 100 mg P.O. 60 to 90 minutes before surgery.
Children: 2 to 6 mg/kg. Maximum, 100 mg/dose.

Pharmacodynamics
Sedative-hypnotic action: The exact site and mechanism of action are unknown. Butabarbital acts throughout the CNS as a nonselective depressant with an intermediate onset and duration of action. The reticular activating system, which controls CNS arousal, is especially sensitive to butabarbital. The drug decreases both presynaptic and postsynaptic membrane excitability by facilitating the action of GABA.

Pharmacokinetics
Absorption: Butabarbital is well absorbed after oral administration. Action begins in 45 to 60 minutes. Levels peak in 3 to 4 hours. Serum levels needed for sedation and hypnosis are 2 to 3 mcg/ml and 25 mcg/ml, respectively.
Distribution: Drug is distributed throughout body tissues and fluids.
Metabolism: Drug is metabolized extensively in the liver by oxidation. Duration of action is 6 to 8 hours.
Excretion: Inactive metabolites of butabarbital are excreted in urine. Only 1% to 2% of an oral dose is excreted in urine unchanged. Terminal half-life ranges from 30 to 40 hours.

Contraindications and precautions
Contraindicated in patients hypersensitive to barbiturates and in patients with bronchopneumonia, other severe pulmonary insufficiency, or porphyria.

Use cautiously in patients with acute or chronic pain, a history of drug abuse, or renal or hepatic impairment.

Interactions
Drug-drug
Antidepressants, antihistamines, opioids, sedative-hypnotics, tranquilizers: additive or potentiated CNS and respiratory depressant effects. Monitor patient closely.
Benzodiazepines, corticosteroids, digitoxin (not digoxin), doxorubicin, doxycycline, estrogens (including oral contraceptives), quinidine, verapamil, xanthines (including theophylline): enhanced hepatic metabolism of some drugs. Monitor patient's response to treatment.
Disulfiram, MAO inhibitors, valproic acid: decreased butabarbital metabolism and possible increased toxicity. Monitor patient for signs of toxicity.
Griseofulvin: impaired griseofulvin effectiveness from decreased GI absorption. Monitor patient's response.
Rifampin: may decrease butabarbital levels by increasing hepatic metabolism. Monitor patient's response to treatment.
Warfarin and other oral anticoagulants: enhanced enzymatic degradation of anticoagulants. Monitor patient's coagulation studies, and increase dosage as needed.

Drug-lifestyle
Alcohol use: may add to or potentiate CNS and respiratory depressant effects. Discourage concurrent use.

Effects on diagnostic tests
Drug may alter EEG pattern (low-voltage, fast activity) for some time after therapy stops.

Adverse reactions
CNS: *drowsiness, hangover, lethargy,* paradoxical excitement in elderly patients, physical and psychological dependence, somnolence.
GI: nausea, vomiting.
Hematologic: decreased serum bilirubin levels in neonates, epileptic patients, and patients with congenital nonhemolytic unconjugated hyperbilirubinemia; worsening of porphyria.
Respiratory: *apnea, respiratory depression.*
Skin: rash, *Stevens-Johnson syndrome,* urticaria.
Other: *angioedema.*

Overdose and treatment
Overdose may cause areflexia, coma, confusion, jaundice, pulmonary edema, respiratory depression, slurred speech, somnolence, and an unsteady gait. Patient also may develop hypothermia followed by fever, oliguria, and typical shock syndrome with tachycardia and hypotension may occur.

Maintain and support ventilation and pulmonary function, as needed. Support cardiac function and circulation with vasopressors and I.V. fluids, as needed. If ingestion was recent and patient is conscious with a functioning gag reflex, induce emesis with ipecac syrup. If emesis is contraindicated, make sure patient has a cuffed endotracheal tube in place, and perform gastric lavage. Follow with activated charcoal or a sodium chloride cathartic. Measure intake and output, vital signs, and laboratory parameters. Maintain body temperature. Alkalinization of urine may be helpful in removing drug from the body; hemodialysis may be useful in severe overdose.

Special considerations
▸ Tablet may be crushed and mixed with food or fluid if patient has trouble swallowing it. Capsules may be opened and contents mixed with food or fluids if needed.
▸ Butabarbital doesn't affect pain.
▸ Check patient's cardiopulmonary status frequently; monitor vital signs for significant changes.
▸ Prolonged administration isn't recommended; drug hasn't been shown effective after 14 days. A drug-free interval of at least 1 week is advised between dosing periods.
▸ Periodically evaluate blood counts and renal and hepatic studies for abnormalities and adverse effects.
▸ Monitor patient for possible allergic reaction from tartrazine sensitivity.
▸ Monitor PT and INR carefully when patient receiving butabarbital starts or ends anticoagulant therapy. Anticoagulant dosage may need to be adjusted.
▸ Watch for signs of barbiturate toxicity (coma, pupillary constriction, cyanosis, clammy skin, hypotension). Overdose can be fatal.
▸ Drug may also be used for insomnia.

Breast-feeding patients
▸ Drug passes into breast milk; avoid use in breast-feeding women.

Pediatric patients
▶ Butabarbital may cause paradoxical excitement in children.
▶ Dosage depends on child's age and weight and the degree of sedation needed. Use with caution.

Geriatric patients
▶ Elderly patients are more susceptible to CNS depressant effects of butabarbital. Confusion, disorientation, and excitability may occur.
▶ Elderly patients usually require lower dosages.

Patient teaching
▶ Tell patient to avoid hazardous activities until full effects of drug are known.
▶ Warn patient that prolonged use can cause physical or psychological dependence.
▶ Emphasize the dangers of combining drug with alcohol. Excessive depressant effect is possible, even if drug is taken the evening before ingesting alcohol.

▶ butorphanol tartrate
Stadol, Stadol NS

Pharmacologic classification:
narcotic agonist-antagonist, opioid partial agonist

Therapeutic classification:
adjunct to anesthesia, analgesic

Pregnancy risk category C

How supplied
Available by prescription only
Injection: 1 mg/ml (1-ml vials), 2 mg/ml (1-ml, 2-ml, and 10-ml vials)
Nasal spray: 10 mg/ml

Indications and dosages
Moderate to severe pain
Adults: 1 to 4 mg I.M. q 3 to 4 hours, p.r.n. Or 0.5 to 2 mg I.V. q 3 to 4 hours, p.r.n., or around-the-clock. Alternatively, give 1 mg by nasal spray (1 spray in one nostril). Repeat if pain relief is inadequate after 1 to 1¼ hours. Repeat q 3 to 4 hours, p.r.n.
Pain during labor
Adults: 1 to 2 mg I.M. or I.V. q 4 hours but not 4 hours before delivery.
Preoperative anesthesia
Adults: 2 mg I.M. 60 to 90 minutes before surgery or 2 mg I.V. shortly before induction.
▧ **DOSAGE ADJUSTMENT.** Give half the usual parenteral adult dose at 6-hour intervals, as needed, to patients with hepatic or renal impairment and to elderly patients.

Pharmacodynamics
Analgesic action: The exact mechanisms of action are unknown. Drug is probably a competitive antagonist at some opiate receptors and an agonist at others, thus relieving moderate to severe pain. Like narcotic agonists, it causes respiratory depression, sedation, and miosis.

Pharmacokinetics
Absorption: Butorphanol is well absorbed after I.M. administration. After parenteral administration, onset of analgesia is less than 10 minutes; analgesic effect peaks in 15 minutes to 1 hour. After nasal administration, onset of analgesia is usually within 15 minutes.
Distribution: Drug rapidly crosses the placenta. Neonatal serum levels are 0.4 to 1.4 times maternal levels.

Metabolism: Drug is metabolized extensively in the liver, primarily by hydroxylation, to inactive metabolites.

Excretion: Duration of effect is 3 to 4 hours after parenteral administration and 4 to 5 hours after nasal administration. Butorphanol is excreted in inactive form, mainly in urine. About 11% to 14% of a parenteral dose is excreted in feces.

Contraindications and precautions

Contraindicated in patients hypersensitive to drug or to the preservative benzethonium chloride, in patients receiving repeated narcotic doses, and in patients addicted to a narcotic, because it may cause withdrawal symptoms.

Use cautiously in emotionally unstable patients and in those with acute MI, coronary insufficiency, head injuries, hepatic dysfunction, a history of drug abuse, increased intracranial pressure, renal dysfuction, respiratory disease or depression, or ventricular dysfunction.

Interactions
Drug-drug
Barbiturate anesthetics (such as thiopental): may produce additive CNS and respiratory depressant effects and possible apnea if combined within a few hours. Monitor patient closely.

Cimetidine: may potentiate butorphanol toxicity, causing disorientation, respiratory depression, apnea, and seizures. Be prepared to give a narcotic antagonist if toxicity occurs. Monitor patient closely.

CNS depressants (antidepressants, antihistamines, barbiturates, benzodiazepines, opioid analgesics, phenothiazines, sedative-hypnotics, tricyclic muscle relaxants): may potentiate respiratory and CNS depression, sedation, and hypotensive effects. Reduced butorphanol dosages are usually necessary.

Drugs extensively metabolized in the liver (digitoxin, phenytoin, rifampin): drug accumulation and enhanced effects may result. Avoid concurrent use.

General anesthetics: may cause severe CV depression. Monitor closely.

Opioid antagonists: acute withdrawal syndrome in patients physically dependent on opioids. Use with caution and monitor closely.

Pancuronium: may increase conjunctival changes. Monitor patient for effects.

Drug-lifestyle
Alcohol use: may potentiate respiratory and CNS depression, sedation, and hypotensive effects. Don't use together.

Effects on diagnostic tests
None reported.

Adverse reactions
CNS: anxiety, *confusion, dizziness,* euphoria, hallucinations, headache, ***increased intracranial pressure,*** insomnia, lethargy, nervousness, paresthesia, *somnolence.*
CV: flushing, hypotension, palpitations, vasodilation.
EENT: blurred vision, *nasal congestion* (with nasal spray), tinnitus.
GI: anorexia, *constipation, nausea,* taste perversion, *vomiting.*
Respiratory: ***respiratory depression.***

Skin: *clamminess, excessive diaphoresis,* rash, sensation of heat, urticaria.

Overdose and treatment
No information available.

Special considerations
▶ Drug is recommended for long-term management of chronic pain.
▶ This drug has no advantage over morphine-like agonists for acute pain or cancer pain.
▶ Drug may cause withdrawal symptoms when given to patients on long-term opioid therapy.
▶ Patients who use the nasal form for severe pain may start therapy with 2 mg (one spray in each nostril) provided they remain recumbent. Dose shouldn't be repeated for 3 to 4 hours.
▶ Mild withdrawal symptoms have been reported with long-term use of injectable form.
▶ Give I.V. form by direct injection into a vein or into the tubing of a free-flowing I.V. solution. Compatible solutions include D_5W and normal saline solution.
▶ Drug has the potential for abuse and dependence. Closely supervise emotionally unstable patients and patients with a history of drug abuse when they need long-term therapy.

Breast-feeding patients
▶ Use of drug in breast-feeding women is not recommended.

Pediatric patients
▶ Safety and efficacy in children under age 18 haven't been established.

Geriatric patients
▶ Elderly patients typically need reduced dosages because they may be more sensitive to therapeutic and adverse effects.
▶ Plasma half-life is increased by 25% in patients over age 65.

Patient teaching
▶ Teach patient how to use nasal spray. Instruct her to spray in one nostril unless otherwise directed.
▶ Caution patient to avoid hazardous activities because drug may cause drowsiness.

▶ **caffeine**
Caffedrine, NoDoz, Quick Pep, Vivarin

Pharmacologic classification: *methylxanthine*

Therapeutic classification: *analeptic, CNS stimulant, respiratory stimulant*

Pregnancy risk category C

How supplied
Available without a prescription
Tablets: 150 mg, 200 mg
Tablets (chewable): 100 mg
Available by prescription only
Injection: 250 mg/ml, caffeine (121.25 mg/ml) with sodium benzoate (128.75 mg/ml)

Indications and dosages
CNS depression
Adults: 100 to 200 mg P.O. q 3 to 4 hours, p.r.n. For emergencies, 250 to 500 mg I.M. or I.V.
Infants and children: 4 mg/kg I.M., I.V., or S.C. q 4 hours, p.r.n.

Pharmacodynamics

CNS stimulant action: Caffeine is a xanthine derivative; it increases levels of cAMP by inhibiting phosphodiesterase. It stimulates all levels of the CNS, hastening and clarifying thinking and improving arousal and psychomotor coordination.

Respiratory stimulant action: In respiratory depression and in neonatal apnea (unlabeled use), larger doses of caffeine increase the respiratory rate. Caffeine increases contractile force and decreases skeletal muscle fatigue.

Pharmacokinetics

Absorption: Caffeine is well absorbed from the GI tract; absorption after I.M. injection may be slower.

Distribution: Caffeine is distributed rapidly throughout the body; it crosses the blood-brain barrier and placenta, and is about 17% protein-bound.

Metabolism: Caffeine is metabolized by the liver. Plasma half-life is 3 to 4 hours. In neonates, liver metabolism is much less evident and half-life may approach 80 hours.

Excretion: Caffeine is excreted in urine.

Contraindications and precautions

Contraindicated in patients hypersensitive to drug.

Use cautiously in patients with history of peptic ulcer, symptomatic arrhythmias, or palpitations, and after an acute MI.

Interactions

Drug-drug

Beta agonists, (albuterol, metaproterenol, terbutaline): increased cardiac effects and tremors. Monitor closely.

Cimetidine, disulfiram, fluoroquinolones (such as ciprofloxacin and enoxacin), oral contraceptives: inhibited caffeine metabolism and increased effects. Monitor patient closely.

Xanthine derivatives (including theophylline): may increase stimulant-induced adverse reactions, such as tremor, tachycardia, insomnia, and nervousness. Monitor patient for symptoms.

Drug-lifestyle

Smoking: may enhance caffeine elimination. Discourage smoking.

Effects on diagnostic tests

Caffeine may increase blood glucose levels and cause false-positive urate levels. It also may cause false-positive test results for pheochromocytoma or neuroblastoma by increasing certain urinary catecholamines.

Adverse reactions

CNS: abrupt withdrawal symptoms (headache, irritability), agitation, excitement, headache, *insomnia,* muscle tremor, nervousness, restlessness, twitching.

CV: extrasystoles, *palpitations, tachycardia.*

EENT: tinnitus.

GI: diarrhea, nausea, stomach pain, vomiting.

GU: *diuresis.*

Overdose and treatment

Overdose may cause altered states of consciousness, arrhythmias, diuresis, dyspnea, fever, insomnia, muscle twitching, and seizures. In infants, symptoms may include alternating hypotonicity and hypertonicity, opisthotonoid posture, tremors, bradycardia, hypotension, and severe acidosis.

Treat overdose symptomatically and supportively; gastric lavage and activated charcoal may help. Carefully monitor patient's vital signs, ECG, and fluid and electrolyte balance. Seizures may be treated with diazepam or phenobarbital; diazepam can worsen respiratory depression.

Special considerations
▶ Caffeine may be used with ergotamine tartrate for treating vascular headaches.
▶ Caffeine has been used to relieve headache after lumbar puncture, in topical creams to treat atopic dermatitis, for sore throat, and for oral surgery pain.
▶ Use of caffeine for CNS depression is strongly discouraged by many clinicians.
▶ Drug may be useful in counteracting opioid-induced effects of sedation.
▶ Single I.V. dose shouldn't exceed 1 g. Give I.V. dose slowly.
▶ Doses of 65 mg may increase analgesia when given with a nonopioid drug.
▶ Monitor patient for desired effects and for development of CV side effects.
▶ Restrict caffeine-containing beverages in patients with arrhythmic symptoms or in those who are taking aminophylline or theophylline.
▶ Caffeine content in beverages (mg/cup) is the following: cola drinks, 24 to 64; brewed tea, 20 to 110; instant coffee, 30 to 120;

brewed coffee, 40 to 180; decaffeinated coffee, 3 to 5.
▶ Many OTC pain relievers contain caffeine, but evidence concerning its analgesic effects is conflicting.
▶ Caffeine (30%) may be used in a hydrophilic base or hydrocortisone cream to treat atopic dermatitis.

Breast-feeding patients
▶ Caffeine appears in breast milk. Alternative feeding method is recommended during therapy with caffeine.

Pediatric patients
▶ Unlabeled uses include neonatal apnea. Maintain plasma caffeine level at 5 to 20 mcg/ml.
▶ In neonates, avoid using caffeine products that contain sodium benzoate because they may cause kernicterus.
▶ Adverse CNS effects are usually more severe in children.

Geriatric patients
▶ Elderly patients are more sensitive to caffeine and should take lower doses.

Patient teaching
▶ Advise patient to avoid excessive caffeine consumption, and therefore CNS stimulation, by learning caffeine content of beverages and foods.
▶ Warn patient not to exceed recommended dosage, not to substitute caffeine for needed sleep, and to discontinue drug if dizziness or tachycardia occurs.

▶ calcitonin
human: Cibacalcin
salmon: Calcimar, Miacalcin, Osteocalcin, Salmonine

Pharmacologic classification:
thyroid hormone

Therapeutic classification:
hypocalcemic

Pregnancy risk category C

How supplied
Available by prescription only
Injection: 200 IU/ml, 2-ml vials
(salmon); 0.5 mg/vial (human)
Nasal spray: 200 IU/activation

Indications and dosages
Paget's disease of bone (osteitis deformans)
Adults: initially, 100 IU calcitonin
(salmon) S.C. or I.M. daily or
0.5 mg calcitonin (human) S.C.
Maintenance dosage is 50 to 100 IU
calcitonin (salmon) three times
weekly or 0.5 mg calcitonin (human) two or three times weekly or
0.25 mg calcitonin (human) daily.
Postmenopausal osteoporosis
Adults: 100 IU calcitonin (salmon)
S.C. or I.M. daily, or 200 IU (one
spray) daily in alternating nostril.
Osteogenesis imperfecta*
Adults: 2 IU/kg calcitonin
(salmon) three times weekly with
daily calcium supplementation.

Pharmacodynamics
Hypocalcemic action: Calcitonin
directly inhibits bone resorption
of calcium. This effect is mediated by drug-induced increase of
cAMP level in bone cells, which
alters transport of calcium and
phosphate across the plasma membrane of the osteoclast. A secondary effect occurs in the kidneys,
where calcitonin directly inhibits
tubular resorption of calcium,
phosphate, and sodium, thereby increasing their excretion. A clinical
effect may not be seen for several
months in patients with Paget's
disease.

Pharmacokinetics
Absorption: Drug can be given
parenterally or nasally. Plasma levels of 0.1 to 0.4 mg/ml occur within 15 minutes of a 200-IU S.C.
dose. Maximum effect occurs in 2
to 4 hours; duration of action may
be 8 to 24 hours for S.C. or I.M.
doses and 30 minutes to 12 hours
for I.V. doses. Plasma levels peak
31 to 39 minutes after using the
nasal form.
Distribution: It is unknown
whether drug enters the CNS or
crosses the placenta.
Metabolism: Rapid metabolism
occurs in the kidneys, with additional activity in the blood and peripheral tissues. Calcitonin salmon
has a longer half-life than calcitonin human, which has a 1-hour
half-life.
Excretion: Calcitonin is excreted
in urine as inactive metabolites.

Contraindications and precautions
Contraindicated in patients who
are hypersensitive to salmon calcitonin. Human calcitonin has no
contraindications.

Interactions
None reported.

Effects on diagnostic tests
None reported.

Adverse reactions

CNS: dizziness, headache, paresthesia, weakness.
CV: chest pressure, edema of feet.
EENT: eye pain, nasal congestion.
GI: abdominal pain, anorexia, diarrhea, epigastric discomfort, *transient nausea,* unusual taste, *vomiting.*
GU: *increased urinary frequency,* nocturia.
Respiratory: shortness of breath.
Skin: *facial flushing, inflammation at injection site,* pruritus of ear lobes, rash, tender palms and soles.
Other: *anaphylaxis,* chills, *hypersensitivity reaction.*

Overdose and treatment

Overdose may cause hypocalcemia and hypocalcemic tetany. This usually will occur in patients at higher risk during the first few doses. Parenteral calcium will correct the symptoms and therefore should be kept readily available.

Special considerations

▶ Calcitonin salmon and calcitonin human are pharmacologically the same, but calcitonin salmon is more potent and has a longer duration of action.
▶ Doses of calcitonin (salmon) are expressed in international units, and calcitonin (human) are expressed in milligrams. Be careful not to confuse units of measurement.
▶ Before starting therapy with calcitonin (salmon), a skin test using calcitonin (salmon) should be considered. If patient has allergic reactions to foreign proteins, test for hypersensitivity before therapy. Systemic allergic reactions are possible because hormone is a protein. Epinephrine should be kept readily available.

▶ To perform the skin test, dilute 10 IU (0.05 ml) of calcitonin to 1 ml with normal saline solution. Give 0.1 ml of the solution intracutaneously to forearm and watch for 15 minutes for wheal formation. If a reaction occurs, calcitonin salmon shouldn't be used.
▶ The S.C. route is the preferred method of administration.
▶ Periodically monitor serum calcium levels during therapy. Keep parenteral calcium available during the first doses in case of hypocalcemic tetany (muscle twitching, tetanic spasms, and seizures if hypocalcemia is severe).
▶ Analgesia may take up to 2 weeks to occur.
▶ Drug may be helpful for neuropathic pain, such as phantom limb and complex regional pain syndrome. It also may be helpful for bone-related pain, such as bone metastases or osteoperosis.
▶ Refrigerate solution. Once activated, nasal spray should be stored upright at room temperature.
▶ Tachyphylaxis to calcitonin may develop after repeated exposure. Some patients may respond to switching from one preparation to the other to overcome this resistance.
▶ Monitor patient for signs of hypercalcemic relapse: bone pain, renal calculi, polyuria, anorexia, nausea, vomiting, thirst, constipation, lethargy, bradycardia, muscle hypotonicity, pathologic fracture, psychosis, and coma. Patients with good initial clinical response to calcitonin who suffer relapse should be evaluated for antibody formation response to the hormone protein.
▶ If patient uses nasal spray, perform periodic nasal examination.

▶ Drug may also be used for hyper-calcemia.

Pediatric patients
▶ There are no data to support the use of the nasal spray in pediatric patients.

Patient teaching
▶ Instruct patient on self-administration of drug, and assist him until he can administer it correctly.
▶ Tell patient to take missed dose as soon as possible. If he misses an every-other-day dose, tell him to take it as soon as possible and then restart the alternating days. Advise against double doses.
▶ Stress the importance of regular follow-up to assess progress.
▶ If given for postmenopausal osteoporosis, remind patient to take adequate calcium and vitamin D supplements.
▶ If patient uses nasal spray, teach him how to activate the pump before first use.
▶ Tell patient to call if nasal irritation occurs.

▶ calcium polycarbophil
Equalactin, Fiberall, FiberCon, Fiber-Lax, Mitrolan

Pharmacologic classification: *hydrophilic*

Therapeutic classification: *antidiarrheal, bulk laxative*

Pregnancy risk category C

How supplied
Available without a prescription
Tablets: 500 mg (FiberCon), 625 mg (Fiber-Lax)

Tablets (chewable): 500 mg (Equalactin, Fiber-Lax, Mitrolan), 1,000 mg (Fiberall)

Indications and dosages
Constipation, acute nonspecific diarrhea with irritable bowel syndrome
Adults: 1 g P.O. q.i.d. as needed. Maximum, 6 g in 24-hour period.
Children ages 6 to 12: 500 mg P.O. one to three times daily as needed. Maximum, 3 g in 24-hour period.
Children ages 3 to 6: 500 mg P.O. one to two times daily as needed. Maximum, 1.5 g in 24-hour period.

Pharmacodynamics
Antidiarrheal action: Calcium polycarbophil absorbs intestinal fluid, thereby restoring normal stool consistency and bulk.
Laxative action: Calcium polycarbophil absorbs water and expands, thereby increasing stool bulk and moisture and promoting normal peristalsis and bowel motility.

Pharmacokinetics
Absorption: None.
Distribution: None.
Metabolism: None.
Excretion: Drug is excreted in feces.

Contraindications and precautions
Contraindicated in patients with GI obstruction because drug may worsen the condition.

Interactions
Drug-drug
Tetracycline: Calcium polycarbophil may impair tetracycline absorption. Monitor patient for effects.

Effects on diagnostic tests
None reported.

Adverse reactions
GI: abdominal fullness, increased flatus, intestinal obstruction.
Other: laxative dependence (with long-term or excessive use).

Overdose and treatment
No information available.

Special considerations
▶ May be helpful in preventing opioid-induced constipation.
▶ Make sure patient fully chews the chewable tablet form before swallowing; give tablets with 8 oz (240 ml) of fluid. Give less fluid for antidiarrheal effect.
▶ If using drug as an antidiarrheal, don't give if patient has a high fever.

Patient teaching
▶ If patient takes chewable tablets, instruct him to chew them thoroughly before swallowing.
▶ If drug is being taken as a laxative, advise patient to drink a full glass (8 oz) of fluid after each tablet. If drug is being taken to treat diarrhea, advise a smaller amount of water.
▶ Warn patient not to take more than 12 tablets in 24-hour period (6 tablets for a child ages 6 to 12; three tablets for a child ages 3 to 6) and to take them for length of time prescribed.
▶ Instruct patient that dose may be taken every 30 minutes for acute diarrhea, but not to exceed maximum daily dosage.
▶ Tell patient that if abdominal discomfort or fullness occurs, he may take smaller doses more frequently

throughout the day, at regular intervals.
▶ If patient is taking drug as laxative, advise him to call promptly and discontinue drug if constipation persists after 1 week or if fever, nausea, vomiting, or abdominal pain occurs.

▶ capsaicin
Dolorac, Zostrix, Zostrix-HP

Pharmacologic classification:
naturally occurring chemical derived from plants of the Solanaceae family

Therapeutic classification:
topical analgesic

Pregnancy risk category NR

How supplied
Available without a prescription
Cream: 0.025% (Zostrix), 0.075% (Zostrix-HP), 0.25% (Dolorac)

Indications and dosages
Temporary pain relief from rheumatoid arthritis, osteoarthritis, and certain neuralgias, such as shingles (herpes zoster) or diabetic neuropathy
Zostrix
Adults and children over age 2: apply to affected areas t.i.d. or q.i.d.
Dolorac
Adults and children over age 12: apply thin film to affected areas b.i.d.

Pharmacodynamics
Analgesic action: Although the precise mechanism of action of capsaicin isn't fully understood, current evidence suggests that drug renders skin and joints insensitive to pain by depleting and pre-

venting reaccumulation of substance P in peripheral sensory neurons. Substance P is probably the principal chemomediator of pain impulses from the periphery to the CNS. In addition, substance P is released into joint tissues and activates inflammatory mediators involved with the pathogenesis of rheumatoid arthritis.

Pharmacokinetics
No information available.

Contraindications and precautions
Contraindicated in patients hypersensitive to drug.

Interactions
None reported.

Effects on diagnostic tests
None reported.

Adverse reactions
Respiratory: cough, irritation.
Skin: redness, *stinging or burning on application.*

Overdose and treatment
No information available.

Special considerations
▶ Transient burning or stinging usually occurs after early applications but disappears in several days.
▶ Applying drug less than 3 times daily (possibly 4 times daily) may not provide optimum pain relief, and the burning sensation may persist.
▶ Therapy may need to last longer than 2 weeks for desired effects to occur.

▶ Capsaicin is for external use only. Avoid contact with eyes and broken or irritated skin.

Patient teaching
▶ Teach patient how to apply cream, stressing the importance of avoiding the eyes and broken or irritated skin.
▶ Instruct patient to wash hands after applying cream, avoiding areas where drug was applied.
▶ Warn patient that transient burning or stinging may occur but should disappear after several days of continued use.
▶ Tell patient not to bandage areas tightly.
▶ Advise patient to discontinue drug and to call if condition worsens or doesn't improve after 28 days.

▶ carbamazepine
Atretol, Carbatrol, Epitol, Tegretol

Pharmacologic classification:
iminostilbene derivative, chemically related to tricyclic antidepressants

Therapeutic classification:
analgesic, anticonvulsant

Pregnancy risk category D

How supplied
Available by prescription only
Capsules (extended-release):
200 mg, 300 mg
Oral suspension: 100 mg/5 ml
Tablets: 200 mg
Tablets (chewable): 100 mg
Tablets (extended-release): 100 mg, 200 mg, 400 mg

Indications and dosages
Trigeminal neuralgia
Adults: 100 mg P.O. b.i.d. with meals on day 1. Increase by 100 mg q 12 hours until pain is relieved. Maintenance, 200 to 1,200 mg P.O. daily. Maximum, 1.2 g daily. For extended-release capsules, 200 mg P.O. day 1. Daily dose may be increased by up to 200 mg/day q 12 hours, p.r.n., to achieve freedom from pain. Maintenance, 400 to 800 mg/day.
Restless legs syndrome*
Adults: 100 to 300 mg h.s.

Pharmacodynamics
Analgesic action: In trigeminal neuralgia, carbamazepine is a specific analgesic through its reduction of synaptic neurotransmission.
Anticonvulsant action: Drug is chemically unrelated to other anticonvulsants, and its mechanism of action is unknown. Anticonvulsant activity appears mainly to involve limitations of seizure propagation by reduction of posttetanic potentiation of synaptic transmissions.

Pharmacokinetics
Absorption: Carbamazepine is absorbed slowly from the GI tract; plasma levels peak at 1½ hours (suspension), 4 to 6 hours (tablets), and 6 hours (extended-release).
Distribution: Drug is distributed widely throughout body; it crosses the placenta and accumulates in fetal tissue. About 75% is protein-bound. Therapeutic serum levels in adults are 4 to 12 mcg/ml; nystagmus can occur above 4 mcg/ml and ataxia, dizziness, and anorexia at or above 10 mcg/ml. Serum levels may be misleading because an unmeasured active metabolite also can cause toxicity. Carbamazepine levels in breast milk approach 60% of serum levels. Plasma levels correlate poorly with dose in children.
Metabolism: Drug is metabolized by the liver to an active metabolite. It may also induce its own metabolism; over time, higher doses are needed to maintain plasma levels. Half-life is initially 25 to 65 hours, 12 to 17 hours with multiple dosing.
Excretion: Drug is excreted in urine (70%) and feces (30%).

Contraindications and precautions
Contraindicated in patients hypersensitive to drug or tricyclic antidepressants, in patients with a history of previous bone marrow suppression, and in patients who have taken an MAO inhibitor within 14 days of therapy. Use cautiously in patients with mixed-type seizure disorders.

Interactions
Drug-drug
Antiretroviral drugs, protease inhibitors: concomitant use may alter metabolism of these drugs. Avoid concurrent use.
Calcium channel blockers (verapamil and possibly diltiazem): may significantly increase serum carbamazepine levels. Carbamazepine dosage should be decreased by 40% to 50% when given with verapamil.
Clarithromycin, cimetidine, erythromycin, isoniazid, propoxyphene, valproic acid: may increase serum carbamazepine levels. Monitor patient for effects.
Ethosuximide, haloperidol, phenytoin, valproic acid, warfarin: increased metabolism of these drugs.

Monitor serum coagulation studies if patient takes warfarin.

Felbamate: may lower serum levels of either drug. Monitor patient for desired effects.

Fluoxetine, fluvoxamine: may increase carbamazepine levels. Monitor patient for effects.

MAO inhibitors: may cause hypertensive crisis. Don't give within 14 days of therapy with MAO inhibitor.

Oral contraceptives, theophylline: may decrease effectiveness of these drugs. Monitor patient for effects.

Phenobarbital, phenytoin, primidone: decreased serum carbamazepine level. Monitor patient for effects.

Drug-herb
Psyllium seed: may inhibit GI absorption; avoid concurrent use.

Effects on diagnostic tests
None reported.

Adverse reactions
CNS: *ataxia,* confusion, *dizziness, drowsiness,* fatigue, headache, syncope, *vertigo,* **worsening of seizures** (usually in patients with mixed-type seizure disorders, including atypical absence seizures).
CV: aggravation of coronary artery disease, **arrhythmias, AV block, heart failure,** hypertension, hypotension.
EENT: blurred vision, conjunctivitis, diplopia, dry mouth and pharynx, nystagmus.
GI: abdominal pain, anorexia, diarrhea, glossitis, *nausea,* stomatitis, *vomiting.*
GU: albuminuria, elevated BUN, glycosuria, impotence, urinary frequency, urine retention.

Hematologic: *agranulocytosis, aplastic anemia,* eosinophilia, leukocytosis, *thrombocytopenia.*
Hepatic: abnormal liver function test results, *hepatitis.*
Metabolic: decreased thyroid function test results, SIADH.
Respiratory: pulmonary hypersensitivity.
Skin: erythema multiforme, excessive diaphoresis, rash, *Stevens-Johnson syndrome,* urticaria.
Other: chills, fever.

Overdose and treatment
Overdose may cause blood pressure changes, irregular breathing, respiratory depression, tachycardia, shock, arrhythmias, impaired consciousness (ranging to deep coma), seizures, restlessness, drowsiness, psychomotor disturbances, nausea, vomiting, anuria, or oliguria.

Treat overdose with repeated gastric lavage, especially if patient ingested alcohol concurrently. Oral activated charcoal and laxatives may hasten excretion. Carefully monitor patient's vital signs, ECG, and fluid and electrolyte balance. Diazepam may control seizures but can worsen respiratory depression.

Special considerations
▶ Drug is indicated as a first-line treatment with tricyclic antidepressants for lancinating, neuropathic pain. It may also be useful for trigeminal neuralgia, diabetic neuropathy, phantom limb, or other intermittent lancinating pain.
▶ For administering drug via nasogastric tube, mix with an equal volume of diluent (D_5W or normal saline solution) and administer; then flush with 100 ml of diluent.

▶ Adjust dosage based on individual response.

▶ Chewable tablets are available for children.

▶ Hematologic toxicity is rare but serious. Routinely monitor patient's hematologic and liver functions.

▶ Carbamazepine is also indicated in seizure activity, bipolar affective disorder, and intermittent explosive disorder.

▶ Unlabeled uses of carbamazepine include hypophyseal diabetes insipidus, certain psychiatric disorders, and management of alcohol withdrawal.

Breast-feeding patients

▶ Significant amounts of drug appear in breast milk; an alternative feeding method is recommended during therapy.

Pediatric patients

▶ Safety and efficacy haven't been established for children under age 6 in doses above 35 mg/kg/day.

Geriatric patients

▶ Drug may activate latent psychosis, confusion, or agitation in elderly patients; use with caution.

Patient teaching

▶ Remind patient to store drug in a cool, dry place, and not in the medicine cabinet. Reduced bioavailability has been reported from improperly stored tablets.

▶ Remind patient to shake suspension well before using.

▶ Tell patient, if necessary, that Carbatrol capsule can be opened and contents sprinkled over food (such as a teaspoon of applesauce), but capsule and contents should never be crushed or chewed.

▶ Tell patient that drug may cause GI distress. Urge him to take drug with food at equal intervals.

▶ Warn patient to avoid hazardous activities, especially during first week of therapy or when dosage increases. Drug may cause drowsiness, dizziness, and blurred vision.

▶ Emphasize importance of follow-up laboratory tests and continued medical supervision. Periodic eye examinations are recommended.

▶ Warn patient not to stop drug abruptly.

▶ Encourage patient to promptly report unusual bleeding, bruising, jaundice, dark urine, pale stools, abdominal pain, impotence, fever, chills, sore throat, mouth ulcers, edema, or disturbances in mood, alertness, or coordination.

▶ carisoprodol
Soma

Pharmacologic classification:
carbamate derivative

Therapeutic classification:
skeletal muscle relaxant

Pregnancy risk category NR

How supplied
Available by prescription only
Tablets: 350 mg

Indications and dosages
Acute, painful musculoskeletal conditions (adjunct)
Adults and children over age 12: 350 mg P.O. t.i.d. and h.s.

Pharmacodynamics
Skeletal muscle relaxant action: Carisoprodol doesn't relax skeletal muscle directly but apparently as a

result of its sedative effects. However, the exact mechanism of action is unknown. Animal studies suggest that it modifies the central perception of pain without eliminating peripheral pain reflexes and has slight antipyretic activity.

Pharmacokinetics
Absorption: Onset of action occurs within 30 minutes and persists 4 to 6 hours.
Distribution: Drug is widely distributed throughout the body.
Metabolism: Drug is metabolized in the liver. Drug may induce microsomal enzymes in the liver; half-life is 8 hours.
Excretion: Drug is excreted mainly in urine as metabolites; less than 1% of a dose is excreted unchanged. Drug may be removed by hemodialysis or peritoneal dialysis.

Contraindications and precautions
Contraindicated in patients hypersensitive to related compounds (for example, meprobamate or tybamate) or intermittent porphyria.

Use cautiously in patients with impaired renal or hepatic function.

Interactions
Drug-drug
CNS depressants, such as antipsychotics, anxiolytics, general anesthetics, opioid analgesics, tricyclic antidepressants: may produce additive effects. Take care to avoid overdose if using together.
MAO inhibitors, tricyclic antidepressants: may increase CNS depression, respiratory depression, and hypotensive effects. Monitor patient closely if drugs must be used together. Dosage adjustments

(reduction of one or both) are needed.

Drug-lifestyle
Alcohol use: produces additive CNS depression. Discourage use.

Effects on diagnostic tests
None reported.

Adverse reactions
CNS: agitation, ataxia, depressive reactions, *dizziness, drowsiness,* headache, insomnia, irritability, tremor, vertigo.
CV: facial flushing, orthostatic hypotension, tachycardia.
GI: epigastric distress, hiccups, nausea, vomiting.
Hematologic: eosinophilia.
Respiratory: asthmatic episodes.
Skin: *erythema multiforme,* pruritus, rash.
Other: *anaphylaxis, angioedema,* fever.

Overdose and treatment
Overdose may cause exaggerated CNS depression, stupor, coma, shock, and respiratory depression.

Treatment of a conscious patient requires emptying the stomach by emesis or gastric lavage; activated charcoal may be used after gastric lavage to adsorb any remaining drug. If patient is comatose with a cuffed endotracheal tube in place, perform gastric lavage. Provide supportive therapy by maintaining adequate airway and assisting ventilation. CNS stimulants and pressor agents should be used cautiously. Monitor patient's vital signs, fluid and electrolyte levels, and neurologic status closely.

Monitor urine output, and avoid overhydration. Forced diuresis using mannitol, peritoneal dialysis, or hemodialysis may be beneficial. Continue to monitor patient for relapse from incomplete gastric emptying and delayed absorption.

Special considerations
▶ Although traditionally used for chronic musculoskeletal pain, drug has minimal effectiveness. Drug isn't useful for muscle spasm pain.
▶ Initially, allergic or idiosyncratic reactions may occur (first to the fourth dose). Symptoms usually subside after several hours; treat with supportive and symptomatic measures.
▶ Psychological dependence may follow long-term use.
▶ Withdrawal symptoms (abdominal cramps, insomnia, chilliness, headache, and nausea) may occur with abrupt termination of drug after prolonged use of higher-than-recommended doses.
▶ Commercially available form may contain sodium metabisulfite, to which some patients have an allergic reaction.
▶ Monitor patient closely for sedative effects if combination therapy is needed with opioids.

Breast-feeding patients
▶ Carisoprodol may be distributed into breast milk at two to four times maternal plasma levels.

Pediatric patients
▶ Safety and efficacy haven't been established in children under age 12. However, some clinicians suggest 25 mg/kg or 750 mg/m^2 divided q.i.d. for children age 5 and older.

Geriatric patients
▶ Elderly patients may be more sensitive to drug effects.

Patient teaching
▶ Tell patient that he may take drug with food to avoid GI upset.
▶ Inform patient that drug may cause dizziness and faintness. Urge him to change positions slowly. Tell him to report persistent symptoms.
▶ Tell patient to avoid alcoholic beverages and to use caution when taking cough or cold medications. Patient should also avoid other CNS depressants (effects may be additive) unless prescribed.
▶ Warn patient to avoid hazardous activities until full effects of drug are known; it may cause drowsiness.
▶ Advise patient to discontinue drug immediately and to notify prescriber if rash, diplopia, dizziness, or other unusual signs or symptoms appear.
▶ Instruct patient to take a missed dose if he remembers it within the hour. If he remembers it later, patient should skip that dose and go back to regular schedule. Warn against doubling the dose.
▶ Tell patient to store drug away from heat and direct light (not in bathroom medicine cabinet).

▶ **celecoxib**
Celebrex

Pharmacologic classification:
cyclooxygenase-2 (COX-2) inhibitor

Therapeutic classification:
NSAID

Pregnancy risk category C

How supplied
Available by prescription only
Capsules: 100 mg, 200 mg

Indications and dosages

Osteoarthritis
Adults: 200 mg P.O. daily as a single dose or divided equally twice daily.

Rheumatoid arthritis
Adults: 100 to 200 mg P.O. twice daily.

⊠ DOSAGE ADJUSTMENT. If patient weighs less than 110 lb (50 kg), start with lowest recommended dosage. If patient has moderate hepatic impairment (Child-Pugh Class II), start with reduced dosage.

Pharmacodynamics

Anti-inflammatory, analgesic, and antipyretic actions: Celecoxib probably selectively inhibits COX-2, resulting in decreased prostaglandin synthesis specific to inflammatory pathways. The relative sparing effect on COX-1 inhibition results in preservation of prostaglandin activity responsible for maintaining viability of the GI mucosa and normal platelet clotting.

Pharmacokinetics

Absorption: After oral administration, plasma levels peak in about 3 hours. Steady state plasma levels occur within 5 days if celecoxib is given in multiple doses.
Distribution: Drug is highly protein-bound, primarily to albumin.
Metabolism: Drug is metabolized mainly by cytochrome P-450-2C9.
Excretion: Celecoxib is eliminated primarily by hepatic metabolism; 27% is excreted in urine. Elimination half-life under fasting conditions is about 11 hours.

Adverse reactions

CNS: dizziness, *headache*, insomnia.
EENT: pharyngitis, rhinitis, sinusitis.
GI: abdominal pain, diarrhea, dyspepsia, flatulence, nausea.
GU: elevated BUN level.
Hepatic: elevated liver enzymes.
Metabolic: hyperchloremia, hypophosphatemia.
Musculoskeletal: *back pain.*
Respiratory: upper respiratory tract infection.
Skin: rash.
Other: *accidental injury, peripheral edema.*

Interactions
Drug-drug

ACE inhibitors: reduced antihypertensive effects. Monitor patient's blood pressure.
Aluminum and magnesium antacids: may decrease plasma celecoxib levels. Give drugs at least 1 hour apart.
Aspirin: increased risk of ulcers, although low aspirin dosages can be used safely for prevention of CV events. Assess patient for evidence of GI bleeding.
Fluconazole: increased celecoxib levels. Reduce celecoxib dosage to minimum effective level.
Furosemide: NSAIDs can reduce sodium excretion with diuretics, leading to sodium retention. Monitor patient for edema and increased blood pressure.
Lithium: increased lithium levels. Monitor plasma lithium levels closely during treatment.
Warfarin: increased risk of bleeding, although direct interaction hasn't been reported. Monitor patient for evidence of bleeding.

Drug-lifestyle
Alcohol use: increased risk of GI irritation or bleeding with chronic use. Monitor patient for evidence of bleeding.

Effects on diagnostic tests
None reported.

Overdose and treatment
Overdose may cause lethargy, drowsiness, nausea, vomiting, epigastric pain, and GI bleeding. Other possible symptoms include hypertension, acute renal failure, respiratory depression, and coma.

No antidote is available, but symptomatic and supportive care is usually sufficient. If overdose occurred within 4 hours, induce emesis, give activated charcoal, give an osmotic cathartic, or apply some combination of these treatments. Because of the high protein-binding, dialysis is unlikely to be effective.

Contraindications and precautions
Contraindicated in patients hypersensitive to celecoxib, sulfonamides, aspirin, or other NSAIDs; in patients with severe hepatic impairment; and during the third trimester of pregnancy.

Use cautiously in patients with a history of ulcers or GI bleeding, advanced renal disease, anemia, symptomatic liver disease, hypertension, edema, heart failure, or asthma. Also use cautiously in patients who smoke or use alcohol chronically, in those taking oral corticosteroids or anticoagulants, and in elderly or debilitated patients.

Special considerations
▶ This drug is recommended over other NSAIDs because it has fewer reported GI effects.
▶ Drug may rarely cause renal insufficiency with long-term use.
▶ Don't combine with aspirin or any other NSAID.
▶ Patients with a history of ulcers or GI bleeding have a higher risk of GI bleeding. Monitor patient for signs and symptoms of overt and occult bleeding. Other risk factors for GI bleeding include treatment with corticosteroids or anticoagulants, longer duration of NSAID treatment, smoking, alcoholism, older age, and poor overall health.
▶ Watch for evidence of allergic reaction because patients may be allergic to celecoxib if they have an allergy to sulfonamides, aspirin, or other NSAIDs.
▶ Assess patient for evidence of hepatic and renal toxicity, especially if the patient is dehydrated. As with any NSAID, drug may cause renal insufficiency (rare) with long-term use.

Breast-feeding patients
▶ It is unknown whether celecoxib is excreted in human breast milk; however, it has been excreted in animal milk. Assess risks and benefits before continuing celecoxib in nursing mothers.

Pediatric patients
▶ Drug hasn't been studied in patients under age 18.

Geriatric patients
▶ Dosage adjustment isn't necessary unless patient weighs less than 110 lb (50 kg); however, elderly patients experience more adverse effects overall.

Patient teaching
▶ If patient takes an antacid that contains aluminum or magnesium, tell him to separate doses by at least 1 hour.
▶ Instruct patient to take drug with food if stomach upset occurs.
▶ Inform patient that it may take several days before he feels consistent pain relief. Urge him to notify prescriber if he feels no relief.
▶ Advise patient to immediately report swelling, excessive fatigue, yellowing of the skin, flulike symptoms, signs of bleeding, or trouble breathing.

▶ chloral hydrate
Aquachloral Supprettes, Novo-Chlorhydrate ◊

Pharmacologic classification: *general CNS depressant*

Therapeutic classification: *sedative-hypnotic*

Controlled substance schedule IV

Pregnancy risk category C

How supplied
Available by prescription only
Capsules: 250 mg, 500 mg
Suppositories: 325 mg, 500 mg, 650 mg
Syrup: 250 mg/5 ml, 500 mg/5 ml

Indications and dosages
Sedation
Adults: 250 mg P.O. t.i.d. after meals.
Children: 8 mg/kg P.O. t.i.d. Maximum, 500 mg t.i.d.
Hypnosis
Children: 50 mg/kg P.O. or 1.5 g/m^2 as a single dose. Maximum dose, 1 g.

▣ Dosage adjustment. Decrease dosage in elderly patients.

Pharmacodynamics
Sedative-hypnotic action: Chloral hydrate has CNS depressant activities similar to those of the barbiturates. Nonspecific CNS depression occurs at hypnotic doses; however, respiratory drive is only slightly affected. Drug's primary site of action is the reticular activating system, which controls arousal. The cellular sites of action aren't known.

Pharmacokinetics
Absorption: Chloral hydrate is absorbed well after oral and rectal use. Sleep starts 30 to 60 minutes after a 500-mg to 1-g dose.
Distribution: Drug and its active metabolite, trichloroethanol, are distributed throughout the body tissue and fluids. Trichloroethanol is 35% to 41% protein-bound.
Metabolism: Drug is metabolized rapidly and nearly completely in the liver and erythrocytes to the active metabolite trichloroethanol. It's further metabolized in the liver and kidneys to trichloroacetic acid and other inactive metabolites.
Excretion: Inactive metabolites of drug hydrate are excreted primarily in urine. Minor amounts are excreted in bile. Trichloroethanol half-life is 8 to 10 hours.

Contraindications and precautions
Contraindicated in patients with impaired hepatic or renal function, severe cardiac disease, or hypersensitivity to drug. Oral administration contraindicated in patients with gastric disorders.

Use with extreme caution in patients with mental depression, suicidal tendencies, or history of drug abuse.

Interactions
Drug-drug
CNS depressants, such as antihistamines, narcotics, sedative-hypnotics, tranquilizers, or tricyclic antidepressants: additive to or potentiated effects. Monitor patient closely.

Furosemide I.V.: administration of drug followed by furosemide I.V. may cause a hypermetabolic state by displacing thyroid hormone from binding sites, resulting in sweating, hot flashes, tachycardia, and variable blood pressure. Avoid using together, if possible. If drugs must be used together, monitor patient closely.

Oral anticoagulants (such as warfarin): chloral hydrate may displace other drugs from protein-binding sites, increased hypoprothrombinemic effects. Monitor patient's coagulation studies.

Phenytoin: phenytoin elimination may be increased. Monitor serum phenytoin levels.

Drug-lifestyle
Alcohol use: may cause vasodilation, tachycardia, sweating, and flushing in some patients. Avoid using together.

Effects on diagnostic tests
Drug therapy may produce false-positive results for urine glucose with tests using cupric sulfate, such as Benedict's reagent and possibly Clinitest. It doesn't interfere with Chemstrip uG, Diastix, or glucose enzymatic test strip results.

Drug interferes with fluorometric tests for urine catecholamines; don't use drug for 48 hours before the test. Drug may also interfere with Reddy-Jenkins-Thorn test for urinary 17-hydroxycorticosteroids. It also may cause a false-positive phentolamine test.

Adverse reactions
CNS: ataxia, confusion, delirium, dizziness, disorientation, drowsiness, hallucinations, hangover, light-headedness, malaise, nightmares, paradoxical excitement, physical and psychological dependence, somnolence, vertigo.
GI: *diarrhea,* flatulence, *nausea, vomiting.*
Hematologic: eosinophilia, *leukopenia.*
Skin: *hypersensitivity reactions* (rash, urticaria).

Overdose and treatment
Overdose may cause stupor, coma, respiratory depression, pinpoint pupils, hypotension, and hypothermia. Esophageal stricture may follow gastric necrosis and perforation. GI hemorrhage has also been reported. Hepatic damage and jaundice may occur.

Treatment involves supporting respiration (including mechanical ventilation if needed), blood pressure, and body temperature. If patient is conscious, induce emesis or use gastric lavage. Hemodialysis will remove drug and its metabolite. Peritoneal dialysis may be effective.

Special considerations
▶ Chloral hydrate isn't a first-line drug because of the risk of adverse or toxic effects.

▶ Check patient's level of consciousness before giving drug to ensure appropriate baseline level.

▶ Give drug capsules with a full glass (8 oz [240 ml]) of water to lessen GI upset; dilute syrup in a half glass of water or juice before administration to improve taste.

▶ Chloral hydrate may produce a hangover effect.

▶ Drug shouldn't be used as a replacement for analgesics because it has minimal analgesic properties.

▶ Monitor vital signs frequently because chloral hydrate has a long half-life, especially in children.

▶ Store in dark container away from heat and moisture to prevent breakdown. Refrigerate suppositories.

▶ Some brands contain tartrazine, to which some patients may be allergic.

▶ Drug is also used for alcohol withdrawal symptoms, insomnia, and as a premedication for EEG.

Breast-feeding patients

▶ Small amounts pass into breast milk and may cause drowsiness in breast-fed infants; avoid use in breast-feeding women.

Pediatric patients

▶ Drug is safe and effective in children as a premedication for EEG and other procedures.

▶ Half-life may be prolonged in children. Careful monitoring is needed.

Geriatric patients

▶ Elderly patients may be more susceptible to CNS depressant effects because of decreased elimination. Lower doses are indicated.

Patient teaching

▶ Advise patient to take drug with a full glass (8 oz [24 ml]) of water and to dilute syrup with juice or water before use.

▶ Instruct patient in proper administration of drug form prescribed.

▶ Warn patient not to attempt tasks that require mental alertness or physical coordination until the CNS effects of drug are known.

▶ Tell patient to avoid alcohol and other CNS depressants.

▶ Instruct patient to call before using OTC allergy or cold preparations.

▶ Warn patient not to increase dose or stop drug except as prescribed.

▶ chloroprocaine hydrochloride
Nesacaine, Nesacaine-MPF

Pharmacologic classification:
ester local anesthetic

Therapeutic classification:
local anesthetic

Pregnancy risk category C

How supplied
Available by prescription only
Injection: 1%, 2%, 3%

Indications and dosages
Dosages given are for the drug without epinephrine.
Mandibular block
Adults: 40 to 60 mg (2 to 3 ml) of a 2% solution.
Infraorbital nerve block
Adults: 10 to 20 mg (0.5 to 1 ml) of a 2% solution.
Brachial plexus block
Adults: 600 to 800 mg (30 to 40 ml) of a 2% solution.

Interdigital block
Adults: 30 to 40 mg (3 to 4 ml) of a 1% solution.
Pudendal block
Adults: 400 mg (10 ml on each side) of a 2% solution.
Paracervical block
Adults: up to 120 mg (3 ml per each of 4 sites) of a 1% solution.
Caudal epidural block
Adults: initially, 15 to 25 ml of a 2% or 3% solution. Repeated doses may be given at 40- to 60-minute intervals.
Lumbar epidural block
Adults: 2 to 2.5 ml per segment of a 2% or 3% solution. The usual total volume of Nescaine MPF Injection is from 15 to 25 ml. Repeated doses 2 to 6 ml less than the original dose may be given at 40- to 50-minute intervals.
Maximum single recommended doses in adults: without epinephrine, 11 mg/kg or 800 mg; with epinephrine (1:200,000) 14 mg/kg or 1,000 mg.
Children age 3 and older: maximum, 11 mg/kg. Concentrations of 0.5% to 1% are suggested for infiltration and 1% to 1.5% for nerve block.
◻ Dosage adjustment. Dosage differs depending on anesthetic procedure, area to be anesthetized, vascularity of area, number of neuronal segments to be blocked, degree of block, duration of anesthesia desired, and individual patient conditions and tolerance. Always use incremental doses. Give reduced dosage to debilitated, elderly, acutely ill patients; children; and patients with cardiac or hepatic disease.

Pharmacodynamics
Local anesthetic action: Drug blocks the generation and conduction of nerve impulses by increasing the threshold for electrical excitation in the nerve, by slowing propagation of the nerve impulse, and by reducing the rate of the action potential.

Pharmacokinetics
Absorption: Depends on dose, concentration, and route of administration because absorption from the site of administration is affected by vascularity of tissue. Onset of action is 6 to 12 minutes.
Distribution: Drug is distributed to some extent to all tissues.
Metabolism: Metabolized primarily in the liver by pseudocholinesterase.
Excretion: Chloroprocaine is mostly excreted in urine.

Contraindications and precautions
Contraindicated in patients with hypersensitivity to chloroprocaine or to any local anesthetic of the PABA ester group.
    Use cautiously for lumbar or caudal epidural anesthesia in patients with neurologic disease, spinal deformities, septicemia, and severe hypertension. Caution should also be used in patients with impaired CV function, hypotension, heart block, or hepatic disease.

Interactions
Drug-drug
Bupivacaine: may lessen bupivacaine's action. Monitor for effect.
CNS depressants: may cause additive CNS effects. Reduce dosage of CNS depressants.
MAO inhibitors, phenothiazines, tricyclic antidepressants: severe, prolonged hypertension or hypotension when used with chloropro-

---

Reactions may be *common,* uncommon, *life-threatening,* or COMMON AND LIFE-THREATENING.

caine and epinephrine. Avoid concurrent use.

Other local anesthetics: may add to toxicity. Use together cautiously

Sulfonamides: para-aminobenzoic acid (metabolite of chloroprocaine) inhibits the action of sulfonamides. Don't use in conditions where a sulfonamide drug is needed.

Adverse reactions

CNS: anxiety, nervousness, *seizures* followed by dizziness, drowsiness, tremors.
CV: *arrhythmias, bradycardia, cardiac arrest,* edema, hypotension, myocardial depression.
EENT: blurred vision, tinnitis.
GI: nausea, vomiting.
Respiratory: *respiratory arrest, status asthmaticus.*
Skin: eryhtema, pruritus, urticaria.
Other: *anaphylaxis, angioneurotic edema.*

Overdose and treatment

Acute emergencies are typically related to high plasma levels. Toxic reactions usually involve the CNS and CV systems. To treat toxic reactions, immediately establish a patent airway or controlled ventilation with oxygen. If necessary, use drugs to treat seizures. Supportive treatment of circulatory depression may require the administration of I.V. fluids and/or appropriate vasopressor agents. If difficulty is encountered in maintaining a patent airway or prolonged ventilatory support is necessary, endotracheal intubation may be indicated.

Special considerations

◗ Local anesthetics should only be administered by clinicians experienced in the diagnosis and management of drug-related toxicity and other acute emergencies.

◗ Keep resuscitative equipment, drugs, and oxygen immediately available.

◗ Chloroprocaine can be given by single injection or continuously through an indwelling catheter.

◗ A test dose, preferably with epinephrine, should be given before epidural anesthesia with chloroprocaine (3 ml of 3% or 5 ml of 2% Nesacaine-MPF injection), and the patient monitored for CNS and CV toxicity and for signs of unintended intrathecal administration before proceeding.

◗ Aspiration should be performed before and during injection of chloroprocaine to avoid intravascular injection.

◗ Intravascular injection is still possible even if aspirations for blood are negative.

◗ Check solution for particles, and don't use if discolored.

◗ Administer the smallest dose and concentration needed to produce the desired result.

◗ Discard partially used bottles of preservative-free drug.

◗ Continuously monitor CV and respiratory status and patient's state of consciousness after each injection. Restlessness, anxiety, incoherent speech, light-headedness, numbness and tingling of mouth and lips, metallic taste, tinnitus, dizziness, blurred vision, tremors, twitching, depression or drowsiness may be early signs of CNS toxicity.

Breast-feeding patients

◗ No data exist to demonstrate whether drug appears in breast milk. Use cautiously in nursing women.

Geriatric patients
▶ Dosage reductions are recommended.

Patient teaching
▶ Advise patient that anesthetized area may have temporary loss of sensation and movement.

▶ chlorzoxazone
Paraflex, Parafon Forte DSC, Remular-S

Pharmacologic classification: *benzoxazole derivative*

Therapeutic classification: *skeletal muscle relaxant*

Pregnancy risk category C

How supplied
Available by prescription only
Caplets (film-coated): 250 mg, 500 mg
Tablets: 250 mg, 500 mg

Indications and dosages
Acute, painful musculoskeletal conditions (adjunct)
Adults: 250, 500, or 750 mg P.O. t.i.d. or q.i.d. Reduce to lowest effective dose after response occurs.
Children: 20 mg/kg or 600 mg/m^2 P.O. daily divided t.i.d. or q.i.d., or 125 to 500 mg t.i.d. or q.i.d., depending on age and weight.

Pharmacodynamics
Skeletal muscle relaxant action: Chlorzoxazone doesn't relax skeletal muscle directly, but apparently through sedation. it may modify perception of pain without eliminating peripheral pain reflexes.

Pharmacokinetics
Absorption: Drug is rapidly and completely absorbed from the GI tract. Action starts within 1 hour and lasts 3 to 4 hours.
Distribution: Drug is widely distributed in the body.
Metabolism: Drug is metabolized in the liver to inactive metabolites. Half-life is 66 minutes.
Excretion: Drug is excreted in urine as glucuronide metabolite.

Contraindications and precautions
Contraindicated in patients hypersensitive to drug and in patients with impaired hepatic function.

Interactions
Drug-drug
CNS depressants (such as antipsychotics, anxiolytics, general anesthetics, opioid analgesics, tricyclic antidepressants): additive CNS depression. Monitor patient closely.
MAO inhibitors, tricyclic antidepressants: increased CNS depression, respiratory depression, and hypotensive effects. Reduce dosage of one or both drugs. Monitor patient closely.

Drug-lifestyle
Alcohol use: increased CNS depression. Discourage alcohol use.

Effects on diagnostic tests
None reported.

Adverse reactions
CNS: *dizziness, drowsiness,* headache, *light-headedness,* malaise, overstimulation, tremor.
GI: abdominal distress, anorexia, constipation, diarrhea, heartburn, nausea, vomiting.

GU: urine discoloration (orange or purple-red).
Hepatic: hepatic dysfunction.
Skin: bruising, petechiae, pruritus, redness, urticaria.
Other: *anaphylaxis, angioedema.*

Overdose and treatment

Overdose may cause nausea, vomiting, diarrhea, drowsiness, dizziness, light-headedness, headache, malaise, or sluggishness, then loss of muscle tone, decreased or absent deep tendon reflexes, respiratory depression, and hypotension.

To treat, induce emesis or perform gastric lavage followed by activated charcoal. Monitor vital signs and neurologic status. Give support, including maintenance of adequate airway and assisted ventilation. Use caution if administering pressor agents.

Special considerations

▶ Drug doesn't relieve muscle spasm pain.
▶ Find out whether patient takes other CNS depressants because of cumulative effects.
▶ Monitor patient for drowsiness.
▶ Monitor liver function tests in patients receiving long-term therapy.

Breast-feeding patients

▶ No data exist to demonstrate whether drug appears in breast milk. No problems are known.

Pediatric patients

▶ Tablets may be crushed and mixed with food, milk, or fruit juice for children.

Geriatric patients

▶ Elderly patients may be more sensitive to drug's effects.

Patient teaching

▶ Caution patient to avoid hazardous activities until CNS effects of drug are known.
▶ Warn patient to avoid alcoholic beverages and to use caution when taking cough and cold preparations that contain alcohol.
▶ Advise patient to store drug away from direct heat or light.
▶ Tell patient to take missed dose only if remembered within 1 hour of scheduled time. If beyond 1 hour, patient should skip dose and go back to regular schedule. Patient should not double the dose.
▶ Tell patient not to stop taking drug without specific instructions.
▶ Tell patient that urine may turn orange or reddish purple.

▶ choline magnesium trisalicylates
Tricosal, Trilisate

▶ choline salicylate
Arthropan

Pharmacologic classification: *salicylate*

Therapeutic classification: *anti-inflammatory, antipyretic, nonnarcotic analgesic*

Pregnancy risk category C

How supplied

Available by prescription only
Tablets: 500 mg, 750 mg, 1,000 mg of salicylate (as choline and magnesium salicylate)
Solution: 500 mg of salicylate/ 5 ml (as choline and magnesium salicylate); 870 mg/5 ml (as choline salicylate)

Indications and dosages
Rheumatoid arthritis, osteoarthritis
Adults: 1,500 mg P.O. b.i.d. or 3,000 mg h.s.

◩ DOSAGE ADJUSTMENT. In elderly patients, give 750 mg t.i.d.
Mild arthritis, antipyresis
Adults: 2,000 to 3,000 mg P.O. daily in divided doses b.i.d.
Mild to moderate pain and fever
Children who weigh 12 to 13 kg (26 to 28.5 lb): 500 mg/day P.O., divided and given b.i.d.
Children who weigh 14 to 17 kg (30 to 37.5 lb): 750 mg/day P.O., divided and given b.i.d.
Children who weigh 18 to 22 kg (39 to 48.5 lb): 1,000 mg/day P.O., divided and given b.i.d.
Children who weigh 23 to 27 kg (50 to 59.5 lb): 1,250 mg/day P.O., divided and given b.i.d.
Children who weigh 28 to 32 kg (61 to 70.5 lb): 1,500 mg/day P.O., divided and given b.i.d.
Children who weigh 33 to 37 kg (73 to 81.5 lb): 1,750 mg/day P.O., divided and given b.i.d.

Pharmacodynamics
Analgesic action: Choline salicylates produce analgesia by an ill-defined effect on the hypothalamus (central action) and by blocking generation of pain impulses (peripheral action). The peripheral action may involve inhibition of prostaglandin synthesis.
Anti-inflammatory action: These drugs exert their anti-inflammatory effect by inhibiting prostaglandin synthesis; they may also inhibit the synthesis or action of other inflammation mediators.
Antipyretic action: Choline salicylates relieve fever by acting on the hypothalamic heat-regulating center to produce peripheral vasodilation. This increases peripheral blood supply and promotes sweating, which leads to loss of heat and to cooling by evaporation. These drugs do not affect platelet aggregation and should not be used to prevent thrombosis.

Pharmacokinetics
Absorption: These salicylate salts are absorbed rapidly and completely from the GI tract. Peak therapeutic effect occurs in 2 hours.
Distribution: Protein-binding depends on concentration and ranges from 75% to 90%, decreasing as serum level increases. Severe toxic effects may occur at serum levels above 400 mcg/ml.
Metabolism: Drug is hydrolyzed to salicylate in the liver.
Excretion: Metabolites are excreted in urine.

Contraindications and precautions
Contraindicated in patients hypersensitive to drug, in patients who consume three or more alcoholic beverages daily, and in patients with hemophilia, bleeding ulcers, and hemorrhagic states.

Use cautiously in patients with impaired renal or hepatic function, peptic ulcer disease, or gastritis. Do not give to children or teenagers with chickenpox or flu-like illnesses.

Interactions
Drug-drug
Ammonium chloride and other urine acidifiers: may increase choline salicylate blood levels. Monitor choline salicylate blood levels and thus toxicity.

Reactions may be *common*, uncommon, **life-threatening**, or COMMON AND LIFE-THREATENING.

Antacids and other urine alkalizers: in high doses, decreased choline salicylate absorption and blood levels. Monitor patient for decreased salicylate effect.

Corticosteroids: enhanced salicylate elimination. Monitor patient for decreased effect.

GI-irritant drugs, such as antibiotics, other NSAIDs: adverse effects may be potentiated. Use together with caution.

Highly protein-bound drugs, such as phenytoin, sulfonylureas, warfarin: may displace either drug and cause adverse effects. Monitor therapy closely for both drugs.

Lithium: choline salicylates decrease renal clearance of lithium carbonate, thus increasing serum lithium levels and the risk of adverse effects. Monitor serum lithium levels.

Methotrexate: may displace bound methotrexate and inhibit renal excretion. Monitor patient closely.

Sulfonylureas: may enhance hypoglycemic effects. Monitor serum glucose levels.

Warfarin: salicylates enhance hypoprothrombinemic effects. Monitor coagulation studies.

Drug-food
Food: delays and decreases absorption of choline salicylates. Give on an empty stomach.

Effects on diagnostic tests
Choline salicylates may interfere with urinary glucose analysis performed via Chemstrip uG, Diastix, glucose enzymatic test strip, Clinitest, and Benedict's solution. These drugs also interfere with urinary 5-hydroxyindoleacetic acid and vanillylmandelic acid.

Adverse reactions
EENT: hearing loss, tinnitus.
GI: GI distress, nausea, vomiting.
GU: *acute tubular necrosis with renal failure.*
Metabolic: elevated free T_4 levels.
Skin: rash.
Other: *anaphylaxis, hypersensitivity reactions, Reye's syndrome.*

Overdose and treatment
Overdose may cause metabolic acidosis with respiratory alkalosis, hyperpnea, and tachypnea from increased carbon dioxide production and direct stimulation of the respiratory center.

To treat overdose of choline salicylates, empty stomach immediately by inducing emesis with ipecac syrup, if patient is conscious, or by gastric lavage. Administer activated charcoal via nasogastric tube. Provide symptomatic and supportive measures (respiratory support and correction of fluid and electrolyte imbalances). Monitor laboratory parameters and vital signs closely. Hemodialysis is effective in removing choline salicylates but is used only in severe poisoning. Forced diuresis with alkalinizing agent accelerates salicylate excretion.

Special considerations
▸ Use of choline salicylates may be effective as an adjunct in cancer patients with pain, where traditional NSAIDs would be contraindicated because of the antiplatelet effects.
▸ Unlike other NSAIDs, there is no effect on platelet aggregation.
▸ Has a longer duration of action than aspirin.
▸ Do not mix choline salicylates with antacids.

▶ Administer oral solution of choline salicylate mixed with fruit juice. Follow with an 8-oz (240 ml) glass of water to ensure passage into stomach.
▶ Monitor serum magnesium levels to prevent possible magnesium toxicity.

Pregnant patients
▶ Use of choline salicylates should be avoided in the third trimester of pregnancy.

Breast-feeding patients
▶ Salicylates are distributed into breast milk. Avoid use in breast-feeding women.

Pediatric patients
▶ Safety of long-term drug use in children under age 14 hasn't been established.
▶ Because they raise the risk of Reye's syndrome, don't give salicylates to children with chickenpox or flulike symptoms.
▶ Febrile, dehydrated children can develop toxicity rapidly. Usually, they shouldn't receive more than five doses in 24 hours.

Geriatric patients
▶ Patients over age 60 may be more susceptible to toxic effects of these drugs.

Patient teaching
▶ Teach patient proper administration of drug.
▶ Instruct patient not to use OTC antacids.

▶ cimetidine
Tagamet, Tagamet HB

Pharmacologic classification:
H$_2$-receptor antagonist

Therapeutic classification:
antiulcer drug

Pregnancy risk category B

How supplied
Available by prescription only
Injection: 150 mg/ml, 300 mg/ 50 ml (premixed)
Liquid: 300 mg/5 ml
Tablets: 200 mg, 300 mg, 400 mg, 800 mg
Available without a prescription
Tablets: 100 mg

Indications and dosages
Duodenal ulcer (short-term treatment)
Adults: 800 mg h.s. for maximum of 8 weeks. Alternatively, give 400 mg P.O. b.i.d. or 300 mg P.O. q.i.d. with meals and h.s. When healing occurs, stop treatment or give h.s. dose only to control nocturnal hypersecretion. For parenteral administration, give 300 mg diluted to 20 ml with normal saline solution or other compatible I.V. solution by I.V. push over 5 minutes q 6 hours. Or 300 mg diluted in 50 ml dextrose 5% solution or other compatible I.V. solution by I.V. infusion over 15 to 20 minutes q 6 to 8 hours. Or 300 mg I.M. q 6 to 8 hours (no dilution necessary). To increase dose, give more frequently to maximum daily dose of 2,400 mg.
Duodenal ulcer prophylaxis
Adults: 400 mg h.s.

Active benign gastric ulcer
Adults: 800 mg h.s., or 300 mg
q.i.d. with meals and h.s. for up to
8 weeks.
Pathologic hypersecretory conditions (such as Zollinger-Ellison syndrome, systemic mastocytosis, and multiple endocrine adenomas)
Short-bowel syndrome*
Adults: 300 mg P.O. q.i.d. with
meals and h.s.; adjust to patient
needs. Maximum, 2,400 mg daily.
For parenteral administration, give
300 mg diluted to 20 ml with normal saline solution or other compatible I.V. solution by I.V. push
over 5 minutes q 6 to 8 hours. Or
300 mg diluted in 50 ml dextrose
5% solution or other compatible
I.V. solution by I.V. infusion over
15 to 20 minutes q 6 to 8 hours. To
increase dosage, give 300 mg doses more frequently to maximum
daily dose of 2,400 mg.
Gastroesophageal reflux symptoms
Adults: 800 mg P.O. b.i.d. or 400 mg
q.i.d., before meals and h.s.
Active upper-GI bleeding*, peptic esophagitis*, stress ulcer*
Adults: 1 to 2 g I.V. or P.O. daily, in
four divided doses.
Children: 20 to 40 mg/kg daily in
divided doses.
Continuous infusion for patients unable to tolerate oral medication
Adults: 37.5 mg/hour (900 mg/
day) by continuous I.V. infusion.
Use an infusion pump if total volume is below 250 ml/day.
Heartburn, acid indigestion, sour stomach
Adults: 200 mg P.O. up to a maximum of b.i.d. (400 mg).
☒ Dosage adjustment. In patients
with renal failure, recommended
dosage is 300 mg P.O. or I.V. q 8 to

12 hours at end of dialysis. Dosage
may be decreased further if hepatic
failure is also present.

Pharmacodynamics
Antiulcer action: Cimetidine competitively inhibits the action of histamine at H_2 receptors in gastric
parietal cells, inhibiting basal and
nocturnal gastric acid secretion
(such as from stimulation by food,
caffeine, insulin, histamine, betazole, or pentagastrin). Cimetidine
may also enhance gastromucosal
defense and healing.
   A 300-mg oral or parenteral
dose inhibits about 80% of gastric
acid secretion for 4 to 5 hours.

Pharmacokinetics
Absorption: About 60% to 75% of
oral dose is absorbed. Rate (but
not extent) may be affected by
food.
Distribution: Drug is distributed to
many body tissues. About 15% to
20% of drug is protein-bound.
Cimetidine apparently crosses the
placenta, and it appears in breast
milk.
Metabolism: About 30% to 40% of
dose is metabolized in the liver.
Drug has a half-life of 2 hours in
patients with normal renal function; half-life increases with decreasing renal function.
Excretion: Drug is excreted primarily in urine (48% of oral dose,
75% of parenteral dose); 10% of
oral dose is excreted in feces. Some
drug is excreted in breast milk.

Contraindications and precautions
Contraindicated in patients hypersensitive to drug. Use with caution
in elderly or debilitated patients.

◇ Available in Canada only   *Unlabeled use

Interactions
Drug-drug
Beta blockers (such as propranolol), benzodiazepines, carmustine, disulfiram, ferrous salts, indomethacin, isoniazid, ketoconazole, lidocaine, metronidazole, oral contraceptives, phenytoin, procainamide, quinidine, tetracyclines, triamterene, tricyclic antidepressants, warfarin, xanthines: by altering gastric pH, cimetidine decreases metabolism of these drugs, thus increasing potential toxicity and possibly necessitating dosage reduction. Adjust dose as necessary, and monitor patient.
Digoxin: decreased serum digoxin levels. Monitor serum levels.
Flecainide: increased serum flecainide levels and increased effects. Monitor patient closely.
Protease inhibitors: adverse effects on protease inhibitor metabolism. Avoid concurrent use.

Drug-herb
Pennyroyal: may change the rate of formation of toxic metabolites of pennyroyal. Avoid use together.
Yerba maté methylxanthines: may decrease clearance and cause toxicity. Use together cautiously.

Drug-lifestyle
Smoking: may increase gastric acid secretion and worsen disease. Discourage smoking.

Effects on diagnostic tests
Cimetidine may antagonize pentagastrin's effect during gastric acid secretion tests; it may cause false-negative results in skin tests using allergen extracts.

FD&C blue dye #2 used in Tagamet tablets may impair interpretation of Hemoccult and Gastroccult tests on gastric content aspirate. Be sure to wait at least 15 minutes after tablet administration before drawing the sample, and follow test manufacturer's instructions closely.

Adverse reactions
CNS: confusion, dizziness, hallucinations, headache, peripheral neuropathy, somnolence.
GI: *mild and transient diarrhea.*
GU: impotence, mild gynecomastia if used for over 1 month, transient elevations in serum creatinine levels.
Hematologic: *neutropenia.*
Musculoskeletal: arthralgia, muscle pain.
Other: *hypersensitivity reactions.*

Overdose and treatment
Overdose may cause respiratory failure and tachycardia. Overdose is rare; intake of up to 10 g has caused no untoward effects.

Support respiration and maintain a patent airway. Induce emesis or use gastric lavage; follow with activated charcoal to prevent further absorption. Treat tachycardia with propranolol if necessary.

Special considerations
▶ Cimetidine may be useful in combination with NSAIDs to lessen adverse GI effects.
▶ Drug enhances the action of benzodiazepines, especially in the elderly.
▶ Drug must be diluted before direct injection and given over 5 minutes. A rapid I.V. injection may result in arrhythmias and hypotension. Some authorities recommend infusing drug over at least 30 minutes to minimize risk of adverse cardiac effects. Sometimes given

as continuous I.V. infusion. Use infusion pump if given in a total volume of 250 ml over 24 hours or less.
▶ Dilute I.V. solutions with normal saline solution, D_5W, $D_{10}W$ (or a combination of these), lactated Ringer's solution, or 5% sodium bicarbonate injection. Don't dilute with sterile water for injection. Cimetidine is also commonly added to total parenteral nutrition solutions with or without fat emulsions.
▶ For I.M. administration, drug may be given undiluted. Injection may be painful.
▶ After administration of the liquid via nasogastric tube, tube should be flushed to clear it and ensure drug's passage to stomach.
▶ Hemodialysis removes drug; schedule dose after dialysis session.

Breast-feeding patients
▶ Drug appears in breast milk. Avoid use in breast-feeding women.

Geriatric patients
▶ Use caution when administering cimetidine to elderly patients because of the potential for adverse reactions affecting the CNS.
▶ Monitor elderly patients closely for changes in CNS status; cimetidine increases the action of benzodiazepines.

Patient teaching
▶ Warn patient to take drug as directed and to continue taking it even after pain subsides, to allow for adequate healing.
▶ Urge patient to avoid smoking, because it may increase gastric acid secretion and worsen disease.

▶ clomipramine hydrochloride
Anafranil

Pharmacologic classification:
tricyclic antidepressant

Therapeutic classification:
antiobsessional

Pregnancy risk category C

How supplied
Available by prescription only
Capsules: 25 mg, 50 mg, 75 mg

Indications and dosages
Obsessive-compulsive disorder
Adults: initially, 25 mg P.O. daily, gradually increasing to 100 mg P.O. daily (in divided doses, with meals) during the first 2 weeks. Maximum dosage, 250 mg daily. After titration, entire daily dose may be given h.s.
Children and adolescents: initially, 25 mg P.O. daily, gradually increased to a maximum of 3 mg/kg or 100 mg P.O. daily, whichever is smaller (in divided doses, with meals) over the first 2 weeks. Maximum daily dosage is 3 mg/kg or 200 mg, whichever is smaller. After titration, entire daily dose may be given h.s.

Pharmacodynamics
Antiobsessional action: A selective inhibitor of serotonin (5-HT) reuptake into neurons within the CNS. It may also have some blocking activity at postsynaptic dopamine receptors. The exact mechanism by which clomipramine treats obsessive-compulsive disorder is unknown.

◇ Available in Canada only   *Unlabeled use

Pharmacokinetics

Absorption: Clomipramine is well absorbed from GI tract, but extensive first-pass metabolism limits bioavailablity to about 50%.

Distribution: Drug distributes well into lipophilic tissues; the volume of distribution is about 12 L/kg; 98% is bound to plasma proteins.

Metabolism: Metabolism is primarily hepatic. Several metabolites have been identified; desmethyl-clomipramine is the primary active metabolite.

Excretion: About 66% of drug is excreted in urine, the rest in feces. Mean elimination half-life of the parent compound is about 36 hours; the elimination half-life of desmethylclomipramine has a mean of 69 hours. After multiple doses, the half-life may increase.

Contraindications and precautions

Contraindicated in patients with hypersensitivity to drug or other TCAs, in those who have taken MAO inhibitors within the previous 14 days, and in patients during acute recovery period after MI.

Use cautiously in patients with urine retention, suicidal tendencies, glaucoma, increased intraocular pressure, brain damage, or seizure disorders and in those taking medications that may lower the seizure threshold. Also use cautiously in patients with impaired renal or hepatic function, hyperthyroidism, or tumors of the adrenal medulla and in those undergoing elective surgery or receiving thyroid medication or electroconvulsive treatment.

Interactions
Drug-drug

Barbiturates: increased activity of hepatic microsomal enzymes with repeated doses, and possible decrease in tricyclic antidepressant levels. Monitor for decreased effectiveness.

CNS depressants: may cause exaggerated depressant effect when used with tricyclic antidepressants. Monitor patient closely.

Epinephrine, norepinephrine: may increase hypertensive effect. Monitor blood pressure.

Methylphenidate: may increase antidepressant blood levels. Monitor patient for adverse effects.

MAO inhibitors: may cause hyperpyretic crisis, seizures, coma, and death. Avoid concomitant use.

Drug-lifestyle

Alcohol use: may exaggerate depressant effect. Discourage concomitant use.

Effects on diagnostic tests

None reported.

Adverse reactions

CNS: *dizziness, EEG changes, fatigue, headache, insomnia, myoclonus, nervousness,* **seizures,** *somnolence, tremor.*

CV: palpitations, orthostatic hypotension, tachycardia.

EENT: *pharyngitis, rhinitis, visual changes.*

GI: *abdominal pain, anorexia, constipation,* diarrhea, *dyspepsia, dry mouth, increased appetite, nausea.*

GU: *altered libido, dysmenorrhea, ejaculation failure, impotence, urinary hesitancy,* urinary tract infection.

Hematologic: anemia, purpura.

Reactions may be *common,* uncommon, *life-threatening,* or COMMON AND LIFE-THREATENING.

Metabolic: *weight gain.*
Musculoskeletal: *myalgia.*
Skin: diaphoresis, dry skin, pruritus, rash.

Overdose and treatment

Overdose may cause sinus tachycardia, intraventricular block, hypotension, irritability, fixed and dilated pupils, drowsiness, delirium, stupor, hyperreflexia, and hyperpyrexia.

Treatment should include gastric lavage with large quantities of fluid. Lavage should be continued for 12 hours because the anticholinergic effects of the drug slow gastric emptying. Hemodialysis, peritoneal dialysis, and forced diuresis are ineffective because of the high degree of plasma protein binding. Support respirations and monitor cardiac function. Treat shock with plasma expanders or corticosteroids; treat seizures with diazepam.

Special considerations

▶ Drug may be effective for neuropathic pain.
▶ Monitor patient for urine retention and constipation. Suggest stool softener or high-fiber diet, as needed, and encourage adequate fluid intake.
▶ Drug may increase opioid level if added to a morphine regimen.
▶ To minimize risk of overdose, dispense drug in small quantities.
▶ Don't withdraw drug abruptly.
▶ Activation of mania or hypomania may occur with clomipramine therapy.

Breast-feeding patients

▶ No data exist to demonstrate whether drug appears in breast milk. Use with caution in breast-feeding women.

Patient teaching

▶ Tell patient that adverse GI effects can be minimized by taking drug with meals during the dosage adjustment period. Later, the entire daily dose may be taken at bedtime to limit daytime drowsiness.
▶ Instruct patient to avoid alcohol and other CNS depressants.
▶ Warn patient to avoid hazardous activities that require alertness or good psychomotor coordination until adverse CNS effects are known. This is especially important early in therapy, when daytime sedation and dizziness may occur.
▶ Suggest a saliva substitute or sugarless candy or gum to relieve dry mouth.
▶ Inform patient to avoid using OTC medications, particularly antihistamines and decongestants, unless recommended by physician or pharmacist.
▶ Encourage patient to continue therapy, even if adverse reactions are troublesome. Advise patient not to stop taking it without notifying caregiver.

▶ clonazepam
Klonopin, Rivotril◇

Pharmacologic classification:
benzodiazepine

Therapeutic classification:
anticonvulsant

Controlled substance schedule IV

Pregnancy risk category C

How supplied
Available by prescription only
Tablets: 0.5 mg, 1 mg, 2 mg

Indications and dosages
*Neuralgia**
Adults: 2 to 4 mg/day P.O.

Pharmacodynamics
Analgesic action: Unknown.
Anticonvulsant action: Unknown; drug appears to act in the limbic system, thalamus, and hypothalamus.

Pharmacokinetics
Absorption: Clonazepam is well absorbed from the GI tract; action begins in 20 to 60 minutes and persists for 6 to 8 hours in infants and children and up to 12 hours in adults.
Distribution: Drug is distributed widely throughout the body; it is about 85% protein-bound.
Metabolism: Clonazepam is metabolized by the liver to several metabolites. The half-life of drug is 18 to 39 hours.
Excretion: Drug is excreted in urine.

Contraindications and precautions
Contraindicated in patients with significant hepatic disease; in those with sensitivity to benzodiazepines; and in patients with acute angle-closure glaucoma.

Use cautiously in children and in patients with mixed-type seizures, respiratory disease, or glaucoma.

Interactions
Drug-drug
CNS depressants (anxiolytics, barbiturates, narcotics, tranquilizers) and other anticonvulsants: additive CNS depressant effects. Avoid using together.
Rifabutin, rifampin: enhanced clonazepam clearance and reduced efficacy. Monitor patient for decreased effectiveness.
Ritonavir: may significantly increase clonazepam levels. Monitor patient for adverse effects.
Valproic acid: may induce absence seizures. Monitor patient closely.

Drug-lifestyle
Alcohol use: produces additive CNS depressant effects. Don't use together.

Effects on diagnostic tests
None reported.

Adverse reactions
CNS: agitation, *ataxia, behavioral disturbances* (especially in children), confusion, *drowsiness,* psychosis, slurred speech, tremor.
CV: palpitations.
EENT: abnormal eye movements, nystagmus, sore gums.
GI: anorexia, change in appetite, constipation, diarrhea, gastritis, nausea.
GU: dysuria, enuresis, nocturia, urine retention.
Hematologic: eosinophilia, *leukopenia, thrombocytopenia.*
Hepatic: increased liver function test results.
Respiratory: *respiratory depression,* chest congestion, shortness of breath.
Skin: rash.

Overdose and treatment
Overdose may cause ataxia, confusion, coma, decreased reflexes, and hypotension.

Treat overdose with gastric lavage and supportive therapy. Flumazenil, a specific benzodiazepine antagonist, may be useful. Vasopressors should be used to treat hypotension. Carefully monitor vital signs, ECG, and fluid and electrolyte balance. Clonazepam is not dialyzable.

Special considerations
▶ Clonazepam appears to be more effective than diazepam for musculoskeletal pain.
▶ Drug is also indicated in seizure activity.
▶ It may be effective for trigeminal neuralgia, phantom limb, and other neuropathic pain.
▶ Drug may be helpful in controlling myoclonus related to high-dose opioids.
▶ Clonazepam is also used to treat myoclonic, atonic, and absence seizures resistant to other anticonvulsants and to suppress or eliminate attacks of sleep-related nocturnal myoclonus (restless legs syndrome).
▶ Monitor CBC and liver function tests periodically.
▶ Abrupt withdrawal may cause status epilepticus; after long-term use, lower dosage gradually.
▶ Use with barbiturates or other CNS depressants may impair patient's ability to perform tasks that require mental alertness.
▶ Watch for oversedation, especially in elderly patients.
▶ Drug may also be used for parkinsonian dysarthria, acute manic episodes, and multifocal tic disorders.

Breast-feeding patients
▶ Alternative feeding method is recommended during clonazepam therapy.

Pediatric patients
▶ Long-term safety in children hasn't been established.

Geriatric patients
▶ Elderly patients may require lower doses because of diminished renal function.
▶ Elderly patients have an increased risk of oversedation from CNS depressants.

Patient teaching
▶ Explain rationale for therapy and risks and benefits that may be anticipated.
▶ Teach patient signs and symptoms of adverse reactions and the need to report them promptly.
▶ Tell patient to avoid alcohol and other sedatives to prevent added CNS depression.
▶ Warn patient not to discontinue drug or change dosage unless prescribed.
▶ Advise patient to avoid hazardous tasks until full sedative effects of drug are known.

▶ clonidine hydrochloride
Catapres, Catapres-TTS, Dixarit◊, Duraclon

Pharmacologic classification: *selective alpha$_2$ agonist*

Therapeutic classification: *antihypertensive*

Pregnancy risk category C

How supplied
Available by prescription only
Injection: 100 mcg/ml (preservative-free)
Tablets: 0.1 mg, 0.2 mg, 0.3 mg
Transdermal: TTS-1 (releases 0.1 mg/24 hours), TTS-2 (releases 0.2 mg/24 hours), TTS-3 (releases 0.3 mg/24 hours)

Indications and dosages

Intractable cancer pain
Adults: 30 mg/hr by continuous epidural infusion.

Opioid withdrawal
Adults: test dose 0.005 to 0.006 mg/kg P.O.; then 0.017 mg/kg/day divided into 3 or 4 doses daily for about 10 days.

Prophylaxis for vascular headache*
Adults: 0.025 mg P.O. b.i.d. to q.i.d. up to 0.15 mg P.O. daily in divided doses.

Menopausal symptoms (adjunct)*
Adults: 0.025 to 0.075 mg P.O. b.i.d.

Ulcerative colitis*
Adults: 0.3 mg P.O. t.i.d.

Neuralgia*
Adults: 0.2 mg P.O. daily.

Pharmacodynamics

Analgesic action: Clonidine produces analgesic effects by mimicking the activation of descending pain-suppressing pathways arising from supraspinal control centers and teminating in the dorsal horn of the spinal cord.

Antihypertensive action: Clonidine decreases peripheral vascular resistance by stimulating central alpha-adrenergic receptors, thus decreasing cerebral sympathetic outflow; drug may also inhibit renin release. Initially, clonidine may stimulate peripheral alpha-adrenergic receptors, producing transient vasoconstriction.

Pharmacokinetics

Absorption: Clonidine is absorbed well from the GI tract when administered orally; after oral administration, blood pressure begins to decline in 30 to 60 minutes, with maximal effect occurring in 2 to 4 hours. Clonidine is absorbed well percutaneously after transdermal topical administration; transdermal therapeutic plasma levels are achieved 2 to 3 days after initial application.

Distribution: Clonidine is distributed widely into the body.

Metabolism: Drug is metabolized in the liver, where nearly 50% is transformed to inactive metabolites.

Excretion: About 65% of a given dose is excreted in urine; 20% is excreted in feces. Half-life of clonidine ranges from 6 to 20 hours in patients with normal renal function. After oral administration, the antihypertensive effect lasts up to 8 hours; after transdermal application, the antihypertensive effect persists for up to 7 days.

Contraindications and precautions

Contraindicated in patients hypersensitive to drug. Transdermal form is contraindicated in patients hypersensitive to any component of the adhesive layer.

Use cautiously in patients with severe coronary disease, recent MI, cerebrovascular disease, and impaired hepatic or renal function.

Interactions
Drug-drug

Barbiturates and other sedatives: may increase CNS depressant effects. Monitor patient closely.

Beta blockers, such as propranolol: may have an additive effect, producing bradycardia. Rebound hypertension may occur with withdrawal. Monitor patient's vital signs closely.

MAO inhibitors, tolazoline, tricyclic antidepressants: may inhibit antihypertensive effects. Monitor blood pressure.

Drug-herb
Capsicum: may reduce antihypertensive effectiveness. Avoid use together.

Drug-lifestyle
Alcohol use: may increase CNS depressant effects. Discourage use together.

Effects on diagnostic tests
Clonidine may decrease urine excretion of vanillylmandelic acid and catecholamines; it may slightly increase blood or serum glucose levels and may cause a weakly positive Coombs' test.

Adverse reactions
CNS: agitation, depression, *dizziness, drowsiness,* fatigue, malaise, *sedation, weakness.*
CV: *bradycardia,* orthostatic hypotension, *severe rebound hypertension.*
GI: anorexia, *constipation, dry mouth,* nausea, vomiting.
GU: impotence, loss of libido, urine retention.
Metabolic: possible slight increase in serum glucose levels, weight gain.
Skin: *dermatitis* (with transdermal patch), *pruritus,* rash.

Overdose and treatment
Overdose may cause bradycardia, CNS depression, respiratory depression, hypothermia, apnea, seizures, lethargy, agitation, irritability, diarrhea, and hypotension; hypertension has also been reported.

After overdose with oral clonidine, do not induce emesis because rapid onset of CNS depression can lead to aspiration. After adequate airway is assured, empty stomach by gastric lavage followed by administration of activated charcoal. If overdose occurs in patients receiving transdermal therapy, remove transdermal patch. Further treatment is usually symptomatic and supportive.

Special considerations
▸ As an alpha$_2$ agonist, drug is useful as a multipurpose analgesic. It also is beneficial for chronic pain that is less responsive to opioids, such as chronic headache or neuropathic pain.
▸ Give drug 4 to 6 hours before scheduled surgery.
▸ Monitor patient's weight daily at the start of therapy to detect fluid retention.
▸ Monitor pulse and blood pressure frequently; dosage is usually adjusted to patient's response and tolerance.
▸ Therapeutic plasma levels are achieved 2 or 3 days after applying transdermal form. Patient may need oral antihypertensive therapy during this interim period.
▸ Don't discontinue abruptly; reduce dosage gradually over 2 to 4 days to prevent severe rebound hypertension.
▸ Patients with renal impairment may respond to smaller doses of drug.
▸ Remove transdermal systems when attempting defibrillation or synchronized cardioversion because of electrical conductivity.
▸ Drug is twice as effective when given epidurally as when given I.V.
▸ Clonidine may be used to lower blood pressure quickly in some hypertensive emergencies.

▶ Clonidine is also indicated in hypertension, Tourette syndrome, growth delay in children, testing for pheochromocytoma, nicotine withdrawal, and diabetic diarrhea.

Breast-feeding patients
▶ Clonidine appears in breast milk. An alternate feeding method is recommended during treatment.

Pediatric patients
▶ Efficacy and safety in children haven't been established; use drug only if potential benefit outweighs risk.

Geriatric patients
▶ Elderly patients may need lower doses because they may be more sensitive to hypotensive effects. Monitor renal function closely.

Patient teaching
▶ Explain disease and rationale for therapy; emphasize importance of follow-up visits in establishing therapeutic regimen.
▶ Advise taking last dose at bedtime to ensure nighttime blood pressure control.
▶ Tell patient to rotate transdermal patch site weekly.
▶ Warn patient to avoid hazardous activities that require mental alertness until tolerance develops to sedation, drowsiness, and other CNS effects.
▶ Advise patient to avoid sudden position changes to minimize orthostatic hypotension.
▶ Inform patient that ice chips, hard candy, or gum will relieve dry mouth.
▶ Warn patient to call for specific instructions before taking OTC cold preparations.

▶ Teach patient signs and symptoms of adverse effects and need to report them; patient should also report excessive weight gain (more than 5 lb [2.27 kg] weekly).
▶ Tell patient not to discontinue drug suddenly; rebound hypertension may develop.

▶ cocaine hydrochloride

Pharmacologic classification:
ester topical local anesthetic

Therapeutic classification:
topical local anesthetic

Controlled substance schedule II

Pregnancy risk category C

How supplied
Available by prescription only
Topical solution: 4% and 10% in 10-ml multidose vials, 5 g and 25 g powder

Indications and dosages
Topical anesthesia for mucous membranes of the oral, laryngeal and nasal cavities
Adults: maximum single dose, 1 mg/kg. Dose varies with vascularity of the area to be anesthetized, individual tolerance, and technique of anesthesia. Give lowest dose needed to provide effective anesthesia.
◩ DOSAGE ADJUSTMENT. Debilitated, elderly, pediatric, and acutely ill patients should receive reduced dosages.

Pharmacodynamics
Topical local anesthetic action: Cocaine inhibits conduction of nerve impulses from sensory

nerves. It also inhibits the uptake of norepinephrine, which potentiates the effects of catecholamines; this results in vasoconstriction and mydriasis.

Pharmacokinetics
Absorption: Absorbed from all sites of application. Following topical application to mucous membranes, peak effects occur in 1 to 5 minutes and persist for 30 minutes or longer depending on dose and concentration. Absorption is enhanced by inflammation.
Distribution: Not clearly defined.
Metabolism: Cocaine is hydrolyzed by plasma esterases and partially demethylated in the liver.
Excretion: Cocaine and its metabolites are excreted in the urine; less than 10% to 20% is excreted in urine unchanged. Cocaine has a half-life of about 75 minutes.

Contraindications and precautions
Contraindicated in patients hypersensitive to drug or components of the topical solution. Topical solutions aren't intended for systemic or ophthalmologic use.

Use with caution in patients with hypertension, thyrotoxicosis, severe CV disease, in patients receiving drugs that also potentiate catecholamines and in patients with severely traumatized mucosa and sepsis in the region of application.

Interactions
Drug-drug
Anesthetics (chloroform, cyclopropane, halothane, trichlorethylene): administration of cocaine before or shortly after anesthesia may increase the risk of ventricular arrhythmias. Use cautiously if concurrent use is necessary.
Beta blockers: cocaine may inhibit beta blocker effects. Use cautiously.
Cholinesterase inhibitors: reduced cocaine metabolism and increased risk of toxicity. Monitor patient closely.
Levodopa, methyldopa: increased risk of cardiac arrhythmias. Use cautiously, reduce dosage, and monitor patient.
MAO inhibitors: may prolong or intensify vasopressor and cardiac stimulant effects of cocaine. Don't use cocaine within 14 days of an MAO inhibitor.
Sympathomimetics: increased CNS stimulation, CV effects, and adverse effects. Use together cautiously.

Effects on diagnostic tests
None reported

Adverse reactions
CNS: euphoria, hallucinations, nervousness, restlessness, *seizures,* tremors.
CV: *bradycardia* with small doses, hypertension with moderate doses, tachycardia.
GI: vomiting.
Respiratory: *respiratory failure,* tachypnea.

Overdose and treatment
A fatal dose is about 500 mg to 1.2 g. Severe toxic effects have occurred with doses as low as 20 mg. Initially, overdose may cause restlessness, anxiety, excitability, hallucinations, confusion, dizziness, tachycardia, dilated pupils, blurred vision, vomiting, abdominal pain, numbness and muscle spasm, followed by irregular respirations,

seizures, coma, and circulatory failure. CV effects include increased blood pressure, increased heart rate, irregular heartbeat, and vasoconstriction. Chronic poisoning may be similar but includes mental deterioration, weight loss, change of character, and possible perforated nasal septum from snorting.

Treatment includes symptomatic and supportive therapy. Maintain airway and respiration. If ingested, give activated charcoal, perform gastric lavage, or induce emesis. Absorption from an injection site can be limited by tourniquet. Give drugs to control seizures and blood pressure as needed.

Special considerations
▶ Cocaine hydrochloride topical solution can be administered by means of cotton applicators or packs, instilled into a cavity, or as a spray.
▶ Keep resuscitative equipment and drugs on hand when using drug as a local anesthetic.
▶ Monitor patient's vital signs.
▶ Concentrations above 4% aren't recommended because of the possible increase in systemic effects.
▶ Continued exposure to the drug can cause psychological dependence.
▶ Prolonged intranasal use can perforate the septum.

Breast-feeding patients
▶ Safety for nursing mothers hasn't been established. Use caution when giving drug to a nursing woman. Because of the potential for serious adverse reactions, it is recommended that nursing be discontinued during cocaine use.

Pediatric patients
▶ Safety and efficacy haven't been established.

Geriatric patients
▶ Reduce dosage in elderly patients.

Patient teaching
▶ Instruct patient to not ingest food for 1 hour after topical anesthetic use in mouth or throat. Topical anesthetics may impair swallowing and increase the risk of aspiration and bite trauma.
▶ Reassure patient that cocaine used as a local anesthetic isn't likely to cause psychological dependence.
▶ Because cocaine is excreted in urine, drug tests will be positive for a few days after use.
▶ Loss of sense or taste may occur after application to the nose or mouth.

▶ **codeine phosphate**

▶ **codeine sulfate**

Pharmacologic classification:
opioid

Therapeutic classification:
analgesic, antitussive

Controlled substance schedule II

Pregnancy risk category C

How supplied
Available by prescription only
Injection: 15 mg/ml, 30 mg/ml, 60 mg/ml codeine phosphate
Oral solution: 15 mg/5 ml codeine phosphate
Tablets: 15 mg, 30 mg, 60 mg; 15 mg, 30 mg, 60 mg (soluble)

Indications and dosages
Mild to moderate pain
Adults: 15 to 60 mg P.O. or 15 to 60 mg (phosphate) S.C. or I.M. q 4 to 6 hours, p.r.n., or around the clock.
Children: 0.5 mg/kg (or 15 mg/m^2) q 4 to 6 hours. (Don't use I.V. route.)

Pharmacodynamics
Analgesic action: Codeine (methylmorphine) has analgesic properties that result from its agonist activity at the opiate receptors.
Antitussive action: Codeine has a direct suppressant action on the cough reflex center.

Pharmacokinetics
Absorption: Codeine is well absorbed after oral or parenteral administration. It is about two-thirds as potent orally as parenterally. After oral or S.C. administration, action occurs in less than 30 minutes. Duration of action is 4 to 6 hours.
Distribution: Drug is distributed widely throughout the body; it crosses the placenta and enters breast milk.
Metabolism: Codeine is metabolized mainly in the liver, by demethylation, or conjugation with glucuronic acid.
Excretion: Drug is excreted mainly in the urine as norcodeine and free and conjugated morphine.

Contraindications and precautions
Contraindicated in patients hypersensitive to drug.

Use cautiously in patients with impaired renal or hepatic function, head injuries, increased intracranial pressure, increased CSF pressure, hypothyroidism, Addison's disease, acute alcoholism, CNS depression, bronchial asthma, COPD, respiratory depression, or shock, and in elderly or debilitated patients.

Interactions
Drug-drug
Anticholinergics: may cause paralytic ileus. Monitor patient closely.
Cimetidine: may increase respiratory and CNS depression, causing confusion, disorientation, apnea, or seizures. Avoid using together or, if necessary, monitor patient closely.
CNS depressants (antihistamines, barbiturates, benzodiazepines, general anesthetics, MAO inhibitors, muscle relaxants, opioid analgesics, phenothiazines, sedative-hypnotics, tricyclic antidepressants): potentiate respiratory and CNS depression, sedation, and hypotensive effects. Avoid using together.
Drugs extensively metabolized in the liver (digitoxin, phenytoin, rifampin): drug accumulation and enhanced effects. Monitor patient for effects.
Drugs that induce cytochrome P-450 isoenzymes: increased codeine clearance. Monitor patient for decreased codeine effects.
General anesthetics: possible severe CV depression. Monitor patient closely.
Opioid antagonists: acute withdrawal syndrome in patients physically dependent on codeine.

Drug-lifestyle
Alcohol use: potentiates respiratory and CNS depression, sedation, and hypotensive effects. Discourage alcohol use.

Effects on diagnostic tests

Drug may increase plasma amylase and lipase levels, delay gastric emptying, increase biliary tract pressure resulting from contraction of the sphincter of Oddi, and may interfere with hepatobiliary imaging studies.

Adverse reactions

CNS: clouded sensorium, dizziness, euphoria, light-headedness, physical dependence, sedation.
CV: *bradycardia, hypotension,* flushing.
GI: *constipation, dry mouth,* ileus, *nausea, vomiting.*
GU: *urine retention.*
Respiratory: *respiratory depression.*
Skin: *diaphoresis,* pruritus.

Overdose and treatment

Overdose may cause CNS depression, respiratory depression, and miosis (pinpoint pupils). Other acute toxic effects include hypotension, bradycardia, hypothermia, shock, apnea, cardiopulmonary arrest, circulatory collapse, pulmonary edema, and seizures.

To treat acute overdose, first establish adequate respiratory exchange via a patent airway and ventilation as needed; administer narcotic antagonist (naloxone) to reverse respiratory depression. (Because the duration of action of codeine is longer than that of naloxone, repeated naloxone dosing is necessary.) Naloxone should not be given unless the patient has clinically significant respiratory or CV depression. Monitor vital signs closely.

If ingestion was within 2 hours, empty the stomach immediately by inducing emesis (ipecac syrup) or performing gastric lavage. Use caution to avoid aspiration. Give activated charcoal via nasogastric tube for further removal of drug in an oral overdose.

Provide symptomatic and supportive treatment (continued respiratory support, correction of fluid or electrolyte imbalance). Monitor laboratory parameters, vital signs, and neurologic status closely.

Special considerations

▶ Codeine and aspirin have additive analgesic effects. Give together for maximum pain relief.
▶ A dose of 30 to 32 mg P.O. equals about 650 mg of aspirin.
▶ When codeine is combined with a nonopioid analgesic, it has limited usefulness for chronic pain because of the ceiling effect.
▶ Codeine has much less abuse potential than morphine.
▶ Give drug very slowly by direct injection into a large vein.
▶ Avoid I.M. route because it has unpredictable absorption and a high adverse effect profile.
▶ Monitor patient for desired effects and adverse effects.
▶ Drug causes more GI toxicity (nausea, vomiting) than other opioids.
▶ Drug may also be used for nonproductive cough.

Breast-feeding patients

▶ Drug appears in breast milk; assess risks and benefits before administering.

Pediatric patients

▶ Administer cautiously to children. Codeine-containing cough medicines may be hazardous in young children.

▶ Use a calibrated measuring device, and don't exceed recommended daily dose.

Geriatric patients
▶ Lower doses are usually indicated for elderly patients, who may be more sensitive to therapeutic and adverse effects.

Patient teaching
▶ Inform patient that codeine may cause drowsiness, dizziness, or blurred vision; tell him to use caution while driving or performing tasks that require mental alertness.
▶ Advise patient to avoid alcohol and other CNS depressants and to take drug with food if GI upset occurs.

▶ cortisone acetate
Cortone

Pharmacologic classification:
glucocorticoid, mineralocorticoid

Therapeutic classification:
anti-inflammatory, replacement therapy

Pregnancy risk category NR

How supplied
Available by prescription only
Injection (I.M. use): 50 mg/ml suspension
Tablets: 5 mg, 10 mg, 25 mg

Indications and dosages
Inflammation
Adults: 25 to 300 mg P.O. or 20 to 300 mg I.M. daily or on alternate days. Dosage highly individualized depending on severity of disease.
Children: 20 to 300 mg/m²/day P.O. in four divided doses or 7 to 37.5 mg/m² I.M. once or twice daily. Dosage is highly individualized.

Pharmacodynamics
Adrenocorticoid replacement: Cortisone acetate is an adrenocorticoid with glucocorticoid and mineralocorticoid properties. It has only about 80% of the anti-inflammatory activity of an equal weight of hydrocortisone. The drug is a potent mineralocorticoid, however, having twice the potency of prednisone. Cortisone (or hydrocortisone) is usually the drug of choice for replacement therapy in patients with adrenal insufficiency. It usually isn't used for anti-inflammatory or immunosuppressant action because of the extremely large doses that must be used and because of the unwanted mineralocorticoid effects. The injectable form has a slow onset but a long duration of action. It usually is used only when the oral route can't be used.

Pharmacokinetics
Absorption: Cortisone is absorbed readily after oral administration, and effects peak in about 1 to 2 hours. The suspension for injection has a variable onset of 24 to 48 hours.
Distribution: Drug is distributed rapidly to muscle, liver, skin, intestines, and kidneys. Cortisone is extensively bound to plasma proteins (transcortin and albumin). Only the unbound portion is active. Cortisone is distributed into breast milk and through the placenta.
Metabolism: Drug is metabolized in the liver to the active metabolite hydrocortisone, which in turn is metabolized to inactive glucuro-

nide and sulfate metabolites. Duration of hypothalamic-pituitary-adrenal axis suppression is 1¼ to 1½ days.

Excretion: Inactive metabolites and small amounts of unmetabolized drug are excreted by the kidneys. Insignificant quantities of the drug are also excreted in feces. Biological half-life of cortisone is 8 to 12 hours.

Contraindications and precautions

Contraindicated in patients hypersensitive to drug or its ingredients and in patients with systemic fungal infection.

Use cautiously in patients with renal disease, recent MI, GI ulcer, hypertension, osteoporosis, diabetes mellitus, hypothyroidism, cirrhosis, diverticulitis, ulcerative colitis, recent intestinal anastomosis, thromboembolic disorders, seizures, myasthenia gravis, heart failure, tuberculosis, ocular herpes, emotional instability, or psychotic tendencies.

Interactions
Drug-drug

Amphotericin B, diuretics: increased hypokalemia and risk of toxicity in patients receiving cardiac glycosides. Monitor serum potassium levels.

Antacids, cholestyramine, colestipol: decreased cortisone absorption and effects. Monitor patient for desired effects.

Barbiturates, phenytoin, rifampin: decreased corticosteroid effects because of increased hepatic metabolism. Monitor patient for effects.

Estrogens: reduced cortisone metabolism from increased transcortin level. Monitor patient for adverse effects.

Inactivated vaccines, toxoids: diminished response to cortisone. Monitor patient for decreased effects.

Insulin, oral antidiabetic drugs: increased risk of hyperglycemia. Monitor serum glucose levels, and adjust dosages accordingly.

Isoniazid, salicylates: increased metabolism of these drugs. Monitor patient for desired effects.

Oral anticoagulants: decreased anticoagulant effects (rare). Monitor coagulation studies.

Ulcerogenic drugs (such as NSAIDs): prolonged cortisone half-life because of increased protein-binding and consequent increased risk of GI ulceration. Avoid use together.

Effects on diagnostic tests

Drug therapy suppresses reactions to skin tests; causes false-negative results in the nitroblue tetrazolium test for systemic bacterial infections; and decreases ^{131}I uptake and protein-bound iodine levels in thyroid function tests.

Adverse reactions

CNS: euphoria, headache, insomnia, paresthesia, pseudotumor cerebri, psychotic behavior, *seizures,* vertigo.
CV: *arrhythmias,* edema, *heart failure,* hypertension, thrombophlebitis, *thromboembolism.*
EENT: cataracts, glaucoma.
GI: GI irritation, increased appetite, nausea, *pancreatitis, peptic ulcer,* vomiting.

GU: increased urine glucose and calcium levels, menstrual irregularities.

Metabolic: *acute adrenal insufficiency may follow increased stress (infection, surgery, trauma) or abrupt withdrawal after long-term therapy;* decreased serum potassium, calcium, thyroxine, and triiodothyronine levels; growth suppression in children; increased hypercholesterolemia; possible hypokalemia, hyperglycemia, and carbohydrate intolerance.

Musculoskeletal: muscle weakness, osteoporosis.

Skin: acne, atrophy at I.M. injection sites, delayed wound healing, various skin eruptions.

Other: cushingoid symptoms (moonface, buffalo hump, central obesity), hirsutism, susceptibility to infections.

Overdose and treatment

Acute ingestion, even in massive doses, is rarely a clinical problem. Toxic signs and symptoms rarely occur if the drug is used for less than 3 weeks, even at large dosage ranges. However, chronic use causes adverse physiologic effects, including suppression of the HPA axis, cushingoid appearance, muscle weakness, and osteoporosis.

Special considerations

▶ Cortisone is a multipurpose analgesic useful for bone pain (such as bone metastasis), neuropathic pain, or headache pain.

▶ Cortisone may be useful in palliative care because it stimulates appetite, provides euphoria, and improves quality of life.

▶ Monitor patient for adverse effects.

▶ Avoid using with aspirin or NSAIDs.

▶ Monitor serum glucose levels if patient has diabetes, and adjust treatment regimen as needed.

▶ Most adverse reactions are dose- or duration-dependent.

▶ Abrupt withdrawal may cause anorexia, arthralgia, depression, dizziness, dyspnea, fainting, fatigue, fever, hypoglycemia, lethargy, orthostatic hypotension, rebound inflammation, weakness.

▶ After prolonged use, abrupt withdrawal may be fatal.

▶ To discontinue long-term use, consider tapering drug for weeks or months to prevent adrenal insufficiency.

▶ Drug may also be used for adrenal insufficiency and for allergies.

Pediatric patients

▶ Long-term use of cortisone in children and adolescents may delay growth and maturation.

Geriatric patients

▶ Use cautiously in elderly patients because they're more likely to develop osteoporosis.

Patient teaching

▶ Inform patient about possible adverse reactions.

*Unlabeled use

▶ cyclizine hydrochloride
Marezine

▶ cyclizine lactate
Marezine, Marzine ◇

Pharmacologic classification:
piperazine-derivative antihistamine

Therapeutic classification:
antiemetic, antivertigo

Pregnancy risk category B

How supplied
Available with or without a prescription
cyclizine hydrochloride
Tablets: 50 mg
cyclizine lactate
Injection: 50 mg/ml

Indications and dosages
Motion sickness (prophylaxis and treatment)
Adults and children over age 12: 50 mg P.O. (hydrochloride) 30 minutes before travel, and then q 4 to 6 hours, p.r.n. Maximum, 200 mg daily or 50 mg I.M. (lactate) q 4 to 6 hours, p.r.n.
Children ages 6 to 12: 25 mg P.O. up to t.i.d. under medical supervision.

Pharmacodynamics
Antiemetic action: Cyclizine probably inhibits nausea and vomiting by centrally depressing sensitivity of the labyrinth apparatus that relays stimuli to the chemoreceptor trigger zone and thus stimulates the vomiting center in the brain.
Antivertigo action: Drug depresses conduction in vestibular-cerebellar pathways and reduces labyrinth excitability.

Pharmacokinetics
Absorption: Not well characterized; onset of action is between 30 and 60 minutes.
Distribution: Drug is well distributed throughout the body.
Metabolism: Cyclizine is metabolized in the liver.
Excretion: Unknown; drug effect lasts 4 to 6 hours.

Contraindications and precautions
Contraindicated in patients hypersensitive to drug.
Use cautiously in patients with heart failure and who have recently had surgery, benign prostatic hypertrophy or asthma.

Interactions
Drug-drug
CNS depressants, such as antianxiety drugs, barbiturates, sleeping aids, tranquilizers: additive sedative and CNS depressant effects. Avoid using together.
Ototoxic drugs, such as aminoglycosides, carboplatin, cisplatin, loop diuretics, salicylates, vancomycin: signs of ototoxicity are masked. Avoid using together.

Drug-lifestyle
Alcohol use: additive sedative and CNS depressant effects. Discourage alcohol use.

Effects on diagnostic tests
Discontinue cyclizine 4 days before diagnostic skin testing, to avoid preventing, reducing, or masking test response.

Adverse reactions
CNS: auditory and visual hallucinations, *drowsiness,* excitation, nervousness, restlessness.

Reactions may be *common*, uncommon, *life-threatening*, or **COMMON AND LIFE-THREATENING**.

CV: hypotension, palpitations, tachycardia.
EENT: blurred vision, diplopia, dry nose and throat, tinnitus.
GI: anorexia, cholestatic jaundice, constipation, diarrhea, dry mouth, nausea, vomiting.
GU: urinary frequency, urine retention.
Skin: rash, urticaria.

Overdose and treatment

Overdose and treatment for cyclizine is not documented; however, symptoms may be like those of other antihistamine H_1-receptor antagonists. Signs and symptoms of overdose may include either CNS depression (sedation, reduced mental alertness, apnea, and CV collapse) or CNS stimulation (insomnia, hallucinations, tremors, or seizures). Anticholinergic symptoms, such as dry mouth, flushed skin, fixed and dilated pupils, and GI symptoms, are common, especially in children.

Treat overdose with gastric lavage to empty stomach contents; inducing emesis with ipecac syrup may be ineffective. Treat hypotension with vasopressors and control seizures with diazepam or phenytoin. Do not give stimulants.

Special considerations

▶ Drug may be useful in treating opioid-induced nausea and vomiting; however, haldol or vistaril make better choices.
▶ Injectable cyclizine is for I.M. use only. When giving drug I.M., aspirate carefully for blood return. Inadvertent I.V. administration can cause anaphylactic reaction.
▶ Injectable solution is incompatible with many drugs; check com-

patibility before mixing in same syringe.
▶ Monitor patient for desired effects.
▶ Store drug in a cool place. At room temperature, injection may turn slightly yellow, but change doesn't indicate loss of potency.

Breast-feeding patients

▶ Antihistamines such as cyclizine should not be used during breast-feeding. Most are secreted in breast milk, raising the risk of unusual excitability in infant. Premature infants are at particular risk for seizures. Cyclizine also may inhibit lactation.

Pediatric patients

▶ Drug isn't indicated for children under age 6. They may experience paradoxical hyperexcitability.
▶ Safety and efficacy of I.M. administration in children haven't been established and, therefore, aren't recommended.

Geriatric patients

▶ Elderly patients are usually more sensitive to adverse effects of antihistamines and are especially likely to experience a greater degree of dizziness, sedation, hyperexcitability, dry mouth, and urine retention than younger patients.

Patient teaching

▶ Instruct patient to position himself in places of minimal motion (such as in the middle, not the front or back, of a ship), to avoid excessive intake of food or drink, and not to read while in motion.
▶ Tell patient to avoid hazardous activities until full CNS effects of drug are known.

▶ cyclobenzaprine hydrochloride
Flexeril

Pharmacologic classification:
tricyclic antidepressant derivative

Therapeutic classification:
skeletal muscle relaxant

Pregnancy risk category B

How supplied
Available by prescription only
Tablets: 10 mg

Indications and dosages
Acute, painful musculoskeletal conditions (adjunct)
Adults: 20 to 40 mg P.O. divided b.i.d. to q.i.d. Maximum, 60 mg daily. Drug shouldn't be given for more than 2 weeks.
Fibrositis*
Adults: 10 to 40 mg/day P.O.

Pharmacodynamics
Anticholinergic action: Drug also potentiates the effects of norepinephrine and exhibits anticholinergic effects similar to those of tricyclic antidepressants, including central and peripheral antimuscarinic actions, sedation, and an increase in heart rate.
Skeletal muscle relaxant action: Cyclobenzaprine relaxes skeletal muscles through an unknown mechanism of action. It's a CNS depressant.

Pharmacokinetics
Absorption: Drug is almost completely absorbed during first pass through GI tract. Onset of action occurs within 1 hour, with peak levels in 3 to 8 hours. Duration of action is 12 to 24 hours.
Distribution: About 93% is plasma protein-bound.
Metabolism: During first pass through GI tract and liver, drug and metabolites undergo enterohepatic recycling. The half-life of cyclobenzaprine is 1 to 3 days.
Excretion: Drug is excreted primarily in urine as conjugated metabolites; also in feces via bile as unchanged drug.

Contraindications and precautions
Contraindicated in patients who have received MAO inhibitors within 14 days; during acute recovery phase of MI; and in patients with hyperthyroidism, hypersensitivity to drug, heart block, arrhythmias, conduction disturbances, or heart failure. Use cautiously in elderly or debilitated patients and in those with increased intraocular pressure, glaucoma, or urine retention.

Interactions
Drug-drug
Antidyskinetics, antimuscarinics (especially atropine and related compounds): potentiated antimuscarinic effects. Monitor patient closely.
CNS depressants (including antipsychotics, anxiolytics, opioids, parenteral magnesium salts, tricyclic antidepressants): potentiated CNS depressant effects. Monitor patient closely.
Guanadrel, guanethidine: decreased or blocked antihypertensive effects. Monitor patient's blood pressure.
MAO inhibitors: hyperpyretic crisis, severe seizures, and death have resulted from tricyclic

---

Reactions may be *common*, uncommon, *life-threatening*, or COMMON AND LIFE-THREATENING.

antidepressant-like effect of cyclobenzaprine. Wait 14 days after MAO inhibitor stops before starting cyclobenzaprine; wait 5 to 7 days after cyclobenzaprine stops before starting an MAO inhibitor.

Drug-lifestyle
Alcohol use: potentiated CNS depressant effects. Discourage alcohol use.

Effects on diagnostic tests
None reported.

Adverse reactions
CNS: asthenia, confusion, depression, *dizziness, drowsiness,* fatigue, headache, insomnia, nervousness, paresthesia, *seizures,* syncope, visual disturbances.
CV: *arrhythmias,* hypotension, palpitations, tachycardia, vasodilation.
EENT: blurred vision, *dry mouth.*
GI: abnormal taste, constipation, dyspepsia, nausea.
GU: urinary frequency, urine retention.
Skin: pruritus, rash, urticaria.

Overdose and treatment
Overdose may cause drowsiness, troubled breathing, syncope, seizures, tachycardia, arrhythmias, hallucinations, increase or decrease in body temperature, and vomiting.

To treat overdose, induce emesis or perform gastric lavage. Give 20 to 30 g activated charcoal every 4 to 6 hours for 24 to 48 hours. Take ECG and monitor cardiac functions for arrhythmias. Monitor vital signs, especially body temperature and ECG. Maintain adequate airway and fluid intake. If needed, 1 to 3 mg I.V. physostigmine may be given to combat severe life-threatening antimuscarinic effects. Provide supportive therapy for arrhythmias, cardiac failure, circulatory shock, seizures, and metabolic acidosis as necessary.

Special considerations
▶ Drug may cause effects and adverse reactions similar to those of tricyclic antidepressants.
▶ Antimuscarinic effect may inhibit saliva, raising the risk of dental caries, periodontal disease, oral candidiasis, and mouth discomfort.
▶ Drug is intended for short-term treatment (2 to 3 weeks) because risk of prolonged use isn't known.
▶ Spasmolytic effect usually starts in 1 or 2 days; pain may decline, range of motion may increase, and ability to perform activities of daily living may improve.
▶ Monitor patient for drug effects and GI problems.
▶ Drug doesn't relieve muscle spasm pain.

Pediatric patients
▶ Drug isn't recommended for children under age 15.

Geriatric patients
▶ Elderly patients are more sensitive to potent sedative and anticholinergic effects. Therefore, use in elderly patients is discouraged.

Patient teaching
▶ Warn patient to avoid hazardous activities until full effects of drug are known. It may cause drowsiness and dizziness.
▶ Instruct patient to avoid alcohol and other CNS depressants (unless prescribed), because combined use can cause additive effects.
▶ Suggest that patient relieve dry mouth with frequent clear water

rinses, extra fluid intake, or with sugarless gum or candy.
▶ Tell patient to use cough and cold preparations cautiously because some products contain alcohol.
▶ Instruct patient to check with dentist to minimize risk of dental disease (tooth decay, fungal infections, or gum disease) if treatment lasts longer than 2 weeks.

▶ **cyproheptadine hydrochloride**
Periactin

Pharmacologic classification:
piperidine-derivative antihistamine

Therapeutic classification:
antihistamine (H_1-receptor antagonist), antipruritic

Pregnancy risk category B

How supplied
Available by prescription only
Syrup: 2 mg/5 ml
Tablets: 4 mg

Indications and dosages
Vascular cluster headaches
Adults: 4 mg P.O. t.i.d. or q.i.d. Maximum, 0.5 mg/kg/day.
Children ages 7 to 14: 4 mg P.O. b.i.d. or t.i.d. Maximum, 16 mg/day.
Children ages 2 to 6: 2 mg P.O. b.i.d. or t.i.d. Maximum, 12 mg/day.

Pharmacodynamics
Antihistamine action: Drug competes with histamine for histamine H_1-receptor sites on smooth muscle of the bronchi, GI tract, uterus, and large blood vessels; it binds to cellular receptors, preventing access by histamine, thereby suppressing histamine-induced allergic symptoms. It doesn't directly alter histamine or its release.
Drug also displays significant anticholinergic and antiserotonin activity.

Pharmacokinetics
Absorption: Drug is well absorbed from the GI tract; peak action occurs in 6 to 9 hours.
Distribution: Unknown.
Metabolism: Drug appears to be almost completely metabolized in the liver.
Excretion: Metabolites are excreted primarily in urine; unchanged drug isn't excreted in urine. Small amounts of unchanged cyproheptadine and metabolites are excreted in feces.

Contraindications and precautions
Contraindicated in patients hypersensitive to drug or other drugs of similar chemical structure and in patients with acute asthma, angle-closure glaucoma, stenosing peptic ulcer, symptomatic prostatic hyperplasia, bladder neck obstruction, and pyloroduodenal obstruction. Also, contraindicated in concurrent therapy with MAO inhibitors, in neonates or premature infants, in elderly or debilitated patients, and in breast-feeding patients.
Use cautiously in patients with increased intraocular pressure, hyperthyroidism, CV disease, hypertension, or bronchial asthma.

Interactions
Drug-drug
CNS depressants (antianxiety drugs, barbiturates, sleeping aids,

---

tranquilizers): potentiated sedative effects. Avoid use together.

MAO inhibitors: interfere with detoxification of antihistamines and thus prolong and intensify central depressant and anticholinergic effects. Avoid use together.

Thyrotropin-releasing hormone: may increase serum amylase and prolactin levels. Monitor serum levels.

Drug-lifestyle

Alcohol use: concomitant effects produce additive sedative effects. Discourage alcohol use.

Effects on diagnostic tests

Discontinue drug 4 days before diagnostic skin tests. Antihistamines can prevent, reduce, or mask positive skin test response.

Adverse reactions

CNS: confusion, *drowsiness,* dizziness, fatigue, headache, incoordination, insomnia, nervousness, restlessness, sedation, *seizures,* sleepiness, tremor.
CV: hypotension, palpitations, tachycardia.
GI: constipation, diarrhea, *dry mouth,* epigastric distress, nausea, vomiting.
GU: urinary frequency, urine retention.
Hematologic: *agranulocytosis,* hemolytic anemia, *leukopenia, thrombocytopenia.*
Metabolic: weight gain.
Respiratory: *anaphylactic shock.*
Skin: photosensitivity, rash, urticaria.

Overdose and treatment

Overdose may cause either CNS depression (sedation, reduced mental alertness, apnea, and CV collapse) or CNS stimulation (insomnia, hallucinations, tremors, or seizures). Anticholinergic symptoms, such as dry mouth, flushed skin, fixed and dilated pupils, and GI symptoms, are common, especially in children.

Treat overdose by inducing emesis with ipecac syrup (in conscious patient), followed by activated charcoal to reduce further drug absorption. Use gastric lavage if patient is unconscious or ipecac fails. Treat hypotension with vasopressors, and control seizures with diazepam or phenytoin. Do not give stimulants.

Special considerations

▶ Drug is also used as a treatment for Cushing's syndrome and has been used experimentally to stimulate appetite and promote weight gain in children.
▶ Drug may be useful for migraine prophylaxis in children, by blocking serotonin.
▶ Give drug with food.
▶ Syrup form is available for children.
▶ Monitor patient's weight because drug can cause weight gain.
▶ In some patients, sedative effect disappears in 3 or 4 days.
▶ Drug may also be used for allergy symptoms, pruritus, cold urticaria, and allergic conjunctivitis.

Breast-feeding patients

▶ Antihistamines such as cyproheptadine should not be used during breast-feeding. Many of these drugs are secreted in breast milk, raising the risk of unusual excitability. Premature infants are at particular risk for seizures.

Pediatric patients
▶ CNS stimulation (agitation, confusion, tremors, hallucinations) is more common in children and may require dosage reduction.
▶ Drug is not indicated for use in newborn or premature infants.

Geriatric patients
▶ Elderly patients are more susceptible to sedative effects.
▶ Elderly patients may experience dizziness or hypotension more readily than younger patients.

Patient teaching
▶ Instruct patient to change positions slowly.
▶ Inform patient about potential adverse reactions.

▶ dantrolene sodium
Dantrium

Pharmacologic classification:
hydantoin derivative

Therapeutic classification:
skeletal muscle relaxant

Pregnancy risk category C

How supplied
Available by prescription only
Capsules: 25 mg, 50 mg, 100 mg
Injection: 20 mg parenteral (contains 3 g mannitol)

Indications and dosages
Spasticity from upper motor neuron disorders
Adults: 25 mg/day P.O., increased by 25 mg at 4- to 7-day intervals, up to 100 mg b.i.d. to q.i.d. Maximum, 400 mg daily.

Children over age 5: 0.5 mg/kg P.O. b.i.d., increased to t.i.d. and then q.i.d. Increase dosage further, p.r.n., by 0.5 mg/kg up to 3 mg/kg b.i.d. to q.i.d. Maximum, 100 mg q.i.d.
Succinylcholine-induced muscle fasciculations and postoperative muscle pain*
Adults under 45 kg (99 lb): 100 mg P.O. 2 hours before succinylcholine.
Adults over 45 kg (99 lb): 150 mg P.O. 2 hours before succinylcholine.

Pharmacodynamics
Skeletal muscle relaxant action: A hydantoin derivative, dantrolene is chemically and pharmacologically unrelated to other skeletal muscle relaxants. It directly affects skeletal muscle, reducing muscle tension. It interferes with the release of calcium ions from the sarcoplasmic reticulum, resulting in decreased muscle contraction. This mechanism is of particular importance in malignant hyperthermia when increased myoplasmic calcium ion concentrations activate acute catabolism in the skeletal muscle cell. Dantrolene prevents or reduces the increase in myoplasmic calcium levels associated with malignant hyperthermia crises.

Pharmacokinetics
Absorption: 35% of oral dose is absorbed through GI tract, with serum half-life reached 8 to 9 hours after oral administration and 5 hours after I.V. administration. Therapeutic effect in patients with upper motor neuron disorders may take 1 week or more.
Distribution: Dantrolene is substantially plasma protein-bound, mainly to albumin.

Metabolism: Drug is metabolized in the liver to its less active 5-hydroxy derivatives and to its amino derivative by reductive pathways.
Excretion: Drug is excreted in urine as metabolites.

Contraindications and precautions

Contraindicated when spasticity maintains motor function in upper motor neuron disorders, for spasms in rheumatic disorders, in patients with active hepatic disease, and in breast-feeding patients. Also contraindicated in combination with verapamil in managing malignant hyperthermia.

Use cautiously in women (especially those taking estrogen), in patients over age 35, and in patients with hepatic disease or severely impaired cardiac or pulmonary function.

Interactions
Drug-drug

CNS depressants (antipsychotics, anxiolytics, opioids, tricyclic antidepressants): increased CNS depression. Reduce dosage of one or both if used concurrently.
Estrogen: may increase the risk of hepatotoxicity in women over age 35. Monitor hepatic function.
Verapamil: cardiac collapse (rare). If concomitant use is necessary, monitor patient closely.

Drug-lifestyle

Alcohol use: increased CNS depression. Avoid use together.

Effects on diagnostic tests
None reported.

Adverse reactions

CNS: *confusion, drowsiness, dizziness, fatigue, headache, insomnia, light-headedness, malaise, muscle weakness, nervousness, seizures.*
CV: blood pressure changes, tachycardia.
EENT: altered taste, diplopia, excessive lacrimation, speech disturbance, visual disturbances.
GI: anorexia, constipation, cramping, dysphagia, GI bleeding, metallic taste, severe diarrhea.
GU: crystalluria, difficult erection, dysuria, hematuria, incontinence, nocturia, urinary frequency, urine retention.
Hepatic: altered liver function test results, *hepatitis.*
Musculoskeletal: back pain, myalgia.
Respiratory: pleural effusion with pericarditis.
Skin: abnormal hair growth, diaphoresis, eczematous eruption, photosensitivity and extravasation with I.V. administration, pruritus, urticaria.
Other: chills, fever.

Overdose and treatment

Overdose may cause exaggeration of adverse reactions, particularly CNS depression, and nausea and vomiting.

Treatment includes supportive measures, gastric lavage, and observation of symptoms. Maintain adequate airway, have emergency ventilation equipment on hand, monitor ECG, and administer large quantities of I.V. solutions to prevent crystalluria. Monitor vital signs closely. The benefit of dialysis is not known.

Special considerations
▶ Before therapy begins, check patient's baseline neuromuscular functions (posture, gait, coordination, range of motion, muscle strength and tone, presence of abnormal muscle movements, and reflexes) for later comparisons.
▶ Perform baseline and regularly scheduled liver function tests (alkaline phosphatase, ALT, AST, and total bilirubin), blood cell counts, and renal function tests.
▶ To reconstitute for I.V. use, add 60 ml sterile water for injection to 20-mg vial. Don't use bacteriostatic water, D_5W, or normal saline for injection. Reconstituted solution should be stored away from direct sunlight at room temperature, and should be discarded after 6 hours.
▶ To prepare suspension for single oral dose, dissolve contents of appropriate number of capsules in fruit juice or other suitable liquid.
▶ Improvement may require 1 week or more of drug therapy.
▶ Drug may cause muscle weakness and impaired walking ability. Use with caution and carefully supervise patients receiving drug for prophylactic treatment for malignant hyperthermia.
▶ Walking should be supervised until patient's reaction to drug is known. With relief of spasticity, patient may lose ability to maintain balance.
▶ Because of the risk of hepatic injury, discontinue drug if improvement is not evident within 45 days.
▶ If used with other central-acting drugs, additive effects may be seen.
▶ Risk of hepatotoxicity may be greater in women, patients over age 35, and in those taking other medications (especially estrogen) or high dantrolene doses (400 mg or more daily) for prolonged periods. Monitor hepatic function closely.
▶ Drug may be useful in treating extrapyramidal effects of neuroleptics. It also is indicated in prevention and treatment of malignant hyperthermia.

Pediatric patients
▶ Drug isn't recommended for long-term use in children under age 5.

Geriatric patients
▶ Administer drug with extreme caution to elderly patients.

Patient teaching
▶ Warn patient to avoid hazardous activities that require alertness until CNS depressant effects are determined. Drug may cause drowsiness.
▶ Advise patient to avoid excessive or unnecessary exposure to sunlight and to use protective clothing and a sunscreen agent because photosensitivity reactions may occur.
▶ Warn patient to avoid OTC medications, alcoholic beverages, and other CNS depressants except as prescribed because hepatotoxicity occurs more commonly after concurrent use of other drugs with dantrolene.
▶ If patient misses a dose, tell her to take it within 1 hour; otherwise, she should omit the dose and return to regular dosing schedule. Tell her not to double the dose.
▶ Advise patient to report adverse reactions immediately.
▶ Instruct patient to report promptly the onset of jaundice: yellow skin or sclerae, dark urine, clay-colored stools, itching, and abdominal discomfort. Hepatotoxicity oc-

curs more frequently between the third and twelfth month of therapy.

▶ Advise patient susceptible to malignant hyperthermia to wear medical identification (for example, Medic Alert) indicating diagnosis, physician's name and telephone number, drug causing reaction, and treatment used.

▶ Tell patient to store drug away from heat and direct light (not in bathroom medicine cabinet). Keep out of reach of children.

▶ desipramine hydrochloride
Norpramin

Pharmacologic classification:
dibenzazepine tricyclic antidepressant

Therapeutic classification:
antidepressant

Pregnancy risk category NR

How supplied
Available by prescription only
Tablets: 10 mg, 25 mg, 50 mg, 75 mg, 100 mg, 150 mg

Indications and dosages
Neuropathic pain
Adults: 25 mg/day P.O. h.s. May increase dose by 25 mg/day until desired therapeutic effects occur or you reach maximum dose of 200 mg/day.

Pharmacodynamics
Analgesic action: Unknown.
Antidepressant action: Drug probably exerts antidepressant effects by inhibiting reuptake of norepinephrine and serotonin in CNS nerve terminals (presynaptic neurons), which results in increased levels and enhanced activity of these neurotransmitters in the synaptic cleft. Desipramine inhibits reuptake of norepinephrine more strongly than serotonin; it has a lesser incidence of sedative effects and less anticholinergic and hypotensive activity than its parent compound, imipramine.

Pharmacokinetics
Absorption: Drug is absorbed rapidly from the GI tract after oral administration.
Distribution: Drug is distributed widely into the body, including the CNS and breast milk. Drug is 90% protein-bound. Effects peak in 4 to 6 hours; steady state occurs in 2 to 11 days, and full therapeutic effect occurs in 2 to 4 weeks. Proposed therapeutic plasma levels (parent drug and metabolite) range from 125 to 300 ng/ml.
Metabolism: Desipramine is metabolized by the liver; a significant first-pass effect may explain variability of serum levels in different patients taking the same dosage.
Excretion: Drug is excreted primarily in urine.

Contraindications and precautions
Contraindicated in patients hypersensitive to drug, in patients who have taken an MAO inhibitor within 14 days, and in patients in the acute recovery phase of MI.

Use with extreme caution in patients with history of seizure disorders or urine retention, CV or thyroid disease, or glaucoma, and in those taking thyroid medication.

Interactions
Drug-drug
Antiarrhythmics (disopyramide, procainamide, quinidine), pimozide, thyroid hormones: may increase risk of cardiac arrhythmias and conduction defects. Monitor patient's cardiac status closely if concomitant use necessary.

Anticholinergics (antihistamines, antiparkinsonians, atropine, meperidine, phenothiazines): may produce oversedation, paralytic ileus, visual changes, and severe constipation. Monitor patient closely.

Barbiturates: induces desipramine metabolism. Monitor patient for decreased therapeutic efficacy.

Beta blockers, cimetidine, methylphenidate, oral contraceptives, propoxyphene: may inhibit desipramine metabolism, increasing plasma levels and toxicity. Monitor patient for side effects.

Central-acting antihypertensives (clonidine, guanabenz, guanadrel, guanethidine, methyldopa, reserpine): may decrease hypotensive effects. Monitor blood pressure.

Cimetidine, fluoxetine, fluvoxamine, paroxetine, sertraline: may increase serum desipramine levels. Monitor patient for adverse effects.

CNS depressants (analgesics, anesthetics, barbiturates, opioids, tranquilizers): additive effects. Avoid using together. If necessary to use together, monitor closely.

Disulfiram, ethchlorvynol: possible delirium and tachycardia. Avoid using together.

Haloperidol, phenothiazines: decreases desipramine metabolism. Monitor patient for decreased therapeutic efficacy.

MAO inhibitors: may cause severe excitation, hyperpyrexia, or seizures, usually with high dosage. Avoid using together. If necessary for concomitant use, monitor patient closely.

Metrizamide: may increase the risk of seizures. Avoid using together.

Selective serotonin-reuptake inhibitors: patient may have toxic reaction to tricyclic antidepressant at much reduced dosages. Use together with caution.

Sympathomimetics (clonidine, ephedrine, epinephrine, norepinephrine, phenylephrine, phenylpropanolamine): may increase blood pressure. Monitor blood pressure.

Warfarin: may increase PT and the risk of bleeding. Monitor patient's PT and INR.

Drug-lifestyle
Alcohol use: may enhance CNS depression. Avoid use together.

Heavy smoking: may lower plasma desipramine levels. Discourage smoking.

Sun exposure: may increase risk of photosensitivity. Take precautions.

Effects on diagnostic tests
None reported.

Adverse reactions
CNS: agitation, confusion, anxiety, *dizziness, drowsiness,* EEG changes, excitation, extrapyramidal reactions, headache, nervousness, restlessness, ***seizures,*** tremor, weakness.

CV: *ECG changes,* hypertension, orthostatic hypotension, *tachycardia.*

EENT: *blurred vision,* mydriasis, tinnitus.

GI: anorexia, *constipation, dry mouth,* nausea, paralytic ileus, vomiting,

GU: *urine retention.*

Reactions may be *common*, uncommon, *life-threatening*, or COMMON AND LIFE-THREATENING.

Hematologic: decreased WBC counts.
Hepatic: elevated liver function tests.
Metabolic: hyperglycemia, hypoglycemia.
Skin: *diaphoresis,* photosensitivity, rash, urticaria,
Other: *hypersensitivity reaction, sudden death* (in children).

Overdose and treatment

The first 12 hours after acute ingestion are a stimulatory phase characterized by excessive anticholinergic activity (agitation, irritation, confusion, hallucinations, parkinsonian symptoms, hyperthermia, seizures, urine retention, dry mucous membranes, pupillary dilatation, constipation, and ileus). This is followed by CNS depressant effects, including hypothermia, decreased or absent reflexes, sedation, hypotension, cyanosis; and cardiac irregularities, including tachycardia, conduction disturbances, and quinidine-like effects on the ECG.

Severity of overdose is best indicated by widening of the QRS complex, which usually represents a serum level in excess of 1,000 ng/ml; serum levels are generally not helpful. Metabolic acidosis may follow hypotension, hypoventilation, and seizures.

Treatment is symptomatic and supportive, including maintaining airway, stable body temperature, and fluid and electrolyte balance. Induce emesis with ipecac if patient is conscious; follow with gastric lavage and activated charcoal to prevent further absorption. Dialysis is of little use. Physostigmine may be used with caution to reverse CV abnormalities or coma;

too rapid administration may cause seizures. Treat seizures with parenteral diazepam or phenytoin; arrhythmias, with parenteral phenytoin or lidocaine; and acidosis, with sodium bicarbonate. Do not give barbiturates; these may enhance CNS and respiratory depressant effects.

Special considerations

▶ Desipramine is useful for many types of neuropathic pain. As with other tricyclic antidepressants, it is useful as an adjunct for chronic pain, especially when pain is accompanied by insomnia.
▶ Check standing and sitting blood pressure to assess orthostasis before administering desipramine.
▶ Drug has a lesser risk of sedative effects and fewer anticholinergic and hypotensive effects than its parent compound imipramine.
▶ Tolerance usually develops to the sedative effects of the drug during initial weeks of therapy.
▶ Because patients have used drug to commit suicide, dispense drug in the smallest possible quantities to depressed outpatients.
▶ Discontinue drug at least 48 hours before surgical procedures.
▶ Monitor patient closely when discontinuing drug. Taper it gradually over 3 to 6 weeks.
▶ Abrupt withdrawal of therapy may cause headache, malaise, and nausea, which don't indicate addiction.
▶ Drug may also be used for depression.
▶ Drug therapy in depressed patients with bipolar illness may induce hypomania.

Breast-feeding patients
▶ Drug appears in breast milk at levels equal to those in maternal serum. The potential benefit to the mother should outweigh the risks for infant.

Pediatric patients
▶ Drug isn't recommended for patients under age 12.

Geriatric patients
▶ Elderly patients may be more susceptible to adverse CV and anticholinergic effects.

Patient teaching
▶ Tell patient to take the full dose at bedtime to alleviate daytime sedation.
▶ Explain that full effects of drug may not become apparent for 4 weeks or more after initiation of therapy.
▶ Tell patient to take the medication exactly as prescribed and not to double the dose for missed ones.
▶ To prevent dizziness, advise patient to lie down for about 30 minutes after each dose at start of therapy and to avoid sudden postural changes, especially when rising to upright position.
▶ Warn patient not to stop taking drug suddenly.
▶ Encourage patient to report unusual or troublesome effects, especially confusion, movement disorders, rapid heartbeat, dizziness, fainting, or difficulty urinating.
▶ Tell patient sugarless chewing gum or hard candy or ice may alleviate dry mouth.
▶ Stress importance of regular dental hygiene to avoid caries.
▶ Tell patient to store drug safely away from children.

▶ dexamethasone (systemic)
Decadron, Deronil◇, Dexasone◇, Dexone, Hexadrol

▶ dexamethasone acetate
Dalalone D.P., Decadron-LA, Decaject-L.A., Dexasone-L.A., Dexone L.A., Solurex LA

▶ dexamethasone sodium phosphate
AK-Dex, Dalalone, Decadrol, Decadron, Decaject, Dexameth, Dexasone, Dexone, Hexadrol Phosphate, Oradexon◇, Solurex

Pharmacologic classification: *glucocorticoid*

Therapeutic classification: *anti-inflammatory, immunosuppressant*

Pregnancy risk category NR

How supplied
Available by prescription only
dexamethasone
Elixir: 0.5 mg/5 ml
Oral solution: 0.5 mg/0.5 ml, 0.5 mg/5 ml
Tablets: 0.25 mg, 0.5 mg, 0.75 mg, 1 mg, 1.5 mg, 2 mg, 4 mg, 6 mg
dexamethasone acetate
Injection: 8 mg/ml, 16 mg/ml suspension
dexamethasone sodium phosphate
Injection: 4 mg/ml, 10 mg/ml, 20 mg/ml, 24 mg/ml

Indications and dosages
Cerebral edema
dexamethasone sodium phosphate
Adults: initially, 10 mg I.V., then 4 mg I.M. q 6 hours for 2 to 4 days, then taper over 5 to 7 days.

Inflammatory conditions, allergic reactions, neoplasias
Adults: 0.75 to 9 mg P.O. daily divided b.i.d., t.i.d., or q.i.d.
Children: 0.024 to 0.34 mg/kg P.O. daily in four divided doses.

dexamethasone acetate
Adults: 4 to 16 mg intra-articularly or into soft tissue q 1 to 3 weeks; 0.8 to 1.6 mg into lesions q 1 to 3 weeks; or 8 to 16 mg I.M. q 1 to 3 weeks, p.r.n.

dexamethasone sodium phosphate
Adults: 0.2 to 6 mg intra-articularly, intralesionally, or into soft tissue; or 0.5 to 9 mg I.M.

dexamethasone sodium phosphate
Adults: 0.5 to 9 mg I.M. or I.V. daily.
Children: 0.235 to 1.25 mg/m I.M. or I.V. once daily or b.i.d.

Prevention of chemotherapy-induced nausea and vomiting*
Adults: 10 to 20 mg I.V. before administration of chemotherapy. Additional doses (individualized for each patient and usually lower than initial dose) may be administered I.V. or P.O. for 24 to 72 hours following chemotherapy, if needed.

Pharmacodynamics

Anti-inflammatory action: Dexamethasone and other corticosteroids have instrinsic anti-inflammatory effects. It causes suppression of the immune system by reducing activity and volume of the lymphatic system, producing lymphocytopenia (primarily T-lymphocytes), decreasing passage of immune complexes through basement membranes, and possibly by depressing reactivity of tissue to antigen-antibody interactions.

Drug is a long-acting synthetic adrenocorticoid with strong anti-inflammatory activity and minimal mineralocorticoid properties. It is 25 to 30 times more potent than an equal weight of hydrocortisone.

The acetate salt is a suspension and should not be used I.V. It is particularly useful as an anti-inflammatory agent in intra-articular, I.D., and intralesional injections.

The sodium phosphate salt is highly soluble and has a more rapid onset and a shorter duration of action than does the acetate salt. It is most commonly used for cerebral edema and unresponsive shock. It can also be used in intra-articular, intralesional, or soft tissue inflammation. Other uses for dexamethasone are symptomatic treatment of bronchial asthma, chemotherapy-induced nausea, and as a diagnostic test for Cushing's syndrome.

Pharmacokinetics

Absorption: After oral administration, drug is absorbed readily, and peak effects occur in about 1 to 2 hours. The suspension for injection has a variable onset and duration of action (ranging from 2 days to 3 weeks), depending on whether it is injected into an intra-articular space, a muscle, or the blood supply to the muscle. After I.V. injection, dexamethosone is rapidly and completely absorbed into the tissues.
Distribution: Drug is removed rapidly from the blood and distributed to muscle, liver, skin, intestines, and kidneys. Dexamethasone is bound weakly to plasma proteins (transcortin and albumin). Only the unbound portion is active. Adreno-

---

corticoids are distributed into breast milk and through the placenta.

Metabolism: Metabolized in the liver to inactive glucuronide and sulfate metabolites.

Excretion: The inactive metabolites and small amounts of unmetabolized drug are excreted by the kidneys. Insignificant quantities of drug are also excreted in feces; biological half-life is 36 to 54 hours.

Contraindications and precautions

Contraindicated in patients hypersensitive to any component of drug and in those with systemic fungal infections.

Use cautiously in patients with recent MI, GI ulcer, renal disease, hypertension, osteoporosis, diabetes mellitus, hypothyroidism, cirrhosis, diverticulitis, nonspecific ulcerative colitis, recent intestinal anastomoses, thromboembolic disorders, seizures, myasthenia gravis, heart failure, tuberculosis, ocular herpes simplex, emotional instability, and psychotic tendencies. Because some formulations contain sulfite preservatives, also use cautiously in patients sensitive to sulfites.

Interactions
Drug-drug

Amphotericin B, diuretics: may enhance hypokalemia, which may increase the risk of toxicity in patients concurrently receiving cardiac glycosides. Monitor serum potassioum levels.

Antacids, cholestyramine, colestipol: may decrease corticosteroid absorption. Monitor patient for decreased therapeutic effects.

Barbiturates, phenytoin, rifampin: may decrease corticosteroid effects because of increased hepatic metabolism. Monitor patient for decreased therapeutic effects.

Estrogens: may reduce dexamethasone metabolism by increasing transcortin level. Corticosteroid half-life is then prolonged because of increased protein-binding. Monitor patient for adverse effects.

Insulin, oral antidiabetic drugs: may cause hyperglycemia. Monitor serum glucose levels, and adjust dosage accordingly.

Isoniazid, salicylates: may increase metabolism of these drugs. Use together cautiously.

Oral anticoagulants: may decrease anticoagulant effects (rare). Monitor coagulation studies.

Skin-test antigens: decreased skin response. Defer skin testing until therapy is completed.

Toxoids, vaccines: may decrease antibody response and increase risk of neurologic complications. Defer until therapy is completed.

Ulcer-causing drugs (aspirin, NSAIDs): may increase the risk of GI ulceration. Avoid using together.

Drug-lifestyle

Alcohol use: increased risk of gastric irritation and GI ulceration. Discourage alcohol use.

Effects on diagnostic tests

Dexamethasone causes false-negative results in the nitroblue tetrazolium test for systemic bacterial infections and decreases ^{131}I uptake and protein-bound iodine levels in thyroid function tests.

Adverse reactions

CNS: *euphoria,* headache, *insomnia,* paresthesia, pseudotumor cerebri, psychotic behavior, *seizures,* vertigo.

CV: *arrhythmias,* edema, *heart failure,* hypertension, *thromboembolism,* thrombophlebitis.
EENT: cataracts, glaucoma.
GI: GI irritation, increased appetite, nausea, *pancreatitis, peptic ulceration,* vomiting.
GU: menstrual irregularities,
Metabolic: *acute adrenal insufficiency may follow increased stress (infection, surgery, or trauma) or abrupt withdrawal after long-term therapy;* carbohydrate intolerance; decreased levels of thyroxine, and triiodothyronine, and increased urine glucose and calcium levels; hyperglycemia; hypocalcemia; hypokalemia.
Musculoskeletal: myopathy, osteoporosis.
Skin: acne, delayed wound healing, various skin eruptions; atrophy at I.M. injection sites, hirsutism.
Other: cushingoid state (moonface, buffalo hump, central obesity), susceptibility to infections, growth suppression in children.

Overdose and treatment
Acute ingestion, even in massive doses, rarely poses a clinical problem. Toxic signs and symptoms rarely occur if drug is used for less than 3 weeks, even at large dosage ranges. However, chronic use causes adverse physiologic effects, including suppression of the hypothalamic-pituitary-adrenal axis, cushingoid appearance, muscle weakness, and osteoporosis.

Special considerations
▶ Most adverse reactions to corticosteroids are dose- or duration-dependent.
▶ Drug is classified as a multipurpose analgesic. It is useful for bone cancer, headache pain, and spinal cord compression. In palliative care, it may stimulate appetite and mood.
▶ When administering as direct I.V injection, inject undiluted over at least 1 minute. When administering as an intermittent or continuous infusion, dilute solution according to the manufacturer's instructions and give over the prescribed duration. If used for continuous infusion, change solution every 24 hours.
▶ Monitor patient for therapeutic efficacy and adverse effects.
▶ Monitor serum gluocse levels in patients with diabetes, and adjust dosage accordingly.
▶ Abrupt withdrawal may cause anorexia, arthralgia, depression, dizziness, dyspnea, fainting, fatigue, fever, hypoglycemia, lethargy, rebound inflammation, orthostatic hypotension, weakness.
▶ After prolonged use, sudden withdrawal may be fatal.
▶ Drug is being used investigationally to prevent hyaline membrane disease (respiratory distress syndrome) in premature infants. The suspension (phosphate salt) is administered I.M. to the mother two or three times daily for 2 days before delivery.

Pediatric patients
▶ Long-term use of drug in children and adolescents may delay growth and maturation.

Patient teaching
▶ Instruct patient on proper administration of drug.
▶ Urge patient to report any unusual effects.

▶ dextroamphetamine sulfate
Dexedrine, Ferndex

Pharmacologic classification:
amphetamine

Therapeutic classification:
CNS stimulant, short-term adjunctive anorexigenic, sympathomimetic amine

Controlled substance schedule II

Pregnancy risk category C

How supplied
Available by prescription only
Capsules (sustained-release): 5 mg, 10 mg, 15 mg
Elixir: 5 mg/5 ml
Tablets: 5 mg, 10 mg, 20 mg

Indications and dosages
Narcolepsy
Adults: 5 to 60 mg/day P.O. in divided doses. Long-acting dosage forms allow once-daily dosing.
Children over age 12: 10 mg/day P.O., increased by 10 mg weekly, as indicated.
Children ages 6 to 12: 5 mg/day P.O., increased by 5 mg weekly, as indicated.
Attention deficit hyperactivity disorder
Children age 6 and older: 5 mg once daily or b.i.d., increased by 5 mg weekly, p.r.n. Total daily dose should rarely exceed 40 mg.
Children ages 3 to 5: 2.5 mg/day P.O., increased by 2.5 mg weekly, as needed. Not recommended for children under age 3.

Pharmacodynamics
Anorexigenic action: Anorexigenic effects are thought to occur in the hypothalamus, where decreased smell and taste acuity decreases appetite. They may be tried for short-term control of refractory obesity, with caloric restriction and behavior modification.
CNS stimulant action: Amphetamines are sympathomimetic amines with CNS stimulant activity; in hyperactive children, they have a paradoxical calming effect.

The cerebral cortex and reticular activating system appear to be the primary sites of activity; amphetamines release nerve terminal stores of norepinephrine, promoting nerve impulse transmission. At high dosages, effects are mediated by dopamine.

Amphetamines are used to treat narcolepsy and as adjuncts to psychosocial measures in attention deficit disorder in children. Their precise mechanism of action in these conditions is unknown.

Pharmacokinetics
Absorption: Drug is rapidly absorbed from the GI tract; serum levels peak 2 to 4 hours after oral dose; long-acting capsules are absorbed more slowly and have a longer duration of action.
Distribution: Drug is distributed widely throughout the body. Pulmonary hypertension and cardiac valvular damage are possible.
Metabolism: Unknown.
Excretion: Drug is excreted in urine.

Contraindications and precautions
Contraindicated in patients with hypersensitivity or idiosyncrasy to the sympathomimetic amines, within 14 days of MAO inhibitor therapy, and in those with hyper-

thyroidism, moderate to severe hypertension, pulmonary hypertension, symptomatic CV disease, history of cardiac valve damage, glaucoma, advanced arteriosclerosis, and history of drug abuse.

Use cautiously in patients with motor and phonic tics, Tourette syndrome, and agitated states.

Interactions
Drug-drug
Acetazolamide, alkalizing drugs, antacids, sodium bicarbonate: enhances dextroamphetamine reabsorption and prolongs duration of action. Monitor patient for adverse effects.

Acidifying drugs, ascorbic acid, ammonium chloride: enhances dextroamphetamine excretion and shortens duration of action. Monitor patient for decreased effects.

Adrenergic blockers: inhibited by amphetamines. Avoid concurrent use.

Antihypertensives: may antagonize antihypertensive effects. Monitor blood pressure closely.

Barbiturates: antagonizes dextroamphetamine by CNS depression. Avoid using together.

Chlorpromazine: inhibits central stimulant effects of amphetamines. Can be used to treat amphetamine poisoning.

CNS stimulants, haloperidol, phenothiazines, theophylline, tricyclic antidepressants: increases CNS effects. Monitor patient for effects if used together.

Insulin, oral antidiabetic drugs: may alter requirements. Monitor serum glucose and adjust dosage accordingly.

Lithium carbonate: may inhibit antiobesity and stimulating effects of amphetamines. Monitor patient for effects.

MAO inhibitors or drugs with MAO-inhibiting activity (such as furazolidone): use within 14 days may cause hypertensive crisis. Avoid using together; if necessary, monitor blood pressure closely.

Meperidine: potentiates analgesic effect. Avoid using together. If necessary to use together, monitor patient closely.

Methenamine therapy: increases urinary excretion of amphetamine. Watch for reduced efficacy.

Norepinephrine: enhances adrenergic effects. Avoid using together.

Phenobarbital, phenytoin: may produce synergistic anticonvulsant action. Avoid using together.

Drug-food
Caffeine: may increase amphetamine and related amine effects. Discourage caffeine intake.

Effects on diagnostic tests
Drug may elevate plasma corticosteroid levels and may interfere with urinary steroid determinations.

Adverse reactions
CNS: chills, dizziness, dysphoria, euphoria, headache, *insomnia,* overstimulation, *restlessness,* tremor.

CV: *arrhythmias, cardiac valve damage,* hypertension, *palpitations, tachycardia.*

GI: anorexia, constipation, diarrhea, dry mouth, other GI disturbances, unpleasant taste.

GU: impotence, altered libido.

Metabolic: weight loss.

Respiratory: *pulmonary hypertension.*

Skin: urticaria.

Overdose and treatment

Individual responses to overdose vary widely. Toxic symptoms may occur at 15 mg and 30 mg and can cause severe reactions; however, doses of 400 mg or more have not always proved fatal.

Overdose may cause restlessness, tremor, hyperreflexia, tachypnea, confusion, aggressiveness, hallucinations, and panic; fatigue and depression usually follow excitement stage. Other symptoms may include arrhythmias, shock, alterations in blood pressure, nausea, vomiting, diarrhea, and abdominal cramps; death is usually preceded by seizures and coma.

Treat overdose symptomatically and supportively: if ingestion is recent (within 4 hours), use gastric lavage or emesis and sedate with a barbiturate; monitor vital signs and fluid and electrolyte balance. Urine acidification may enhance excretion. Saline catharsis (magnesium citrate) may hasten GI evacuation of unabsorbed sustained-release drug.

Special considerations

▶ Dextroamphetamine may produce additive analgesia when combined with opioids postoperatively.
▶ Drug is useful when pain is accompanied by sedation, such as in palliative care.
▶ Give drug 30 to 60 minutes before meals when using it for anorexigenic effects. To minimize insomnia, avoid giving drug within 6 hours of bedtime.
▶ When tolerance to anorexigenic effect develops, dosage should be discontinued, not increased.

▶ For narcolepsy, patient should take first dose on awakening.
▶ Monitor patient's vital signs regularly, and watch for signs of excessive stimulation.
▶ Monitor blood and urine glucose levels. Drug may alter daily insulin requirement in patients with diabetes.

Breast-feeding patients

▶ Safety hasn't been established. Alternative feeding method is recommended during therapy with dextroamphetamine sulfate.

Pediatric patients

▶ Drug isn't recommended for treatment of obesity in children under age 12.

Geriatric patients

▶ Use lower doses in elderly patients.
▶ Avoid using drug in elderly patients with CV, CNS, or GI disturbances.

Patient teaching

▶ Instruct patient to take drug early in the day to minimize insomnia.
▶ Tell patient not to crush sustained-release forms or to increase dosage.
▶ Warn patient to avoid hazardous activities that require alertness until CNS response is determined.
▶ Teach parents to provide drug-free periods for children with attention deficit disorder, especially during periods of reduced stress.

Reactions may be *common*, uncommon, *life-threatening*, or COMMON AND LIFE-THREATENING.

❱ dezocine
Dalgan

Pharmacologic classification:
opioid (narcotic) agonist-antagonist

Therapeutic classification:
analgesic

Pregnancy risk category C

How supplied
Available by prescription only
Injection: 5 mg/ml, 10 mg/ml,
15 mg/ml

Indications and dosages
Moderate to severe pain
Adults: 5 to 20 mg I.M. every 3 to
6 hours or 2.5 mg to 10 mg I.V.
every 2 to 4 hours. Maximum
concentration single I.M. dose is
20 mg, with a maximum daily
dosage of 120 mg. Maximum
dosage for I.V. use has not been
determined.

◲ **DOSAGE ADJUSTMENT.** Limited studies suggest that drug should be
used with caution and in lower
doses if patient has renal or hepatic
dysfunction. Half-life increases in
hepatic failure. The primary means
of drug elimination is renal excretion of the metabolite.

Pharmacodynamics
Analgesic action: A synthetic opioid agonist-antagonist, dezocine
produces postoperative analgesia
qualitatively similar to morphine.

Pharmacokinetics
Absorption: The drug is rapidly
and completely absorbed after I.M.
administration. Levels peak 10 to
90 minutes after I.M. administration. Peak analgesic effects appear
to lag blood levels by 20 to 60
minutes.
Distribution: After a 10-mg I.M.
injection, peak serum levels average 19 ng/ml. The average volume
of distribution is 10.1 L/kg and is
increased by hepatic disease. The
degree of serum protein-binding is
not known.
Metabolism: Probably hepatic. A
glucuronide conjugate has been
identified.
Excretion: About 66% of a dose
appears in the urine. About 1% is
unchanged drug; the remainder is
the metabolite. Half-life is about
2½ hours, longer with hepatic disease.

Contraindications and precautions
Contraindicated in patients hypersensitive to drug and in those
physically dependent on narcotics.
    Use very cautiously in patients
with head injury because drug's
CNS depressant effects may obscure clinical signs. Related drugs
have caused elevations of CSF
pressure in patients with head injury. Use cautiously and in lower
doses in patients with chronic respiratory disease and in patients undergoing biliary surgery. Related
drugs have caused significant increases in pressure within the common bile duct.

Interactions
Drug-drug
Opioids: patients may experience
withdrawal effects after receiving
dezocine. Monitor patient.

Drug-lifestyle
Alcohol use: concomitant use may
cause additive effects. Discourage
use of alcohol.

◇ Available in Canada only   *Unlabeled use

Effects on diagnostic tests
None reported.

Adverse reactions
CNS: anxiety, *dizziness,* headache, *sedation,* sleep disturbances, *vertigo.*
CV: chest pain, edema, flushing, hypertension, hypotension, irregular heartbeat, thrombophlebitis.
EENT: dry mouth.
GI: abdominal distress, constipation, diarrhea, *nausea, vomiting.*
Hematologic: anemia.
Respiratory: *respiratory depression.*
Skin: diaphoresis, *irritation at injection site,* pruritus, rash.
Other: chills.

Overdose and treatment
Dezocine overdose hasn't been reported. However, based on animal studies, it may be expected to cause respiratory depression, delirium, and CV dysfunction.

Treat overdose with naloxone hydrochloride to reverse the respiratory depressant effects. Continuous CV monitoring is recommended, with measures to maintain a patent airway. Vasopressors, I.V. fluids, oxygen, and controlled ventilation may be needed.

Special considerations
▶ Give drug by direct injection into a vein or into the tubing of a free-flowing I.V. solution.
▶ Mixed opioid agonist-antagonists tend to have less potential for abuse than agonists, and dezocine isn't a controlled substance. However, patients with a history of opiate use or dependence are at risk for abuse of this drug.

▶ Dezocine has limited risk of physical dependence; tolerance and physical dependence haven't been reported in humans.
▶ Currently, drug isn't recommended for patients with chronic pain because of limited experience and because the drug can precipitate an abstinence syndrome in patients with substantial tolerance to opiates.
▶ Monitor patient closely during withdrawal.

Breast-feeding patients
▶ No data exist to demonstrate whether drug appears in breast milk. Breast-feeding isn't recommended during therapy with dezocine.

Pediatric patients
▶ Safety and efficacy in children under age 18 haven't been established.

Geriatric patients
▶ Like other potent analgesics, dezocine should be administered with caution to the elderly.

Patient teaching
▶ Warn the patient to move about cautiously because the drug may cause dizziness.

Reactions may be *common,* uncommon, *life-threatening,* or COMMON AND LIFE-THREATENING.

◗ diazepam
Apo-Diazepam ◊ **, Diastat, Dizac,
Novodipam** ◊ **, Valium, Vivol** ◊ **,
Zetran**

Pharmacologic classification:
benzodiazepine

Therapeutic classification:
*antianxiety, skeletal muscle relaxant,
amnesic, anticonvulsant, sedative-
hypnotic*

Controlled substance schedule IV

Pregnancy risk category D

How supplied
Available by prescription only
Capsules (extended-release): 15 mg
Disposable syringe: 2-ml Tel-E-
Ject
Injection: 5 mg/ml in 2-ml am-
pules or 10-ml vials
Oral solution: 5 mg/ml; 5 mg/5 ml
Oral suspension: 5 mg/5 ml
Rectal gel: 2.5 mg, 5.0 mg, 10.0 mg,
15.0 mg, 20.0 mg Twin Packs
Tablets: 2 mg, 5 mg, 10 mg

Indications and dosages
Muscle spasm
Adults: 2 to 10 mg P.O. b.i.d. to
q.i.d.; or 15 to 30 mg extended-
release capsules once daily.
Alternatively, 5 to 10 mg I.M. or
I.V. q 3 to 4 hours, p.r.n.
Tetanus
Children age 5 and older: 5 to
10 mg I.M. or I.V. slowly q 3 to 4
hours, p.r.n.
*Infants over age 30 days to chil-
dren age 5:* 1 to 2 mg I.M. or I.V.
slowly, repeated q 3 to 4 hours.

Pharmacodynamics
Amnesic action: The exact mechanism of action is unknown.

Anticonvulsant action: Diazepam
suppresses the spread of seizure
activity produced by epileptogenic
foci in the cortex, thalamus, and
limbic structures by enhancing
presynaptic inhibition.
*Anxiolytic and sedative-hypnotic
actions:* Diazepam depresses the
CNS at the limbic and subcortical
levels of the brain. It produces an
anti-anxiety effect by influencing
the effect of the neurotransmitter
GABA on its receptor in the ascending reticular activating system, which increases inhibition
and blocks cortical and limbic
arousal.
Skeletal muscle relaxant action:
The exact mechanism is unknown,
but it is believed to involve inhibiting polysynaptic afferent pathways.

Pharmacokinetics
Absorption: When administered
orally, drug is absorbed through
the GI tract. Onset of action occurs
within 30 to 60 minutes, with peak
action in 1 to 2 hours. I.M. administration results in erratic absorption of the drug; onset of action
usually occurs in 15 to 30 minutes.
After I.V. administration, rapid onset occurs 1 to 5 minutes after injection. Drug is well absorbed rectally and reaches peak plasma levels in 1¼ hours.
Distribution: Drug is distributed
widely throughout the body. About
85% to 95% of a dose is bound to
plasma protein.
Metabolism: Drug is metabolized
in the liver to the active metabolite
desmethyldiazepam.
Excretion: Most metabolites of
diazepam are excreted in urine,
with only small amounts excreted
in feces. Half-life of desmethyl-

diazepam is 30 to 200 hours. Duration of sedative effect is 3 hours; this may be prolonged up to 90 hours in elderly patients and in patients with hepatic or renal dysfunction. Anticonvulsant effect occurs 30 to 60 minutes after I.V. administration.

Contraindications and precautions

Contraindicated in patients with hypersensitivity or angle-closure glaucoma; in patients experiencing shock, coma, or acute alcohol intoxication (parenteral form); and in children under age 6 months (oral form). Use cautiously in the elderly, in debilitated patients, and in those with impaired hepatic or renal function, depression, or chronic open-angle glaucoma. Avoid use in pregnant women, especially during the first trimester.

Interactions
Drug-drug

Antacids: may decrease rate of diazepam absorption. Avoid using together.
Antidepressants, antihistamines, barbiturates, general anesthetics, MAO inhibitors, opioids, phenothiazines: potentiates CNS depressant effects. Avoid using together.
Cimetidine, possibly disulfiram: diminished hepatic metabolism of diazepam, which increases plasma level. Monitor patient for side effects.
Digoxin: decreased digoxin clearance. Monitor patient for digoxin toxicity, and monitor serum digoxin levels.
Haloperidol: may change seizure patterns of patients treated with diazepam; benzodiazepines also may reduce serum haloperidol levels. If

necessary to use together, monitor patient closely, and monitor serum haloperidol levels.
Levodopa: may inhibit levodopa effects. Monitor patient for decreased efficacy if concomitant use is necessary.
Nondepolarizing neuromuscular blockers (pancuronium, succinylcholine): intensified and prolonged respiratory depression. If necessary to use together, monitor patient closely.
Oral contraceptives: may impair diazepam metabolism. Counsel patient for another form of birth control.
Theophylline: may antagonize sedative effects. Monitor patient for decreased efficacy.

Drug-lifestyle

Alcohol use: potentiates CNS depressant effects. Discourage alcohol consumption.
Heavy smoking: accelerates diazepam metabolism, thus lowering clinical effectiveness. Discourage smoking.

Effects on diagnostic tests
None reported.

Adverse reactions
CNS: *acute withdrawal syndrome* after sudden discontinuation in physically dependent persons, ataxia, changes in EEG patterns, *drowsiness,* fatigue, hallucinations, headache, insomnia, paradoxical anxiety, physical or psychological dependence, slurred speech, transient amnesia, tremor.
CV: **bradycardia, CV collapse,** hypotension.
EENT: blurred vision, diplopia, *dysarthria,* nystagmus.
GI: constipation, nausea.

Reactions may be *common,* uncommon, *life-threatening,* or COMMON AND LIFE-THREATENING.

GU: altered libido, incontinence, urine retention.
Hematologic: *neutropenia.*
Hepatic: elevated liver function tests, *jaundice.*
Respiratory: *respiratory depression.*
Skin: *pain, phlebitis* (at injection site), rash.

Overdose and treatment

Overdose may cause somnolence, confusion, coma, hypoactive reflexes, dyspnea, labored breathing, hypotension, bradycardia, slurred speech, and unsteady gait or impaired coordination.

Support blood pressure and respiration until drug effects subside; monitor vital signs. Mechanical ventilatory assistance via endotracheal tube may be needed to maintain a patent airway and support adequate oxygenation. Flumazenil, a specific benzodiazepine antagonist, may be useful, but should not be administered during status epilepticus. Use I.V. fluids and vasopressors such as dopamine and phenylephrine to treat hypotension as needed. If the patient is conscious, induce emesis; use gastric lavage if ingestion was recent, but only if an endotracheal tube is present to prevent aspiration. After emesis or lavage, administer activated charcoal with a cathartic as a single dose. Dialysis is of limited value.

Special considerations

▶ I.V. route is preferred because of rapid and more uniform absorption.
▶ For I.V. administration, drug should be infused slowly, directly into a large vein, at a rate not exceeding 5 mg/minute for adults or 0.25 mg/kg of body weight over 3 minutes for children. Do not inject diazepam into small veins to avoid extravasation into S.C. tissue. Observe infusion site for phlebitis. If direct I.V. administration is not possible, inject diazepam directly into I.V. tubing at point closest to vein insertion site to prevent extravasation.
▶ Administration by continuous I.V. infusion is not recommended.
▶ Do not mix diazepam with other drugs in a syringe or infusion container.
▶ Parenteral forms of diazepam may be diluted in normal saline solution; a slight precipitate may form, but the solution can still be used.
▶ Diazepam interacts with plastic. Do not store diazepam in plastic syringes or administer it in plastic administration sets, which will decrease availability of the infused drug.
▶ To enhance taste, oral solution can be mixed with liquids or semi-solid foods, such as applesauce or puddings, immediately before administration.
▶ Extended-release capsule should be swallowed whole; do not let patient crush or chew it.
▶ Shake oral suspension well before administering.
▶ When prescribing with opiates for endoscopic procedures, reduce opiate dose by at least one-third.
▶ Inject I.M. dose deep into deltoid muscle. Aspirate for backflow to prevent inadvertent intra-arterial administration. Use I.M. route only if I.V. or oral routes are unavailable.
▶ Patient should remain in bed under observation for at least 3 hours after parenteral administration of

diazepam to prevent potential hazards; keep resuscitation equipment nearby.

▶ Monitor patient closely when discontinuing drug. Do not discontinue drug suddenly; decrease dosage slowly over 8 to 12 weeks after long-term therapy.

▶ During prolonged therapy, periodically monitor blood counts and liver function studies.

▶ Assess gag reflex after endoscopy and before resuming oral intake to prevent aspiration.

▶ Lower doses are effective in patients with renal or hepatic dysfunction.

▶ Diastat rectal gel should be used to treat no more than five episodes per month and no more than one episode every 5 days.

▶ Diazepines aren't effective as analgesics except for muscle spasm.

▶ Opioid doses may need to be decreased if using with benzodiazepines due to sedative and respiratory depressant effects.

▶ Not recommended for long-term use.

▶ Monitor patients with a history of renal or hepatic dysfunction.

▶ Diazepam is also indicated as an adjunct to endoscopic procedures and cardioversion, in status epilepticus, and as an adjunct to the medical regimen in seizure control.

▶ It also is used for anxiety and acute alcohol withdrawal.

Breast-feeding patients

▶ Diazepam appears in breast milk. The breast-fed infant of a mother who uses diazepam may become sedated, have trouble feeding, or lose weight. Avoid use of drug in breast-feeding women.

Pediatric patients

▶ Safe use of oral diazepam in infants under age 6 months has not been established. Safe use of parenteral diazepam in infants under age 30 days has not been established.

▶ Closely observe neonates whose mothers took diazepam for a prolonged period during pregnancy; the infants may show withdrawal symptoms. Use of diazepam during labor may cause neonatal flaccidity.

Geriatric patients

▶ Elderly patients are more sensitive to the CNS depressant effects of diazepam. Use with caution.

▶ Lower doses are usually effective in elderly patients because of decreased elimination.

▶ Elderly patients who receive this drug require assistance with walking and activities of daily living during initiation of therapy or after an increase in dose.

▶ Parenteral administration of this drug is more likely to cause apnea, hypotension, and bradycardia in elderly patients.

Patient teaching

▶ Advise patient of the potential for physical and psychological dependence with chronic use.

▶ Warn patient that sudden changes of position can cause dizziness. Advise patient to dangle legs for a few minutes before getting out of bed to prevent falls and injury.

▶ Encourage patient to avoid or limit smoking to prevent increased diazepam metabolism.

▶ Warn woman to call immediately if she becomes pregnant.

▶ Caution patient to avoid alcohol while taking diazepam.

Reactions may be *common*, uncommon, *life-threatening*, or COMMON AND LIFE-THREATENING.

▶ Advise patient not to suddenly discontinue drug.
▶ Teach patient's caregiver when to use rectal gel (to control bouts of increased seizure activity) and how to monitor and record patient's clinical response.
▶ Teach patient's caregiver how to administer rectal gel.

▶ **diclofenac potassium**
Cataflam

▶ **diclofenac sodium**
Voltaren, Voltaren Ophthalmic, Voltaren-XR

Pharmacologic classification:
NSAID

Therapeutic classification:
antiarthritic, anti-inflammatory

Pregnancy risk category B

How supplied
Available by prescription only
Ophthalmic solution: 0.1%
Tablets: 25 mg, 50 mg
Tablets (enteric-coated): 25 mg, 50 mg, 75 mg, 100 mg

Indications and dosages
Osteoarthritis
Adults: 50 mg P.O. b.i.d. or t.i.d., or 75 mg P.O. b.i.d. (diclofenac sodium only).
Ankylosing spondylitis
Adults: 25 mg P.O. q.i.d. An additional 25 mg dose may be needed h.s.
Rheumatoid arthritis
Adults: 50 mg P.O. t.i.d. or q.i.d. Alternatively, 75 mg P.O. b.i.d. (diclofenac sodium only).

Analgesia and primary dysmenorrhea
Adults: 50 mg (diclofenac potassium only) P.O. t.i.d. Alternatively, 100 mg (diclofenac potassium only) P.O. initially, followed by 50 mg doses, up to a maximum dose of 200 mg in first 24 hours; subsequent dosing should follow 50 mg t.i.d. regimen.
Inflammation after cataract removal
Adults: 1 drop in the conjunctival sac q.i.d., beginning 24 hours after surgery and continuing throughout the first 2 weeks of the postoperative period.

Pharmacodynamics
Anti-inflammatory action: Drug exerts its anti-inflammatory and antipyretic actions through an unknown mechanism that may involve inhibition of prostaglandin synthesis.

Pharmacokinetics
Absorption: After oral administration, diclofenac is rapidly and almost completely absorbed, with peak plasma levels occurring in 1 to 3 hours for tablets and 10 to 30 minutes for oral solution. Absorption is delayed by food, with peak plasma levels occurring in 5 to 6 hours; however, bioavailability is unchanged.
Distribution: Drug is highly (nearly 100%) protein-bound.
Metabolism: Drug undergoes first-pass metabolism, with 60% of unchanged drug reaching systemic circulation. The principal active metabolite, 48-hydroxydiclofenac, has about 3% of the activity of the parent compound. Mean terminal half-life is about 1 to 2 hours after an oral dose.

Excretion: About 40% to 60% of diclofenac is excreted in the urine; the balance is excreted in the bile. The 4'-hydroxy metabolite accounts for 20% to 30% of the dose excreted in the urine; the other metabolites account for 10% to 20%; 5% to 10% is excreted unchanged in the urine. More than 90% is excreted within 72 hours. Moderate renal impairment does not alter the elimination rate of unchanged diclofenac but may reduce the elimination rate of the metabolites. Hepatic impairment does not appear to affect the pharmacokinetics of diclofenac.

Contraindications and precautions

Oral form is contraindicated in patients with hypersensitivity to drug and in those with hepatic porphyria or a history of asthma, urticaria, or other allergic reactions after taking aspirin or other NSAIDs. Avoid use during late pregnancy or while breast-feeding. Ophthalmic solution is contraindicated in patients with hypersensitivity to any component of the drug and in those wearing soft contact lenses; also avoid use during late pregnancy.

Use oral form cautiously in patients with history of peptic ulcer disease, hepatic or renal dysfunction, cardiac disease, hypertension, or conditions associated with fluid retention.

Use ophthalmic solution cautiously in patients with hypersensitivity to aspirin, phenylacetic acid derivatives, and other NSAIDs and in surgical patients with known bleeding tendencies or in those receiving medications that may prolong bleeding time.

Interactions
Drug-drug
Aspirin: lowers plasma diclofenac level. Avoid concurrent use.
Beta blockers: may blunt antihypertensive effects. Monitor blood pressure.
Cyclosporine, digoxin, methotrexate: may increase toxicity of these drugs. Monitor serum levels when possible, and monitor patient for toxicity.
Diuretics: may inhibit diuretic action. Monitor for decreased diuretic effect.
Insulin, oral antidiabetic drugs: may alter patient's response to these drugs. Monitor serum glucose levels, and adjust dosages accordingly.
Lithium: decreases renal lithium clearance and increases plasma levels. Monitor patient for lithium toxicity.
Phenytoin: may increase serum phenytoin levels. Monitor serum levels.
Potassium-sparing diuretics: may increase serum potassium levels. Monitor serum levels.
Warfarin: altered platelet function. Close monitoring of coagulation studies and anticoagulant dosage is recommended.

Drug-lifestyle
Sun exposure: may cause photosensitivity reactions. Take precautions.

Effects on diagnostic tests
None reported.

Adverse reactions
Unless otherwise noted, the following adverse reactions refer to oral administration of drug.

Reactions may be *common,* uncommon, *life-threatening,* or COMMON AND LIFE-THREATENING.

CNS: anxiety, depression, dizziness, drowsiness, headache, insomnia, irritability.
CV: edema, *heart failure,* hypertension.
EENT: anterior chamber reaction, blurred vision, epistaxis, eye pain, *increased intraocular pressure, keratitis,* laryngeal edema, night blindness, ocular allergy (with ophthalmic solution), reversible hearing loss, swelling of the lips and tongue, taste disorder, *tinnitus, transient stinging and burning.*
GI: abdominal distention, *abdominal pain or cramps,* appetite change, *bleeding,* bloody diarrhea, colitis, *constipation, diarrhea,* flatulence, *indigestion,* melena, *nausea,* peptic ulceration, vomiting.
GU: *acute renal failure,* fluid retention, interstitial nephritis, *nephrotic syndrome,* oliguria, papillary necrosis, proteinuria.
Hematologic: increased platelet aggregation time.
Hepatic: elevated liver enzymes, *hepatitis, hepatotoxicity,* jaundice.
Metabolic: hyperglycemia, hypoglycemia.
Musculoskeletal: back, leg, or joint pain.
Respiratory: asthma.
Skin: allergic purpura, alopecia, bullous eruption, dermatitis, eczema, photosensitivity, pruritus, rash, urticaria.
Other: *anaphylaxis, angioedema,* viral infection (with ophthalmic solution).

Overdose and treatment
No information available. There is no special antidote. Supportive and symptomatic treatment may include induction of vomiting or gastric lavage. Treatment with activated charcoal or dialysis may also be appropriate.

Special considerations
▶ Concurrent administration with other drugs, such as glucocorticoids, that produce adverse GI effects may aggravate such effects.
▶ Cataflam is immediate release and used most often for acute pain. Voltaren-XR is extended release and used most often for chronic pain.
▶ Drug may be less expensive than other NSAIDs.
▶ Some studies report that this drug has lower risk of GI effects than most other NSAIDs, but GI bleeding is still a concern.
▶ Monitor renal function during treatment. Use with caution and at reduced dosage in patients with renal impairment.
▶ Periodic ophthalmologic examinations are recommended during prolonged therapy.
▶ Monitor liver function during therapy. Abnormal liver function test results and severe hepatic reactions may occur.
▶ Periodic evaluation of hematopoietic function is recommended because bone marrow abnormalities have occurred. Regular check of hemoglobin level is important to detect toxic effects on the GI tract.
▶ Because the anti-inflammatory, antipyretic, and analgesic effects of diclofenac may mask the usual signs of infection, monitor carefully for infection.

Breast-feeding patients
▶ Low levels of diclofenac have been measured in breast milk. Risk-to-benefit ratio must be considered.

Pediatric patients
▶ Drug is not recommended for use in children.

Geriatric patients
▶ Use with caution in elderly patients. Elderly patients may be more susceptible to adverse reactions, especially GI toxicity and nephrotoxicity. Reduce dosage to lowest level that controls symptoms.

Patient teaching
▶ Advise patient to take drug with meals or milk to avoid GI upset.
▶ Teach patient to restrict salt intake because diclofenac may cause edema, especially if patient is hypertensive.
▶ Instruct patient to report symptoms that may be related to GI ulceration, such as epigastric pain and black or tarry stools, as well as other unusual symptoms such as skin rash, pruritus or significant edema or weight gain.

▶ difenoxin hydrochloride (with atropine sulfate)
Motofen

Pharmacologic classification:
opioid agonist

Therapeutic classification:
antidiarrheal

Controlled substance schedule IV

Pregnancy risk category C

How supplied
Available by prescription only
Tablets: 1 mg (with atropine sulfate 0.025 mg)

Indications and dosages
Acute nonspecific diarrhea, acute exacerbation of chronic functional diarrhea (adjunct)
Adults: initially 2 mg P.O. Then 1 mg P.O. after each loose bowel movement or 1 mg every 3 to 4 hours, p.r.n. Maximum, 8 mg daily. Not recommended for use longer than 2 days.

Pharmacodynamics
Antidiarrheal action: Difenoxin exerts a direct effect on the intestinal wall to slow motility. Atropine sulfate has been added to the formulation to minimize the potential for drug abuse.

Pharmacokinetics
Absorption: Rapidly absorbed after oral administration.
Distribution: Peak levels occur about 1 hour after a dose.
Metabolism: Metabolized to an inactive hydroxylated metabolite and conjugates.
Excretion: In urine and feces, as parent drug and metabolites. Over 90% of the drug is excreted within 24 hours of a single dose.

Contraindications and precautions
Contraindicated in patients hypersensitive to difenoxin or atropine, in children under age 2, in patients with diarrhea caused by pseudomembranous colitis associated with antibiotics, and in those with jaundice or diarrhea from organisms that may penetrate the intestinal mucosa (including *Escherichia coli, Salmonella,* or *Shigella*).
    Use cautiously in patients with a history of drug abuse or in those currently receiving drugs with a high abuse potential. Use cautious-

---

ly in patients with ulcerative colitis or renal or hepatic impairment.

Interactions
Drug-drug
Barbituates, CNS depressants, opioids, tranquilizers: may produce additive effects. Monitor patient closely if concomitant use is necessary.
MAO inhibitors: may precipitate hypertensive crisis. Monitor patient's blood pressure.

Drug-lifestyle
Alcohol use: may cause additive effects. Discourage alcohol use.

Effects on diagnostic tests
None reported.

Adverse reactions
CNS: confusion, dizziness, drowsiness, fatigue, headache, insomnia, light-headedness, nervousness.
EENT: blurred vision, burning eyes.
GI: constipation, dry mouth, epigastric distress, nausea, vomiting.

Overdose and treatment
Overdose may cause respiratory depression, coma, and death. Patients who overdose with difenoxin should be observed for at least 48 hours. Respiratory depression may occur up to 30 hours after ingestion. Gastric lavage, establishment of a patent airway, and mechanically assisted ventilation are advised. Naloxone will reverse the respiratory depression; however, because difenoxin has a longer duration of action than naloxone, supplemental naloxone injections will be necessary.

Special considerations
▶ Patient may require fluid and electrolyte correction. Difenoxin-induced decreases in peristalsis may result in fluid retention in the colon, with subsequent dehydration and, possibly, delyaed difenoxin intoxication.
▶ Monitor patient's weight, skin turgor, and serum electrolytes.

Breast-feeding patients
▶ Because of the potential for serious adverse effects on neonates, consider discontinuing the drug or recommend discontinuing breast-feeding during therapy.

Pediatric patients
▶ Safety in children under age 12 has not been established. The drug is contraindicated in children under age 2.

Geriatric patients
▶ Use cautiously in elderly patients. The drug may aggravate pre-existing glaucoma, exacerbate blurred vision, or contribute to urine retention.

Patient teaching
▶ Advise patient to avoid hazardous activities that require mental alertness until the CNS effects of the drug are known.
▶ Advise patient to adhere to dosing schedule. Overdose with difenoxin may result in respiratory depression and coma.
▶ Encourage proper storage to keep drug out of the reach of children.

◗ diflunisal
Dolobid

Pharmacologic classification:
NSAID, salicylic acid derivative

Therapeutic classification:
anti-inflammatory, antipyretic, nonnarcotic analgesic

Pregnancy risk category C

How supplied
Available by prescription only
Tablets: 250 mg, 500 mg

Indications and dosages
Mild to moderate pain
Adults: initially, 1 g. Then 500 mg/day in two or three divided doses, usually q 8 to 12 hours. Maximum, 1,500 mg daily.
◨ DOSAGE ADJUSTMENT. In adults over age 65, start at half the usual adult dose.
Rheumatoid arthritis, osteo-arthritis
Adults: 500 to 1,000 mg/day P.O. in two divided doses, usually q 12 hours. Maximum, 1,500 mg daily.
◨ DOSAGE ADJUSTMENT. In adults over age 65, start at half the usual dose.

Pharmacodynamics
Analgesic, antipyretic, and anti-inflammatory actions: Mechanisms of action are unknown, but are probably related to inhibition of prostaglandin synthesis. Diflunisal is a salicylic acid derivative, but is not hydrolyzed to free salicylate in vivo.

Pharmacokinetics
Absorption: Diflunisal is absorbed rapidly and completely via the GI tract. Plasma levels peak in 2 to 3 hours. Analgesia occurs within 1 hour and peaks within 2 to 3 hours.
Distribution: Drug is highly protein-bound.
Metabolism: Diflunisal is metabolized in the liver; it is not metabolized to salicylic acid.
Excretion: Drug is excreted in urine. Half-life is 8 to 12 hours.

Contraindications and precautions
Contraindicated in patients hypersensitive to drug or in whom aspirin or other NSAIDs cause acute asthma attacks, urticaria, or rhinitis.

Use cautiously in patients with GI bleeding, history of peptic ulcer disease, renal impairment, and compromised cardiac function, hypertension, or other conditions predisposing patient to fluid retention. Because of the epidemiologic association with Reye's syndrome, the Centers for Disease Control and Prevention recommends not giving salicylates to children and teenagers with chickenpox or influenza-like illness.

Interactions
Drug-drug
Acetaminophen: may increase serum acetaminophen levels by up to 50%, increasing the risk of hepatotoxicity and nephrotoxicity. Use together cautiously and monitor renal and hepatic function.
Antacids: delays and decreases diflunisal absorption. Instruct patient to avoid antacids with drug.
Anticoagulants, thrombolytics: may potentiate anticoagulant effects by platelet-inhibiting effect of diflunisal. Monitor coagulation studies.
Antihypertensives: may decrease effect on blood pressure. Monitor blood pressure.

Aspirin: may decrease bioavailability of diflunisal. Monitor patient for effectiveness.

Cyclosporine, diuretics, gold compounds: may enhance nephrotoxicity. Monitor renal status.

Furosemide: may decrease furosemide's hyperuricemic effect. Monitor patient for adverse effects.

GI-irritating drugs (antibiotics, other NSAIDs, steroids): may potentiate adverse GI effects of diflunisal. Use together with caution.

Highly protein-bound drugs (phenytoin, sulfonylureas, warfarin): may cause displacement of either drug, along with adverse effects. Monitor therapy closely for both drugs.

Hydrochlorothiazide: may increase plasma hydrochlorothiazide level but decrease its hyperuricemic, diuretic, antihypertensive, and natriuretic effects. Monitor patient closely for decreased effectiveness of these drugs.

Indomethacin: possible decreased renal clearance of indomethacin. Fatal GI hemorrhage has also been reported. Avoid using together, or if necessary to use together, monitor patient closely.

Lithium: may increase lithium serum levels. Monitor closely.

Methotrexate, nifedipine, verapamil: may decrease renal excretion of these drugs. Monitor patient for adverse effects.

Probenecid: may decrease renal clearance of diflunisal. Monitor patient for adverse effects.

Sulindac: diflunisal decreases blood levels of sulindac's active metabolite. Monitor patient.

Drug-food
Any food: delayed and decreased absorption of diflunisal. Instruct patient to wait at least 1 hour after eating before taking drug.

Drug-lifestyle
Alcohol use: may potentiate adverse GI effects of diflunisal. Discourage alcohol use.

Effects on diagnostic tests
None reported.

Adverse reactions
CNS: *dizziness,* fatigue, *headache,* insomnia, somnolence.
EENT: *tinnitus.*
GI: constipation, *diarrhea, dyspepsia,* flatulence, *GI pain, nausea,* vomiting.
GU: hematuria, interstitial nephritis, increased serum BUN and creatinine, renal impairment.
Hematologic: prolonged bleeding time.
Hepatic: increased liver function test results.
Metabolic: hyperkalemia, hypouricemia.
Skin: *erythema multiforme,* pruritus, *rash,* **Stevens-Johnson syndrome,** stomatitis, sweating.

Overdose and treatment
Overdose may cause drowsiness, nausea, vomiting, hyperventilation, tachycardia, sweating, tinnitus, disorientation, stupor, and coma.

To treat overdose of diflunisal, empty stomach immediately by inducing emesis with ipecac syrup, if patient is conscious, or by gastric lavage. Administer activated charcoal via nasogastric tube. Provide symptomatic and supportive measures (respiratory support and correction of fluid and electrolyte imbalances). Monitor laboratory parameters and vital signs closely. Hemodialysis has little effect.

Special considerations

▶ Diflunisal is recommended for twice-daily dosing for added patient convenience and compliance.
▶ Don't break, crush, or allow patient to chew diflunisal. Patient should swallow medication whole.
▶ If needed, administer diflunisal with water, milk, or meals to minimize GI upset.
▶ Do not administer concurrently with aspirin, acetaminophen, corticosteroids, or other NSAIDs.
▶ Institute safety measures to prevent injury if patient experiences CNS effects.
▶ Highly protein-bound NSAIDs such as diflunisal may have greater pharmacologic effects, but also have greater toxicities.
▶ Diflunisal has less GI toxicity than aspirin.
▶ Diflunisal is less expensive than other NSAIDs.
▶ Monitor results of laboratory tests, especially renal and liver function studies. Assess presence and amount of peripheral edema. Monitor weight frequently.
▶ Evaluate patient's response to diflunisal therapy as evidenced by a reduction in pain or inflammation. Monitor vital signs frequently, especially temperature.
▶ Monitor patient for signs and symptoms of potential hemorrhage, such as bruising, petechiae, coffee ground emesis, and black, tarry stools.
▶ Monitor renal and hepatic function in patients with renal or hepatic disease.

Breast-feeding patients
▶ Because drug appears in breast milk, breast-feeding isn't recommended.

Pediatric patients
▶ Don't use long-term diflunisal therapy in children under age 14; safe use hasn't been established.

Geriatric patients
▶ Patients over age 60 may be more susceptible to the toxic effects (particularly GI toxicity) of this drug.
▶ The effects of this drug on renal prostaglandins may cause fluid retention and edema, a significant drawback for elderly patients, especially those with heart failure or hypertension.

Patient teaching

▶ Instruct patient in diflunisal regimen and need for compliance. Advise him to report adverse reactions.
▶ Tell patient to take diflunisal with foods to minimize GI upset and to swallow capsule whole.
▶ Caution patient to avoid activities requiring alertness or concentration, such as driving, until CNS effects are known.
▶ Instruct patient in safety measures to prevent injury.

▶ dihydroergotamine mesylate
D.H.E. 45, Migranal

Pharmacologic classification:
ergot alkaloid

Therapeutic classification:
vasoconstrictor

Pregnancy risk category X

How supplied
Available by prescription only
Injection: 1 mg/ml
Nasal spray: 4 mg/ml

Indications and dosages
To prevent or abort vascular headaches, including migraine headaches
Adults: 1 mg I.M. or I.V., repeated at 1-hour intervals, up to total of 3 mg I.M. or 2 mg I.V. Maximum, 6 mg weekly.
Acute migraine headaches with or without aura
Adults: 1 spray (0.5 mg) administered in each nostril, then another spray in each nostril in 15 minutes for a total of 4 sprays (2 mg).

Pharmacodynamics
Vasoconstrictor action: By stimulating alpha-adrenergic receptors, drug causes peripheral vasoconstriction (if vascular tone is low). However, it causes vasodilation in hypertonic blood vessels. At high doses, it is a competitive alpha-adrenergic blocker. In therapeutic doses, drug inhibits the reuptake of norepinephrine. A weak antagonist of serotonin, drug reduces the increased rate of platelet aggregation caused by serotonin.

In the treatment of vascular headaches, drug probably causes direct vasoconstriction of the dilated carotid artery bed while decreasing the amplitude of pulsations. Its serotoninergic and catecholamine effects also appear to be involved.

Effects on blood pressure are minimal. The vasoconstrictor effect is more pronounced on veins and venules than on arteries and arterioles.

Pharmacokinetics
Absorption: Drug is incompletely and irregularly absorbed from the GI tract. Onset of action depends on how promptly after onset of headache the drug is given. After I.M. injection or intranasal administration, onset of action occurs within 15 to 30 minutes, and after I.V. injection, within a few minutes. Duration of action persists 3 to 4 hours after I.M. injection.
Distribution: 90% of dose is plasma protein-bound.
Metabolism: Drug is extensively metabolized, probably in the liver.
Excretion: 10% of dose is excreted in urine within 72 hours as metabolites; the rest in feces.

Contraindications and precautions
Contraindicated in patients with hypersensitivity to drug, in pregnant or breast-feeding patients, and in those with peripheral and occlusive vascular disease, coronary artery disease, uncontrolled hypertension, sepsis, hemiplegic or basilar migraine, and severe hepatic or renal dysfunction. Avoid use of drug in patients with uncontrolled hypertension or within 24 hours of 5-HT$_5$ agonists, ergotamine-containing or ergot-type medications, or methysergide.

Interactions
Drug-drug
Antihypertensives: may antagonize antihypertensive effects. Monitor patient's blood pressure.
Beta blockers (propranolol): block natural pathway for vasodilation in patients receiving ergot alkaloids and may cause excessive vasoconstriction and cold limbs. Monitor patient closely.
Erythromycin, other macrolides: may cause ergot toxicity. Monitor patient for effects.
Vasodilators: concomitant use may result in pressor effects and

dangerous hypertension. Avoid using together. If concomitant use necessary, monitor blood pressure closely.

Effects on diagnostic tests
None reported.

Adverse reactions
CV: increased arterial pressure, localized edema, numbness and tingling in fingers and toes, precordial distress and pain, transient tachycardia or *bradycardia.*
GI: *nausea, vomiting.*
Musculoskeletal: muscle pain in limbs, weakness in legs.
Skin: itching.

Overdose and treatment
Overdose may cause symptoms of ergot toxicity, including peripheral ischemia, paresthesia, headache, nausea, and vomiting.

Treatment requires prolonged and careful monitoring. Provide respiratory support, treat seizures if necessary, and apply warmth (not direct heat) to ischemic extremities if vasospasm occurs. Administer vasodilators, if needed.

Special considerations
▶ Drug is most effective when used at first sign of migraine, or as soon after onset as possible. It may also be helpful for acute cluster headaches.
▶ If migraine is severe and lasting longer than 3 days, D.H.E. I.V. may be recommended.
▶ Directly inject solution into the vein over 3 minutes. Continuous and intermittent infusion are not recommended.
▶ Protect ampules from heat and light. Discard if solution is discolored.

▶ If severe vasospasm occurs, keep limbs warm. Provide supportive treatment to prevent tissue damage. Give vasodilators if needed.
▶ For short-term use only. Do not exceed recommended dose.
▶ Monitor vital signs routinely if patient has a history of hypertension.
▶ Patient may self-administer using S.C. or I.M. route.
▶ Ergotamine rebound or an increase in frequency or duration of headaches may occur when drug is stopped.
▶ Drug has also been used to treat orthostatic hypotension as an unlabeled use.
▶ There are less potent vasoconstricting effects than ergotamine.

Breast-feeding patients
▶ Breast-feeding isn't recommended during therapy.

Geriatric patients
▶ Use drug cautiously in elderly patients. Safety and efficacy haven't been established.

Patient teaching
▶ Advise patient to lie down and relax in a quiet, darkened room after dose is administered.
▶ Urge patient to report immediately feelings of numbness or tingling in fingers and toes, or red or violet blisters on hands or feet.
▶ Warn patient to avoid alcoholic beverages during drug therapy.
▶ Caution patient to avoid smoking during drug therapy because the adverse effects of drug may be increased.
▶ Tell patient to avoid prolonged exposure to very cold temperatures while taking this medication. Cold may increase adverse reactions.

▶ Advise patient to report illness or infection, which may increase sensitivity to drug reactions.
▶ Instruct patient to prime the pump before using nasal spray.
▶ Instruct patient to discard nasal spray applicator once it has been prepared together with unused drug after 8 hours.
▶ For women of childbearing age, discuss birth control methods with patient, as this drug is absolutely contraindicated in pregnancy.

▶ diltiazem hydrochloride
Cardizem, Cardizem CD, Cardizem SR, Dilacor XR, Tiazac

Pharmacologic classification: *calcium channel blocker*

Therapeutic classification: *antianginal*

Pregnancy risk category C

How supplied
Available by prescription only
Capsules (extended-release):
120 mg, 180 mg, 240 mg, 300 mg (extended-release Cardizem CD only); 360 mg (extended-release Tiazac only)
Capsules (sustained-release):
60 mg, 90 mg, 120 mg (Cardizem SR)
Injection: 5 mg/ml 5-ml vials, Lyo-Ject 25 mg syringe
Tablets: 30 mg, 60 mg, 90 mg, 120 mg

Indications and dosages
Prinzmetal's (variant) angina, chronic stable angina
Adults: 30 mg P.O. q.i.d. before meals and h.s. Increase gradually to maximum of 360 mg/day divided into three or four doses, as indicated. Alternatively, give 120 or 180 mg (extended-release) P.O. once daily. Titrate over a 7- to 14-day period as needed and tolerated up to a maximum dose of 480 mg daily.

Pharmacodynamics
Antianginal and antihypertensive actions: By dilating systemic arteries, diltiazem decreases total peripheral resistance and afterload, slightly reduces blood pressure, and increases cardiac index, when given in high doses (over 200 mg). Afterload reduction, which occurs at rest and with exercise, and the resulting decrease in myocardial oxygen consumption account for diltiazem's effectiveness in controlling chronic stable angina.

Diltiazem also decreases myocardial oxygen demand and cardiac work by reducing heart rate, relieving coronary artery spasm (through coronary artery vasodilation), and dilating peripheral vessels. These effects relieve ischemia and pain. In patients with Prinzmetal's angina, diltiazem inhibits coronary artery spasm, increasing myocardial oxygen delivery.
Antiarrhythmic action: By impeding the slow inward influx of calcium at the AV node, diltiazem decreases conduction velocity and increases refractory period, thereby decreasing the impulses transmitted to the ventricles in atrial fibrillation or flutter. The end result is a decreased ventricular rate.

Pharmacokinetics
Absorption: About 80% of a dose is absorbed rapidly from the GI tract. However, only about 40% of drug enters systemic circulation because of a significant first-pass

---

effect in the liver. Serum levels peak in about 2 to 3 hours.
Distribution: About 70% to 85% of circulating drug is bound to plasma proteins.
Metabolism: Diltiazem is metabolized in the liver.
Excretion: About 35% of drug is excreted in the urine and about 65% in the bile as unchanged drug and inactive and active metabolites. Elimination half-life is 3 to 9 hours. Half-life may increase in elderly patients; however, renal dysfunction does not appear to affect half-life.

Contraindications and precautions
Contraindicated in patients with sick sinus syndrome or second- or third-degree AV block in the absence of an artificial pacemaker, in supraventricular tachycardias associated with a bypass tract such as in Wolfe-Parkinson-White syndrome or Lown-Ganong-Levine syndrome, in patients with left ventricular failure, hypotension (systolic blood pressure below 90 mm Hg), hypersensitivity to the drug, acute MI, and pulmonary congestion (documented by X-ray).

Use cautiously in the elderly and in patients with heart failure or impaired hepatic or renal function.

Interactions
Drug-drug
Anesthetics: may potentiate anesthetic effects. Monitor patient closely.
Beta blockers: may cause combined effects that result in heart failure, conduction disturbances, arrhythmias, and hypotension. Use together cautiously, and monitor patient closely.

Cimetidine: may increase diltiazem's plasma level. Patient should be carefully monitored for a change in diltiazem's effects when starting and stopping therapy with cimetidine.
Cyclosporine: may increase serum cyclosporine levels and subsequent cyclosporine-induced nephrotoxicity. If necessary to use together, monitor renal status.
Digoxin: may increase serum digoxin levels. Monitor serum levels.
Furosemide: forms a precipitate when mixed with diltiazem injection. Avoid mixing together.

Effects on diagnostic tests
None reported.

Adverse reactions
CNS: asthenia, dizziness, *headache,* somnolence.
CV: abnormal ECG, ***arrhythmias, AV block, bradycardia,*** conduction abnormalities, *edema,* flushing, ***heart failure,*** hypotension.
GI: abdominal discomfort, *constipation, nausea.*
Hepatic: acute hepatic injury.
Skin: *rash.*

Overdose and treatment
Clinical effects of overdose primarily are extensions of drug's adverse reactions. Heart block, asystole, and hypotension are the most serious effects and require immediate attention.

Treatment may involve I.V. isoproterenol, norepinephrine, epinephrine, atropine, or calcium gluconate administered in usual doses. Adequate hydration must be ensured. Inotropic agents, including dobutamine and dopamine, may be used, if necessary. If the patient develops severe conduction

---

disturbances (such as heart block and asystole) with hypotension that does not respond to drug therapy, cardiac pacing and resuscitation should be started immediately, as indicated.

Special considerations
▶ Diltiazem may be useful for acute migraine or cluster headaches, but verapamil is the calcium channel blocker of choice.
▶ The initial bolus dose is 0.25 mg/kg over 2 minutes (20 mg is a reasonable dose for the average patient). After 15 minutes, a second bolus dose of 0.35 mg/kg may be given over 2 minutes.
▶ Monitor patient for desired effects and adverse effects.
▶ If diltiazem is added to therapy of patient receiving digoxin, monitor serum digoxin levels and observe patient closely for signs of toxicity, especially elderly patients, those with unstable renal function, and those with serum digoxin levels in the upper therapeutic range.
▶ S.L. nitroglycerin may be administered concomitantly, as needed, if patient has acute angina symptoms.
▶ Drug is also used for hypertension, atrial fibrillation or flutter, and paroxysmal supraventricular tachycardia.
▶ Diltiazem has been used investigationally to prevent reinfarction after non-Q-wave MI; as an adjunct in the treatment of peripheral vascular disorders; and in the treatment of several spastic smooth muscle disorders, including esophageal spasm.

Breast-feeding patients
▶ Drug appears in breast milk; women should stop breast-feeding during diltiazem therapy.

Geriatric patients
▶ Use drug with caution in elderly patients because the half-life may be prolonged.
▶ If diltiazem is given with analgesics, it may decrease metabolism of the drug.

Patient teaching
▶ Tell patient that nitrate therapy prescribed during titration of diltiazem dosage may cause dizziness. Urge patient to continue compliance.
▶ Inform patient of proper use, dose, and adverse effects associated with diltiazem use.
▶ Instruct patient to continue taking drug even when feeling better.
▶ Tell patient to report feelings of light-headedness or dizziness and to avoid sudden position changes.

▶ **dimenhydrinate**
Apo-Dimenhydrinate◊, Calm-X, Dimetabs, Dinate, Dommanate, Dramamine, Dramocen, Dramoject, Dymenate, Gravol◊, Hydrate, PMS-Dimenhydrinate◊

Pharmacologic classification: *ethanolamine-derivative antihistamine*

Therapeutic classification: *antiemetic, antihistamine (H₁-receptor antagonist), antivertigo drug*

Pregnancy risk category B

How supplied
Available with or without a prescription
Capsules: 50 mg
Injection: 50 mg/ml

Liquid: 12.5 mg/4 ml, 15 mg/5 ml ◇
Tablets: 50 mg

Indications and dosages
Prophylaxis and treatment of nausea, vomiting, dizziness from motion sickness
Adults and children age 12 and older: 50 to 100 mg q 4 to 6 hours P.O., I.V., or I.M. For I.V. administration, dilute each 50-mg dose in 10 ml of normal saline solution and inject slowly over 2 minutes. Maximum, 400 mg/24 hours.
Children: 1.25 mg/kg/day or 37.5 mg/m²/day P.O. or I.M. q.i.d. (maximum, 300 mg/day) or according to following schedule:
Children ages 6 to 12: 25 to 50 mg P.O. q 6 to 8 hours; maximum, 150 mg/day.
Children ages 2 to 6: 12.5 to 25 mg P.O. q 6 to 8 hours; maximum, 75 mg/day.
Meniere's disease*
Adults: 50 mg I.M. for acute attack. Maintenance, 25 to 50 mg P.O. t.i.d.

Pharmacodynamics
Antiemetic and antivertigo actions: Dimenhydrinate probably inhibits nausea and vomiting by centrally depressing sensitivity of the labyrinth apparatus that relays stimuli to the chemoreceptor trigger zone and stimulates the vomiting center in the brain.

Pharmacokinetics
Absorption: Drug is well absorbed. Action begins within 15 to 30 minutes after oral administration, 20 to 30 minutes after I.M. administration, and almost immediately after I.V. administration. Its duration of action is 3 to 6 hours.

Distribution: Drug is well distributed throughout the body and crosses the placenta.
Metabolism: Dimenhydrinate is metabolized in the liver.
Excretion: Metabolites are excreted in urine.

Contraindications and precautions
Contraindicated in patients hypersensitive to drug or its components. I.V. product contains benzyl alcohol, which has been associated with a fatal "gasping syndrome" in premature infants and low birth weight infants.

Use cautiously in patients with seizures, acute angle-closure glaucoma, or enlarged prostate gland and in those receiving ototoxic drugs.

Interactions
Drug-drug
CNS depressants (antianxiety drugs, barbiturates, sleeping aids, tranquilizers): may produce additive CNS sedation and depression. Monitor patient closely.
Ototoxic drugs (aminoglycosides, cisplatin, loop diuretics, salicylates, vancomycin): may mask signs of ototoxicity. Avoid using together. If use together is necessary, monitor hearing status closely.

Drug-lifestyle
Alcohol use: may cause additive CNS depression. Discourage alcohol use.

Effects on diagnostic tests
Dimenhydrinate may alter or confuse test results for xanthines (caffeine, aminophylline) because of its 8-chlorotheophylline content; discontinue dimenhydrinate 4 days

before diagnostic skin tests to avoid preventing, reducing, or masking test response.

Adverse reactions

CNS: confusion, dizziness, *drowsiness,* excitation, headache, insomnia (especially in children), lassitude, nervousness, vertigo, tingling and weakness of hands.
CV: hypotension, palpitations, tachycardia, tightness of chest.
EENT: blurred vision, diplopia, dry respiratory passages, nasal congestion.
GI: anorexia, constipation, diarrhea, dry mouth, epigastric distress, nausea, vomiting.
Respiratory: wheezing, thickened bronchial secretions.
Skin: photosensitivity, rash, urticaria.
Other: *anaphylaxis.*

Overdose and treatment

Overdose may cause either CNS depression (sedation, reduced mental alertness, apnea, and CV collapse) or CNS stimulation (insomnia, hallucinations, tremors, or seizures). Anticholinergic symptoms, such as dry mouth, flushed skin, fixed and dilated pupils, and GI symptoms, are likely to occur, especially in children.

Use gastric lavage to empty stomach contents; emetics may be ineffective. Diazepam or phenytoin may be used to control seizures. Provide supportive treatment.

Special considerations

▶ Dimenhydrinate may be helpful for opioid-induced nausea related to vertigo.
▶ Incorrectly administered or undiluted I.V. solution is irritating to veins and may cause sclerosis.

▶ Parenteral solution is incompatible with many drugs; do not mix other drugs in the same syringe.
▶ Before administration, dilute each ml of drug with 10 ml of sterile water for injection, D_5W, or normal saline for injection.
▶ Give by direct injection over 2 minutes.
▶ Most I.V. products contain benzyl alcohol, which has been linked to fatal gasping syndome in premature infants.
▶ Advise safety measures for all patients; dimenhydrinate has a high incidence of drowsiness. Tolerance to CNS depressant effects usually develops within a few days.
▶ To prevent motion sickness, patient should take medication 30 minutes before traveling and again before meals and at bedtime.
▶ Antiemetic effect may diminish with prolonged use.

Breast-feeding patients

▶ Avoid use of antihistamines during breast-feeding. Many of these drugs, including dimenhydrinate, are secreted in breast milk, exposing the infant to risks of unusual excitability; premature infants are at particular risk for seizures.

Pediatric patients

▶ Safety in neonates has not been established. Infants and children under age 6 may experience paradoxical hyperexcitability. I.V. dosage for children has not been established.

Geriatric patients

▶ Elderly patients are usually more sensitive to adverse effects of antihistamines than younger patients and are especially likely to experience a greater degree of dizziness, sedation, hyperexcitability, dry mouth, and urine retention.

Patient teaching
▶ Tell patient to avoid hazardous activities, such as driving or operating heavy machinery, until adverse CNS effects of drug are known.
▶ Tell patient to take drug for motion sickness 30 minutes before exposure.

▶ diphenhydramine hydrochloride
Benadryl, Benadryl Allergy, Compoz, Diphen AF, Diphen Cough, Diphenadryl Children's Elixir, Hydramine, Nervine Nighttime Sleep-Aid, Nytol, Nytol QuickCaps, Sleep-eze 3, Sominex, Tusstat, Twilite

Pharmacologic classification: *ethanolamine-derivative antihistamine*

Therapeutic classification: *antihistamine (H$_1$-receptor antagonist), antiemetic, antivertigo, antitussive, sedative-hypnotic, topical anesthetic, antidyskinetic (anticholinergic)*

Pregnancy risk category B

How supplied
Available with or without a prescription
Capsules: 25 mg, 50 mg
Capsules (chewable): 12.5 mg
Cream: 1%, 2%
Elixir: 12.5 mg/5 ml (14% alcohol)
Gel: 1%, 2%
Injection: 50 mg/ml

Spray: 1%, 2%
Syrup: 12.5 mg/5 ml (5% alcohol)
Tablets: 25 mg, 50 mg

Indications and dosages
Sedation
Adults: 25 to 50 mg P.O., or deep I.M., p.r.n.
Nausea and vomiting
Adults: 25 to 50 mg I.V. every 6 hours, p.r.n.

Pharmacodynamics
Anesthetic action: Drug is structurally related to local anesthetics, which prevent initiation and transmission of nerve impulses; this is the probable source of its topical and local anesthetic effects.
Antihistamine action: Drug competes for H$_1$-receptor sites on the smooth muscle of the bronchi, GI tract, uterus, and large blood vessels; by binding to cellular receptors, it prevents access by histamine and suppresses histamine-induced allergic symptoms, even though it doesn't prevent release.
Antitussive action: Drug suppresses the cough reflex by a direct effect on the cough center.
Antivertigo, antiemetic, and antidyskinetic actions: Central antimuscarinic actions of antihistamines probably are responsible for these effects of diphenhydramine.
Sedative action: Mechanism of the CNS depressant effects of diphenhydramine is unknown.

Pharmacokinetics
Absorption: Drug is well absorbed from the GI tract. Action begins within 15 to 30 minutes and peaks in 1 to 4 hours.
Distribution: Drug is distributed widely throughout the body, including the CNS; drug crosses the

placenta and is excreted in breast milk. Drug is about 82% protein-bound.

Metabolism: About 50% to 60% of an oral dose of diphenhydramine is metabolized by the liver before reaching the systemic circulation (first-pass effect); virtually all available drug is metabolized by the liver within 24 to 48 hours.

Excretion: Plasma elimination half-life of drug is about 2½ to 9 hours; drug and metabolites are excreted primarily in urine.

Contraindications and precautions

Contraindicated in patients with hypersensitivity to drug, in patients having acute asthmatic attacks, and in newborns, premature neonates, or breast-feeding patients.

Use with extreme caution in patients with angle-closure glaucoma, prostatic hyperplasia, pyloroduodenal and bladder neck obstruction, asthma or COPD, increased intraocular pressure, hyperthyroidism, CV disease, hypertension, and stenosing peptic ulcer.

Interactions
Drug-drug

CNS depressants (antianxiety drugs, barbiturates, sleeping aids, tranquilizers): may result in CNS depression. Monitor patient closely.

Epinephrine: enhanced effects of epinephrine. Monitor patient closely.

Heparin: anticoagulant effects of heparin may be partially counteracted. Monitor patient.

MAO inhibitors: interferes with detoxification of diphenhydramine and prolongs central depressant and anticholinergic effects.

Monitor patient closely if concomitant use necessary.

Sulfonylureas: diminish sulfonylurea effects. Monitor patient closely.

Drug-lifestyle

Alcohol use: may cause additive CNS depression. Discourage use.

Sun exposure: may cause photosensitivity reactions. Take precautions.

Effects on diagnostic tests

Discontinue drug 4 days before diagnostic skin tests; antihistamines can prevent, reduce, or mask positive skin test response.

Adverse reactions

CNS: confusion, *dizziness, drowsiness,* fatigue, headache, *incoordination,* insomnia, nervousness, restlessness, *sedation,* **seizures,** *sleepiness,* tremor, vertigo.

CV: hypotension, palpitations, tachycardia.

EENT: blurred vision, diplopia, tinnitus.

GI: anorexia, constipation, diarrhea, *dry mouth, epigastric distress, nausea,* vomiting.

GU: dysuria, urinary frequency, urine retention.

Hematologic: *agranulocytosis,* hemolytic anemia, ***thrombocytopenia.***

Respiratory: nasal congestion, *thickening of bronchial secretions.*

Skin: photosensitivity, rash, urticaria.

Other: ***anaphylactic shock.***

Overdose and treatment

Drowsiness is the usual symptom of overdose. Seizures, coma, and respiratory depression may occur with profound overdose. Anti-

---

cholinergic symptoms, such as dry mouth, flushed skin, fixed and dilated pupils, and GI symptoms, are common, especially in children.

Treat overdose by inducing emesis with ipecac syrup (in conscious patient), followed by activated charcoal to reduce further drug absorption. Use gastric lavage if patient is unconscious or ipecac fails. Treat hypotension with vasopressors, and control seizures with diazepam or phenytoin. Do not give stimulants.

Special considerations
▶ Diphenhydramine is the drug of choice for pruritus caused by patient-controlled analgesia and epidural opioids.
▶ Diphenhydramine injection is compatible with most I.V. solutions but is incompatible with some drugs; check compatibility before mixing in the same I.V. line.
▶ Make sure that I.V. site is patent. Drug infiltrate causes extravasation with perivascular tissue irritation.
▶ Alternate injection sites to prevent irritation. Administer deep I.M. into large muscle.
▶ Injectable and elixir solutions are light-sensitive; protect them from light.
▶ Drowsiness is the most common adverse effect during initial therapy but usually disappears with continued use of drug.
▶ Diphenhydramine is useful for treating phenothiazine extrapyramidal symptoms.
▶ Drug is also used for rhinitis, allergy symptoms, motion sickness, Parkinson's disease, nonproductive cough, and insomnia.

Breast-feeding patients
▶ Avoid use of antihistamines during breast-feeding. Many of these drugs appear in breast milk, exposing the infant to risks of unusual excitability; premature infants are at particular risk for seizures.

Pediatric patients
▶ Drug should not be used in premature infants or neonates. Infants and children, especially those under age 6, may experience paradoxical hyperexcitability.

Geriatric patients
▶ Elderly patients are usually more sensitive to adverse effects of antihistamines than younger patients and are especially likely to experience a greater degree of dizziness, sedation, hyperexcitability, dry mouth, and urine retention. Symptoms usually respond to a decrease in medication dosage.

Patient teaching
▶ Advise patient that drowsiness is very common initially, but may be reduced with continued use of drug.
▶ Warn patient to avoid alcohol during therapy.
▶ Advise patient undergoing skin testing for allergies to notify physician of current drug therapy.

▶ **docusate calcium**
Pro-Cal-Sof, Surfak

▶ **docusate potassium**
Dialose, Diocto-K, Kasof

▶ **docusate sodium**
Colace, Diocto, Dioeze, Diosuccin, Disonate, DOK, D.O.S, Doxinate, D-S-S, Duosol, Modane Soft, Pro-Sof, Regulax SS, Regulex◊, Regutol

Pharmacologic classification: *surfactant*

Therapeutic classification: *emollient laxative*

Pregnancy risk category C

How supplied
Available without a prescription
Capsules: 50 mg, 60 mg, 100 mg, 120 mg, 240 mg, 250 mg, 300 mg
Liquid: 150 mg/15 ml
Solution: 50 mg/ml
Syrup: 50 mg/15 ml, 60 mg/15 ml
Tablets: 50 mg, 100 mg

Indications and dosages
Stool softener
docusate sodium
Adults and children age 12 and older: 50 to 200 mg/day P.O. until bowel movements are normal. Alternatively, add 50 to 100 mg to saline or oil retention enema to treat fecal impaction.
Children ages 6 to 12: 40 to 120 mg/day P.O.
Children ages 3 to 6: 20 to 60 mg/day P.O.
Children under age 3: 10 to 40 mg/day P.O.
docusate calcium or potassium
Adults: 240 mg (calcium) or 100 to 300 mg (potassium) P.O. daily un-til bowel movements are normal. Higher doses are for initial therapy. Adjust dose to individual response.
Children age 6 and older: 50 to 150 mg (calcium) or 100 mg (potassium) P.O. daily.

Pharmacodynamics
Laxative action: Docusate salts act as detergents in the intestine, reducing surface tension of interfacing liquids; this promotes incorporation of fat and additional liquid, softening the stool.

Pharmacokinetics
Absorption: Docusate salts are absorbed minimally in the duodenum and jejunum; drug acts in 1 to 3 days.
Distribution: Docusate salts are distributed primarily locally, in the gut.
Metabolism: None.
Excretion: Docusate salts are excreted in feces.

Contraindications and precautions
Contraindicated in patients hypersensitive to drug and in those with intestinal obstruction, undiagnosed abdominal pain, vomiting or other signs of appendicitis, fecal impaction, or acute surgical abdomen.

Interactions
Drug-drug
Mineral oil: may increase absorption of mineral salts. Monitor patient for adverse effects.

Effects on diagnostic tests
None reported.

Adverse reactions
GI: bitter taste, diarrhea, laxative dependence (with long-term or ex-

cessive use), mild abdominal cramping.

Overdose and treatment
No information available.

Special considerations
▶ Drug is useful as prophylaxis for opioid-induced constipation.
▶ Liquid or syrup must be given in 6 to 8 oz (180 to 240 ml) of milk or fruit juice or in infant's formula to prevent throat irritation.
▶ Avoid using docusate sodium in sodium-restricted patients.
▶ Docusate salts are available in combination with casanthranol (Peri-Colace), senna (Senokot, Gentlax), and phenolphthalein (Femilax, Unilax Softgel).
▶ Docusate salts are the preferred laxative for most patients who must avoid straining at stool, such as those recovering from MI or rectal surgery. They also are used commonly to treat patients with postpartum constipation.

Breast-feeding patients
▶ Because absorption of docusate salts is minimal, they presumably pose no risk to breast-feeding infants.

Geriatric patients
▶ Docusate salts are good choices for elderly patients because they rarely cause laxative dependence, they produce fewer adverse effects, and they're gentler than some other laxatives.

Patient teaching
▶ Docusate salts lose their effectiveness over time; advise patient to report failure of medication.

▶ Encourage patients to drink plenty of liquids and add high fiber foods to their diet.

▶ **dolasetron mesylate**
Anzemet

Pharmacologic classification:
selective serotonin 5-HT₃ receptor antagonist

Therapeutic classification:
antinauseant, antiemetic

Pregnancy risk category B

How supplied
Available by prescription only
Injection: 20 mg/ml as 12.5 mg/0.625 ml ampules or 100 mg/5 ml vials
Tablets: 50 mg, 100 mg

Indications and dosages
Prevention of nausea and vomiting from chemotherapy
Adults: 100 mg P.O. given as a single dose 1 hour before chemotherapy, or 1.8 mg/kg as a single I.V. dose given 30 minutes before chemotherapy, or a fixed dose of 100 mg I.V. given 30 minutes before chemotherapy.
Children ages 2 to 16: 1.8 mg/kg P.O. given 1 hour before chemotherapy, or 1.8 mg/kg as a single I.V. dose given 30 minutes before chemotherapy. Injectable form can be mixed with apple or apple-grape juice and given P.O. 1 hour before chemotherapy. Maximum, 100 mg/day.
Prevention of postoperative nausea and vomiting
Adults: 100 mg P.O. within 2 hours before surgery; 12.5 mg as a single

I.V. dose about 15 minutes before cessation of anesthesia.

Children ages 2 to 16: 1.2 mg/kg P.O. given within 2 hours before surgery, up to maximum of 100 mg; or 0.35 mg/kg (up to 12.5 mg) given as a single I.V. dose about 15 minutes before the cessation of anesthesia. Injectable form (1.2 mg/kg up to 100-mg dose) can be mixed with apple or apple-grape juice and administered P.O. 2 hours before surgery.

Postoperative nausea and vomiting (I.V. form only)

Adults: 12.5 mg as a single I.V. dose as soon as nausea or vomiting presents.

Children ages 2 to 16: 0.35 mg/kg, up to a maximum dose of 12.5 mg, given as a single I.V. dose as soon as nausea or vomiting occurs.

Pharmacodynamics

Antinauseant and antiemetic actions: A selective serotonin 5-HT$_3$ receptor antagonist that blocks the action of serotonin. 5-HT$_3$ receptors are located on the nerve terminals of the vagus nerve in the periphery and in the central chemoreceptor trigger zone. Blocking the activity of the serotonin receptors prevents serotonin from stimulating the vomiting reflex.

Pharmacokinetics

Absorption: Orally administered dolasetron, injection, the I.V. solution, and tablets are bioequivalent. Oral dolasetron is well absorbed, although parent drug is rarely detected in plasma due to rapid and complete metabolism to the most clinically relevant metabolite, hydrodolasetron.

Distribution: Drug is widely distributed in the body, with a mean apparent volume of distribution of 5.8 L/kg; 69% to 77% of hydrodolasetron is bound to plasma protein.

Metabolism: A ubiquitous enzyme, carbonyl reductase, mediates the reduction of dolasetron to hydrodolasetron. Cytochrome P-450 (CYP)2D6 and CYP3A are responsible for subsequent hydroxylation and N-oxidation of hydrodolasetron, respectively.

Excretion: Two-thirds of dose is excreted in the urine and one-third in the feces. Mean elimination half-life of hydrodolasetron is about 8 hours.

Contraindications and precautions

Contraindicated in patients hypersensitive to drug.

Use drug cautiously in patients with, or at risk for developing, prolonged cardiac conduction intervals, particularly QTc. These include patients taking antiarrhythmic drugs or other drugs which lead to QT prolongation; hypokalemia or hypomagnesemia; a potential for electrolyte abnormalities, including those receiving diuretics; congenital QT syndrome; and those who have received cumulative high-dose anthracycline therapy.

Interactions
Drug-drug

Drugs that induce cytochrome P-450 isoenzymes (such as rifampin): may decrease hydrodolasetron levels. Monitor patient for decreased efficacy of antiemetic.

Drugs that inhibit the cytochrome P-450 isoenzymes: can increase hydrodolasetron levels. Monitor patient for adverse effects.

Drugs that prolong ECG intervals (such as antiarrhythmics): may increase the risk of arrhythmias. Monitor patient closely.

Effects on diagnostic tests

None reported.

Adverse reactions

CNS: dizziness, drowsiness, fatigue, *headache.*
CV: *arrhythmias, bradycardia,* ECG changes, hypertension, hypotension, tachycardia.
GI: abdominal pain, anorexia, constipation, *diarrhea,* dyspepsia.
GU: oliguria, urine retention.
Hepatic: elevation of liver function test results.
Skin: chills, fever, pain at injection site, pruritus, rash.

Overdose and treatment

There is no specific antidote for dolasetron overdose; provide supportive care. It is not known if drug is removed by hemodialysis or peritoneal dialysis.

Special considerations

❯ Dolasetron and other 5-HT$_3$ antagonists are only marginally effective for delayed chemotherapy-induced nausea and vomiting (i.e., greater than 24 hours following completion of chemotherapy).
❯ Dolasetron does not produce analgesia.
❯ Injection can be infused as rapidly as 100 mg/30 seconds or diluted in 50 ml compatible solution and infused over 15 minutes.
❯ Safety and efficacy of multiple drug doses have not been evaluated. Efficacy studies have all been conducted with single doses of drug.

❯ Injection for oral administration is stable in apple or apple-grape juice for 2 hours at room temperature.
❯ Oral and I.V. dosage forms are equivalent for acute chemotherapy-induced nausea and vomiting.

Breast-feeding patients

❯ No data exist to demonstrate whether drug appears in breast milk. Use caution when giving drug to breast-feeding women.

Pediatric patients

❯ Clinical experience is lacking with this drug in patients under age 2.
❯ Efficacy information in patients ages 2 to 17 receiving chemotherapy are consistent with those obtained in adults.
❯ No efficacy information was collected in pediatric postoperative nausea and vomiting studies.

Geriatric patients

❯ Dosage adjustment isn't needed in patients over age 65.
❯ Effectiveness in prevention of nausea and vomiting in elderly patients was no different from that in younger age groups.

Patient teaching

❯ Inform patient that oral doses of drug must be taken 1 to 2 hours before surgery or 1 hour before chemotherapy to be effective.
❯ Teach patient about potential adverse effects.
❯ Instruct patient not to mix injection in juice for oral administration until just before dosing.
❯ Tell patient to report if nausea or vomiting occurs.

▶ doxacurium chloride
Nuromax

Pharmacologic classification:
nondepolarizing neuromuscular blocker

Therapeutic classification:
skeletal muscle relaxant

Pregnancy risk category C

How supplied
Available by prescription only
Injection: 1 mg/ml

Indications and dosages
To provide skeletal muscle relaxation for endotracheal intubation and during surgery as an adjunct to general anesthesia
Adults: dosage is highly individualized; 0.05 mg/kg rapid I.V. produces adequate conditions for endotracheal intubation in 5 minutes in about 90% of patients when used as part of a thiopental-narcotic induction technique. Lower doses may require longer delay before intubation is possible. Neuromuscular blockade at this dose lasts an average of 100 minutes.
Children over age 2: dosage is highly individualized; an initial dose of 0.03 mg/kg I.V. administered during halothane anesthesia produces effective blockade in 7 minutes and has a duration of 30 minutes. Under the same conditions, 0.05 mg/kg produces a blockade in 4 minutes and lasts 45 minutes.
Maintenance of neuromuscular blockade during long procedures
Adults and children over age 2: initial dose of 0.05 mg/kg I.V. Maintenance dosage of 0.005 and 0.01 mg/kg will prolong neuromuscular blockade for an average of 30 minutes and 45 minutes, respectively. Children usually require more frequent administration of maintenance dosages.
◫ DOSAGE ADJUSTMENT. Adjust dosage to ideal body weight in obese patients (patients whose weight is 30% or more above their ideal weight) to avoid prolonged neuromuscular blockade.

Pharmacodynamics
Skeletal muscle relaxant action:
Doxacurium binds competitively to cholinergic receptors on the motor end-plate to antagonize the action of acetylcholine, resulting in a block of neuromuscular transmission.

Pharmacokinetics
Absorption: First signs of neuromuscular blockade occur within about 2 minutes following I.V. administration. Maximum effects occur in about 3 to 6 minutes.
Distribution: Plasma protein-binding of drug is about 30% in human plasma.
Metabolism: Doxacurium is thought not to be metabolized.
Excretion: Drug is primarily eliminated as unchanged drug in urine and bile.

Contraindications and precautions
Contraindicated in patients with hypersensitivity to drug and in neonates. Drug contains benzyl ethanol, which has been associated with death in newborns.

Use cautiously, perhaps at a reduced dose, in debilitated patients; in patients with metastatic cancer, severe electrolyte disturbances, or neuromuscular diseases; and in those in whom potentiation or difficulty in reversal of neuromuscular blockade is anticipated. Patients with myasthenia gravis or myasthenic syndrome (Eaton-Lambert syndrome) are particularly sensitive to the effects of nondepolarizing relaxants. Shorter-acting agents are recommended for use in such patients.

Interactions
Drug-drug
Alkaline solutions: precipitate may form. Don't mix together.
Antibiotics (aminoglycosides [gentamycin, kanamycin, neomycin, streptomycin], bacitracin, clindamycin, colistimethate sodium, colistin, lincomycin, polymyxins, tetracyclines), lithium, local anesthetics, magnesium salts, procainamide, and quinidine: neuromuscular blocking action of doxacurium may be enhanced. Monitor patient closely.
Carbamazepine, phenytoin: may delay onset of neuromuscular blockade and shorten its duration. Monitor patient for desired effects.
Enflurane, halothane, isoflurane: may decrease the ED_{50} (effective dose needed to produce a 50% suppression of the response to ulnar nerve stimulation) of doxacurium by 30% to 45%. These drugs also may prolong doxacurium duration of action by up to 25%. If necessary to use together, dosage adjustment may be necessary.

Effects on diagnostic tests
None reported.

Adverse reactions
Musculoskeletal: prolonged muscle weakness.

Respiratory: dyspnea, *respiratory depression, respiratory insufficiency or apnea.*

Overdose and treatment
Overdose with neuromuscular blocking agents such as doxacurium may result in neuromuscular block beyond the time needed for surgery and anesthesia. The primary treatment is maintenance of a patent airway and controlled ventilation until recovery of normal neuromuscular function is assured. Once initial evidence of recovery is observed, further recovery may be facilitated by administration of an anticholinesterase agent (such as neostigmine or edrophonium) in conjunction with an appropriate anticholinergic agent.

Special considerations
▶ Drug may be useful in facilitating passage of tubes (i.e., endotracheal, endoscopes, etc.).
▶ All times of onset and duration of neuromuscular blockade are averages; considerable individual variation in dosages is normal.
▶ Drug should be used only under direct medical supervision by personnel skilled in the use of neuromuscular blockers and techniques for maintaining a patent airway. Do not use unless facilities have equipment for mechanical ventilation, oxygen therapy, and intubation, and an antagonist are within reach.
▶ To avoid patient distress, do not give drug until patient's consciousness is obtunded by general anesthetic. Drug has no effect on consciousness or pain threshold.
▶ Prepare drug for I.V. use with D_5W, normal saline solution for injection, dextrose 5% in normal

saline solution for injection, lactated Ringer's solution, and dextrose 5% in lactated Ringer's solution.

▶ Administer drug immediately after reconstitution. Diluted solutions are stable for 24 hours at room temperature; however, because reconstitution dilutes the preservative, risk of contamination increases. Discard unused solutions after 8 hours.

▶ As with other nondepolarizing neuromuscular blocking agents, a reduction in dosage of doxacurium must be considered in cachectic or debilitated patients; in patients with neuromuscular diseases, severe electrolyte abnormalities, or carcinomatosis; and in other patients in whom potentiation of neuromuscular block or difficulty with reversal is anticipated. Increased doses of doxacurium may be needed in burn patients.

▶ Drug has no effect on consciousness or pain threshold. To avoid distress to the patient, it should not be administered until patient's consciousness is obtunded by general anesthetic.

▶ Drug may prolong neuromuscular block in patients undergoing renal transplantation; onset and duration of the block may vary with patients undergoing liver transplantation.

▶ Use drug only under direct medical supervision by caregivers familiar with use of neuromuscular blocking agents and in airway management. Do not use unless facilities and equipment for mechanical ventilation, oxygen therapy, and intubation and an antagonist are within reach.

▶ Use of a peripheral nerve stimulator will permit the most advantageous use of doxacurium, mini-mize the possibility of overdosage or underdosage, and assist in the evaluation of recovery.

Breast-feeding patients
▶ No data exist to demonstrate whether drug appears in breast milk. Use cautiously when administrating to breast-feeding women.

Pediatric patients
▶ Drug use hasn't been studied in children younger than age 2.

Geriatric patients
▶ Elderly patients may be more sensitive to the drug's effects. They may experience a slower onset of the blockade and a longer duration.

Patient teaching
▶ Instruct patient on effects of drugs before administration.

▶ **doxepin hydrochloride**
Adapin, Sinequan, Triadapin ◊

Pharmacologic classification:
tricyclic antidepressant

Therapeutic classification:
antidepressant

Pregnancy risk category NR

How supplied
Available by prescription only
Capsules: 10 mg, 25 mg, 50 mg, 75 mg, 100 mg, 150 mg
Oral concentrate: 10 mg/ml

Indications and dosages
Analgesic adjunct for phantom limb pain*, chronic pain (migraine, chronic tension headache, diabetic neuropathy, tic douloureux, cancer pain, periph-

---

eral neuropathy with pain, post-herpetic neuralgia, arthritic pain)*
Adults: 30 to 300 mg/day.
⚠ **Dosage adjustment.** Reduce dosage in elderly, debilitated, or adolescent patients and in those receiving certain other drugs (especially anticholinergics).

Pharmacodynamics
Analgesic action: Unknown.
Antidepressant action: Doxepin is thought to exert its antidepressant effects by inhibiting reuptake of norepinephrine and serotonin in CNS nerve terminals (presynaptic neurons), which results in increased levels and enhanced activity of these neurotransmitters in the synaptic cleft. Doxepin more actively inhibits reuptake of serotonin than norepinephrine. Anxiolytic effects of this drug usually precede antidepressant effects. Doxepin also may be used as an anxiolytic. Doxepin has the greatest sedative effect of all tricyclic antidepressants; tolerance to this effect usually develops in a few weeks.

Pharmacokinetics
Absorption: Drug is absorbed rapidly from the GI tract after oral administration.
Distribution: Doxepin is distributed widely into the body, including the CNS and breast milk. Drug is 90% protein-bound. Peak effect occurs in 2 to 4 hours; steady state is achieved within 7 days. Therapeutic levels (parent drug and metabolite) are thought to range from 150 to 250 ng/ml.
Metabolism: Drug is metabolized by the liver to the active metabolite desmethyldoxepin. A significant first-pass effect may explain vari-

ability of serum levels in different patients on the same dosage.
Excretion: Drug is mostly excreted in urine.

Contraindications and precautions
Contraindicated in patients with hypersensitivity to drug, glaucoma, or tendency to retain urine.

Interactions
Drug-drug
Antiarrhythmics (disopyramide, procainamide, quinidine), pimozide, thyroid hormones: may increase risk of cardiac arrhythmias and conduction defects. Monitor cardiac status closely.
Anticholinergics (antihistamines, atropine, meperidine, phenothiazines), antiparkinsonians, CNS depressants (analgesics, anesthetics, opioids, tranquilizers): may produce additive effects, which include oversedation, paralytic ileus, visual changes, and severe constipation. Monitor patient closely.
Barbiturates: may induce doxepin metabolism. Monitor patient for decreased therapeutic efficacy.
Beta blockers, cimetidine, fluoxetine, methylphenidate, oral contraceptives, propoxyphene, sertraline: may inhibit doxepin metabolism, increasing plasma levels and toxicity. Monitor patient for adverse effects.
Central-acting antihypertensives (clonidine, guanabenz, guanadrel, guanethidine, methyldopa, reserpine): may decrease hypotensive effects. Monitor blood pressure.
Clonidine: increases hypertensive effect. Monitor blood pressure.
Disulfiram, ethchlorvynol: may cause delirium and tachycardia. Monitor patient's response.

Reactions may be *common*, uncommon, *life-threatening*, or COMMON AND LIFE-THREATENING.

Haloperidol, phenothiazines: decreased doxepin metabolism. Adjust dosages of both drugs when given together.

MAO inhibitors: may cause severe excitation, hyperpyrexia, or seizures, usually at high dosage. Monitor patient closely, and adjust dosages accordingly.

Metrizamide: may produce additive effects, including an increased risk of seizures. Use together cautiously, and monitor patient closely.

Sympathomimetics (such as ephedrine, epinephrine, norepinephrine, phenylephrine, phenylpropanolamine): may increase blood pressure. Monitor blood pressure.

Warfarin: may increase PT, INR, and risk of bleeding. Monitor lab values closely.

Drug-food

Carbonated beverages, grape juice: don't give together. Drug is incompatible with these liquids.

Drug-lifestyle

Alcohol use: induces doxepin metabolism, decreases therapeutic efficacy, and enhances CNS depression. Discourage alcohol intake.

Heavy smoking: induces doxepin metabolism and decreases therapeutic efficacy. Discourage smoking.

Sun exposure: increases risk of photosensitivity reactions. Take precautions.

Effects on diagnostic tests

Doxepin may prolong conduction time (elongation of QT and PR intervals, flattened T waves on ECG); it also may elevate liver function test results, decrease WBC counts, and decrease or increase serum glucose levels.

Adverse reactions

CNS: ataxia, confusion, *dizziness, drowsiness,* extrapyramidal reactions, hallucinations, headache, numbness, paresthesia, **seizures,** weakness.

CV: ECG changes, *orthostatic hypotension, tachycardia.*

EENT: *blurred vision,* tinnitus.

GI: anorexia, *constipation, dry mouth,* nausea, vomiting.

GU: urine retention.

Hematologic: *bone marrow depression,* eosinophilia.

Hepatic: elevated liver function tests.

Metabolic: hyperglycemia, hypoglycemia.

Skin: *diaphoresis,* photosensitivity, rash, urticaria.

Other: *hypersensitivity reaction.*

After abrupt withdrawal of long-term therapy: headache, malaise (does not indicate addiction), nausea.

Overdose and treatment

The first 12 hours after acute ingestion are a stimulatory phase characterized by excessive anticholinergic activity (agitation, irritation, confusion, hallucinations, hyperthermia, parkinsonian symptoms, seizures, urine retention, dry mucous membranes, pupillary dilation, constipation, and ileus). This is followed by CNS depressant effects, including hypothermia, decreased or absent reflexes, sedation, hypotension, cyanosis, and cardiac irregularities, including tachycardia, conduction disturbances, and quinidine-like effects on the ECG.

Severity of overdose is best indicated by widening of QRS complex. Usually, this represents a serum level in excess of 1,000 ng/ml. Serum levels are usually not helpful. Metabolic acidosis may follow hypotension, hypoventilation, and seizures.

Treatment is symptomatic and supportive, including maintaining airway, stable body temperature, and fluid and electrolyte balance. Induce emesis with ipecac if patient is conscious; follow with gastric lavage and activated charcoal to prevent further absorption. Dialysis is little use. Physostigmine may be cautiously used to reverse central anticholinergic effects. Treat seizures with parenteral diazepam or phenytoin; arrhythmias with parenteral phenytoin or lidocaine; and acidosis with sodium bicarbonate. Do not give barbiturates: these may enhance CNS and respiratory depressant effects.

Special considerations
▶ As with all tricyclics, administer full dose at bedtime.
▶ Full therapeutic effects may not be seen for 7 to 10 days after initiation of treatment.
▶ Drug is also used for depression and anxiety.
▶ Smaller doses are sufficient for pain management (as opposed to doses needed for depression management).

Breast-feeding patients
▶ Drug appears in breast milk. Avoid use of drug in breast-feeding patients, especially at high doses.

Pediatric patients
▶ Doxepin is rarely used for treating anxiety in children.

Geriatric patients
▶ Elderly patients are more likely to develop adverse CNS reactions, orthostatic hypotension, and GI and GU disturbances.

Patient teaching
▶ Teach patient to dilute oral concentrate with 120 ml water, milk, or juice (grapefruit, orange, pineapple, prune, or tomato). Drug is incompatible with carbonated beverages.
▶ Tell patient to use ice chips, sugarless gum or hard candy, or saliva substitutes to treat dry mouth.
▶ Warn patient to avoid taking other drugs while taking doxepin unless they have been prescribed.
▶ Instruct patient to take full dose at bedtime.

▶ droperidol
Inapsine

Pharmacologic classification:
butyrophenone derivative

Therapeutic classification:
tranquilizer

Pregnancy risk category C

How supplied
Available by prescription only
Injection: 2.5 mg/ml

Indications and dosages
Anesthetic premedication
Adults: 2.5 to 10 mg I.M. 30 to 60 minutes before induction of general anesthesia.
Children ages 2 to 12: 0.088 to 0.165 mg/kg I.V. or I.M.
Induction of general anesthesia (adjunct)
Adults: 0.22 to 0.275 mg/kg I.V. (preferably) or I.M. concomitantly with an analgesic or general anesthetic.

Children: 0.088 to 0.165 mg/kg
I.V. or I.M.
Maintenance of general anesthesia (adjunct)
Adults: 1.25 to 2.5 mg I.V.
For use without a general anesthetic during diagnostic procedures
Adults: 2.5 to 10 mg I.M. 30 to 60
minutes before the procedure.
Additional doses of 1.25 to 2.5 mg
I.V. are given, p.r.n.
Regional anesthesia (adjunct)
Adults: 2.5 to 5 mg I.M. or slow
I.V. injection.
Antiemetic in conjunction with chemotherapy
Adults: 6.25 mg I.M. or by slow
I.V. injection.

Pharmacodynamics
Tranquilizer action: Droperidol
produces marked sedation by directly blocking subcortical receptors. Droperidol also blocks CNS
receptors at the chemoreceptor
trigger zone, producing an
antiemetic effect.

Pharmacokinetics
Absorption: Drug is well absorbed
after I.M. injection. Sedation begins in 3 to 10 minutes, peaks at
30 minutes, and lasts for 2 to 4
hours; some alteration of consciousness may persist for 12
hours.
Distribution: Not well understood;
drug crosses the blood-brain barrier and is distributed in the CSF. It
also crosses the placenta.
Metabolism: Droperidol is metabolized by the liver to *p*-fluorophenylacetic acid and *p*-hydroxypiperidine.
Excretion: Drug and metabolites
are excreted in urine and feces.

Contraindications and precautions
Contraindicated in patients with
known hypersensitivity or intolerance to drug. Use cautiously in patients with hypotension and other
CV disease because of its vasodilatory effects, in patients with hepatic
or renal disease in whom drug clearance may be impaired, and in patients taking other CNS depressants,
including alcohol, opiates, and sedatives, because droperidol may potentiate the effects of these drugs.

Interactions
Drug-drug
*CNS depressants (barbiturates,
sedative-hypnotics, tranquilizers):*
potentiates CNS depressant effects.
When used concurrently, the dosage
of both drugs should be reduced.
Fentanyl citrate: may cause hypertension and respiratory depression.
Monitor patient's vital signs closely.
Opiates, other analgesics: potentiates CNS depressant effects.
Monitor closely.

Drug-lifestyle
Alcohol use: potentiates CNS depressant effects. Discourage alcohol intake.

Effects on diagnostic tests
None reported.

Adverse reactions
CNS: akathisia, altered consciousness, dystonia, extrapyramidal reactions, fine tremors of limbs, postoperative hallucinations, *sedation,*
temporarily altered EEG pattern.
CV: *bradycardia,* decreased pulmonary artery pressure, *hypotension* with rebound tachycardia.
Respiratory: *respiratory depression.*

Overdose and treatment
Overdose may cause extension of the drug's pharmacologic actions. Treat overdose symptomatically and supportively.

Special considerations
▶ If opiates are needed during recovery from anesthesia to prevent potentiation of respiratory depression, they should be used initially in reduced dosages (as low as one-fourth to one-third of the usual recommended dosage).
▶ Administer I.V. doses slowly.
▶ Monitor patient for postoperative hallucinations or emergence delirium and drowsiness.
▶ Be prepared to treat severe hypotension.
▶ Monitor patient's vital signs, and watch carefully for extrapyramidal reactions. Droperidol is related to haloperidol and is more likely than other antipsychotics to cause extrapyramidal symptoms.
▶ Discontinue drug if patient shows signs of dystonia, hypersensitivity, paradoxical hypertension, respiratory depression, or severe persistent hypotension.

Breast-feeding patients
▶ No data exist to demonstrate whether droperidol appears in breast milk.

Pediatric patients
▶ Safety and efficacy in children under age 2 haven't been established.

Geriatric patients
▶ Drug should be used with caution. Elderly patients are more prone to extrapyramidal symptoms, CNS disturbances, and adverse CV effects.

Patient teaching
▶ Advise patient of possible postoperative effects.

---

ergotamine tartrate
Cafergot, Ergomar, Ergostat, Gynergen, Medihaler Ergotamine, Wigraine

Pharmacologic classification: *ergot alkaloid*

Therapeutic classification: *vasoconstrictor*

Pregnancy risk category X

How supplied
Available by prescription only
Aerosol inhaler: 360 mcg/metered spray
Suppositories: 2 mg (with 100 mg of caffeine)
Tablets: 1 mg◊ (with 100 mg of caffeine)
Tablets (S.L.): 2 mg

Indications and dosages
To prevent or abort vascular headache, including migraine and cluster headaches
Adults: initially, 2 mg S.L. or P.O. Then 1 to 2 mg S.L. or P.O. q 30 minutes. Maximum, 6 mg/attack, 6 mg/24 hours, and 10 mg/week. For inhaler, give 1 inhalation. If headache isn't relieved in 5 minutes, repeat 1 inhalation. May repeat inhalations at least 5 minutes apart to maximum of 6 inhalations/24 hours or 15 inhalations/week. For rectal suppositories, give 2 mg P.R. at start of attack. Repeat in 1

hour, p.r.n. Maximum, 2 suppositories/attack or 5 suppositories/week. *Children:* 1 mg S.L. in older children and adolescents. If no improvement, may give another 1-mg dose in 30 minutes.

Pharmacodynamics
Vasoconstricting action: By stimulating alpha-adrenergic receptors, ergotamine causes peripheral vasoconstriction if vascular tone is low and vasodilation if vascular tone is high. It probably relieves vascular headaches by causing direct vasoconstriction of dilated carotid artery beds while decreasing the amplitude of pulsations. Drug also inhibits norepinephrine reuptake, which increases its vasoconstricting activity. And it weakly antagonizes serotonin, thus reducing the increased rate of platelet aggregation caused by serotonin. These catecholamine and serotoninergic effects seem to affect headaches as well. At high doses, the drug is a competitive alpha-adrenergic blocker.

Pharmacokinetics
Absorption: Drug is rapidly absorbed after inhalation and variably absorbed after oral administration. Levels peak in 30 minutes to 3 hours. Caffeine may increase the rate and extent of absorption. Drug undergoes first-pass metabolism after oral administration.
Distribution: Drug is widely distributed throughout the body.
Metabolism: Drug is extensively metabolized in the liver.
Excretion: About 4% of a dose is excreted in urine within 96 hours; the rest is probably excreted in feces. Ergotamine is dialyzable. Onset of action depends on how promptly drug is given after onset of headache.

Contraindications and precautions
Contraindicated in pregnant patients and those with peripheral and occlusive vascular diseases, coronary artery disease, hypertension, hepatic or renal dysfunction, severe pruritus, sepsis, or hypersensitivity to ergot alkaloids.

Interactions
Drug-drug
Beta blockers, such as propranolol: may cause excessive vasoconstriction by blocking natural pathway for vasodilation during ergot alkaloid administration. Avoid concomitant use.
Macrolides, such as erythromycin: may cause ergot toxicity (severe peripheral vasospasm with possible ischemia, cyanosis, and numbness). As needed, give a vasodilator, such as nifedipine, nitroprusside, or prazosin.

Drug-food
Caffeine: may increase rate and extent of absorption. Monitor caffeine intake.

Drug-lifestyle
Smoking: may increase adverse drug effects. Urge smoking cessation.

Effects on diagnostic tests
None reported.

Adverse reactions
CNS: numbness and tingling in fingers and toes.
CV: angina, increased arterial pressure, localized edema, peripheral vasoconstriction, precordial

distress and pain, ***transient brady-cardia,*** transient tachycardia.
GI: nausea, vomiting.
Musculoskeletal: muscle pain in limbs, weakness in legs.
Skin: pruritus.

Overdose and treatment

Overdose may cause vasospastic effects, nausea, vomiting, lassitude, impaired mental function, delirium, severe dyspnea, hypotension or hypertension, rapid or weak pulse, unconsciousness, spasms of the limbs, seizures, and shock.

Treatment is supportive, with prolonged and careful monitoring. If patient is conscious and ingestion was recent, induce emesis or gastric lavage. If patient is comatose with a cuffed endotracheal tube in place, perform gastric lavage. Activated charcoal and a saline (magnesium sulfate) cathartic may be used. Provide respiratory support. Apply warmth (not direct heat) to ischemic limbs if vasospasm occurs. As needed, give vasodilators (nitroprusside, prazosin, or tolazoline) and, if necessary, I.V. diazepam for seizures. Dialysis may be helpful.

Special considerations

▶ Drug is most effective when used in prodromal stage of headache or as soon as possible after onset.
▶ Consider giving an antiemetic 30 minutes before drug to prevent nausea.
▶ S.L. tablet is preferred during early stage of attack because of its rapid absorption.
▶ Suppositories may be cut in half or quarters to find lowest effective dosing.
▶ Provide quiet, low-light environment to relax patient after dose is administered.

▶ If patient develops severe vasoconstriction with tissue necrosis, give sodium nitroprusside I.V. or intra-arterial tolazoline. To prevent vascular stasis and thrombosis, consider giving heparin I.V. and 10% dextran 40 in D_5W injection.
▶ Overuse can result in chronic daily headache syndrome.
▶ Rebound headache or increased duration or frequency of headache may occur when drug is stopped.
▶ Drug isn't effective for muscle contraction headaches.
▶ Store drug in light-resistant container.
▶ Obtain a detailed history to detect a possible relationship between diet and onset of headache.

Breast-feeding patients

▶ Drug appears in breast milk. Use cautiously in breast-feeding women.
▶ Excessive drug amounts or prolonged administration may inhibit lactation.

Pediatric patients

▶ Safety and efficacy in children haven't been established.

Geriatric patients

▶ Give cautiously to elderly patients.

Patient teaching

▶ Teach patient to use inhaler correctly. Instruct him to gargle and rinse his mouth after each dose to help prevent hoarseness and irritation.
▶ Tell patient not to eat, drink, or smoke while S.L. tablet is dissolving.
▶ Urge patient not to exceed recommended dosage.
▶ Caution patient to avoid alcoholic beverages during therapy be-

---

Reactions may be *common*, uncommon, ***life-threatening***, or COMMON AND LIFE-THREATENING.

cause alcohol may worsen headache.
▶ Tell patient to avoid smoking because it may increase adverse drug effects.
▶ Warn patient to avoid prolonged exposure to very cold temperatures because they may increase adverse drug effects.
▶ Urge patient to immediately report numbness or tingling in fingers or toes, red or violet blisters on hands or feet, and chest, muscle, or abdominal pain.
▶ If patient uses an inhaler, tell him to promptly notify prescriber if condition worsens or if he develops mouth, throat, or lung infection.
▶ Advise patient to report nausea and vomiting.

▶ **etanercept**
Enbrel

Pharmacologic classification:
tumor necrosis factor (TNF) blocker

Therapeutic classification:
antirheumatic

Pregnancy risk category B

How supplied
Available by prescription only
Injection: 25 mg single-use vial

Indications and dosages
Moderate to severe rheumatoid arthritis symptoms in patients who don't respond to one or more disease-modifying antirheumatic drugs, or with methotrexate in patients who do not respond adequately to methotrexate alone
Adults: 25 mg S.C. twice weekly.

Children ages 4 to 17: 0.4 mg/kg S.C. twice weekly for 3 months. Maximum, 25 mg/dose.

Pharmacodynamics
Antirheumatic action: Binds to TNF and blocks its action with cell surface TNF receptors, reducing inflammatory and immune responses found in rheumatoid arthritis.

Pharmacokinetics
Absorption: Serum levels peak in 72 hours.
Distribution: Not reported.
Metabolism: Not reported.
Excretion: Elimination half-life is 115 hours.

Contraindications and precautions
Contraindicated in patients with sepsis or hypersensitivity to etanercept or any of its components.
    Use cautiously in patients with a history of active or chronic infection or with an underlying disease that raises the risk of infection, such as diabetes or heart failure.

Interactions
None reported.

Effects on diagnostic tests
None reported.

Adverse reactions
CNS: asthenia, dizziness, *headache.*
EENT: pharyngitis, *rhinitis,* sinusitis.
GI: abdominal pain, dyspepsia.
Respiratory: cough, respiratory disorder, *upper respiratory tract infections.*
Skin: *injection site reaction,* rash.
Other: *infections, malignancies.*

Special considerations
▶ Response to drug may begin in 1 or 2 weeks, but full effects may take up to 3 months.
▶ Reconstitute aseptically with 1 ml of supplied sterile bacteriostatic water for injection, USP (0.9% benzyl alcohol). Don't filter reconstituted solution during preparation or administration. Inject diluent slowly into vial. Minimize foaming by gently swirling during dissolution rather than shaking. Dissolution takes less than 5 minutes.
▶ Reconstituted solution should be clear and colorless. Don't use if solution is discolored, cloudy, or if particulate matter remains.
▶ Don't add other drugs or diluents to reconstituted solution.
▶ Use reconstituted solution as soon as possible; it may be refrigerated in vial for up to 6 hours at 36° to 46° F (2° to 8° C).
▶ Injection site should be at least 1″ from an old site and preferably on the thigh, abdomen, or upper arm. Don't inject drug into tender, bruised, red, or hard skin areas. Rotate sites regularly.
▶ The needle cover of the diluent syringe contains latex and shouldn't be handled by anyone sensitive to latex.
▶ Patient may develop positive antinuclear antibodies or positive anti-double-stranded DNA antibodies, as measured by radioimmunoassay and *Crithidia lucilae* assay.
▶ Because drug may alter defenses against infection, monitor patient and stop therapy if serious infection occurs.
▶ Expect arthritis symptoms to return within 1 month of stopping treatment.

Breast-feeding patients
▶ Advise patient not to breast-feed during therapy.

Pediatric patients
▶ If possible, bring children up-to-date with all vaccinations before starting drug. Don't give live-virus vaccines during therapy.
▶ Safety and effectiveness haven't been studied in children under age 4.
▶ Children with juvenile rheumatoid arthritis are more prone to certain adverse effects (abdominal pain and vomiting) than adults.

Geriatric patients
▶ Although no data exist to suggest it, elderly patients may have increased sensitivity to drug effects.

Patient teaching
▶ If patient will administer drug, teach injection techniques and recommend that he rotate injection sites.
▶ Instruct patient to use a puncture-resistant container for disposal of needles and syringes.
▶ Explain that injection site reactions, if they occur, typically do so during the first month of therapy and then decrease.
▶ Stress the importance of avoiding live-virus vaccines during therapy, and of telling other health care providers about therapy.
▶ Instruct patient to promptly report signs and symptoms of infection.

▶ethyl chloride
(chloroethane)
Ethyl Chloride

Pharmacologic classification:
halogenated hydrocarbon

Therapeutic classification:
counterirritant, local anesthetic

Pregnancy risk category C

How supplied
Available by prescription only
Topical liquid spray: 3-oz, 3.5-oz
bottles

Indications and dosages
Local anesthesia in minor operative procedures; pain caused by insect stings, burns, bruises, contusions, abrasions, swelling, and minor sports-related sprains; tinea lesions; creeping eruption
Adults and children: dosage varies. Use smallest amount needed to produce desired effect. For local anesthesia, use fine-spray nozzle, hold container about 12″ (30 cm) from area, and spray downward until a light frosting appears.
Infants: saturate cotton ball and hold against area for a few seconds.
Counterirritant to relieve myofascial and visceral pain syndromes
Adults, children, infants: dosage varies. Use smallest amount needed to produce desired effect. Using large-sized nozzle, hold container about 24″ (60 cm) from skin and spray at an acute angle in one direction in a sweeping motion until area has been covered.

Pharmacodynamics
Anesthetic action: Rapid vaporization of ethyl chloride freezes superficial tissues, producing insensitivity of peripheral nerve endings and local anesthesia. Anesthesia lasts for up to 1 minute.

Pharmacokinetics
Absorption: Limited with topical use.
Distribution: None.
Metabolism: None.
Excretion: None.

Contraindications and precautions
Ethyl chloride is contraindicated for use near eyes or on broken skin or mucous membranes; it shouldn't be inhaled. Freezing and thawing process may damage epithelial cells; avoid repeated use over long periods. Ethyl chloride is highly flammable and explosive; it shouldn't be used near open fire and should be stored away from heat or open flame.

Interactions
None reported.

Effects on diagnostic tests
None reported.

Adverse reactions
Musculoskeletal: muscle spasm.
Skin: burning, frostbite, inflammation, pain from excessive cooling; rash, skin lesions, stinging, tenderness, tissue necrosis with prolonged use; urticaria.

Overdose and treatment
No cases of poisoning have been reported from long-term use.

Special considerations
▶ Don't apply drug to broken skin or mucous membranes.

◇ Available in Canada only   *Unlabeled use

▶ Protect adjacent skin with petroleum jelly to prevent tissue damage.

▶ When using ethyl chloride as a counterirritant, avoid frosting the skin because excessive cooling may increase spasms and pain.

▶ Rewarm the muscle with moist heat for 10 to 15 minutes after the trigger point is inactivated.

▶ Monitor patient for adequate pain relief during procedure.

▶ Monitor skin for adverse reactions.

▶ Discontinue drug if sensitization develops.

Breast-feeding patients
▶ Clean drug from breast area before patient breast-feeds.

Pediatric patients
▶ Use smaller amounts of drug.

Patient teaching
▶ Advise patient that drug will produce a temporary numbness.

▶ **etidocaine hydrochloride**
Duranest, Duranest MPF

Pharmacologic classification:
amide local anesthetic

Therapeutic classification:
local anesthetic

Pregnancy risk category B

How supplied
Available by prescription only
Injection: 1% and 1.5%

Indications and dosages
Dosage differs depending on anesthetic procedure, area to be anesthetized, vascularity of area, number of neuronal segments to be blocked, and individual patient conditions and tolerance. Maximum, 400 mg per injection with epinephrine, 300 mg per injection without epinephrine. Doses may be repeated at 2- to 3-hour intervals.

Central neural block, peripheral nerve block, lumbar peridural block
Adults: 50 to 400 mg (5 to 40 ml) of a 1% solution.

Caudal nerve block
Adults: 100 to 300 mg (10 to 30 ml) of a 1% solution.

Retrobulbar nerve block
Adults: 20 to 60 mg (2 to 4 ml) of a 1% or 1.5% solution.

Maxillary infiltration and/or inferior alveolar nerve block
Adults: 15 to 75 mg (1 to 5 ml) of a 1.5% solution.

Intra-abdominal or pelvic surgery, lower limb surgery, caesarean section
Adults: 100 to 300 mg (10 to 30 ml) of a 1% solution or 150 to 300 mg (10 to 20 ml) of a 1.5% solution.

◩ DOSAGE ADJUSTMENT. Reduce dosage in children, elderly, debilitated, and acutely ill patients and in those with severe renal disease, shock, or heart block.

Pharmacodynamics
Anesthetic action: Drug stabilizes the neuronal membrane by inhibiting the ionic fluxes needed for initiation and conduction of impulses, thereby causing local anesthesia.

Pharmacokinetics
Absorption: Completely absorbed following parenteral administration. The rate of absorption depends on site of administration and the presence or absence of a vaso-

constrictor. Onset of action is 3 to 5 minutes.
Distribution: Plasma protein-binding is 95%. Etidocaine crosses the blood-brain barrier and placenta.
Metabolism: Rapidly metabolized in the liver.
Excretion: Metabolites and unchanged drug are excreted in urine, less than 10% as unchanged drug. Elimination half-life is about 2½ hours after bolus I.V. injection. Duration of action is 5 to 10 hours.

Contraindications and precautions

Contraindicated in patients hypersensitive to local anesthetics of the amide type.

Use cautiously in patients with severe shock, heart block, hepatic disease, impaired CV function. Also, use cautiously in patients with known drug sensitivities. Lumbar and caudal epidurals should be used with extreme caution in patients with existing neurologic disease, spinal deformities, septicemia, and severe hypertension.

Interactions
Drug-drug

CNS depressants: may cause additive CNS effects; reduce dosages of CNS depressants.
MAO inhibitors, phenothiazines, tricyclic antidepressants: increased risk of severe, prolonged hypotension or hypertension with etidocaine and epinephrine. Use with extreme caution.

Adverse reactions

CNS: apprehension, confusion, dizziness, drowsiness, euphoria, light-headedness, nervousness, *seizures,* tremors, twitching.

CV: *bradycardia, cardiac arrest,* edema, hypotension.
EENT: blurred vision, diplopia, tinnitus, trismus.
GI: vomiting.
Respiratory: *respiratory arrest.*
Skin: urticaria.
Other: *anaphylaxis,* sensations of heat, cold, or numbness.

Overdose and treatment

Toxic reactions may include CNS stimulation, seizures, circulatory depression, apnea, and respiratory depression. High plasma levels or unintended subarachnoid injection may cause acute emergency.

To treat toxic reactions, immediately establish and maintain a patent airway or administer controlled ventilation with oxygen. Endotracheal intubation may be indicated. If necessary, use I.V. barbiturates, anticonvulsants, or muscle relaxants to control seizures. Supportive treatment of circulatory depression may require I.V. fluids, vasopressors, or both. Dialysis has limited value.

Special considerations

▸ Local anesthetics should be administered only by clinicians experienced in diagnosing and managing drug-related toxicity and other acute emergencies.
▸ Keep resuscitative equipment, drugs, and oxygen immediately available.
▸ To avoid intravascular injection, aspirate for blood before injecting etidocaine. (Intravascular injection is still possible even after negative aspiration.)
▸ For epidural anesthesia, don't use a local anesthetic that contains a preservative.

▶ Inspect product for particulate matter before giving it. Discard if it contains precipitate or the color is pinkish or slightly darker than yellow.

▶ Give a test dose of 2 to 5 ml at least 5 minutes before an epidural, preferably with epinephrine. Monitor patient for CNS and CV toxicity.

▶ Give smallest dose and concentration needed to produce the desired result.

▶ Small doses of local anesthetics injected into the head and neck area may produce adverse reactions similar to systemic toxicity caused by unintentional intravascular injections of larger doses.

▶ Continuously monitor CV status, respiratory status, and level of consciousness after each injection. Early signs of CNS toxicity include anxiety, blurred vision, depression, dizziness, drowsiness, incoherent speech, light-headedness, metallic taste, numbness and tingling of mouth and lips, restlessness, tinnitus, tremors, twitching.

Pregnant patients
▶ Local anesthetics rapidly cross the placenta and can cause maternal, fetal, and neonatal toxicity. Adverse reactions may involve alterations in the CNS, peripheral vascular tone, and cardiac function, including maternal hypotension and fetal bradycardia. Monitor fetal heart rate continuously.

Breast-feeding patients
▶ Some local anesthetics appear in breast milk. Use with caution in breast-feeding women.

Pediatric patients
▶ No information is currently available on appropriate pediatric doses.

Geriatric patients
▶ Reduce dosages in elderly patients.

Patient teaching
▶ Tell patient that anesthetized part of body may have temporary loss of sensation and motor activity.
▶ If patient receives drug for dental anesthesia, caution against chewing solid foods or testing the area by biting or probing while still anesthetized.

▶ **etidronate disodium**
Didronel

Pharmacologic classification:
pyrophosphate analogue

Therapeutic classification:
antihypercalcemic

Pregnancy risk category C

How supplied
Available by prescription only
Injection: 50 mg/ml (300-mg ampule)
Tablets: 200 mg, 400 mg

Indications and dosages
Symptomatic Paget's disease
Adults: 5 mg/kg/day P.O. as a single dose with water or juice 2 hours before a meal. Patient shouldn't eat, consume milk or milk products, or take antacids or vitamins with mineral supplements for 2 hours after dose. May give up to 10 mg/kg/day in severe cases,

not to exceed 6 months. Maximum, 20 mg/kg/day for 3 months.
Heterotopic ossification in spinal cord injuries
Adults: 20 mg/kg/day P.O. for 2 weeks, followed by 10 mg/kg/day for 10 weeks.
Heterotopic ossification after total hip replacement
Adults: 20 mg/kg/day P.O. for 1 month before total hip replacement and for 3 months afterward.

Pharmacodynamics
Bone-metabolism inhibitor action: Although its exact mechanism isn't known, drug acts on bone by adsorbing to hydroxyapatite crystals, thereby inhibiting their growth and dissolution. It also decreases the number of osteoclasts in bone, thereby slowing excessive remodeling of pagetic or heterotopic bone.

Pharmacokinetics
Absorption: Absorption following an oral dose is variable and is decreased in the presence of food. Absorption may also be dose-related.
Distribution: About half the dose is distributed to bone.
Metabolism: Etidronate isn't metabolized.
Excretion: About 50% of drug is excreted within 24 hours in urine.

Contraindications and precautions
Contraindicated in patients hypersensitive to drug or in those with active osteomalacia.
  Use cautiously in patients with impaired renal function.

Interactions
Drug-drug
Antacids that contain calcium, magnesium, or aluminum; mineral supplements that contain calcium, iron, magnesium, or aluminum: inhibited etidronate absorption. Avoid use within 2 hours of dose.

Drug-food
Foods that contain large amounts of calcium (such as milk and dairy products): may prevent absorption of oral etidronate. Avoid use within 2 hours of dose.

Effects on diagnostic tests
None reported.

Adverse reactions
CNS: *seizures.*
CV: fluid overload.
GI: diarrhea, increased frequency of bowel movements, nausea, constipation, stomatitis.
Hepatic: abnormal hepatic function.
Metabolic: *elevated serum phosphate level.*
Musculoskeletal: increased or recurrent bone pain, pain at previously asymptomatic sites, increased risk of fracture.
Respiratory: dyspnea.
Other: fever, *hypersensitivity reactions.*

Overdose and treatment
Overdose may cause diarrhea, nausea, and hypocalcemia. Treat with gastric lavage and induced emesis. Give calcium if needed.

Special considerations
❚ This drug is for use in patients with Paget's disease who have moderate to severe pain, neural

compression, or increased cardiac output as a result of the disease.
▶ In patients with Paget's disease, mild symptoms can be treated with analgesics.
▶ Drug also is used (via I.V. route) for hypercalcemia linked to malignancy.
▶ Monitor renal function before and during therapy.
▶ Dilute daily dose in at least 250 ml of normal saline solution or D_5W and infuse over at least 2 hours. Diluted solution may be stored at room temperature for up to 48 hours.
▶ Adverse reactions in the GI tract are especially likely at 20 mg/kg/day.
▶ Drug should be taken in a single daily dose. However, if nausea occurs, daily amount may be divided.
▶ Monitor drug effect by serum alkaline phosphate and urinary hydroxyproline excretion; both are lowered by effective therapy.
▶ Some patients may receive I.V. drug for up to 7 days, but risk of hypokalemia increases after 3 days.

Patient teaching
▶ Instruct patient to take drug on an empty stomach with water or juice and to avoid food, milk, milk products, antacids, and vitamins with mineral supplements for 2 hours.
▶ Remind patient that improvement may take at least 3 months and may continue even after drug is stopped.

▶ etodolac
Lodine, Lodine XL

Pharmacologic classification:
NSAID

Therapeutic classification:
antiarthritic

Pregnancy risk category C

How supplied
Available by prescription only
Capsules: 200 mg, 300 mg
Tablets: 400 mg
Tablets (extended-release): 400 mg, 1,000 mg

Indications and dosages
Acute pain
Adults: 200 to 400 mg P.O. q 6 to 8 hours, p.r.n. Maximum, 1,200 mg/day. For patients who weigh 60 kg (132 lb) or less, daily dose shouldn't exceed 20 mg/kg.
Acute and chronic osteoarthritis, rheumatoid arthritis
Adults: initially, 800 to 1,200 mg P.O. daily in divided doses. Follow with adjustments of 600 to 1,200 mg in divided doses. For example, 200 mg P.O. t.i.d. or q.i.d.; 300 mg P.O. b.i.d., t.i.d., or q.i.d.; or 400 mg P.O. b.i.d. or t.i.d. Maximum, 1,200 mg/day. For patients who weigh 60 kg or less, daily dose shouldn't exceed 20 mg/kg (400 to 1,000 mg P.O. daily for extended-release form). Adjust dosage to lowest effective amount based on patient response. Maximum, 1,000 mg daily.

Pharmacodynamics
Analgesic and antiarthritic actions: Mechanism of action is unknown but presumed to be related

to inhibition of prostaglandin biosynthesis.

Pharmacokinetics

Absorption: Etodolac is well-absorbed from GI tract; levels peak in 1 to 2 hours. Analgesic activity begins within 30 minutes and lasts 4 to 6 hours. Antacids don't appear to affect absorption; however, they can decrease peak levels by 15% to 20%. They have no effect once peak levels are reached.

Distribution: Drug is found in liver, lungs, heart, and kidneys.

Metabolism: Drug is extensively metabolized in the liver.

Excretion: Drug is excreted mainly in urine, and mainly as metabolites; 16% is excreted in feces.

Contraindications and precautions

Contraindicated in patients hypersensitive to drug and in patients with a history of aspirin- or NSAID-induced asthma, rhinitis, urticaria, or other allergic reactions.

Use cautiously in patients with impaired renal or hepatic function, history of peptic ulcer disease, cardiac disease, hypertension, or conditions linked to fluid retention.

Interactions

Drug-drug

Antacids: decreased peak etodolac levels. Avoid concurrent use.

Aspirin: reduces etodolac protein-binding without altering its clearance, which may increase GI toxicity. Monitor patient carefully.

Beta blockers, diuretics: may blunt etodolac effects. Monitor patient closely.

Cyclosporine: enhanced nephrotoxicity and altered cyclosporine elimination causes increased cyclosporine levels. Monitor renal function and cyclosporine levels closely.

Digoxin, lithium, methotrexate: etodolac may alter elimination of these drugs, increasing their levels. Monitor serum levels.

Phenytoin: increased serum phenytoin levels. Monitor serum levels and adjust dose as needed.

Warfarin: decreased warfarin protein-binding but no change in clearance. No dosage adjustment is necessary, but monitor INR and watch for bleeding.

Drug-lifestyle

Alcohol use: increased risk of adverse effects. Advise against concurrent use.

Sun exposure: photosensitivity reactions. Urge patient to avoid exposure.

Effects on diagnostic tests

Phenolic metabolites may cause false-positive test for urinary bilirubin.

Adverse reactions

CNS: *asthenia,* depression, *dizziness,* drowsiness, insomnia, *malaise,* nervousness.

CV: edema, fluid retention, flushing, ***heart failure,*** hypertension, palpitations, syncope.

EENT: blurred vision, dry mouth, photophobia, tinnitus.

GI: *abdominal pain,* anorexia, constipation, *diarrhea, dyspepsia, flatulence,* gastritis, melena, *nausea,* peptic ulceration with or without ***GI bleeding or perforation,*** thirst, ulcerative stomatitis, vomiting.

GU: dysuria, ***renal failure,*** urinary frequency.

Hematologic: *agranulocytosis,* hemolytic anemia, *leukopenia, thrombocytopenia.*
Hepatic: elevated liver function test results, *hepatitis.*
Metabolic: decreased serum uric acid levels, weight gain.
Respiratory: asthma.
Skin: pruritus, rash, *Stevens-Johnson syndrome.*
Other: chills, fever.

Overdose and treatment
Overdose may cause lethargy, drowsiness, nausea, vomiting, and epigastric pain. Rare symptoms include GI bleeding, coma, renal failure, hypertension, and anaphylaxis. Treatment is symptomatic and supportive.

Special considerations
▶ Chronic conditions typically respond within 2 weeks. Once patient experiences pain relief, dosage should be evaluated and adjusted.
▶ Use caution when giving diuretics to patients with cardiac, renal, or hepatic failure.
▶ Etodolac 1,200 mg/day causes less GI bleeding than ibuprofen 2,400 mg/day, indomethacin 200 mg/day, naproxen 750 mg/day, or piroxicam 20 mg/day.
▶ Monitor patient for evidence of GI ulceration and bleeding.

Breast-feeding patients
▶ No data exist to demonstrate whether etodolac appears in breast milk. Use cautiously in breast-feeding women.

Pediatric patients
▶ Safety and efficacy haven't been established in children under age 18.

Geriatric patients
▶ Elderly patients typically don't require age-related dosage adjustments; however, they may have a greater risk of NSAID-induced adverse effects. Individual dosing may be necessary.

Patient teaching
▶ Tell patient that drug may be taken with food to avoid stomach upset.
▶ Instruct patient to report adverse GI effects.
▶ Caution patient to avoid use during pregnancy.

▶ famotidine
Pepcid, Pepcid AC

Pharmacologic classification: *H₂-receptor antagonist*

Therapeutic classification: *antiulcer drug*

Pregnancy risk category B

How supplied
Available by prescription only
Injection: 10 mg/ml
Injection, premixed: 20 mg/50 ml normal saline solution
Suspension: 40 mg/5 ml
Tablets: 20 mg, 40 mg
Available without a prescription (Pepcid AC)
Tablets: 10 mg

Indications and dosages
Duodenal and gastric ulcer
Adults: For acute ulcer, 40 mg P.O. h.s. for 4 to 8 weeks. For maintenance therapy, 20 mg P.O. h.s.

Pathologic hypersecretory conditions (such as Zollinger-Ellison syndrome)
Adults: 20 mg P.O. q 6 hours. Maximum, 160 mg q 6 hours.
Short-term treatment of gastroesophageal reflux disease
Adults: 20 to 40 mg P.O. b.i.d. for up to 12 weeks.
Hospitalized patients with intractable ulcers or hypersecretory conditions, patients who can't take oral drug, patients with GI bleeding, to control gastric pH in critically ill patients
Adults: 20 mg I.V. q 12 hours.
Prevention or treatment of heartburn
Pepcid AC
Adults: 10 mg P.O. when symptoms occur or 10 mg P.O. 1 hour before meals to prevent symptoms. Drug can be used b.i.d. if necessary.
◻ DOSAGE ADJUSTMENT. If patient's creatinine clearance is below 10 ml/minute, dosage may be reduced to 20 mg h.s. or interval may be prolonged to 36 to 48 hours to avoid excess accumulation of drug.

Pharmacodynamics
Antiulcer action: Famotidine competitively inhibits histamine's action at H_2 receptors in gastric parietal cells. This inhibits basal and nocturnal gastric acid secretion from stimulation by caffeine, food, pentagastrin, and other substances.

Pharmacokinetics
Absorption: About 40% to 45% of oral dose is absorbed. Action begins within 1 hour and peaks in 1 to 3 hours. After parenteral administration, action peaks in 30 minutes.

Distribution: Drug is distributed widely to many body tissues.
Metabolism: About 30% to 35% of a dose is metabolized by the liver.
Excretion: Most of drug is excreted unchanged in urine. Famotidine has a longer duration of effect than its 2½- to 4-hour half-life suggests.

Contraindications and precautions
Contraindicated in patients hypersensitive to drug.

Interactions
Drug-drug
Enteric-coated drugs: famotidine may cause enteric coatings to dissolve too rapidly because of increased gastric pH. Separate administration times.
Ketoconazole: decreased ketoconazole absorption. Increase ketoconazole dosage as needed.

Effects on diagnostic tests
Drug may antagonize pentagastrin during gastric acid secretion tests. In skin tests using allergen extracts, drug may cause false-negative results.

Adverse reactions
CNS: dizziness, *headache,* malaise, paresthesia, vertigo.
CV: flushing, palpitations.
EENT: orbital edema, taste disorder, tinnitus.
GI: anorexia, constipation, diarrhea, dry mouth.
GU: increased BUN and creatinine levels.
Hepatic: elevated liver enzymes.
Musculoskeletal: musculoskeletal pain.
Skin: acne, dry skin.
Other: fever, transient irritation at I.V. site.

Overdose and treatment
Overdose hasn't been reported. If it occurred, treatment would include gastric lavage or induced emesis, followed by activated charcoal and supportive and symptomatic therapy. Hemodialysis doesn't remove famotidine.

Special considerations
▶ Drug is most effective when given at bedtime.
▶ If needed, patient may take drug with antacid, especially at the start of therapy when pain is more severe.
▶ After administration via nasogastric tube, tube should be flushed to clear it and to ensure passage of drug into stomach.
▶ For I.V. push, dilute with normal saline solution to total volume of 5 to 10 ml and administer over at least 2 minutes. For I.V. infusion, dilute in 100 ml of D_5W and administer over 15 to 30 minutes. Drug is stable at room temperature for 48 hours. Don't use discolored or precipitated solution.
▶ Drug isn't recommended for more than 8 weeks in patients with uncomplicated duodenal ulcer.
▶ Drug appears to cause fewer adverse reactions and interactions than cimetidine.
▶ Monitor patient for blood in emesis, stool, or gastric aspirate.
▶ Mint flavor contains phenylalanine.

Breast-feeding patients
▶ Drug may appear in breast milk. Use with caution in breast-feeding women.

Geriatric patients
▶ Use drug cautiously in elderly patients because of increased risk of adverse reactions, particularly those affecting the CNS.

Patient teaching
▶ Caution patient to take drug only as directed and to continue taking it even after pain subsides, to ensure adequate healing.
▶ Instruct patient to take dose at bedtime.
▶ Advise patient to avoid smoking because it may increase gastric acid secretion.

▶ fenoprofen calcium
Nalfon

Pharmacologic classification:
NSAID

Therapeutic classification:
anti-inflammatory, antipyretic, nonnarcotic analgesic

Pregnancy risk category NR

How supplied
Available by prescription only
Capsules: 200 mg, 300 mg
Tablets: 600 mg

Indications and dosages
Rheumatoid arthritis and osteoarthritis
Adults: 300 to 600 mg P.O. t.i.d. or q.i.d. Maximum, 3.2 g/day.
Mild to moderate pain
Adults: 200 mg P.O. q 4 to 6 hours, p.r.n.
Acute gouty arthritis*
Adults: 200 mg P.O. q 6 hours. Decrease dose based on patient response.

Pharmacodynamics
Analgesic, anti-inflammatory, and antipyretic actions: Mechanisms

of action unknown, but drug probably inhibits prostaglandin synthesis. Fenoprofen decreases platelet aggregation and may prolong bleeding time.

Pharmacokinetics
Absorption: Drug is absorbed rapidly and completely from the GI tract. Analgesic activity starts in 15 to 30 minutes; plasma levels peak in 2 hours. Duration of action is about 4 to 6 hours.
Distribution: About 99% of fenoprofen is protein-bound.
Metabolism: Fenoprofen is metabolized in the liver.
Excretion: Drug is excreted chiefly in urine with a serum half-life of 2½ to 3 hours. A small amount is excreted in feces.

Contraindications and precautions
Contraindicated in pregnant patients, in patients hypersensitive to drug, and in patients with significantly reduced renal function, a history of aspirin- or NSAID-induced asthma, rhinitis, or urticaria.

Use cautiously in elderly patients and patients with a history of GI events, peptic ulcer disease, compromised cardiac function, or hypertension.

Interactions
Drug-drug
Acetaminophen, gold compounds: increased nephrotoxicity. Monitor renal function.
Anticoagulants, thrombolytics: may potentiate anticoagulant effects. Monitor PT and INR.
Antihypertensives, diuretics: fenoprofen may decrease the effectiveness of these drugs. Monitor for clinical effects.

Anti-inflammatory drugs (aspirin, salicylates): increased risk of nephrotoxicity, bleeding problems, and adverse GI reactions, including ulceration and hemorrhage. Use cautiously together, and monitor patient's renal function, PT, and INR.
Aspirin: may decrease fenoprofen bioavailability. Monitor patient for effectiveness.
Cefamandole, cefoperazone, drugs that inhibit platelet aggregation (dextran, dipyridamole, mezlocillin, piperacillin, sulfinpyrazone, ticarcillin, valproic acid), plicamycin: increased risk of bleeding problems. Monitor PT and INR during concurrent use.
Corticosteroids, corticotropin: may increase risk of adverse GI reactions, including ulceration and hemorrhage. Use together with caution.
Diuretics: may increase nephrotoxic potential. Use together with caution.
Highly protein-bound drugs, such as coumarin derivatives, nifedipine, phenytoin, verapamil: these drugs may be displaced from binding sites. Monitor patient for evidence of toxicity.
Insulin, oral antidiabetic drugs: may potentiate hypoglycemic effects. Monitor serum glucose levels.
Lithium, methotrexate: decreased renal clearance of these drugs. Monitor patient for evidence of toxicity.

Drug-lifestyle
Alcohol use: increased risk of adverse GI reactions. Advise against concurrent use.

Effects on diagnostic tests
None reported.

Adverse reactions

CNS: asthenia, confusion, dizziness, fatigue, *headache,* nervousness, *somnolence,* tremor.
CV: palpitations, peripheral edema.
EENT: blurred vision, decreased hearing, nasopharyngitis, tinnitus.
GI: anorexia, constipation, *dyspepsia, epigastric distress,* flatulence, *GI bleeding, nausea,* occult blood loss, peptic ulceration, vomiting.
GU: cystitis, increased BUN and creatinine, hematuria, interstitial nephritis, oliguria, papillary necrosis, proteinuria, reversible renal failure.
Hematologic: anemia, *agranulocytosis, aplastic anemia,* bruising, hemolytic anemia, *hemorrhage,* prolonged bleeding time, *thrombocytopenia.*
Hepatic: elevated liver enzymes, *hepatitis.*
Metabolic: false elevations of free and total serum T_3, hyperkalemia.
Respiratory: dyspnea, upper respiratory tract infections.
Skin: increased diaphoresis, *pruritus,* rash, urticaria.
Other: *anaphylaxis, angioedema.*

Overdose and treatment

Little is known about the acute toxicity of fenoprofen. Nonoliguric renal failure, tachycardia, and hypotension have been observed. Other symptoms include drowsiness, dizziness, confusion and lethargy, nausea, vomiting, headache, tinnitus, and blurred vision. Elevations in serum creatinine and BUN levels have been reported.

To treat fenoprofen overdose, immediately induce emesis with ipecac syrup or perform gastric lavage. Give activated charcoal via nasogastric tube. Provide symptomatic and supportive measures (respiratory support and correction of fluid and electrolyte imbalances). Monitor laboratory values and vital signs closely. Dialysis is of little value.

Special considerations

▶ Fenoprofen has been used to treat fever, acute gouty arthritis, and juvenile arthritis.
▶ Drug is effective in treating pain from inflammation, migraines, other headaches, and dysmenorrhea.
▶ Start at low doses and increase to lowest effective maintenance dose.
▶ Monitor patient for CNS effects, and take safety precautions to prevent injury.
▶ Monitor patient's renal, hepatic, ocular, and auditory function during long-term therapy. Stop drug if abnormalities occur.
▶ Because of antipyretic and anti-inflammatory actions, NSAIDs may mask evidence of infection.
▶ Because NSAIDs impair renal prostaglandin synthesis, they can decrease renal blood flow and lead to reversible renal impairment, especially in patients with pre-existing renal failure, liver dysfunction, or heart failure; in elderly patients; and in patients who take diuretics.
▶ NSAIDs may precipitate asthma.

Breast-feeding patients

▶ Because drug appears in breast milk, avoid use in breast-feeding women.

Pediatric patients

▶ Safe use of fenoprofen in children hasn't been established. Drug isn't recommended for children under age 14.

Reactions may be *common,* uncommon, *life-threatening,* or COMMON AND LIFE-THREATENING.

Geriatric patients
▶ Patients over age 60 may be more susceptible to toxic effects, especially adverse GI reactions. Use with caution.
▶ The effects of drug on renal prostaglandins may cause fluid retention and edema, a significant drawback for elderly patients and those with heart failure.

Patient teaching
▶ Tell patient to avoid hazardous activities until full CNS effects of drug are known.
▶ Instruct patient in safety measures to prevent injury.
▶ Caution patient to consult prescriber before taking OTC analgesics.

▶ **fentanyl citrate**
Sublimaze

▶ **fentanyl transdermal system**
Duragesic-25, Duragesic-50, Duragesic-75, Duragesic-100

▶ **fentanyl transmucosal**
Actiq lozenge on a stick, Fentanyl Oralet

Pharmacologic classification: *opioid agonist*

Therapeutic classification: *adjunct to anesthesia, analgesic, anesthetic*

Controlled substance schedule II

Pregnancy risk category C

How supplied
Available by prescription only
Injection: 50 mcg/ml

Lozenge on a stick: 100 mcg, 200 mcg, 300 mcg, 400 mcg, 600 mcg, 800 mcg, 1200 mcg, 1600 mcg
Transdermal: patches designed to release 25 mcg, 50 mcg, 75 mcg, or 100 mcg of fentanyl/hour.
Transmucosal: 100 mcg, 200 mcg, 300 mcg, 400 mcg

Indications and dosages
Preoperative analgesia
Adults: 50 to 100 mcg I.M. 30 to 60 minutes before surgery. Or one Oralet lozenge (100 mcg, 200 mcg, 300 mcg, or 400 mcg) P.O. 20 to 40 minutes before surgery, which patient sucks until dissolved. Oralet dose is usually 5 mcg/kg for adults and up to 15 mcg/kg for children.
Adjunct to general anesthetic for minor procedures
Adults: 2 mcg/kg I.V.
Adjunct to general anesthetic for major procedures
Adults: initially, 2 to 20 mcg/kg I.V. May give additional doses of 25 to 100 mcg I.V. or I.M., p.r.n.
Adjunct to general anesthetic for complicated procedures
Adults: initially, 20 to 50 mcg/kg. May give additional doses of 25 mcg to half the initial dose, p.r.n.
Adjunct to regional anesthesia
Adults: 50 to 100 mcg I.M. or slow I.V. over 1 to 2 minutes.
Induction and maintenance of anesthesia
Children ages 2 to 12: Reduced dose as low as 2 to 3 mcg/kg.
Postoperative analgesic
Adults: 50 to 100 mcg I.M. q 1 to 2 hours, p.r.n.
Chronic pain in patients for whom lesser drugs have failed
Adults: one transdermal patch applied to the upper torso on an area of skin that isn't irritated and

---

◇ Available in Canada only   *Unlabeled use

hasn't been irradiated. Start with 25-mcg/hour and adjust dosage as needed and tolerated. Each patch may be worn for 72 hours.

Breakthrough cancer pain
Adults: initially, 200-mcg lozenge placed between cheek and lower gum. Patient should suck, not chew, the lozenge over 15 minutes. One more lozenge may be given 30 minutes after the first if needed. Don't give more than 2 lozenges per episode. Re-evaluate pain control every 1 to 2 days.

◙ DOSAGE ADJUSTMENT. Lower doses are usually indicated for elderly patients, who may be more sensitive to therapeutic and adverse effects of drug.

Pharmacodynamics
Analgesic action: Fentanyl binds to opiate receptors as an agonist to alter the perception of painful stimuli, thus providing analgesia for moderate to severe pain. CNS and respiratory depressant effects are similar to those of morphine. Drug has little hypnotic activity and rarely causes histamine release.

Pharmacokinetics
Absorption: Onset of action is immediate after I.V. administration, 7 to 8 minutes after I.M. injection, and 5 to 15 minutes after transmucosal dose. Onset after transdermal delivery may take several hours. Effects peak 3 to 5 minutes after I.V. dose, 20 to 30 minutes after I.M. or transmucosal dose, and 1 to 3 days after transdermal dose.
Distribution: Redistribution has been suggested as the main cause of the brief analgesic effect of fentanyl.

Metabolism: Fentanyl is metabolized in the liver.
Excretion: Fentanyl is excreted in urine as metabolites and unchanged drug. Elimination half-life is about 7 hours after parenteral use, 5 to 15 hours after transmucosal use, and 18 hours after transdermal use.

Contraindications and precautions
Contraindicated in patients intolerant of drug and within 14 days of taking an MAO inhibitor.

Use cautiously in elderly or debilitated patients and in those with head injuries, increased CSF pressure, COPD, decreased respiratory reserve, compromised respirations, arrhythmias, or hepatic, renal, or cardiac disease.

Interactions
Drug-drug
Anticholinergics: may cause paralytic ileus. Monitor patient closely.
Cimetidine: increased respiratory and CNS depression, causing confusion, disorientation, apnea, or seizures. Fentanyl dosage should be reduced by one-quarter to one-third.
CNS depressants, such as antihistamines, barbiturates, benzodiazepines, general anesthetics, muscle relaxants, narcotic analgesics, phenothiazines, sedative-hypnotics, tricyclic antidepressants: potentiates drug's respiratory and CNS depression, sedation, and hypotensive effects. Use together cautiously.
Diazepam: potential CV depression when given with high doses of fentanyl. Use together cautiously.
Droperidol: when used with fentanyl, may cause hypotension and

a decrease in pulmonary artery pressure. (A droperidol-fentanyl combination, Innovar, is available.) Monitor patient closely.

Drugs extensively metabolized in the liver, such as digitoxin, phenytoin, rifampin: drug accumulation and enhanced effects may result from concomitant use of these drugs. Monitor patient for toxicity.

General anesthetics: potentially severe CV depression. Monitor patient closely.

Narcotic antagonists: acute withdrawal syndrome if narcotic antagonist given to a patient physically dependent on fentanyl. Use very cautiously, if necessary.

Spinal anesthesia and some peridural anesthetics: when used to supplement conduction anesthesia, fentanyl can alter respiration by blocking intercostal nerves. Monitor vital signs closely.

Drug-lifestyle

Alcohol use: may cause additive effects. Advise against concurrent use.

Effects on diagnostic tests

None reported.

Adverse reactions

CNS: anxiety, *asthenia, clouded sensorium, confusion,* depression, dizziness, *euphoria,* headache, hallucinations, nervousness, *sedation, somnolence.*
CV: *arrhythmias,* chest pain, hypertension, *hypotension.*
GI: abdominal pain, anorexia, *constipation,* diarrhea, *dry mouth,* dyspepsia, ileus, increased plasma amylase and lipase levels, *nausea, vomiting.*
GU: *urine retention.*

Respiratory: *apnea,* dyspnea, hypoventilation, *respiratory depression.*
Skin: *diaphoresis, pruritus,* reaction at application site (erythema, papules, edema).
Other: physical dependence.

Overdose and treatment

Overdose most often causes extensions of drug actions. They include CNS depression, respiratory depression, and miosis (pinpoint pupils). Other acute toxic effects include hypotension, bradycardia, hypothermia, shock, apnea, cardiopulmonary arrest, circulatory collapse, pulmonary edema, and seizures.

To treat acute overdose, establish adequate respiratory exchange via a patent airway and ventilation as needed. Give naloxone to reverse significant respiratory or CV depression. (Because fentanyl's duration of action is longer than naloxone's, repeated doses may be needed.) Monitor vital signs closely. Also, provide symptomatic and supportive treatment, such as continued respiratory support and correction of fluid or electrolyte imbalance. Monitor laboratory values, vital signs, and neurologic status closely.

Special considerations

▶ For better analgesic effect, give drug before patient has intense pain.
▶ High doses can produce muscle rigidity. This effect can be reversed by naloxone.
▶ Many anesthesiologists use epidural and intrathecal fentanyl as a potent adjunct to epidural anesthesia.

▶ Epidural administration allows for less sedation than systemic opiates and a faster recovery.

▶ Observe patient for delayed onset of respiratory depression. The high lipid solubility of fentanyl may contribute to this potential adverse effect.

▶ Monitor patient's heart rate. Fentanyl may cause bradycardia. Pretreatment with an anticholinergic (such as atropine or glycopyrrolate) may minimize this effect.

▶ Assess patient for constipation, and place on a bowel regimen. Note that drug may be helpful in treating diarrhea caused by chemotherapy or radiation therapy.

Transdermal form

▶ Transdermal fentanyl isn't recommended for postoperative pain.

▶ Dosage equivalent charts are available to calculate the fentanyl transdermal dose based on daily morphine intake. For example, 25 mcg/hour of transdermal fentanyl is needed for every 90 mg of oral morphine or 15 mg of I.M. morphine per 24 hours. Some patients will require alternative means of opiate administration when the dose exceeds 300 mcg/hour.

▶ Dosage adjustments in patients using the transdermal system should be made gradually. Reaching steady state levels of a new dose may take up to 6 days; delay dose adjustment until after at least two applications.

▶ Adjust dose gradually in 25 mcg/hour increments based on breakthrough pain.

▶ Most patients experience good control of pain for 3 days while wearing the transdermal system, although a few may need a new application after 48 hours. Because serum fentanyl level rises for the first 24 hours after application, analgesic effect can't be evaluated for the first day. Make sure patient has adequate supplemental analgesic to prevent breakthrough pain.

▶ When reducing opiate therapy or switching to a different analgesic, withdraw the transdermal system gradually. Because fentanyl's serum level drops very gradually after removal, give half of the equianalgesic dose of the new analgesic 12 to 18 hours after removal.

▶ Actiq pops may be effective in combination with transdermal patches for effective pain relief.

▶ Monitor patients who develop adverse reactions to the transdermal system for at least 12 hours after removal. Serum levels of fentanyl drop very gradually and may take as long as 17 hours to decline by 50%.

Transmucosal form

▶ Remove foil wrapper of fentanyl Oralet just before administration.

▶ Have patient place Oralet in mouth and suck (not chew or swallow) it.

▶ After consumption or if patient shows signs of respiratory depression, remove Oralet from patient's mouth using the handle. Place any remaining portion in the plastic wrapper and discard accordingly for Schedule II drugs.

I.V. administration

▶ Only staff trained to administer I.V. anesthetics and manage their adverse effects should administer I.V. fentanyl.

▶ Fentanyl is commonly used I.V. with droperidol to produce neuroleptanalgesia.

▶ Keep narcotic antagonist (naloxone) and resuscitation equipment available when giving drug I.V.

Breast-feeding patients
▶ Drug appears in breast milk; administer cautiously to breast-feeding women.

Pediatric patients
▶ Safe parenteral use in children under age 2 hasn't been established.
▶ Safe transdermal use in children of all ages hasn't been established.
▶ Safe use of Actiq hasn't been established in children under age 16.
▶ Avoid using Oralet in children who weigh less than 10 kg (22 lbs).

Geriatric patients
▶ Use with caution in elderly patients.

Patient teaching
▶ Teach patient proper application of the transdermal patch: Clip hair at the application site, but don't use a razor, which may irritate the skin. Wash area with clear water if necessary, but not with soaps, oils, lotions, alcohol, or other substances that may irritate the skin or prevent adhesion. Dry area completely before applying the patch.
▶ Tell patient to remove transdermal patch from package just before applying. Hold in place for 10 to 20 seconds, and make sure the edges of the patch adhere to the patient's skin.
▶ For disposal, teach patient to fold patch so adhesive side adheres to itself, and then flush it down the toilet.

▶ If another patch is needed after 72 hours, tell patient to apply it to a new site.
▶ Teach patient to suck, not chew, transmucosal form of drug. Chewing or swallowing may reduce peak levels and shorten pain relief.
▶ Instruct patient that when using Actiq, two units may be used per breakthrough pain episode. If using more than 4 units/day, dosing adjustments may be needed.
▶ Tell patient not to discontinue the drug abruptly.
▶ Tell patient to discard drug out of the reach of children.

▶ flumazenil
Romazicon

Pharmacologic classification: *benzodiazepine antagonist*

Therapeutic classification: *antidote*

Pregnancy risk category C

How supplied
Available by prescription only
Injection: 0.1 mg/ml in 5-ml and 10-ml multiple-dose vials

Indications and dosages
Complete or partial reversal of benzodiazepine sedative effects after anesthesia or short diagnostic procedure (conscious sedation)
Adults: initially, 0.2 mg I.V. over 15 seconds. If patient doesn't reach desired level of consciousness after 45 seconds, repeat dose. Repeat at 1-minute intervals until a cumulative dose of 1 mg has been given (initial dose plus four more doses). Most patients respond after 0.6 to

1 mg of drug. If resedation occurs, dosage may be repeated after 20 minutes, but no more than 1 mg should be given at one time, and patient should not receive more than 3 mg/hour.

Suspected benzodiazepine overdose

Adults: initially, 0.2 mg I.V. over 30 seconds. If patient doesn't reach desired level of consciousness after 30 seconds, administer 0.3 mg over 30 seconds. If patient still doesn't respond adequately, give 0.5 mg over 30 seconds, then repeat 0.5-mg doses at 1-minute intervals until a cumulative dose of 3 mg has been given. Most patients with benzodiazepine overdose respond to cumulative doses between 1 and 3 mg; rarely, patients who respond partially after 3 mg may require additional doses. Don't give more than 5 mg over 5 minutes initially; sedation that persists after this dosage is unlikely to be caused by benzodiazepines. If resedation occurs, dosage may be repeated after 20 minutes, but no more than 1 mg should be given at one time, and patient shouldn't receive more than 3 mg/hour.

Pharmacodynamics

Antidote action: Flumazenil competitively inhibits the actions of benzodiazepines on the GABA-benzodiazepine receptor complex.

Pharmacokinetics

Absorption: Action starts 1 to 2 minutes after injection; 80% response occurs within 3 minutes, and peak effect occurs in 6 to 10 minutes.

Distribution: After administration, drug redistributes rapidly (initial distribution half-life is 7 to 15 minutes). It's about 50% bound to plasma proteins.

Metabolism: Drug is rapidly extracted from blood and metabolized by the liver. Metabolites that have been identified are inactive. Ingestion of food during an I.V. infusion enhances extraction of drug from plasma, probably by increasing hepatic blood flow.

Excretion: About 90% to 95% appears in the urine as metabolites; the rest is excreted in feces. Plasma half-life is about 54 minutes.

Contraindications and precautions

Contraindicated in patients hypersensitive to drug or benzodiazepines, in patients who show evidence of serious tricyclic antidepressant overdose, and in those who received a benzodiazepine to treat a potentially life-threatening condition (such as status epilepticus).

Use cautiously in alcohol-dependent or psychiatric patients, in those at high risk for developing seizures, or in those with head injuries, signs of seizures, or recent high intake of benzodiazepines (such as patients in the ICU).

Interactions
Drug-drug

Antidepressants, drugs that cause seizures or arrhythmias: increased risk of seizures or arrhythmias after flumazenil removes the effects of benzodiazepine overdose. Flumazenil shouldn't be used in mixed overdose, especially if seizures (from any cause) are likely to occur.

Reactions may be *common,* uncommon, *life-threatening,* or COMMON AND LIFE-THREATENING.

Effects on diagnostic tests
None reported.

Adverse reactions
CNS: *abnormal or blurred vision,* agitation, *dizziness,* emotional lability, *headache,* insomnia, *seizures,* tremor.
CV: *arrhythmias,* cutaneous vasodilation, palpitations.
GI: nausea, vomiting.
Respiratory: dyspnea, hyperventilation.
Skin: *diaphoresis.*
Other: *pain at injection site.*

Overdose and treatment
In clinical trials, large doses of flumazenil were administered I.V. to volunteers in the absence of a benzodiazepine agonist. No serious adverse reactions, signs or symptoms, or altered laboratory tests were noted. In patients with benzodiazepine overdose, large doses of flumazenil may produce agitation or anxiety, hyperesthesia, increased muscle tone, or seizures.

Seizures may be treated with barbiturates, phenytoin, or benzodiazepines.

Special considerations
▶ Because flumazenil has a shorter duration of action than benzodiazepines, monitor patient carefully and give additional drug as needed. Duration and degree of effect depend on plasma levels of the sedating benzodiazepine and the dose of flumazenil.
▶ Monitor patient for resedation according to duration of drug being reversed. Monitor closely after long-acting benzodiazepines (such as diazepam) or after high doses of shorter-acting benzodiazepines (such as 10 mg of midazolam).

Usually, serious resedation is unlikely in patients who fail to show signs of it 2 hours after a 1-mg dose of flumazenil.
▶ During I.V. administration, make sure that airway is secure and patent.
▶ Flumazenil can be given by direct injection or diluted with a compatible solution. Discard within 24 hours any unused drug that has been drawn into a syringe or diluted.
▶ Compatible solutions include D_5W, lactated Ringer's injection, and normal saline solution.
▶ To minimize pain at injection site, give drug over 15 to 30 seconds into a free-flowing I.V. solution running into a large vein.
▶ Avoid extravasation into perivascular tissues.

Breast-feeding patients
▶ No data exist to demonstrate whether drug appears in breast milk. Use cautiously in breast-feeding women.

Pediatric patients
▶ Because no data exist regarding risks, benefits, or dosage range in children, manufacturer doesn't recommend its use.

Patient teaching
▶ Because of risk of resedation, advise patient to avoid hazardous activities, alcohol use, CNS depressants, and OTC drugs within 24 hours after receiving drug.

▶ fluoxetine
Prozac, Prozac Pulvules

Pharmacologic classification:
selective serotonin reuptake inhibitor

Therapeutic classification:
antidepressant

Pregnancy risk category B

How supplied
Available by prescription only
Capsules: 10 mg, 20 mg
Oral solution: 20 mg/5 ml

Indications and dosages
Myoclonus*
Adults: 20 mg/day P.O. in the morning. Increase dosage, p.r.n., after several weeks to 40 mg daily with a dose in the morning and midday. Maximum, 80 mg/day.
Daily headaches*, migraine headaches*, tension headaches*
Adults: 20 mg P.O. every other day to 40 mg daily.
Premenstrual syndrome*
Adults: 20 mg P.O. daily.
◨ DOSAGE ADJUSTMENT. Elderly patients, patients with concurrent disease, patients who take several drugs, and patients with renal or hepatic impairment may need a lower dosage or less frequent administration schedule.

Pharmacodynamics
Analgesic action: Unknown.
Antidepressant action: The antidepressant action of fluoxetine is purportedly related to its inhibition of CNS neuronal uptake of serotonin. Fluoxetine blocks uptake of serotonin, but not of norepinephrine. Animal studies suggest it's a much more potent uptake inhibitor of serotonin than of norepinephrine.

Pharmacokinetics
Absorption: Drug is well absorbed after oral administration. Absorption isn't altered by food.
Distribution: Drug is apparently highly protein-bound (about 95%).
Metabolism: Drug is metabolized primarily in the liver to active metabolites.
Excretion: Drug is excreted in urine. Elimination half-life is 2 to 3 days. Norfluoxetine, the primary active metabolite, has an elimination half-life of 7 to 9 days.

Contraindications and precautions
Contraindicated in patients hypersensitive to drug and in patients who took an MAO inhibitor within 14 days.
　Use cautiously in patients at high risk of suicide or in those with a history of seizures, diabetes mellitus, or renal, hepatic, or CV disease.

Interactions
Drug-drug
Carbamazepine, flecainide, vinblastine: may increase serum levels of these drugs. Monitor patient for toxicity.
Insulin, oral antidiabetic drugs: may alter blood glucose levels and possible requirements for antidiabetic drug. Monitor serum glucose and adjust dosage as needed.
Lithium, tricyclic antidepressants: may increase adverse CNS effects. Monitor patient for adverse effects.
Phenytoin: may increase plasma phenytoin levels and risk of toxicity. Monitor patient for toxicity.

Tryptophan: may increase adverse CNS effects (agitation, restlessness) and GI distress. Monitor patient for adverse effects.
Warfarin and other highly protein-bound drugs: may increase plasma levels of fluoxetine or other highly protein-bound drugs. Monitor patient for toxicity, and adjust dosages as needed.

Drug-lifestyle
Alcohol use: may increase CNS depression. Advise against concurrent use.

Effects on diagnostic tests
None reported.

Adverse reactions
CNS: *anxiety, asthenia, dizziness, drowsiness,* fatigue, *headache, insomnia, nervousness, tremor.*
CV: hot flashes, palpitations.
EENT: cough, nasal congestion, pharyngitis, sinusitis.
GI: abdominal pain, *anorexia,* constipation, *diarrhea, dry mouth, dyspepsia,* flatulence, increased appetite, *nausea,* vomiting.
GU: sexual dysfunction.
Metabolic: *weight loss.*
Musculoskeletal: muscle pain.
Respiratory: respiratory distress, upper respiratory infection.
Skin: diaphoresis, *pruritus, rash.*
Other: fever, flulike syndrome.

Overdose and treatment
Overdose may cause agitation, restlessness, hypomania, and other signs of CNS excitation. Higher doses may cause nausea and vomiting as well. About 38 reports of acute fluoxetine overdose include two fatalities; they involved plasma levels of 4.57 mg/L and 1.93 mg/L. One person took 1.8 g

of fluoxetine with an undetermined amount of maprotiline. The other took fluoxetine, codeine, and temazepam. A third person developed two tonic-clonic seizures after taking 3 g of fluoxetine; they stopped spontaneously and didn't require anticonvulsant treatment.

To treat fluoxetine overdose, establish and maintain an airway; ensure adequate oxygenation and ventilation. Induce emesis, perform gastric lavage, or give activated charcoal with or without sorbitol. Monitor patient's cardiac status and vital signs, and provide supportive measures as needed. Fluoxetine-induced seizures that don't subside spontaneously may respond to diazepam. Forced diuresis, dialysis, hemoperfusion, and exchange transfusion are unlikely to help.

Special considerations
▶ Effective migraine prophylaxis may take several months.
▶ Drug is usually used to treat depression.
▶ Consider a depressed patient to have a risk of suicide until depression improves significantly. Supervise high-risk patients closely early in therapy. To reduce risk of suicidal overdose, prescribe the smallest quantity of pulvules consistent with good management.
▶ Full antidepressant effect may not occur for 4 weeks or possibly longer.
▶ Treatment of acute depression usually requires at least several months of continuous drug therapy; optimal duration of therapy hasn't been established.
▶ Because of its long elimination half-life, changes in fluoxetine

dosage won't be reflected in plasma for several weeks.

▶ Fluoxetine therapy may activate mania or hypomania.

▶ Fluoxetine is also used for panic disorder, bipolar disorder, alcohol dependence, cataplexy, obesity, eating disorders, and obsessive-compulsive disorder.

Patient teaching

▶ Caution patient to avoid hazardous activities until full CNS effects of drug are known. Drug may cause dizziness or drowsiness.

▶ Tell patient to avoid alcohol and to consult prescriber before taking other prescribed drugs, OTC medications, or herbal remedies.

▶ Tell patient to promptly report rash or hives, anxiety, nervousness, anorexia (especially in underweight patients), suspicion of pregnancy, or intent to become pregnant.

▶ flurbiprofen
Ansaid

Pharmacologic classification:
NSAID, phenylalkanoic acid derivative

Therapeutic classification:
antiarthritic

Pregnancy risk category B

How supplied

Available by prescription only
Tablets: 50 mg, 100 mg

Indications and dosages
Rheumatoid arthritis, osteoarthritis
Adults: 200 to 300 mg/day P.O. divided b.i.d., t.i.d., or q.i.d.

☒ **DOSAGE ADJUSTMENT.** Flurbiprofen metabolites may accumulate if patient has end-stage renal disease. Monitor patient closely and adjust dosage accordingly.

Pharmacodynamics
Anti-inflammatory action: An NSAID, flurbiprofen interferes with prostaglandin synthesis.

Pharmacokinetics
Absorption: Drug is well absorbed after oral administration; levels peak in about 1 to 1½ hours. Giving drug with food alters rate but not extent of absorption.
Distribution: Flurbiprofen is highly bound (more than 99%) to plasma proteins.
Metabolism: Drug is metabolized primarily in the liver. The major metabolite shows little anti-inflammatory activity.
Excretion: Drug is excreted primarily in the urine. Average elimination half-life is 6 to 10 hours.

Contraindications and precautions
Contraindicated in patients hypersensitive to drug and patients with a history of aspirin- or NSAID-induced asthma, urticaria, or other allergic reactions.

Use cautiously in elderly or debilitated patients and those with a history of peptic ulcer disease, herpes simplex keratitis, impaired renal or hepatic function, cardiac disease, or conditions linked to fluid retention.

Interactions
Drug-drug
Aspirin: may decrease flurbiprofen levels and increase GI toxicity. Monitor patient closely.

Beta blockers: antihypertensive effect may be impaired. Monitor patient's blood pressure.

Cyclosporine: increased risk of nephrotoxicity. Monitor renal function.

Diuretics: decreased diuretic effect. Monitor patient for drug effects.

Lithium: serum lithium levels may be increased. Monitor lithium levels.

Methotrexate: increased risk of methotrexate toxicity. Monitor patient for signs of toxicity.

Oral anticoagulants: increased bleeding tendencies. Monitor PT and INR.

Drug-lifestyle

Alcohol use: increased risk of adverse GI reactions. Advise patient to avoid alcohol.

Sun exposure: may potentiate photosensitivity reactions. Urge precautions.

Effects on diagnostic tests

None reported.

Adverse reactions

CNS: amnesia, anxiety, asthenia, depression, dizziness, drowsiness, *headache,* increased reflexes, insomnia, malaise, tremors.

CV: *edema,* **heart failure,** hypertension, vasodilation.

EENT: epistaxis, rhinitis, tinnitus, visual changes.

GI: *abdominal pain, bleeding,* constipation, *diarrhea, dyspepsia,* flatulence, *nausea,* vomiting.

GU: hematuria, interstitial nephritis, **renal failure,** *symptoms suggesting urinary tract infection.*

Hematologic: anemia, **aplastic anemia, neutropenia, thrombocytopenia.**

Hepatic: *elevated liver enzymes, jaundice.*

Metabolic: weight changes.

Respiratory: asthma.

Skin: **angioedema,** photosensitivity, rash, urticaria.

Overdose and treatment

Overdose may cause lethargy, coma, respiratory depression, epigastric pain and distress.

Treatment should be supportive. Induce emesis or perform gastric lavage, but keep in mind that emptying patient's stomach is of little use if ingestion took place more than an hour before treatment.

Special considerations

▶ Drug may be used for other types of pain; for example, menstrual, headache, or cancer pain.

▶ Start therapy at a low dosage and increase to lowest effective maintenance dose.

▶ Because NSAIDs inhibit platelet aggregation, patients should be monitored for increased bleeding tendencies.

▶ Patients receiving long-term therapy should have periodic liver function studies, ophthalmologic and auditory examinations, and hematocrit determinations.

▶ Because of antipyretic and anti-inflammatory actions, NSAIDs may mask evidence of infection.

▶ Because NSAIDs impair synthesis of renal prostaglandins, they can decrease renal blood flow and lead to reversible renal impairment, especially in patients with renal failure, liver dysfunction, or heart failure. Risk is also increased in elderly patients and in patients who take diuretics. Start these patients at low dosages, and monitor renal function periodically.

▶ NSAIDs may precipitate asthma.

Breast-feeding patients
▶ A breast-feeding woman taking 200 mg of flurbiprofen daily could deliver as much as 0.1 mg to the infant each day. Breast-feeding isn't recommended while using the drug.

Pediatric patients
▶ Safe use in children hasn't been established.

Patient teaching
▶ Tell patient to take drug with food, milk, or antacid to minimize GI upset.
▶ Review the signs and symptoms of GI bleeding, and tell patient to discontinue drug and promptly notify prescriber if they occur.
▶ Caution patient to avoid hazardous activities until full CNS effects of drug are known.
▶ Tell patient to immediately notify prescriber about edema, substantial weight gain, black stools, rash, itching, or visual disturbances.

▶ gabapentin
Neurontin

Pharmacologic classification:
1-amino-methyl cyclohexoneacetic acid

Therapeutic classification:
anticonvulsant

Pregnancy risk category C

How supplied
Available by prescription only
Capsules: 100 mg, 300 mg, 400 mg

Indications and dosages
Partial seizures with or without secondary generalization (adjunct)
Adults: 300 mg P.O. on day 1, 300 mg P.O. b.i.d. on day 2, and 300 mg P.O. t.i.d. on day 3. Increase dosage as needed and tolerated to 1,800 mg daily, in three divided doses. Usual dosage is 300 to 600 mg P.O. t.i.d., although dosages up to 3,600 mg/day have been well tolerated.
◪ DOSAGE ADJUSTMENT. In adult patients with renal failure, give 400 mg P.O. t.i.d. if creatinine clearance is above 60 ml/minute, 300 mg P.O. b.i.d. if creatinine clearance is 31 to 60 ml/minute, 300 mg P.O. daily if creatinine clearance is 15 to 30 ml/minute, and 300 mg P.O. every other day if creatinine clearance is less than 15 ml/minute. Patients on hemodialysis should receive a loading dose of 300 to 400 mg P.O. and then 200 to 300 mg P.O. after hemodialysis.

Pharmacodynamics
Anticonvulsant action: Unknown. Although drug is structurally related to GABA, it doesn't interact with GABA receptors, isn't converted metabolically into GABA or a GABA agonist, and doesn't inhibit GABA uptake or degradation. Gabapentin doesn't exhibit affinity for other common receptor sites.

Pharmacokinetics
Absorption: Drug bioavailability isn't dose proportional. A 400-mg dose, for example, is about 25% less bioavailable than a 100-mg dose. Over the recommended dose range of 300 to 600 mg t.i.d., differences in bioavailability aren't

---

large and bioavailability is about 60%. Food has no effect on the rate or extent of absorption.

Distribution: Gabapentin circulates largely unbound (less than 3%) to plasma protein. It crosses the blood-brain barrier, and about 20% of plasma level appears in CSF.

Metabolism: Drug isn't appreciably metabolized.

Excretion: Gabapentin is eliminated from systemic circulation by renal excretion as unchanged drug. Its elimination half-life is 5 to 7 hours. Drug can be removed from plasma by hemodialysis.

Contraindications and precautions
Contraindicated in patients hypersensitive to drug.

Interactions
Drug-drug
Antacids: decreased gabapentin absorption. Separate drugs by at least 2 hours.

Effects on diagnostic tests
Gabapentin causes false-positive results in the Ames N-Multistix SG dipstick test for urine protein when added to other antiepileptic drugs. The more specific sulfosalicylic acid precipitation procedure is recommended to detect urine protein.

Adverse reactions
CNS: abnormal thinking, amnesia, *ataxia,* depression, *dizziness,* dysarthria, *fatigue,* incoordination, nervousness, *nystagmus, somnolence, tremor,* twitching.

CV: peripheral edema, vasodilation.

EENT: *amblyopia,* coughing, dental abnormalities, *diplopia,* dry throat, pharyngitis, *rhinitis.*

GI: constipation, dry mouth, dyspepsia, increased appetite, nausea, vomiting.

GU: impotence.

Hematologic: *leukopenia.*

Metabolic: weight gain.

Musculoskeletal: back pain, fractures, myalgia.

Skin: abrasion, pruritus.

Overdose and treatment
Acute overdose may cause double vision, slurred speech, drowsiness, lethargy, and diarrhea.

Give supportive care. Gabapentin can be removed by hemodialysis if patient's condition warrants it or patient has significant renal impairment.

Special considerations
▶ Start therapy at a low dosage and gradually increase to minimize side effects.

▶ Drug can also be used to treat neuropathic pain.

▶ In pain management, don't expect immediate results. Several months may be needed to determine drug's effectiveness.

▶ Routine monitoring of plasma drug levels isn't necessary. Drug doesn't appear to alter plasma levels of other anticonvulsants.

▶ Stop drug or substitute another drug gradually over at least 1 week to minimize the risk of seizures. Don't suddenly withdraw other anticonvulsants in patients starting gabapentin.

Breast-feeding patients
▶ No data exist to demonstrate whether drug appears in breast milk. Use in breast-feeding patients only if benefits clearly outweigh risks.

Pediatric patients
▶ Safety and effectiveness in children under age 12 haven't been established.

Patient teaching
▶ Instruct patient to take first dose at bedtime to minimize drowsiness, dizziness, fatigue, and ataxia.
▶ Inform patient that drug can be taken without regard to meals.
▶ Caution patient to avoid hazardous activities until full CNS effects of drug are known.

▶ glycerin (glycerol)
Fleet Babylax, Ophthalgan, Osmoglyn, Sani-Supp

Pharmacologic classification:
ophthalmic osmotic vehicle, trihydric alcohol

Therapeutic classification:
adjunct in treating glaucoma, lubricant, ophthalmic osmotic, osmotic laxative

Pregnancy risk category C

How supplied
Available by prescription only
Ophthalmic solution: 7.5-ml containers
Oral solution: 50% (0.6 g/ml), 75% (0.94 g/ml)
Available without a prescription
Rectal solution: 4 ml/applicator
Suppository: 1.5 g (for infants), 3 g (adults)

Indications and dosages
Constipation
Adults and children age 6 and older: 3 g as a suppository or 5 to 15 ml as an enema.

Children under age 6: 1 to 1.5 g as a suppository or 2 to 5 ml as an enema.

Pharmacodynamics
Laxative action: Glycerin suppositories produce laxative action by causing rectal distention, thereby stimulating the urge to defecate; by causing local rectal irritation; and by triggering a hyperosmolar mechanism that draws water into the colon.
Antiglaucoma action: Orally administered glycerin helps reduce intraocular pressure by increasing plasma osmotic pressure, thereby drawing water into the blood from extravascular spaces. It also reduces intraocular fluid volume independently of routine flow mechanisms, decreasing intraocular pressure; it may cause tissue dehydration and decreased CSF pressure.

Topically applied glycerin produces a hygroscopic (moisture-retaining) effect that reduces edema and improves visualization in ophthalmoscopy or gonioscopy. Glycerin reduces fluid in the cornea via its osmotic action and clears corneal haze.

Pharmacokinetics
Rectal form
Absorption: Glycerin suppositories are absorbed poorly; after rectal administration, laxative effect occurs in 15 to 30 minutes.
Distribution: Glycerin is distributed locally.
Metabolism: Not reported.
Excretion: Drug is excreted in the feces.
Oral form
Absorption: Drug is absorbed rapidly from GI tract. Serum levels

---

peak in 60 to 90 minutes after oral administration. Intraocular pressure decreases in 10 to 30 minutes. Action peaks in 30 minutes to 2 hours, and effects last 4 to 8 hours. Intracranial pressure (ICP) decreases in 10 to 60 minutes and persists 2 to 3 hours.

Distribution: Drug is distributed throughout the blood, but it doesn't enter ocular fluid; drug may enter breast milk.

Metabolism: After oral administration, about 80% of dose is metabolized in the liver, 10% to 20% in the kidneys.

Excretion: Drug is excreted in feces and urine.

Contraindications and precautions

Contraindicated in patients hypersensitive to drug. Rectal administration is contraindicated in those with intestinal obstruction, undiagnosed abdominal pain, vomiting or other signs of appendicitis, fecal impaction, or acute surgical abdomen.

Use oral form cautiously in elderly or dehydrated patients and in those with diabetes or cardiac, renal, or hepatic disease.

Interactions
Drug-drug

Diuretics: may cause additive effects. Monitor patient for increased diuresis. Also, monitor serum electrolytes.

Effects on diagnostic tests

None reported.

Adverse reactions

CNS: dizziness (oral), mild headache.

EENT: eye pain, irritation.

GI: cramping pain, diarrhea (oral), hyperemia of rectal mucosa (rectal), nausea, rectal discomfort, thirst, vomiting.

GU: mild glycosuria.

Metabolic: mild hyperglycemia.

Overdose and treatment

If excess glycerin is administered into eye, irrigate conjunctiva with sterile normal saline solution or water. Systemic effects are not expected.

Special considerations

◗ Routine use of analgesics commonly causes constipation.

◗ Hyperosmolar laxatives are used most commonly to help laxative-dependent patients reestablish normal bowel habits.

◗ Commercially available solutions may be poured over ice and sipped through a straw.

◗ When giving oral glycerin, don't give hypotonic fluids to relieve thirst and headache (from glycerin-induced dehydration) because they'll counteract osmotic effects of drug.

◗ To prevent or relieve headache, have patient remain supine during and after oral administration.

◗ Monitor bowel activity; discontinue or alter dosing as bowel movements become more frequent.

◗ Use topical tetracaine hydrochloride or proparacaine before ophthalmic instillation to prevent discomfort.

◗ Don't touch tip of dropper to eye, surrounding tissues, or tear-film; glycerin will absorb moisture.

◗ Monitor diabetic patients for possible alteration of serum and urine glucose levels; dosage adjustment may be necessary.

▶ Glycerin is also used to reduce intraocular pressure and corneal edema (ophthalmic form) and as an osmotic diuretic.

▶ Drug is also used to reduce ICP in patients with CVA, meningitis, encephalitis, Reye's syndrome, or CNS trauma or tumors. And it's used to reduce brain volume during neurosurgical procedures through oral or I.V. administration, or both.

▶ Stop drug if symptoms of hypersensitivity occur.

Breast-feeding patients
▶ Safety in breast-feeding women hasn't been established; weigh risks against benefits.

Pediatric patients
▶ Safety and effectiveness of ophthalmic glycerin solutions in children haven't been established.

Geriatric patients
▶ Dehydrated elderly patients may experience seizures and disorientation.

Patient teaching
▶ Instruct patient how to insert a suppository.
▶ Tell patient that suppository must be retained for at least 15 minutes and that it usually acts within 1 hour. Entire suppository need not melt to be effective.
▶ Tell patient that onset of action may be rapid. Urge patient to stay near a bathroom.
▶ Tell patient that he may experience irritation around insertion site.
▶ Warn patient about adverse GI reactions.

▶ Instruct patient to call if he experiences severe headache from oral dose.
▶ Teach patient correct way to instill drops and warn him not to touch the dropper to his eye.
▶ Tell patient to lie down during and after taking oral glycerin to prevent or relieve headache.

▶ **haloperidol**
Apo-Haloperidol◇, Haldol, Novo-Peridol◇, Peridol◇

▶ **haloperidol decanoate**
Haldol Decanoate, Haldol Decanoate 100, Haldol LA◇

▶ **haloperidol lactate**
Haldol, Haldol Concentrate, Haloperidol Intensol

Pharmacologic classification: *butyrophenone*

Therapeutic classification: *antipsychotic*

Pregnancy risk category C

How supplied
Available by prescription only
haloperidol
Tablets: 0.5 mg, 1 mg, 2 mg, 5 mg, 10 mg, 20 mg
haloperidol decanoate
Injection: 50 mg/ml, 100 mg/ml
haloperidol lactate
Oral concentrate: 2 mg/ml
Injection: 5 mg/ml

Indications and dosages
Prevention and control of severe nausea and vomiting from opiate therapy*
Adults: give small doses. More studies are needed to determine the efficacy of haloperidol for this use.

Pharmacodynamics

Antiemetic action: Unknown.
Antipsychotic action: Haloperidol probably exerts antipsychotic effects via strong postsynaptic blockade of CNS dopamine receptors, thereby inhibiting dopamine-mediated effects. Its effects are most similar to those of piperazine antipsychotics. Its mechanism of action in Tourette syndrome is unknown.

Haloperidol has many other central and peripheral effects; it produces weak peripheral anticholinergic effects, antiemetic effects, and alpha and ganglionic blockade. And it counteracts histamine- and serotonin-mediated activity. Its most prominent adverse reactions are extrapyramidal.

Pharmacokinetics

Absorption: Rate and extent of absorption vary with route of administration. Oral tablet absorption yields 60% to 70% bioavailability. I.M. dose is 70% absorbed within 30 minutes. Plasma levels peak 2 to 6 hours after oral administration, 30 to 45 minutes after I.M. administration, and 6 to 7 days after I.M. administration of long-acting (decanoate) form.
Distribution: Haloperidol is distributed widely into the body, with high levels in adipose tissue. Drug is 90% to 92% protein-bound.
Metabolism: Drug is metabolized extensively by the liver; there may be only one active metabolite that is less active than parent drug.
Excretion: About 40% of a dose is excreted in urine within 5 days; about 15% is excreted in feces via the biliary tract.

Contraindications and precautions

Contraindicated in patients hypersensitive to drug and in patients with parkinsonism, coma, or CNS depression.

Use cautiously in elderly or debilitated patients; in patients with history of seizures, EEG abnormalities, CV disorders, allergies, angle-closure glaucoma, or urine retention; and in those receiving anticoagulants, anticonvulsants, antiparkinsonians, or lithium.

Interactions
Drug-drug

Antiarrhythmics, such as disopyramide, procainamide, quinidine: increased risk of arrhythmias and conduction defects. Monitor patient closely if given together.
Anticholinergics, such as antidepressants, antihistamines, antiparkinsonians, atropine, MAO inhibitors, meperidine, phenothiazines: oversedation, paralytic ileus, visual changes, and severe constipation. Monitor patient for adverse effects.
Antidiarrheals, aluminum- and magnesium-containing antacids: decreased absorption. Separate administration times by at least 2 hours.
Appetite suppressants, sympathomimetics (such as ephedrine, epinephrine, phenylephrine, phenylpropanolamine): decreased stimulatory and pressor effects. Monitor patient for drug effects.
Beta blockers: may inhibit haloperidol metabolism, increasing plasma levels and toxicity. Monitor patient for toxicity.
Bromocriptine: antagonized prolactin secretion. Monitor patient for drug effect.

Central-acting antihypertensives, such as clonidine, guanabenz, guanadrel, guanethidine, methyldopa, reserpine: haloperidol may inhibit blood pressure response to these drugs. Monitor blood pressure.

CNS depressants (analgesics, barbiturates, epidural anesthetics, general anesthetics, narcotics, spinal anesthetics, tranquilizers), parenteral magnesium sulfate: increased risk of oversedation, respiratory depression, and hypotension. Use together cautiously.

Dopamine: decreased vasoconstricting effects of high-dose dopamine. Monitor vital signs.

Levodopa: decreased effectiveness and increased toxicity of levodopa (by dopamine blockade). Monitor patient for drug effect.

Lithium: decreased response to haloperidol and severe neurologic toxicity with an encephalitis-like syndrome. Avoid using together if possible.

Metrizamide: increased risk of seizures. Monitor patient closely if given together.

Nitrates: hypotension. Monitor blood pressure.

Phenobarbital: enhanced renal excretion of haloperidol. Adjust dosage as needed.

Phenytoin: haloperidol may inhibit phenytoin metabolism and increase risk of toxicity. Monitor phenytoin levels.

Propylthiouracil: increased risk of agranulocytosis. Monitor blood count.

Drug-herb
Nutmeg: may reduce symptom control or disrupt existing therapy for psychiatric illnesses. Avoid concurrent use.

Drug-lifestyle
Alcohol use: additive effects. Advise against concurrent use.
Heavy smoking: increased haloperidol metabolism. Urge smoking cessation.

Effects on diagnostic tests
None reported.

Adverse reactions
CNS: confusion, drowsiness, headache, insomnia, lethargy, sedation, *seizures, severe extrapyramidal reactions, tardive dyskinesia,* vertigo.
CV: ECG changes, hypertension, hypotension, tachycardia.
EENT: *blurred vision.*
GI: anorexia, constipation, diarrhea, dry mouth, dyspepsia, nausea, vomiting.
GU: gynecomastia, menstrual irregularities, priapism, urine retention.
Hematologic: leukocytosis, *leukopenia.*
Hepatic: altered liver function test results, jaundice.
Skin: diaphoresis, other skin reactions, rash.

Overdose and treatment
Overdose may cause CNS depression with deep, unarousable sleep and possible coma, hypotension or hypertension, extrapyramidal symptoms, dystonia, abnormal involuntary muscle movements, agitation, seizures, arrhythmias, ECG changes (may show QT-interval prolongation and torsades de pointes), hypothermia or hyperthermia, and autonomic nervous system dysfunction. Overdose with long-acting decanoate requires prolonged recovery time.

Reactions may be *common*, uncommon, *life-threatening*, or COMMON AND LIFE-THREATENING.

Treatment is symptomatic and supportive, including maintaining vital signs, airway, stable body temperature, and fluid and electrolyte balance. Ipecac may be used to induce vomiting, keeping in mind the antiemetic properties of haloperidol and the risk of aspiration. Gastric lavage also may be used, followed by activated charcoal and saline cathartics. Dialysis doesn't help.

Regulate patient's body temperature as needed. Treat hypotension with I.V. fluids; don't give epinephrine. Give diazepam or barbiturates for seizures; parenteral phenytoin for arrhythmias (1 mg/kg I.V. [maximum, 50 mg/minute] adjusted to blood pressure with ECG monitoring and repeated every 5 minutes up to 10 mg/kg), and benztropine (1 to 2 mg) or parenteral diphenhydramine (10 to 50 mg) for extrapyramidal reactions.

Special considerations
▶ Drug is used for treating psychotic disorders, alcohol dependence (off label), and control of tics and vocal utterances in Tourette syndrome.
▶ Drug is used as a second-line adjunctive treatment for nausea caused by opiate therapy.
▶ Drug has few adverse CV effects and may be preferred in patients with cardiac disease.
▶ Just before administration, dilute dose with water or a beverage, such as orange juice, apple juice, tomato juice, or cola.
▶ Protect drug from light. Slight yellowing of injection or concentrate is common and doesn't indicate altered potency. Discard markedly discolored solutions.

▶ Don't withdraw drug abruptly except when severe adverse reaction requires it.
▶ Assess patient periodically for abnormal body movements. Tardive dyskinesia may occur after prolonged use. It may not appear until months or years later and may disappear spontaneously or persist for life.
▶ A 2-mg dose is therapeutic equivalent of 100 mg of chlorpromazine.
▶ When changing from tablets to decanoate injection, patient should initially receive 10 to 20 times the oral dose once monthly (maximum, 100 mg). Give drug by deep I.M. injection.
▶ I.V. route is an unlabeled method of administration. Don't give decanoate form by I.V. route.
▶ Consider continuous I.V. infusion if patient needs multiple I.M. injections to control delirium.
▶ Monitor patient's ECG at baseline and periodically during I.V. therapy to detect prolonged QT interval.

Pediatric patients
▶ Children are especially prone to extrapyramidal adverse reactions.
▶ Drug isn't recommended for children under age 3.

Geriatric patients
▶ Drug is especially useful for agitation with senile dementia.
▶ Elderly patients usually require lower initial doses and a more gradual dosage adjustment.

Patient teaching
▶ Instruct patient not to combine drug with alcohol or other depressants.
▶ Caution patient to avoid hazardous activities until full CNS ef-

fects of drug are known. Drowsiness and dizziness usually subside after a few weeks.
▶ Tell patient to report adverse effects, such as extrapyramidal reactions.

▶ **hydrocodone bitartrate and acetaminophen**
Vicodin, Vicodin ES Tablets, Vicodin HP

Pharmacologic classification:
opioid (hydrocodone), para-aminophenol derivative (acetaminophen)

Therapeutic classification:
analgesic

Controlled substance schedule III

Pregnancy risk category C

How supplied
Available by prescription only
Tablets: 5 mg hydrocodone bitartrate with 500 mg acetaminophen, 7.5 mg hydrocodone bitartrate with 750 mg acetaminophen, 10 mg hydrocodone bitartrate with 660 mg acetaminophen

Indications and dosages
Moderate to severe pain
Vicodin
Adults: 1 to 2 tablets P.O. every 4 to 6 hours p.r.n. Maximum, 8 tablets/day.
Vicodin ES
Adults: 1 tablet P.O. every 4 to 6 hours p.r.n. Maximum, 5 tablets/day.
Vicodin HP
Adults: 1 tablet P.O. every 4 to 6 hours p.r.n. Maximum, 6 tablets/day.

Pharmacodynamics
Analgesic action: Unknown, although hydrocodone may alter the perception of pain by acting at opiate receptor sites in the CNS; acetaminophen may inhibit prostaglandin synthesis in the CNS.

Pharmacokinetics
Absorption: Serum hydrocodone levels peak in 1 to 1½ hours. Acetaminophen is rapidly absorbed from the GI tract.
Distribution: Hydrocodone isn't extensively protein-bound. Acetaminophen is widely distributed to most body tissues.
Metabolism: Hydrocodone is metabolized to 6-alpha- and 6-beta-hydroxy-metabolites. Acetaminophen is metabolized in the liver.
Excretion: Acetaminophen, hydrocodone, and their metabolites are excreted in the urine. The half-life is 3⅓ to 4½ hours.

Contraindications and precautions
Contraindicated in patients hypersensitive to hydrocodone or acetaminophen.
    Use cautiously in elderly or debilitated patients, and in patients with severe renal or hepatic impairment, hypothyroidism, Addison's disease, prostatic hypertrophy, or urethral stricture. Use cautiously in the postoperative period and in patients with pulmonary disease because hydrocodone suppresses the cough reflex. Use cautiously in patients with head injuries or other intracranial lesions, or in patients with increased intracranial pressure (ICP) because hydrocodone may further increase ICP.

Interactions
Drug-drug
CNS depressants, including antianxiety drugs, antihistamines, antipsychotics: additive CNS depression. Reduce dosage of one or both drugs.
MAO inhibitors, tricyclic antidepressants: increased effects of either drug. Monitor closely.

Drug-lifestyle
Alcohol use: additive CNS depression. Advise against concurrent use.

Effects on diagnostic tests
Acetaminophen may produce false-positive results in urine 5-hydroxyindoleacetic acid test.

Adverse reactions
CNS: anxiety, *dizziness,* drowsiness, dysphoria, fear, impaired mental and physical performance, lethargy, *light-headedness,* mental clouding, mood changes, psychic dependence, *sedation.*
GI: constipation, *nausea, vomiting.*
GU: ureteral spasm, urine retention.
Hematologic: *agranulocytosis, thrombocytopenia.*
Respiratory: *respiratory depression.*
Skin: rash, pruritus.
Other: *allergic reactions.*

Overdose and treatment
Hydrocodone overdose may cause respiratory depression, extreme somnolence progressing to stupor or coma, skeletal muscle flaccidity, cold and clammy skin, bradycardia and hypotension. In severe overdose, apnea, circulatory collapse, and death may occur. Acetaminophen overdose may cause hepatic necrosis, renal tubular necrosis, hypoglycemic coma, and thrombocytopenia.

Treatment is supportive and symptomatic. Induce vomiting mechanically or by using syrup of ipecac, and then give activated charcoal. In severe cases, peritoneal or hemodialysis may be considered. Naloxone may reverse respiratory depression and coma caused by hydrocodone. Acetylcysteine may be given if the acetaminophen dose was greater than 140 mg/kg. Monitor hepatic enzymes. Treat methemoglobinemia over 30% with methylene blue.

Special considerations
▶ Drug may be habit-forming.
▶ Adjust dose according to pain level and patient response.
▶ Daily acetaminophen dose shouldn't exceed 4 g.
▶ Tolerance may develop with prolonged use.
▶ Assess patient for irregular breathing.
▶ If patient has a head injury, intracranial lesion, or increased ICP, watch for continued increases in ICP.
▶ Some adverse reactions, such as light-headedness, dizziness, sedation, nausea and vomiting, may be less severe if patient is supine.
▶ Monitor liver function in patients with severe hepatic impairment and kidney function in patients with severe renal impairment.
▶ Drug may obscure the diagnosis or clinical course of abdominal conditions.

Breast-feeding patients
▶ No data exist to demonstrate whether hydrocodone appears in

breast milk. Because of risk of adverse reactions, avoid giving drug to nursing mothers.

Pediatric patients
▶ Safety and effectiveness haven't been established.

Geriatric patients
▶ Use cautiously and start at low end of dosage range.

Patient teaching
▶ Caution patient that drug may be habit-forming, and to take it only as prescribed.
▶ Urge patient to avoid alcohol during therapy.
▶ Inform patient that acetaminophen dosage from all sources shouldn't exceed 4 g/day.
▶ Caution patient to avoid hazardous activities until full CNS effects of drug are known.

▶ **hydrocodone bitartrate and ibuprofen**
Vicoprofen

Pharmacologic classification:
opioid (hydrocodone), NSAID (ibuprofen)

Therapeutic classification:
analgesic

Controlled substance schedule III

Pregnancy risk category C

How supplied
Available by prescription only
Tablets: 7.5 mg hydrocodone bitartrate with 200 mg ibuprofen

Indications and dosages
Acute pain (short-term management)
Adults: 1 tablet every 4 to 6 hours p.r.n. for up to 10 days. Do not exceed 5 tablets daily.

Pharmacodynamics
Analgesic action: Unknown, although hydrocodone probably alters pain perception by acting at opiate receptor sites in the CNS; ibuprofen probably inhibits cyclooxygenase and prostaglandin synthesis.

Pharmacokinetics
Absorption: Plasma hydrocodone levels peak in 1.7 hours. Ibuprofen levels peak at 1.8 hours.
Distribution: Hydrocodone isn't extensively protein-bound. Ibuprofen is about 99% protein-bound.
Metabolism: Hydrocodone is metabolized to 6-alpha- and 6-beta-hydroxy-metabolites. Ibuprofen undergoes interconversion in the plasma to two primary metabolites.
Excretion: Hydrocodone, ibuprofen and their metabolites are excreted in urine.

Contraindications and precautions
Contraindicated in patients hypersensitive to hydrocodone or ibuprofen. Also contraindicated in patients who have experienced asthma, urticaria, or allergic reactions after taking aspirin or other NSAIDs.
    Use cautiously in elderly or debilitated patients, and in patients with severe renal or hepatic impairment, hypothyroidism,

---

Addison's disease, prostatic hypertrophy, or urethral stricture. Use cautiously in the postoperative period and in patients with pulmonary disease because hydrocodone suppresses the cough reflex. Use cautiously in patients with head injuries or other intracranial lesions, or in patients with increased intracranial pressure (ICP) because hydrocodone may further increase it. Use cautiously in patients with history of ulcer disease or GI bleeding, and in dehydrated patients. Use cautiously in patients with coagulation disorders, because drug may prolong bleeding time. Use cautiously in patients with history of cardiac decompensation, hypertension, or heart failure because drug may cause fluid retention and edema. Use cautiously in patients with asthma, who may be sensitive to aspirin.

Interactions
Drug-drug
ACE inhibitors: reduced effectiveness of ACE inhibitors and increased risk of renal toxicity. Use together cautiously.
Anticholinergics: increased risk of paralytic ileus. Monitor patient closely.
Anticoagulants, corticosteroids: increased risk of GI bleeding. Use together cautiously.
Aspirin: possible increased adverse effects. Avoid concomitant use.
CNS depressants, including antianxiety drugs, antihistamines, antipsychotics, opioids: additive CNS depression. Reduce dosage of one or both drugs.
Diuretics, such as furosemide and thiazides: increased risk of renal

toxicity. Use together cautiously. Monitor patient for renal failure.
Lithium: elevated lithium levels and decreased lithium clearance. Monitor patient for toxicity.
MAO inhibitors, tricyclic antidepressants: increased effects of either drug. Monitor patient closely.
Methotrexate: increased risk of methotrexate toxicity. Use together cautiously.
Warfarin: increased risk of GI bleeding. Monitor patient closely.

Drug-lifestyle
Alcohol use: additive CNS depression. Advise against concurrent use.
Chronic alcoholism, smoking: increased risk of GI bleeding. Advise patient of danger.

Effects on diagnostic tests
None reported.

Adverse reactions
CNS: anxiety, asthenia, confusion, *dizziness, headache,* hypertonia, insomnia, nervousness, paresthesia, *somnolence,* thinking abnormalities.
CV: palpitations, edema, vasodilation.
EENT: pharyngitis, rhinitis, tinnitus.
GI: abdominal pain, anorexia, *constipation,* diarrhea, dry mouth, *dyspepsia,* flatulence, gastritis, melena, mouth ulcers, *nausea,* thirst, vomiting.
GU: urinary frequency.
Hepatic: *elevated liver enzymes.*
Respiratory: dyspnea, hiccups.
Skin: prutitus, sweating.
Other: fever, flulike syndrome, infection, pain.

Overdose and treatment
Hydrocodone overdose may cause respiratory depression, extreme somnolence progressing to stupor or coma, skeletal muscle flaccidity, cold and clammy skin, bradycardia and hypotension. Severe overdose may lead to apnea, circulatory collapse, cardiac arrest, and death.

Ibuprofen overdose may cause GI irritation, kidney, liver or heart damage, hemolytic anemia, agranulocytosis, thrombocytopenia, aplastic anemia, and meningitis.

Treatment is supportive and symptomatic. Naloxone may reverse respiratory depression and coma caused by hydrocodone.

Special considerations
▶ Adjust dosage according to pain level and patient response.
▶ Drug may be habit-forming.
▶ Tolerance may develop with prolonged use.
▶ Drug increases the risk of GI toxicity, including inflammation, bleeding, ulceration, and perforation of the stomach, small intestine, and large intestine.
▶ Rehydrate a severely dehydrated patient before starting drug.
▶ Monitor patient for GI ulceration and bleeding, for evidence of liver dysfunction, and for irregular or periodic breathing.
▶ Monitor kidney function in patients with renal disease and liver function in patients with hepatic disease.
▶ Discontinue drug if liver dysfunction persists or worsens.
▶ If patient has a head injury, intracranial lesion, or increased ICP, watch for continued increases in ICP.
▶ Drug may obscure the diagnosis and clinical course of abdominal conditions.

Breast-feeding patients
▶ No data exist to demonstrate whether hydrocodone appears in breast milk. Because of risk of adverse reactions, avoid giving drug to nursing mothers.

Pediatric patients
▶ Safety and effectiveness in children under age 16 haven't been established.

Geriatric patients
▶ Elderly patients are at increased risk for GI bleeding. Use lowest effective dose for shortest period of time.

Patient teaching
▶ Caution patient that drug may be habit-forming and to take it only as prescribed.
▶ Advise patient to avoid alcohol while taking drug.
▶ Caution patient to avoid hazardous activities until full CNS effects of drug are known.
▶ Tell patient to notify prescriber about evidence of GI bleeding, blurred vision, rash, weight gain, or edema.

▶ **hydrocortisone (systemic)**
**Cortef, Cortenema, Hycort◇,
Hydrocortone**

▶ **hydrocortisone acetate**
Cortifoam

▶ **hydrocortisone cypionate**
Cortef

▶ **hydrocortisone sodium
phosphate**
Hydrocortone Phosphate

▶ **hydrocortisone sodium
succinate**
A-Hydrocort, Solu-Cortef

Pharmacologic classification:
glucocorticoid, mineralocorticoid

Therapeutic classification:
adrenocorticoid replacement

Pregnancy risk category C

How supplied
Available by prescription only
hydrocortisone
Enema: 100 mg/60 ml
Injection: 25 mg/ml, 50 mg/ml
suspension
Tablets: 5 mg, 10 mg, 20 mg
hydrocortisone acetate
Enema: 10% aerosol foam (provides 90 mg/application)
Injection: 25 mg/ml, 50 mg/ml
suspension
hydrocortisone cypionate
Oral suspension: 10 mg/5 ml
**hydrocortisone sodium phos-
phate**
Injection: 50 mg/ml solution
hydrocortisone sodium succinate
Injection: 100 mg/vial, 250 mg/
vial, 500 mg/vial, 1,000 mg/vial

Indications and dosages
Severe inflammation
hydrocortisone
Adults: 5 to 30 mg P.O. b.i.d., t.i.d.,
or q.i.d. (as much as 80 mg P.O.
q.i.d. may be given in acute situations).
Children: 2 to 8 mg/kg or 60 to
240 mg/m² P.O. daily.
hydrocortisone acetate
Adults: 10 to 75 mg into joints or
soft tissue at 2- or 3-week intervals. Dose varies with size of joint.
In many cases, local anesthetics
are injected with dose.
**hydrocortisone sodium phos-
phate**
Adults: 15 to 240 mg S.C., I.M., or
I.V. daily in divided doses q 12
hours.
hydrocortisone sodium succinate
Adults: initially, 100 to 500 mg
I.M. or I.V., then 50 to 100 mg
I.M. as indicated.

Pharmacodynamics
*Adrenocorticoid replacement ac-
tion:* Hydrocortisone is an adrenocorticoid with both glucocorticoid
and mineralocorticoid properties.
It's a weak anti-inflammatory but a
strong mineralocorticoid, with potency similar to that of cortisone
and twice that of prednisone.

Hydrocortisone (or cortisone) is
usually the drug of choice for replacement therapy in patients with
adrenal insufficiency. It's usually
not used for immunosuppressant
activity because of the extremely
large doses needed and the unwanted mineralocorticoid effects.

Pharmacokinetics
Absorption: Drug is absorbed
readily after oral administration.
After oral and I.V. administration,
effects peak in about 1 to 2 hours.

---

*Unlabeled use

The acetate suspension for injection has a variable absorption over 24 to 48 hours, depending on whether it is injected into an intra-articular space or a muscle, and the blood supply to that muscle.

Distribution: Hydrocortisone is removed rapidly from the blood and distributed to muscle, liver, skin, intestines, and kidneys. It's bound extensively to plasma proteins (transcortin and albumin). Only the unbound portion is active. Adrenocorticoids are distributed into breast milk and through the placenta.

Metabolism: Drug is metabolized in the liver to inactive glucuronide and sulfate metabolites.

Excretion: The inactive metabolites and small amounts of unmetabolized drug are excreted by the kidneys. Insignificant quantities of drug are excreted in feces. Biological half-life of hydrocortisone is 8 to 12 hours.

Contraindications and precautions

Contraindicated in patients allergic to any component of the formulation, in those with systemic fungal infections, and in premature infants (hydrocortisone sodium succinate).

Use hydrocortisone sodium phosphate or succinate cautiously in patients with a recent MI, GI ulcer, renal disease, hypertension, osteoporosis, diabetes mellitus, hypothyroidism, cirrhosis, diverticulitis, ulcerative colitis, recent intestinal anastomosis, thromboembolic disorders, seizures, myasthenia gravis, heart failure, tuberculosis, ocular herpes simplex, emotional instability, and psychotic tendencies.

Interactions
Drug-drug

Antacids, cholestyramine, colestipol: decreased corticosteroid effect from adsorption to corticosteroid, thereby decreasing the amount absorbed. Do not administer together.

Barbiturates, phenytoin, rifampin: decreased corticosteroid effects because of increased hepatic metabolism. Monitor patient for drug effects.

Cardiac glycosides: if hypokalemia occurs, may increase the risk of toxicity. Monitor serum digoxin level.

Amphotericin B, diuretics: enhanced hypokalemia. Monitor serum potassium level.

Estrogens: reduced metabolism of corticosteroids by increasing the level of transcortin. Monitor patient for adverse effects and toxicity.

Isoniazid, salicylates: increased metabolism of these drugs. Monitor patient for this effect.

Oral anticoagulants: decreased anticoagulant effects. Monitor PT and INR.

Ulcer-causing drugs, such as NSAIDs: increased risk of GI ulceration. Use together cautiously.

Effects on diagnostic tests

Hydrocortisone suppresses reactions to skin tests, causes false-negative results in the nitroblue tetrazolium tests for systemic bacterial infections, and decreases uptake and protein-bound iodine levels in thyroid function tests.

Adverse reactions

CNS: *euphoria,* headache, *insomnia,* paresthesia, psychotic behavior, pseudotumor cerebri, **seizures,** vertigo.

CV: *arrhythmias*, edema, *heart failure*, hypertension, thrombophlebitis, *thromboembolism*.
EENT: cataracts, glaucoma.
GI: GI irritation, increased appetite, nausea, *pancreatitis, peptic ulceration,* vomiting.
GU: menstrual irregularities.
Metabolic: hyperglycemia (requiring dosage adjustment in diabetics), possible hypokalemia.
Musculoskeletal: growth suppression in children, muscle weakness, osteoporosis.
Skin: acne, delayed wound healing, easy bruising, various skin eruptions.
Other: *acute adrenal insufficiency* with increased stress (such as infection, surgery, trauma, or abrupt withdrawal after long-term therapy), carbohydrate intolerance, cushingoid state (moonface, buffalo hump, central obesity), hirsutism, susceptibility to infections.

Overdose and treatment
Acute ingestion, even in massive doses, rarely causes much problem. Toxic signs and symptoms rarely occur if drug is used for less than 3 weeks, even at large doses. However, chronic use causes adverse physiologic effects, including suppression of the hypothalamic-pituitary-adrenal axis, cushingoid appearance, muscle weakness, and osteoporosis.

Special considerations
▶ Drug can be used to relieve pain from bony metastasis, nerve compression, and spinal cord compression.
▶ Drug is also used to treat adrenal insufficiency, shock, ulcerative colitis (adjunct), and proctitis (adjunct).

▶ Hydrocortisone and hydrocortisone cypionate may be administered orally. Hydrocortisone sodium phosphate may be administered by I.M., S.C., or I.V. injection or by I.V. infusion, usually at 12-hour intervals. Hydrocortisone sodium succinate may be administered by I.M. or I.V. injection or I.V. infusion every 2 to 10 hours, depending on the clinical situation. Hydrocortisone acetate is a suspension that may be administered by intra-articular, intrasynovial, intrabursal, intralesional, or soft tissue injection. It has a slow onset but a long duration of action. Injectable forms are usually used only when oral forms can't be used.
▶ For better results and less toxicity, give a daily dose in the morning.
▶ Always adjust to lowest effective dose.
▶ High-dose therapy usually isn't continued beyond 48 hours.
▶ Give oral dose with food when possible. Patient may require medication to prevent GI irritation.
▶ Hydrocortisone sodium phosphate may be added directly to D_5W, normal saline solution, or half-normal saline solution for I.V. administration.
▶ Reconstitute hydrocortisone sodium succinate with bacteriostatic water or bacteriostatic sodium chloride solution before adding to I.V. solutions. When giving by direct I.V. injection, inject over 30 seconds to 10 minutes. For infusion, dilute with D_5W, normal saline solution, or dextrose 5% in normal or half-normal saline solution to yield 1 mg/ml or less.
▶ Don't use the acetate or suspension form for I.V. delivery. When giving as a direct injection, inject

directly into vein or an I.V. line with free-flowing compatible solution over 30 seconds to several minutes. When giving an intermittent or continuous infusion, dilute solution according to manufacturer's instructions, and give over prescribed duration. If used for continuous infusion, change solution every 24 hours.

▶ Don't use injectable forms for alternate-day therapy.

▶ Monitor patient's weight, blood pressure, and serum electrolyte levels.

▶ Drug may increase appetite in patients with cancer.

▶ Gradually reduce dosage after long-term therapy. Reduction may affect patient's sleep.

▶ Drug may mask or exacerbate infections.

▶ Don't confuse Solu-Cortef with Solu-Medrol.

▶ Most adverse reactions to corticosteroids are dose- or duration-dependent.

▶ Observe patient for depression or psychotic episodes, especially during high-dose therapy.

▶ Inspect patient's skin for petechiae.

▶ Monitor serum glucose in diabetic patients.

▶ After abrupt withdrawal, patient may develop rebound inflammation, fatigue, weakness, arthralgia, fever, dizziness, lethargy, depression, fainting, orthostatic hypotension, dyspnea, anorexia, hypoglycemia. Abrupt withdrawal after prolonged use may be fatal.

Pediatric patients

▶ Long-term use of hydrocortisone in children and adolescents may delay growth and maturation. Assess growth and development periodically during high-dose or prolonged therapy in children.

Patient teaching

▶ Instruct patient to take oral form with milk or food.

▶ Warn patient about easy bruising.

▶ Tell patient not to discontinue drug abruptly or without consulting prescriber.

▶ Advise patient on long-term therapy to have periodic ophthalmic examinations and to consider exercise, physical therapy, or vitamin D or calcium supplement.

▶ Urge patient to avoid exposure to persons infected with chickenpox or measles, and to notify prescriber if such exposure occurs.

▶ Inform patient on long-term therapy about cushingoid symptoms and the need to notify prescriber about sudden weight gain or swelling.

▶ hydromorphone hydrochloride
Dilaudid, Dilaudid-HP, Hydrostat IR

Pharmacologic classification: *opioid*

Therapeutic classification: *analgesic, antitussive*

Controlled substance schedule II

Pregnancy risk category C

How supplied
Available by prescription only
Injection: 1 mg/ml, 2 mg/ml, 3 mg/ml, 4 mg/ml, 10 mg/ml
Oral liquid: 5 mg/5 ml
Suppository: 3 mg

Tablets: 1 mg, 2 mg, 3 mg, 4 mg, 8 mg

Indications and dosages
Moderate to severe pain
Adults: 2 to 10 mg P.O. q 3 to 6 hours, p.r.n., or around the clock; 2 to 4 mg I.M., S.C., or I.V. q 4 to 6 hours, p.r.n., or around the clock. Give I.V. dose over 3 to 5 minutes. Or give 3 mg rectal suppository q 6 to 8 hours, p.r.n., or around the clock. Give 1 to 14 mg Dilaudid-HP S.C. or I.M. q 4 to 6 hours.

Pharmacodynamics
Analgesic action: Hydromorphone has analgesic properties related to opiate receptor affinity. Unlike other opioids, there's no intrinsic limit to analgesic effects of hydromorphone,
Antitussive action: Hydromorphone acts directly on the cough center in the medulla to produce an antitussive effect.

Pharmacokinetics
Absorption: Drug is well absorbed after oral, rectal, or parenteral administration. Action starts in 15 to 30 minutes and lasts 4 to 5 hours.
Distribution: Unknown.
Metabolism: Drug is metabolized primarily in the liver, where it undergoes conjugation with glucuronic acid.
Excretion: Drug is excreted primarily in urine as the glucuronide conjugate.

Contraindications and precautions
Contraindicated in patients hypersensitive to drug, in patients with intracranial lesions with increased intracranial pressure, and in patients with depressed respiratory function, as in status asthmaticus, COPD, cor pulmonale, emphysema, and kyphoscoliosis.

Use cautiously in elderly or debilitated patients and in those with hepatic or renal disease, Addison's disease, hypothyroidism, prostatic hyperplasia, or urethral strictures.

Interactions
Drug-drug
Anticholinergics: may cause paralytic ileus. Monitor patient for abdominal pain.
Antihistamines, barbiturates, benzodiazepines, general anesthetics, muscle relaxants, opioid analgesics, phenothiazines, sedative-hypnotics, tricyclic antidepressants: potentiated respiratory and CNS depression, sedation, and hypotensive effects. Use together very cautiously.
Cimetidine: increased respiratory and CNS depression, causing confusion, disorientation, apnea, or seizures. Requires reduced dosage of hydromorphone.
Drugs extensively metabolized in the liver, such as digitoxin, phenytoin, rifampin: drug accumulation and enhanced effects may result. Monitor patient closely.
General anesthetics: severe CV depression. Monitor vital signs closely.
Narcotic antagonists: patients who become physically dependent on drug may experience acute withdrawal syndrome if given a narcotic antagonist. Avoid concurrent use if possible.

Drug-lifestyle
Alcohol use: may potentiate CNS effects. Advise against concurrent use.

Effects on diagnostic tests

Increased biliary tract pressure resulting from contraction of the sphincter of Oddi may interfere with hepatobiliary imaging studies.

Adverse reactions

CNS: clouded sensorium, dizziness, euphoria, sedation, somnolence.
CV: *bradycardia*, hypotension.
EENT: blurred vision, diplopia, nystagmus.
GI: constipation, ileus, nausea, vomiting.
GU: urine retention.
Respiratory: *respiratory depression, bronchospasm.*
Other: induration with repeated S.C. injections, physical dependence.

Overdose and treatment

Hydromorphone overdose may cause CNS depression, respiratory depression, and miosis. Other acute toxic effects include hypotension, bradycardia, hypothermia, shock, apnea, cardiopulmonary arrest, circulatory collapse, pulmonary edema, and seizures.

To treat an acute overdose, first establish adequate respiration via a patent airway and ventilate as needed; administer a narcotic antagonist such as naloxone, to reverse respiratory depression. Because the duration of action of hydromorphone is longer than that of naloxone, repeated dosing is necessary. Naloxone should not be given unless patient has clinically significant respiratory or CV depression. Monitor vital signs closely.

If patient presents within 2 hours of ingestion of an oral overdose, empty the stomach immediately by inducing emesis with ipecac syrup or using gastric lavage. Use caution to minimize risk of aspiration. Administer activated charcoal via nasogastric tube for further removal of an oral overdose.

Provide symptomatic and supportive treatment such as continued respiratory support, and correction of fluid or electrolyte imbalance. Monitor laboratory values, vital signs, and neurologic status closely.

Contact the local or regional poison control center for further information.

Special considerations

▶ Give hydromorphone hydrochloride in the smallest effective dose to minimize tolerance and physical dependence. Dosage must be individually adjusted based on pain level and patient's age and size.
▶ Assess patient's pain (as with a pain scale from 0 to 10) and adjust dosage accordingly.
▶ Discard parenteral products if they contain particulates or have extreme yellow discoloration.
▶ For I.V. use, give drug by direct injection over at least 2 minutes. For infusion, drug may be mixed in D_5W, normal saline solution, dextrose 5% in normal or half-normal saline solution, or Ringer's or lactated Ringer's solutions.
▶ Respiratory depression and hypotension can occur with I.V. administration. Give drug very slowly, and monitor patient constantly. Keep resuscitation equipment available.
▶ Patient-controlled analgesia is effective in managing chronic cancer pain, along with continuous nighttime infusion. Stop infusion in the

---

Reactions may be *common,* uncommon, *life-threatening,* or COMMON AND LIFE-THREATENING.

morning to establish sleep/wake pattern.

▶ Dilaudid-HP, a highly concentrated form (10 mg/ml), allows smaller-volume injections to prevent the discomfort of large-volume injections.

▶ For better analgesic effect, give drug before patient has intense pain.

▶ Oral dosage form is particularly convenient for patients with chronic pain because tablets are available in several strengths, enabling patient to adjust dosage precisely as needed.

▶ With long-term use, expect dose tolerance and physical dependence.

▶ Drug can be given via intrathecal route for cancer pain and spinal compression pain.

▶ Monitor patient's respiratory status, circulatory status, and bowel function during therapy.

▶ Drug is also used to relieve cough.

▶ Drug may worsen or mask gallbladder pain.

Breast-feeding patients
▶ No data exist to demonstrate whether drug appears in breast milk. Use cautiously in breast-feeding women.

Geriatric patients
▶ Lower doses are usually indicated for elderly patients because they may be more sensitive to drug effects.

Patient teaching
▶ Instruct patient to take or ask for drug before pain becomes intense.

▶ Tell patient to refrigerate suppositories.

▶ Encourage coughing or deep breathing to avoid postoperative atelectasis.

▶ Caution patient to avoid hazardous activities until full CNS effects or drug are known.

▶ Advise patient to avoid alcohol.

▶ hydroxyzine hydrochloride
Anxanil, Apo-Hydroxyzine◊, Atarax, Hydroxacen, Hyzine-50, Multipax◊, Novo-Hydroxyzin◊, Quiess, Vistacon-50, Vistazine 50

▶ hydroxyzine pamoate
Vistaril

Pharmacologic classification:
antihistamine (piperazine derivative)

Therapeutic classification:
antianxiety drug, antiemetic, antipruritic, antispasmodic, sedative

Pregnancy risk category C

How supplied
Available by prescription only
hydroxyzine hydrochloride
Capsules: 10 mg, 25 mg, 50 mg
Injection: 25 mg/ml, 50 mg/ml
Syrup: 10 mg/5 ml
Tablets: 10 mg, 25 mg, 50 mg, 100 mg
hydroxyzine pamoate
Capsules: 25 mg, 50 mg, 100 mg
Oral suspension: 25 mg/5 ml

Indications and dosages
Preoperative and postoperative sedation (adjunct), control of emesis
Adults: 50 to 100 mg P.O. or 25 to 100 mg I.M. q 4 to 6 hours.
Children: 0.6 mg/kg P.O. or 1.1 mg/kg I.M. q 4 to 6 hours.

Pharmacodynamics

Antipruritic action: Drug is a direct competitor of histamine for binding at cellular receptor sites.
Anxiolytic and sedative actions: Hydroxyzine produces sedative and antianxiety effects by suppressing activity at subcortical levels; analgesia occurs at high doses.
Other actions: Hydroxyzine is used as a preoperative and postoperative adjunct for its sedative, antihistaminic, and anticholinergic activity.

Pharmacokinetics

Absorption: Drug is absorbed rapidly and completely after oral administration. Serum levels peak within 4 hours. Sedation and other clinical effects are usually noticed within 30 minutes.
Distribution: Not well understood.
Metabolism: Drug is metabolized almost completely in the liver.
Excretion: Drug metabolites are excreted primarily in urine; small amounts of drug and metabolites are found in feces. Half-life of drug is 3 hours. Sedative effects can last for 4 to 6 hours, and antihistaminic effects can persist up to 4 days.

Contraindications and precautions

Contraindicated in patients hypersensitive to drug and during early pregnancy.

Use cautiously and adjust dosage as needed in elderly or debilitated patients.

Interactions

Drug-drug
Anticholinergics: additive anticholinergic effects. Use together cautiously.

CNS depressants, such as barbiturates, opioids, tranquilizers: hydroxyzine may add to or potentiate the effects of these drugs. Dose of CNS depressant should be reduced by half.
Epinephrine: hydroxyzine may block vasopressor action of epinephrine. If a vasoconstrictor is needed, use norepinephrine or phenylephrine.

Drug-lifestyle
Alcohol use: potentiated effects. Advise against concurrent use.

Effects on diagnostic tests

Drug therapy causes falsely elevated urine 17-hydroxycorticosteroid levels. It also may cause false-negative skin allergen tests by attenuating or inhibiting the cutaneous response to histamine.

Adverse reactions

CNS: *drowsiness,* involuntary motor activity.
GI: *dry mouth.*
Other: *hypersensitivity reactions* (wheezing, dyspnea, chest tightness), marked discomfort at I.M. injection site.

Overdose and treatment

Overdose may cause excessive sedation and hypotension; seizures may occur.

Treatment is supportive. For recent oral ingestion, induce emesis or perform gastric lavage. Correct hypotension with fluids and vasopressors (phenylephrine or metaraminol). Don't give epinephrine because hydroxyzine may counter its effect.

Special considerations
▶ Drug can be used to treat postoperative muscle spasms not relieved by opiates and also for anxiety, tension, hyperkinesias, and (as an adjunct) asthma.
▶ Analgesic action occurs with parenteral use but not with oral use.
▶ Inject deep I.M. only; avoid I.V., intra-arterial, or S.C. use. Aspirate injection carefully to prevent inadvertent intravascular administration.
▶ Observe patients for excessive sedation, especially those receiving other CNS depressants.

Breast-feeding patients
▶ No data exist to demonstrate whether drug appears in breast milk. Safe use hasn't been established in breast-feeding women.

Geriatric patients
▶ Elderly patients may experience greater CNS depression and anticholinergic effects. Use lower dosage.

Patient teaching
▶ Caution patient to avoid hazardous activities until full CNS effects of drug are known.
▶ Urge patient to avoid alcohol and other CNS depressants unless prescribed.
▶ Tell patient to consult prescriber before taking OTC cold or allergy medications that contain antihistamine, because it may potentiate hydroxyzine effects.
▶ Suggest sugarless gum or candy to help relieve dry mouth and plenty of water to ease dry mouth or constipation.

ibuprofen
Advil, Children's Advil, Medipren, Motrin, Motrin IB, Nuprin, Rufen, Trendar

Pharmacologic classification:
NSAID

Therapeutic classification:
nonnarcotic analgesic, antipyretic, anti-inflammatory

Pregnancy risk category B (D in third trimester)

How supplied
Available by prescription only
Oral drops: 40 mg/ml
Oral suspension: 100 mg/5 ml
Tablets: 100 mg, 300 mg, 400 mg, 600 mg, 800 mg
Available without a prescription
Oral suspension: 100 mg/5 ml
Tablets: 200 mg
Tablets (chewable): 50 mg, 100 mg

Indications and dosages
Arthritis, gout, and postextraction dental pain
Adults: 300 to 800 mg P.O. t.i.d. or q.i.d. Maximum, 3,200 mg/day.
Primary dysmenorrhea
Adults: 400 mg P.O. q 4 to 6 hours.
Mild to moderate pain
Adults: 400 mg P.O. q 4 to 6 hours.
Children: 10 mg/kg P.O. q 6 to 8 hours. Maximum dose, 40 mg/kg.
Juvenile rheumatoid arthritis
Children: 20 to 40 mg/kg/day P.O., divided into three or four doses. For mild disease, 20 mg/kg/day in divided doses.

Pharmacodynamics
Analgesic, antipyretic, and anti-inflammatory actions: Unknown, although ibuprofen is thought to inhibit prostaglandin synthesis.

Pharmacokinetics
Absorption: 80% of an oral dose is absorbed from the GI tract.
Distribution: Ibuprofen is highly protein-bound.
Metabolism: Drug undergoes biotransformation in the liver.
Excretion: Drug is excreted mainly in urine, with some biliary excretion. Plasma half-life ranges from 2 to 4 hours.

Contraindications and precautions
Contraindicated in patients hypersensitive to drug and in those who have the syndrome of reaction to aspirin or other NSAIDs (nasal polyps, angioedema, bronchospastic reaction).

Use cautiously in patients with impaired renal or hepatic function, GI disorders, peptic ulcer disease, cardiac decompensation, hypertension, or known coagulation defects. Because chewable tablets contain aspartame, use cautiously in patients with phenylketonuria.

Interactions
Drug-drug
ACE inhibitors: ibuprofen may reduce the blood pressure response to ACE inhibitors and may result in an acute reduction in renal function. Monitor blood pressure and renal function closely if used together.
Acetaminophen, anti-inflammatory drugs, gold compounds: increased nephrotoxicity. Monitor renal function.
Antacids: may decrease ibuprofen absorption. Separate administration times by at least 2 hours.
Anticoagulants, thrombolytics: may potentiate anticoagulant effects. Monitor PT and INR.

Antihypertensives: ibuprofen may decrease effectiveness of these drugs. Monitor patient for drug effect.
Anti-inflammatory drugs, corticosteroids, corticotropin, salicylates: may increase adverse GI effects, including ulceration and hemorrhage. Monitor patient closely
Aspirin: may decrease ibuprofen bioavailability. Avoid using together.
Diuretics: may increase nephrotoxicity and decrease diuretic effectiveness. Monitor renal function and drug effect.
Drugs that inhibit platelet aggregation, such as anti-inflammatory drugs, aspirin, parenteral carbenicillin, cefamandole, cefoperazone, dextran, dipyridamole, mezlocillin, piperacillin, plicamycin, salicylates, sulfinpyrazone, ticarcillin, valproic acid: increased risk of bleeding problems. Monitor patient for bleeding tendencies and bruising.
Highly protein-bound drugs, such as coumarin derivatives, nifedipine, phenytoin, verapamil: ibuprofen may displace these drugs from binding sites and increase risk of toxicity. Monitor patient for evidence of toxicity.
Insulin, oral antidiabetics: may potentiate hypoglycemic effects. Monitor serum glucose.
Lithium, methotrexate: decreased renal clearance of these drugs. Monitor patient for toxicity.

Drug-lifestyle
Alcohol use: may increase adverse GI effects, including ulceration and hemorrhage. Avoid alcohol use.

Effects on diagnostic tests
None reported.

Reactions may be *common,* uncommon, *life-threatening,* or COMMON AND LIFE-THREATENING.

Adverse reactions

CNS: aseptic meningitis, *dizziness, headache,* nervousness.
CV: edema, fluid retention, *peripheral edema.*
EENT: *tinnitus.*
GI: constipation, decreased appetite, diarrhea, dyspepsia, *epigastric distress,* flatulence, heartburn, *nausea, occult blood loss, peptic ulceration.*
GU: *acute renal failure,* azotemia, cystitis, hematuria.
Hematologic: *agranulocytosis,* anemia, *aplastic anemia, leukopenia, neutropenia, pancytopenia,* prolonged bleeding time, *thrombocytopenia.*
Hepatic: elevated liver enzymes.
Respiratory: *bronchospasm.*
Skin: pruritus, *rash, Stevens-Johnson syndrome,* urticaria.

Overdose and treatment

Overdose may cause dizziness, drowsiness, paresthesia, vomiting, nausea, abdominal pain, headache, sweating, nystagmus, apnea, and cyanosis.

To treat overdose, induce emesis with ipecac syrup or perform gastric lavage. Give activated charcoal via nasogastric tube. Provide symptomatic and supportive measures (respiratory support and correction of fluid and electrolyte imbalances). Monitor laboratory values and vital signs closely. Alkaline diuresis may enhance renal excretion. Dialysis has little value because ibuprofen is strongly protein-bound.

Special considerations

▶ Give drug on an empty stomach, 1 hour before or 2 hours after meals for maximum absorption. To lessen GI upset, it may be given with meals.
▶ Maximum results in arthritis may require 1 to 2 weeks of continuous therapy. Improvement may start within 7 days.
▶ Drug is very effective against cramping after cesarean section if regular doses are given.
▶ Drug is also used to reduce fever.
▶ Antipyretic effects may mask or reduce fever caused by infection.
▶ Combination NSAID therapy causes gastric irritation.
▶ Establish safety measures, including raised side rails and supervised walking, to prevent possible injury from CNS effects.
▶ Monitor cardiopulmonary status and vital signs, especially heart rate and blood pressure.
▶ Observe patient for possible fluid retention.
▶ Monitor auditory and ophthalmic functions periodically during ibuprofen therapy. Monitor renal and liver function in long-term therapy.

Breast-feeding patients

▶ Drug doesn't enter breast milk in significant quantities. However, manufacturer recommends alternative feeding methods during ibuprofen therapy.

Pediatric patients

▶ Safety and efficacy in children under age 6 months haven't been established.

Geriatric patients

▶ Patients over age 60 may be more susceptible to the toxic effects of ibuprofen, especially adverse GI reactions. Use lowest effective dosage.
▶ The effect of drug on renal prostaglandins may cause fluid re-

tention and edema, a significant drawback for elderly patients and those with heart failure.

Patient teaching
▶ Encourage patient to adhere to prescribed drug regimen, and stress importance of medical follow-up.
▶ Caution patient to avoid hazardous activities until full CNS effects of drug are known.
▶ Tell patient to consult prescriber before taking other OTC medications.
▶ Advise patient not to self-medicate with ibuprofen for longer than 10 days for analgesic use and not to exceed maximum dose of six tablets (1,200 mg) daily. Caution patient not to take drug if fever lasts longer than 3 days, unless prescribed.
▶ Tell patient to report adverse reactions; they're usually dose-related.

▶ imipramine hydrochloride
Apo-Imipramine◇, Impril◇, Novopramine◇, Tofranil

▶ imipramine pamoate
Tofranil-PM

Pharmacologic classification: *dibenzazepine tricyclic antidepressant*

Therapeutic classification: *antidepressant*

Pregnancy risk category B

How supplied
Available by prescription only
imipramine hydrochloride
Injection: 25 mg/2 ml

Tablets: 10 mg, 25 mg, 50 mg
imipramine pamoate
Capsules: 75 mg, 100 mg, 125 mg, 150 mg

Indications and dosages
Chronic neuropathic pain, migraine prophylaxis
Adults: 25 to 200 mg/day P.O.
Adjunctive analgesia for arthritis pain*, cancer pain*, chronic tension headache*, diabetic neuropathy*, migraine headaches*, phantom limb pain*, peripheral neuropathy with pain*, postherpetic neuralgia*, tic douloureux*
Adults: 75 to 300 mg/day P.O.
◪ **DOSAGE ADJUSTMENT.** For elderly patients, recommended dosage is 30 to 40 mg/day P.O. Start with 10 mg/day and adjust slowly. Maximum, 100 mg/day.

Pharmacodynamics
Analgesic action: Unknown.
Antidepressant action: Imipramine probably inhibits reuptake of norepinephrine and serotonin in CNS nerve terminals (presynaptic neurons), which results in increased levels and enhanced activity of these neurotransmitters in the synaptic cleft. Drug also has anticholinergic activity and is used to treat nocturnal enuresis in children over age 6.

Pharmacokinetics
Absorption: Drug is absorbed rapidly from the GI tract and muscle tissue after oral and I.M. administration.
Distribution: Imipramine is distributed widely into the body, including the CNS and breast milk. Drug is 90% protein-bound. Effect peaks within 2 hours; steady state occurs in 2 to 5 days. Therapeutic

plasma levels (parent drug and metabolite) are thought to range from 150 to 300 ng/ml.
Metabolism: Drug is metabolized by the liver to the active metabolite desipramine. A significant first-pass effect may explain the variability of serum levels in different patients taking the same dosage.
Excretion: Drug is mostly excreted in urine.

Contraindications and precautions

Contraindicated in patient hypersensitive to drug, in patients taking an MAO inhibitor, and during the acute recovery phase of MI.

Use cautiously in patients at risk for suicide; in patients with impaired renal or hepatic function, history of urine retention, angle-closure glaucoma, increased intraocular pressure, CV disease, hyperthyroidism, seizure disorders, or allergy to sulfites (injectable form); and in patients receiving thyroid medications.

Interactions
Drug-drug

Antiarrhythmics (disopyramide, procainamide, quinidine), pimozide, thyroid hormones: increased risk of arrhythmias and conduction defects. Use together very cautiously.
Anticholinergics, such as antihistamines, antiparkinsonians, atropine, meperidine, phenothiazines: increased risk of oversedation, paralytic ileus, visual changes, and severe constipation. Monitor patient closely.
Barbiturates: induced imipramine metabolism and decreased therapeutic efficacy. Monitor patient for drug effects.

Beta blockers, cimetidine, methylphenidate, oral contraceptives, propoxyphene: may inhibit imipramine metabolism, increasing plasma levels and toxicity. Monitor patient for toxicity.
Central-acting antihypertensives, such as clonidine, guanabenz, guanadrel, guanethidine, methyldopa, reserpine: decreased hypotensive effects. Monitor blood pressure.
CNS depressants, including analgesics, anesthetics, barbiturates, narcotics, tranquilizers: increased risk of oversedation. Monitor patient closely.
Disulfiram, ethchlorvynol: may cause delirium and tachycardia. Monitor patient closely.
Haloperidol, phenothiazines: decreased imipramine metabolism, decreasing therapeutic efficacy. Monitor patient for drug effects.
Metrizamide: increased risk of seizures. Avoid concomitant use.
Sympathomimetics, including ephedrine, epinephrine, phenylephrine, phenylpropanolamine: may increase blood pressure. Monitor blood pressure.
Warfarin: may prolong PT and cause bleeding. Monitor patient's PT and INR.

Drug-lifestyle

Alcohol use: additive effects. Advise against concurrent use.
Heavy smoking: induces imipramine metabolism and decreases efficacy. Advise patient to avoid heavy smoking.

Effects on diagnostic tests
None reported.

Adverse reactions
CNS: anxiety, ataxia, confusion, *drowsiness, dizziness,* EEG

changes, excitation, hallucinations, paresthesia, nervousness, *seizures,* tremor.
CV: *arrhythmias, CVA,* ECG *changes,* **heart block,** hypertension, *MI, orthostatic hypotension, precipitation of heart failure, tachycardia.*
EENT: blurred vision, mydriasis, tinnitus.
GI: abdominal cramps, anorexia, *constipation, dry mouth,* nausea, paralytic ileus, vomiting.
GU: altered libido, galactorrhea and breast enlargement in females, gynecomastia in males, impotence, testicular swelling, *urine retention.*
Metabolic: hyperglycemia, hypoglycemia, SIADH.
Skin: *diaphoresis,* photosensitivity, pruritus, rash, urticaria.
Other: *hypersensitivity reaction.*

Overdose and treatment

Overdose usually is life-threatening, particularly when drug is combined with alcohol. The first 12 hours after acute ingestion are a stimulatory phase characterized by excessive anticholinergic activity (agitation, irritation, confusion, hallucinations, hyperthermia, parkinsonian symptoms, seizure, urine retention, dry mucous membranes, pupillary dilatation, constipation, and ileus). This is followed by CNS depressant effects, including hypothermia, decreased or absent reflexes, sedation, hypotension, cyanosis, and cardiac irregularities, including tachycardia, conduction disturbances, and quinidine-like effects on the ECG.

Severity of overdose is best indicated by widening of the QRS complex, which usually represents a serum level in excess of 1,000 ng/ml; serum levels are usually not

helpful. Metabolic acidosis may follow hypotension, hypoventilation, and seizures.

Treatment is symptomatic and supportive, including maintaining airway, stable body temperature, and fluid and electrolyte balance. Induce emesis if patient is conscious; follow with gastric lavage and activated charcoal to prevent further absorption. Dialysis is of little use.

Treat seizures with parenteral diazepam or phenytoin and arrhythmias with parenteral phenytoin or lidocaine. Quinidine, procainamide, and atropine are not to be used during an overdose. Treat acidosis with sodium bicarbonate. Don't give barbiturates; these may enhance CNS and respiratory depressant effects.

Special considerations

▶ Drug can be used as adjuvant analgesic to opioid therapy by blocking reuptake of serotonin and norepinephrine at CNS synapses. It traditionally is used to treat depression. It may be used to treat nocturnal enuresis in children, and it's effective for patients who complain of chronic fatigue.
▶ Analgesic effect is independent of mood effects.
▶ Imipramine commonly causes orthostatic hypotension. Check sitting and standing blood pressures after first dose.
▶ Tolerance to drug's sedative effects usually develops over several weeks.
▶ Drug should be discontinued at least 48 hours before surgical procedures.
▶ Drug shouldn't be withdrawn abruptly, but tapered gradually over time. Abrupt withdrawal of

long-term therapy can cause nausea, headache, and malaise (which don't indicate addiction).

Breast-feeding patients
▶ Low levels of imipramine appear in breast milk. Make sure potential benefits to mother outweigh possible risks to infant.

Pediatric patients
▶ Drug isn't recommended for depression in patients under age 12.
▶ Don't use pamoate salt for enuresis in children.

Geriatric patients
▶ Elderly patients may be at greater risk for adverse cardiac and anticholinergic effects.

Patient teaching
▶ Tell patient to take drug exactly as prescribed.
▶ Explain that full effects of drug may take up to 6 weeks.
▶ Advise patient to take drug with food or milk if it causes stomach upset.
▶ Suggest relieving dry mouth with sugarless chewing gum or hard candy.
▶ Tell patient to change positions slowly.
▶ Warn patient not to stop drug abruptly, not to share drug with others, and not to drink alcoholic beverages while taking drug.
▶ Encourage patient to report unusual or troublesome effects immediately, including confusion, movement disorders, rapid heartbeat, dizziness, fainting, or difficulty urinating.

▶ indomethacin, indomethacin sodium trihydrate
Apo-Indomethacin◇, Indameth, Indocid◇, Indocin, Indocin SR, Novomethacin◇

Pharmacologic classification:
NSAID

Therapeutic classification:
anti-inflammatory, antipyretic, nonnarcotic analgesic

Pregnancy risk category NR

How supplied
Available by prescription only
Capsules: 25 mg, 50 mg
Capsules (sustained-release): 75 mg
Injection: 1-mg vials
Suppositories: 50 mg
Suspension: 25 mg/5 ml

Indications and dosages
Moderate to severe arthritis, ankylosing spondylitis
Adults: 25 mg P.O. b.i.d. or t.i.d. with food or antacids, increased by 25 to 50 mg/day q 7 days as needed up to 200 mg/day. Or give 50 mg P.R. q.i.d. For sustained-release capsules, give 75 mg to start, morning or h.s., followed by 75 mg b.i.d. if needed.
Acute gouty arthritis
Adults: 50 mg t.i.d. Reduce dosage and stop drug as soon as possible. Don't use sustained-release capsules for this condition.
Acute shoulder pain
Adults: 75 to 150 mg P.O. b.i.d. or t.i.d. with food or antacids. Treatment usually lasts 7 to 14 days.

Dysmenorrhea*
Adults: 25 mg P.O. t.i.d. with food or antacids.

Pharmacodynamics
Analgesic, antipyretic, and anti-inflammatory actions: Exact mechanisms of action are unknown; drug probably produces its analgesic, antipyretic, and anti-inflammatory effects by inhibiting prostaglandin synthesis and possibly by inhibiting phosphodiesterase.
Closure of patent ductus arteriosus: Mechanism of action is unknown, but it's believed to be through inhibition of prostaglandin synthesis.

Pharmacokinetics
Absorption: Drug is absorbed rapidly and completely from the GI tract.
Distribution: Drug is highly protein-bound.
Metabolism: Drug is metabolized in the liver.
Excretion: Drug is excreted mainly in urine, with some biliary excretion.

Contraindications and precautions
Contraindicated in patients hypersensitive to drug, in patients who are pregnant or breast-feeding, and in patients with a history of aspirin- or NSAID-induced asthma, rhinitis, or urticaria. Also, contraindicated in infants with untreated infection, active bleeding, coagulation defects or thrombocytopenia, congenital heart disease in those where patency of the ductus arteriosus is necessary for satisfactory pulmonary or systemic blood flow, necrotizing enterocolitis, or impaired renal function.

Suppositories are contraindicated in patients with a history of proctitis or recent rectal bleeding.

Use cautiously in elderly patents and those with a history of GI disease, impaired renal or hepatic function, epilepsy, parkinsonism, CV disease, infection, mental illness, or depression.

Interactions
Drug-drug
Acetaminophen, anti-inflammatory drugs, gold compounds: increased nephrotoxicity. Monitor renal function.
Antacids: may decrease indomethacin absorption. Separate administration times by at least 2 hours.
Anticoagulants, thrombolytics: may potentiate anticoagulant effects. Monitor PT and INR.
Antihypertensives, diuretics: indomethacin may decrease effectiveness of these drugs. Monitor patient for drug effect.
Anti-inflammatory drugs, corticosteroids, corticotropin, salicylates: may increase adverse GI effects, including ulceration and hemorrhage. Monitor patient closely.
Aspirin: may decrease indomethacin bioavailability. Avoid concurrent use.
Diuretics, such as triamterene: potential nephrotoxicity. Avoid concomitant use if possible.
Drugs that inhibit platelet aggregation, such as aspirin, carbenicillin (parenteral), cefamandole, cefoperazone, dextran, dipyridamole, mezlocillin, piperacillin, plicamycin, salicylates, sulfinpyrazone, ticarcillin, valproic acid: bleeding problems may occur. Monitor patient for bleeding tendencies and bruising.

Reactions may be *common*, uncommon, *life-threatening*, or **COMMON AND LIFE-THREATENING**.

Highly protein-bound drugs, such as coumarin derivatives, nifedipine, phenytoin, verapamil: indomethacin may displace these drugs from binding sites. Monitor patient for evidence of toxicity.

Insulin, oral antidiabetic drugs: may potentiate hypoglycemic effects. Monitor serum glucose.

Lithium, methotrexate: decreased renal clearance of these drugs. Monitor patient for toxicity.

Drug-herb
Senna: may block senna's effects. Avoid concomitant use.

Drug-lifestyle
Alcohol use: may increase adverse GI effects. Discourage alcohol use.

Effects on diagnostic tests
Drug may interfere with dexamethasone suppression test results. It may also interfere with urine 5-hydroxyindoleacetic acid determinations.

Adverse reactions
CNS: confusion, depression, *dizziness,* drowsiness, fatigue, *headache,* peripheral neuropathy, psychic disturbances, somnolence, *seizures,* syncope, *vertigo.*
CV: *edema,* **heart failure**, hypertension.
EENT: blurred vision, corneal and retinal damage, hearing loss, tinnitus.
GI: anorexia, constipation, *diarrhea,* dyspepsia, **GI bleeding**, nausea, **pancreatitis,** peptic ulceration.
GU: *acute renal failure,* hematuria, interstitial nephritis, proteinuria.
Hematologic: *agranulocytosis,* **aplastic anemia,** hemolytic anemia, **leukopenia, thrombocytopenic purpura**, iron-deficiency anemia.
Metabolic: hyperkalemia.
Skin: pruritus, *Stevens-Johnson syndrome*, urticaria.
Other: *hypersensitivity* (rash, respiratory distress, **anaphylaxis, angioedema**).

Overdose and treatment
Overdose may cause dizziness, nausea, vomiting, intense headache, mental confusion, drowsiness, tinnitus, sweating, blurred vision, paresthesias, and seizures.

To treat indomethacin overdose, induce emesis with ipecac syrup or by gastric lavage. Administer activated charcoal via nasogastric tube. Provide symptomatic and supportive measures (respiratory support and correction of fluid and electrolyte imbalances). Monitor laboratory parameters and vital signs closely. Dialysis may be of little value because indomethacin is strongly protein-bound.

Special considerations
▶ Drug is also used to close a hemodynamically significant patent ductus arteriosus in premature infants (I.V. form only) and to treat Bartter's syndrome.
▶ Drug has limited usefulness because of the risk of CNS, GI, and hemapoetic toxicity.
▶ Don't mix oral suspension with liquids or antacids before administering.
▶ Patient should retain suppository in the rectum for at least 1 hour after insertion to ensure maximum absorption.
▶ I.V. route should be used only for premature neonates with patent ductus arteriosus.

❱ For I.V. use, reconstitute 1-mg vial with 1 to 2 ml of sterile water for injection or preservative-free normal saline injection. Prepare solution immediately before use.

❱ Don't use discolored or precipitated solution.

❱ Give drug by direct I.V. injection over 5 to 10 seconds. Use a large vein to prevent extravasation.

❱ If ductus arteriosus reopens, a second course of one to three doses may be given. If ineffective, surgery may be necessary. Don't administer a second or third I.V. dose if anuria or marked oliguria exists.

❱ Severe headaches may occur. If they persist, decrease dose.

❱ For maximum effectiveness, give doses on a regular schedule.

❱ Assess patient's cardiopulmonary status for significant changes. Watch for evidence of fluid overload. Check weight and intake and output daily.

❱ Monitor renal function studies before therapy starts and frequently during therapy to prevent adverse effects.

❱ Monitor patient carefully for bleeding and reduced urine output, especially with I.V. administration.

❱ Assess I.V. site for complications.

Breast-feeding patients
❱ Drug appears in breast milk at levels similar to those in maternal plasma; avoid use in breast-feeding women.

Pediatric patients
❱ Use of I.V. indomethacin in premature infants for patent ductus arteriosus is considered an alternative to surgery.

❱ Safety of long-term drug use in children under age 14 hasn't been established.

Geriatric patients
❱ Patients over age 60 may be more susceptible to the toxic effects of indomethacin.

❱ The effect of drug on renal prostaglandins may cause fluid retention and edema, a significant drawback for elderly patients and those with heart failure.

Patient teaching
❱ Instruct patient in proper administration of suppository, sustained-release capsule, or suspension, as prescribed.

❱ Tell patient to take oral form with food to avoid adverse GI effects.

❱ Advise patient to consult prescriber before taking other prescribed or OTC medications.

❱ Caution patient to avoid hazardous activities until full CNS effects of drug are known. Instruct him in safety measures to prevent injury.

❱ Instruct patient to report adverse reactions. Encourage him to adhere to prescribed drug regimen and recommended follow-up.

❱ ipecac syrup

Pharmacologic classification:
alkaloid emetic

Therapeutic classification:
emetic

Pregnancy risk category C

How supplied
Available with and without a prescription
Syrup: 70 mg powdered ipecac/ml

Indications and dosages
To induce vomiting in poisoning
Adults: 15 to 30 ml P.O., followed by 200 to 300 ml of water. May repeat dose once after 20 minutes, if necessary.
Children age 1 or older: 15 ml P.O., followed by about 200 ml of water. May repeat dose once after 20 minutes, if necessary.
Children under age 1: 5 to 10 ml P.O., followed by 100 to 200 ml of water. May repeat dose once after 20 minutes, if necessary.

Pharmacodynamics
Emetic action: Ipecac syrup directly irritates the GI mucosa and directly stimulates the chemoreceptor trigger zone through the effects of emetine and cephalin, its two alkaloids.

Pharmacokinetics
Absorption: Ipecac syrup is absorbed in significant amounts mainly when it doesn't produce emesis. Action typically starts in 20 minutes.
Distribution: Unknown.
Metabolism: Unknown.
Excretion: Emetine is excreted in urine slowly over up to 60 days. Duration of effect is 20 to 25 minutes.

Contraindications and precautions
Contraindicated in semicomatose or unconscious patients and in those with severe inebriation, seizures, shock, or loss of gag reflex. Don't give drug after ingestion of gasoline, kerosene, volatile oils, or caustic substances (such as lye).

Interactions
Drug-drug
Activated charcoal: may inactivate ipecac syrup. Don't administer together; allow time for ipecac syrup to work before giving charcoal.
Antiemetics: may decrease ipecac syrup's therapeutic effectiveness. Don't give together.

Drug-food
Carbonated beverages: may cause abdominal distention. Don't give together.
Milk or milk products: may decrease ipecac syrup's effectiveness. Don't give together.
Vegetable oil: delayed absorption. Don't give together.

Effects on diagnostic tests
None reported.

Adverse reactions
CNS: depression, *drowsiness*.
CV: *arrhythmias,* atrial fibrillation, *bradycardia, fatal myocarditis* (with excessive doses), hypotension.
GI: diarrhea.

Overdose and treatment
Overdose may cause diarrhea, persistent nausea or vomiting longer than 30 minutes, stomach cramps or pain, arrhythmias, hypotension, myocarditis, difficulty breathing, and unusual fatigue or weakness.

Toxicity from chronic ipecac overdose usually involves use of the concentrated fluid extract in dosage appropriate for the syrup. Clinical effects of cardiotoxicity include tachycardia, T-wave depression, atrial fibrillation, depressed myocardial contractility, heart failure, and myocarditis. Other toxic effects include bloody stools and vomitus, hypotension, shock, seizures, and coma. Heart failure is the usual cause of death.

Treatment requires discontinuation of drug followed by symptomatic and supportive care, which may include digoxin and pacemaker therapy to treat cardiotoxic effects. However, no antidote exists for the cardiotoxic effects of ipecac, which may be fatal despite intensive treatment.

Special considerations
▶ Always administer ipecac syrup before giving activated charcoal. Follow ipecac dose with 1 or 2 glasses of water. If vomiting doesn't occur after second dose, give activated charcoal to adsorb both ipecac syrup and ingested poison. Follow with gastric lavage.
▶ In 9 of 10 patients, ipecac syrup empties the stomach completely within 30 minutes; average emptying time is 20 minutes.
▶ Inspect emesis for ingested substances, such as tablets or capsules.
▶ Little if any systemic toxicity occurs with doses of 30 ml or less.
▶ Be careful not to confuse ipecac syrup with ipecac fluid extract, which is rarely used but 14 times more potent. Never store these two drugs together—the wrong drug could be fatal.
▶ In antiemetic toxicity, ipecac syrup is usually effective if less than 1 hour has passed since ingestion of antiemetic.
▶ Drug may be abused by patients with eating disorders, such as bulimia or anorexia nervosa.
▶ Ipecac syrup may be used in small amounts as an expectorant in cough preparations; however, this use has doubtful benefit.

Breast-feeding patients
▶ Safety in breast-feeding infants hasn't been established; possible risks must be weighed against drug's benefits.

Pediatric patients
▶ Advise parents to keep ipecac syrup at home at all times but to keep it out of children's reach.

Patient teaching
▶ Advise patient to seek medical attention immediately in cases of suspected poisoning.
▶ Caution patient to call poison information center before taking ipecac syrup.
▶ Warn patient to avoid drinking milk or carbonated beverages with ipecac syrup because they may decrease its effectiveness; instruct him to take syrup with 1 or 2 glasses of water.
▶ Tell patient that vomiting should begin within 20 minutes and may last 20 to 25 minutes.

▶ ketamine hydrochloride
Ketalar

Pharmacologic classification:
dissociative anesthetic

Therapeutic classification:
I.V. anesthetic

Pregnancy risk category NR

How supplied
Available by prescription only
Injection: 10 mg/ml, 50 mg/ml, 100 mg/ml

Indications and dosages
Induction of general anesthesia, especially for short diagnostic or

---

surgical procedures that don't require skeletal muscle relaxation; adjunct to other general or low-potency anesthetics, such as nitrous oxide
Adults and children: 1 to 4.5 mg/kg I.V. over 60 seconds or 6.5 to 13 mg/kg I.M. To maintain anesthesia, repeat half- to full-size dose.

Pharmacodynamics
Anesthetic action: Ketamine induces a profound sense of dissociation from the environment by direct action on the cortex and limbic system.

Pharmacokinetics
Absorption: Drug is absorbed rapidly after I.M. injection. It induces surgical anesthesia 30 seconds after I.V. administration and lasts 5 to 10 minutes. After I.M. injection, anesthesia begins in 3 to 4 minutes and lasts 12 to 25 minutes.
Distribution: Drug rapidly enters the CNS.
Metabolism: Drug is metabolized by the liver to an active metabolite with one-third the potency of parent drug.
Excretion: Drug is excreted in urine.

Contraindications and precautions
Contraindicated in patients with schizophrenia or other acute psychosis because it may exacerbate the condition, in patients with CV disease in which a sudden rise in blood pressure would be harmful, and in patients allergic to drug.

Interactions
Drug-drug
Barbiturates, narcotics: may prolong recovery time. Monitor patient closely.
Enflurane, halothane: ketamine's CV effects may be blocked by halothane or, to a lesser extent, enflurane. Significant myocardial depression and hypotension may result. Monitor vital signs closely if used together.
Nondepolarizing muscle relaxants, such as tubocurarine: ketamine may increase neuromuscular effects of these drugs, resulting in prolonged respiratory depression. Monitor patient closely.
Thyroid hormones: hypertension and tachycardia. Monitor vital signs.

Effects on diagnostic tests
None reported.

Adverse reactions
CNS: confusion, dreamlike states, excitement, hallucinations, irrational behavior, psychic abnormalities, tonic-clonic movements.
CV: *arrhythmias, bradycardia* if used with halothane, *hypertension,* hypotension, *tachycardia.*
EENT: diplopia, nystagmus.
GI: excessive salivation, mild anorexia, nausea, vomiting.
Respiratory: *apnea* if given too rapidly, laryngospasm, *respiratory depression* in high doses.
Skin: measles-like rash, transient erythema.

Overdose and treatment
Overdose may cause respiratory depression. Support respiration using mechanical ventilation if necessary.

Special considerations

▶ Drug is especially useful in managing minor surgical or diagnostic procedures or in repeated procedures that require large amounts of analgesia, such as the changing of burn dressings.

▶ For direct injection, dilute 100 mg/ml concentration with an equal volume of sterile water for injection, normal saline solution, or D_5W. For continuous infusion, prepare a 1 mg/ml solution by adding 5 ml from the 100 mg/ml vial to 500 ml of D_5W or normal saline solution.

▶ Patients require physical support because of rapid induction; monitor vital signs perioperatively. Blood pressure begins to rise shortly after injection, peaks at 10% to 50% above preanesthetic levels, and returns to baseline within 15 minutes. Effects on blood pressure make this drug particularly useful in hypovolemic patients as an induction drug that supports blood pressure.

▶ Minimize verbal, tactile, and visual stimulation during induction and recovery. Emergence reactions occur in 12% of patients for up to 24 hours postoperatively and may include dreams, visual imagery, hallucinations, and delirium. Reactions may be reduced with a lower ketamine dosage or I.V. diazepam and can be treated with short- or ultrashort-acting barbiturates. They're less common in patients under age 15 or over age 65 and when drug is given I.M.

▶ Dissociative and hallucinatory adverse effects have led to drug abuse.

▶ Barbiturates are incompatible in the same syringe.

▶ Monitor patient's vital signs during administration and through the recovery period.

▶ Discontinue drug if hypersensitivity, laryngospasm, or severe hypotension or hypertension occurs.

Geriatric patients

▶ Use drug with caution, especially in patients with suspected CVA, hypertension, or cardiac disease.

Patient teaching

▶ Warn patient to avoid hazardous activities for 24 hours after anesthesia.

▶ ketoprofen
Actron, Orudis, Orudis KT, Oruvail

Pharmacologic classification:
NSAID

Therapeutic classification:
anti-inflammatory, antipyretic, nonnarcotic analgesic

Pregnancy risk category B

How supplied

Available by prescription only
Capsules: 25 mg, 50 mg, 75 mg
Capsules (extended-release):
100 mg, 150 mg, 200 mg
Available without a prescription
Tablets: 12.5 mg

Indications and dosages

Rheumatoid arthritis, osteoarthritis
Adults: Usual dose is 75 mg t.i.d. or 50 mg q.i.d. P.O. Maximum, 300 mg/day. For extended-release capsules, maximum is 200 mg/day P.O.

Reactions may be *common*, uncommon, *life-threatening*, or COMMON AND LIFE-THREATENING.

Mild to moderate pain, dysmenorrhea
Adults: 25 to 50 mg P.O. q 6 to 8 hours, p.r.n.
Temporary relief of mild aches and pain
Adults: 12.5 mg q 4 to 6 hours. Maximum, 75 mg in a 24-hour period.

Pharmacodynamics
Analgesic, antipyretic, and anti-inflammatory actions: Mechanisms of action are unknown; ketoprofen is thought to inhibit prostaglandin synthesis.

Pharmacokinetics
Absorption: Drug is absorbed rapidly and completely from the GI tract.
Distribution: Drug is highly protein-bound. Extent of body tissue fluid distribution isn't known, but therapeutic levels range from 0.4 to 6 mcg/ml.
Metabolism: Drug is metabolized in the liver.
Excretion: Drug is excreted in urine as parent drug and its metabolites.

Contraindications and precautions
Contraindicated in patients hypersensitive to drug and in patients with a history of aspirin- or NSAID-induced asthma, urticaria, or other allergic-type reactions.

Use cautiously in patients with impaired renal or hepatic function, peptic ulcer disease, heart failure, hypertension, or fluid retention.

Interactions
Drug-drug
Acetaminophen, anti-inflammatory drugs, gold compounds: increased nephrotoxicity. Monitor renal function.
Anticoagulants, thrombolytics: may potentiate anticoagulant effects. Monitor PT and INR.
Antihypertensives: possible decreased antihypertensive effectiveness. Monitor patient for drug effect.
Anti-inflammatory drugs, corticosteroids, corticotropin, salicylates: may increase adverse GI effects, including ulceration and hemorrhage. Monitor patient closely.
Aspirin: may decrease ketoprofen bioavailability. Avoid using together.
Coumarin derivatives, nifedipine, phenytoin, verapamil: ketoprofen may displace highly protein-bound drugs from binding sites. Monitor patient for evidence of toxicity.
Diuretics: ketoprofen may decrease diuretic effectiveness and increase nephrotoxicity. Monitor patient's renal function.
Drugs that inhibit platelet aggregation, such as aspirin, parenteral carbenicillin, cefamandole, cefoperazone, dextran, dipyridamole, mezlocillin, piperacillin, plicamycin, salicylates, sulfinpyrazone, ticarcillin, valproic acid: bleeding problems may occur. Monitor patient for bleeding tendencies and bruising.
Insulin, oral antidiabetic drugs: may potentiate hypoglycemic effects. Monitor serum glucose levels.
Lithium, methotrexate: decreased the renal clearance of these drugs. Monitor patient for toxicity.

Drug-lifestyle
Alcohol use: may increase adverse GI effects, including ulceration and hemorrhage. Advise against alcohol use.

Prolonged sun exposure: increased risk of photosensitivity. Urge precautions.

Effects on diagnostic tests

In vitro interactions with glucose determinations have been reported with glucose oxidase and peroxidase methods. Ketoprofen may interfere with serum iron determination (false increases or decreases depending on method used).

Adverse reactions

CNS: *CNS excitation* or depression, *dizziness, headache.*
CV: peripheral edema.
EENT: tinnitus, visual disturbances.
GI: *abdominal pain,* anorexia, *constipation, diarrhea,* dyspepsia, *flatulence, **GI bleeding**, nausea, peptic ulceration,* stomatitis, vomiting.
GU: elevated BUN, ***nephrotoxicity.***
Hematologic: *agranulocytosis,* prolonged bleeding time, ***thrombocytopenia.***
Hepatic: elevated liver enzymes.
Respiratory: *bronchospasm,* dyspnea, *laryngeal edema.*
Skin: exfoliative dermatitis, photosensitivity, rash.

Overdose and treatment

Overdose may cause nausea and drowsiness. To treat, induce emesis with ipecac syrup or perform gastric lavage; administer activated charcoal via nasogastric tube. Provide symptomatic and supportive measures, such as respiratory support and correction of fluid and electrolyte imbalances. Monitor laboratory values and vital signs closely. Hemodialysis may be useful in removing ketoprofen and assisting in care of renal failure.

Special considerations

▶ Drug is effective for bony and visceral pain.
▶ Drug is also used to treat fever.
▶ Give tablets on an empty stomach either 30 minutes before or 2 hours after meals to ensure adequate absorption. To minimize GI distress, they may be taken with food or antacid.
▶ Refrigerate suppositories.
▶ Monitor CNS effects of drug. Use safety measures, such as assisted walking, raised side rails, and gradual position changes, to prevent injury.
▶ Don't give sustained-release form to patients with acute pain.
▶ NSAIDs may mask evidence of infection because of their antipyretic and anti-inflammatory action.
▶ Watch for possible photosensitivity reactions.
▶ Check renal and hepatic function every 6 months or as indicated.
▶ Monitor laboratory test results for abnormalities.

Breast-feeding patients

▶ Most NSAIDs are distributed into breast milk; however, distribution of ketoprofen is unknown. Avoid use of ketoprofen in breast-feeding women.

Pediatric patients

▶ Safe use in children under age 12 has not been established.

Geriatric patients

▶ Patients over age 60 may be more susceptible to the toxic effects of ketoprofen. Use with caution.

▶ The effects of drug on renal prostaglandins may cause fluid retention and edema, a significant drawback for elderly patients and those with heart failure. The manufacturer recommends that initial dose be reduced by 33% to 50% in geriatric patients.

Patient teaching
▶ Teach patient to take prescribed dosage and form correctly.
▶ Tell patient to take drug with food to avoid adverse GI side effects.
▶ Caution patient to avoid hazardous activities, and teach safety measures to help prevent injury.
▶ Advise patient to avoid alcohol during therapy.
▶ Tell patient about possible photosensitivity reactions, and recommend sunscreen.
▶ Tell patient to consult prescriber before taking other prescribed and OTC medications (especially aspirin and products that contain aspirin).
▶ Instruct patient to report adverse reactions.

▶ ketorolac tromethamine
Toradol

Pharmacologic classification:
NSAID

Therapeutic classification:
analgesic

Pregnancy risk category C

How supplied
Available by prescription only
Injection: 15 mg/ml (1-ml cartridge), 30 mg/ml (1-ml and 2-ml cartridges)
Tablets: 10 mg

Indications and dosages
Short-term management of pain
Adults under age 65: dosage based on patient response. Initially, 60 mg I.M. or 30 mg I.V. as a single dose, or multiple doses of 30 mg I.M. or I.V. q 6 hours. Maximum, 120 mg/day.
⊠ Dosage adjustment. In elderly patients, renally impaired patients, and patients who weigh less than 50 kg (110 lb), start with 30 mg I.M. or 15 mg I.V. as a single dose, or give multiple doses of 15 mg I.M. or I.V. q 6 hours. Maximum, 60 mg/day.
Short-term management of moderately severe, acute pain when switching from parenteral to oral administration
Adults under age 65: 20 mg P.O. as a single dose followed by 10 mg P.O. q 4 to 6 hours. Maximum, 40 mg/day.
⊠ Dosage adjustment. In elderly patients, renally impaired patients, and patients who weigh less than 50 kg (110 lb), give 10 mg P.O. as a single dose, followed by 10 mg P.O. q 4 to 6 hours. Maximum, 40 mg/day.

Pharmacodynamics
Analgesic action: Ketorolac is an NSAID that acts by inhibiting prostaglandin synthesis.

Pharmacokinetics
Absorption: Drug is completely absorbed after I.M. administration. After oral administration, food delays absorption but doesn't decrease total amount of drug absorbed.
Distribution: Mean peak plasma levels occur about 30 minutes after a 50-mg dose and range from 2.2

to 3 mcg/ml. Over 99% of drug is protein-bound.

Metabolism: Drug's metabolism is primarily hepatic; a para-hydroxy metabolite and conjugates have been identified; less than 50% of a dose is metabolized. Liver impairment doesn't substantially alter drug clearance.

Excretion: Primary excretion is in the urine (over 90%), the rest in feces. Terminal plasma half-life is 4 to 6 hours in young adults; it's substantially prolonged in patients with renal failure.

Contraindications and precautions

Contraindicated in patients hypersensitive to drug and in patients with active peptic ulcer disease, recent GI bleeding or perforation, advanced renal impairment, risk of renal impairment from volume depletion, suspected or confirmed cerebrovascular bleeding, hemorrhagic diathesis, incomplete hemostasis, or high risk of bleeding.

Also contraindicated in patients with a history of peptic ulcer disease or GI bleeding, allergic reactions to aspirin or other NSAIDs, and during labor and delivery or breast-feeding. In addition, drug is contraindicated as prophylactic analgesic before major surgery or intraoperatively when hemostasis is critical; in patients receiving aspirin, an NSAID, or probenecid; and in those who need epidural or intrathecal analgesia.

Use cautiously in patients with impaired renal or hepatic function.

Interactions
Drug-drug

Diuretics: may decrease efficacy of diuretic and enhance nephrotoxici-ty. Monitor kidney function and drug effect.

Lithium: increased lithium levels. Monitor patient for toxicity.

Methotrexate: decreased clearance and increased risk of toxicity. Monitor patient for toxicity.

Salicylates, warfarin: ketorolac may increase the levels of free unbound drug in the blood. Clinical significance is unknown. Monitor patient closely.

Effects on diagnostic tests
None reported.

Adverse reactions

CNS: dizziness, *drowsiness, headache, sedation.*

CV: *arrhythmias,* edema, hypertension, palpitations.

GI: constipation, diarrhea, *dyspepsia,* flatulence, *GI bleeding, GI pain, nausea,* peptic ulceration, stomatitis, vomiting.

GU: *renal failure.*

Hematologic: decreased platelet adhesion, purpura, *thrombocytopenia.*

Skin: diaphoresis, pain at injection site, pruritus, rash.

Overdose and treatment

There's no experience with overdose in humans. Withhold drug and provide supportive treatment.

Special considerations

▶ Drug is intended for short-term management of pain. The rate and severity of adverse reactions should be less than that observed in patients taking long-term NSAIDs.

▶ Correct hypovolemia before starting therapy with ketorolac.

▶ Give I.V. drug over 15 seconds or more.

Reactions may be *common,* uncommon, *life-threatening,* or COMMON AND LIFE-THREATENING.

▶ I.M. injections in patients with coagulopathies or those receiving anticoagulants may cause bleeding and hematoma at the site of injection. Monitor these patients carefully.

▶ The combined duration of ketorolac I.M., I.V., or P.O. shouldn't exceed 5 days. Oral use is only for continuation of I.V. or I.M. therapy.

▶ Monitor patient for abdominal pain or signs of increased bleeding.

Breast-feeding patients
▶ Because drug appears in breast milk, its use is contraindicated in breast-feeding patients.

Pediatric patients
▶ Drug isn't recommended for use in children because safety and efficacy haven't been established.

Geriatric patients
▶ In clinical trials, drug's terminal half-life increased in elderly patients. Use with extreme caution in this population.

Patient teaching
▶ Warn patient that GI ulceration, bleeding, and perforation can occur at any time, with or without warning, in anyone taking NSAIDs on a long-term basis. Teach patient how to recognize the signs and symptoms of GI bleeding.

▶ Instruct patient to avoid aspirin, aspirin-containing products, and alcoholic beverages during therapy.

▶ lactulose
Cephulac, Cholac, Chronulac, Constilac, Constulose, Duphalac, Enulose

Pharmacologic classification: *disaccharide*

Therapeutic classification: *laxative*

Pregnancy risk category B

How supplied
Available by prescription only
Rectal solution: 3.33 g/5 ml
Syrup: 10 g/15 ml

Indications and dosages
Constipation
Adults: 15 to 30 ml P.O. daily. May increase to 60 ml if needed.

Pharmacodynamics
Laxative action: Because lactulose is indigestible, it passes through the GI tract to the colon unchanged; there, it's digested by normally occurring bacteria. The weak acids produced in this manner increase the fluid content of stool and cause distention, thus promoting peristalsis and bowel evacuation.

Lactulose also is used to reduce serum ammonia levels in patients with hepatic disease. Lactulose breakdown acidifies the colon; this, in turn, converts ammonia (NH_3) to ammonium (NH_4^+), which is not absorbed and is excreted in the stool. Furthermore, this "ion trapping" effect causes ammonia to diffuse from the blood into the colon, where it's also excreted.

Pharmacokinetics

Absorption: Drug is absorbed minimally.
Distribution: Drug is distributed locally, primarily in the colon.
Metabolism: Drug is metabolized by colonic bacteria (absorbed portion is not metabolized).
Excretion: Drug is mostly excreted in feces; absorbed portion is excreted in urine.

Contraindications and precautions

Contraindicated in patients on a low-galactose diet.

Use cautiously in patients with diabetes mellitus.

Interactions
Drug-drug

Neomycin and other antibiotics: may theoretically decrease lactulose effectiveness by eliminating bacteria needed to digest it into the active form. Monitor patient for clinical effect.
Nonabsorbable antacids: may decrease lactulose effectiveness by preventing a decrease in colon pH. Avoid concomitant use.

Effects on diagnostic tests

None reported.

Adverse reactions

GI: *abdominal cramps, belching, diarrhea* with excessive dosage, *gaseous distention, flatulence,* nausea, vomiting.

Overdose and treatment

No cases of overdose have been reported. Clinical effects include diarrhea and abdominal cramps.

Special considerations

▶ Drug helps to relieve constipation caused by opiate therapy; consider daily dose to maintain regular bowel routine.
▶ Drug is also used to prevent and treat portal-systemic encephalopathy, including hepatic precoma and coma in patients with severe hepatic disease; after barium meal examination; and to restore bowel movements after hemorrhoidectomy.
▶ Drug is recommended for use in patients with irritable bowel syndrome on long-term narcotic therapy.
▶ After giving drug via nasogastric tube, flush tube with water to clear it and ensure drug's passage to stomach.
▶ Dilute drug with water or fruit juice to minimize its sweet taste.
▶ For retention enema, patient should retain drug for 30 to 60 minutes. If retained less than 30 minutes, repeat dose immediately. Begin oral therapy before discontinuing retention enemas.
▶ Don't administer drug with other laxatives because resulting loose stools may falsely indicate adequate dosage of lactulose.
▶ Monitor frequency and consistency of stools.

Geriatric patients

▶ Monitor patient's serum electrolyte levels; elderly patients are more sensitive to possible hypernatremia.

Patient teaching

▶ Advise patient to take drug with juice to improve taste.

▶ lansoprazole
Prevacid

Pharmacologic classification:
acid (proton) pump inhibitor

Therapeutic classification:
antiulcer drug

Pregnancy risk category B

How supplied
Available by prescription only
Capsules (delayed-release): 15 mg, 30 mg

Indications and dosages
Short-term treatment of active duodenal ulcer
Adults: 15 mg/day P.O. before meals for 4 weeks.
Maintenance of healed duodenal ulcer
Adults: 15 mg P.O. once daily.
Short-term treatment of erosive esophagitis
Adults: 30 mg P.O. daily before meals for up to 8 weeks; if healing doesn't occur, an additional 8 weeks of therapy may be needed.
Maintenance of healing of erosive esophagitis
Adults: 15 mg P.O. once daily.
Long-term treatment of pathologic hypersecretory conditions, including Zollinger-Ellison syndrome
Adults: initially, 60 mg P.O. once daily. Increase dosage, p.r.n., to 180 mg/day. Daily amounts exceeding 120 mg should be divided.
Short-term treatment of gastric ulcer
Adults: 30 mg P.O. daily for up to 8 weeks.

Short-term treatment of symptomatic gastroesophageal reflux disease
Adults: 15 mg P.O. daily for up to 8 weeks.
Helicobacter pylori eradication to reduce risk of duodenal ulcer recurrence
Adults: For dual therapy, 30 mg P.O. lansoprazole with 1 g P.O. amoxicillin, each given q 8 hours for 14 days. For triple therapy, 30 mg P.O. lansoprazole with 1 g P.O. amoxicillin and 500 mg P.O. clarithromycin, all given q 12 hours for 10 or 14 days.

Pharmacodynamics
Antiulcer action: Lansoprazole inhibits activity of the acid (proton) pump and binds to hydrogen-potassium ATPase, located at the secretory surface of the gastric parietal cells, to block the formation of gastric acid.

Pharmacokinetics
Absorption: Drug is rapidly absorbed with absolute bioavailability of over 80%.
Distribution: Lansoprazole is 97% bound to plasma proteins.
Metabolism: Drug is extensively metabolized in the liver.
Excretion: About two-thirds of dose is excreted in feces; one-third in urine.

Contraindications and precautions
Contraindicated in patients hypersensitive to drug.

Interactions
Drug-drug
Ampicillin esters, iron salts, ketoconazole: lansoprazole may inter-

fere with absorption of these drugs. Monitor patient closely.
Sucralfate: delays lansoprazole absorption. Give lansoprazole at least 30 minutes before sucralfate.
Theophylline: may cause mild increase in theophylline excretion; use together cautiously. Theophylline dosage may need adjustment when lansoprazole is started or stopped.

Drug-herb
Male fern: inactivated in alkaline stomach environment. Advise against use together.

Effects on diagnostic tests
None reported.

Adverse reactions
CNS: dizziness, headache.
GI: abdominal pain, diarrhea, nausea.

Overdose and treatment
No adverse effects have been reported with drug overdose. If needed, treatment should be supportive. Hemodialysis doesn't remove drug.

Special considerations
▶ Drug may be given concurrently with antacids.
▶ Dosage adjustment isn't necessary in elderly patients or those with renal insufficiency; however, it may be needed by patients with severe liver disease.
▶ If patient has a nasogastric tube, capsules can be opened and intact granules mixed in 40 ml of apple juice and given through tube into the stomach. After giving granules, flush tube with additional apple juice to clear it.

▶ Symptomatic response to lansoprazole therapy doesn't rule out gastric cancer.
▶ Don't use lansoprazole as maintenance therapy for patients with duodenal ulcer or erosive esophagitis.

Breast-feeding patients
▶ No data exist to demonstrate whether lansoprazole appears in breast milk; avoid giving drug during breast-feeding.

Pediatric patients
▶ Safety and effectiveness in children haven't been established.

Geriatric patients
▶ Although initial dosing regimen need not be altered for elderly patients, subsequent doses over 30 mg/day shouldn't be given unless additional gastric acid suppression is necessary.

Patient teaching
▶ Instruct patient to take drug before meals.
▶ Caution patient not to chew or crush capsules but to swallow them whole.
▶ If patient has trouble swallowing capsules, tell him to open them, sprinkle contents over 1 tablespoon of applesauce, and swallow immediately.

⟩ leflunomide
Arava

Pharmacologic classification:
pyrimidine synthesis inhibitor

Therapeutic classification:
antirheumatic

Pregnancy risk category X

How supplied
Available by prescription only
Tablets: 10 mg, 20 mg, 100 mg

Indications and dosages
Active rheumatoid arthritis (to reduce symptoms and retard structural damage seen as erosion and joint space narrowing on X-rays)
Adults: 100 mg P.O. q 24 hours for 3 days, followed by 20 mg (maximum daily dose) P.O. q 24 hours. Dose may be decreased to 10 mg daily if higher dose isn't tolerated well.

Pharmacodynamics
Immunomodulatory action: Drug inhibits dihydroorotate dehydrogenase, an enzyme involved in de novo pyrimidine synthesis, and has antiproliferative activity and anti-inflammatory effects.

Pharmacokinetics
Absorption: Bioavailability is 80%. Plasma levels peak within 12 hours after loading dose. Without loading dose, plasma levels peak in about 2 months.
Distribution: Drug is extensively bound to plasma proteins (over 99%).
Metabolism: Drug is metabolized to an active metabolite (M1), responsible for most of its activity.

Excretion: Leflunomide is eliminated by renal and direct biliary excretion. About 43% is excreted in urine and 48% in feces. Half-life of the active metabolite is about 2 weeks.

Contraindications and precautions
Contraindicated in patients hypersensitive to drug or its components and in women who are or may become pregnant or who are breast-feeding. Drug isn't recommended for patients with hepatic insufficiency, hepatitis B or C, severe immunodeficiency, bone marrow dysplasia, or severe uncontrolled infections.

Vaccination with live vaccines isn't recommended. The long half-life of drug should be considered when contemplating administration of a live vaccine after stopping drug treatment.

Drug isn't recommended for use by men attempting to father a child.

Risk of malignancy, particularly lymphoproliferative disorders, increases with use of some immunosuppressants, including leflunomide. Use cautiously in patients with renal insufficiency.

Interactions
Drug-drug
Charcoal, cholestyramine: decreased plasma leflunomide levels. These drugs are sometimes used for this effect in treating overdose.
Hepatotoxic drugs, such as methotrexate: increased risk of hepatotoxicity. Monitor liver enzymes as appropriate.
NSAIDs, such as diclofenac and ibuprofen: leflunomide increases

levels of these drugs. The clinical significance is unknown.

Rifampin: increased level of active leflunomide metabolite. Use together cautiously.

Tolbutamide: leflunomide increases levels of this drug. Clinical significance is unknown.

Effects on diagnostic tests
None reported.

Adverse reactions
CNS: anxiety, asthenia, depression, dizziness, headache, insomnia, malaise, migraine, neuralgia, neuritis, paresthesia, sleep disorder, vertigo.

CV: angina, chest pain, *hypertension*, increased CK, palpitations, peripheral edema, tachycardia, varicose veins, vasculitis, vasodilation.

EENT: blurred vision, cataracts, conjunctivitis, dry mouth, enlarged salivary glands, epistaxis, eye disorder, gingivitis, mouth ulcer, oral candidiasis, pharyngitis, rhinitis, stomatitis, sinusitis, taste perversion, tooth disorder.

GI: abdominal pain, anorexia, cholelithiasis, colitis, constipation, *diarrhea,* dyspepsia, esophagitis, flatulence, gastritis, gastroenteritis, melena, nausea, vomiting.

GU: albuminuria, cystitis, dysuria, hematuria, menstrual disorder, pelvic pain, prostate disorder, urinary frequency, urinary tract infection, vaginal candidiasis.

Hematologic: anemia, ecchymosis, hyperlipidemia.

Hepatic: elevated liver enzymes.

Metabolic: diabetes mellitus, hyperglycemia, hyperthyroidism, hypokalemia, weight loss.

Musculoskeletal: arthralgia, arthrosis, back pain, bone necrosis, bone pain, bursitis, joint disorder, leg cramps, muscle cramps, myalgia, neck pain, synovitis, tendon rupture, tenosynovitis.

Respiratory: *asthma,* bronchitis, dyspnea, increased cough, lung disorder, pneumonia, *respiratory infection.*

Skin: acne, *alopecia*, contact dermatitis, dry skin, eczema, fungal dermatitis, hair discoloration, hematoma, herpes simplex, herpes zoster, increased sweating, maculopapular rash, nail disorder, pruritus, *rash*, skin disorder, skin discoloration, skin nodule, skin ulcer, S.C. nodule.

Other: abscess, *allergic reaction*, cyst, fever, flulike syndrome, hernia, injury or accident, pain.

Overdose and treatment
No overdose has been reported in humans. Should overdose occur, activated charcoal (50 g every 6 hours for 24 hours) has been shown to reduce plasma levels. Cholestyramine may also be given as 8 g P.O. three times daily for 11 days.

Special considerations
▶ A loading dose of drug is necessary to attain steady state levels quickly.

▶ Aspirin, other NSAIDs, and low-dose corticosteroids may be continued during treatment; however, combined use of drug with antimalarials, I.M. or oral gold, penicillamine, azathioprine, or methotrexate hasn't been adequately studied.

▶ Monitor ALT and AST before starting therapy and monthly thereafter until stable. Frequency can then be decreased based on clinical situation.

▶ Because active metabolite of leflunomide has prolonged half-life, monitor patient closely during dosage reduction; reduction of these levels may take several weeks.

▶ A man planning to father a child should stop drug and follow recommended leflunomide removal protocol (cholestyramine 8 g, P.O. t.i.d. for 11 days).

Pregnant patients
▶ Leflunomide can cause fetal harm when given to pregnant women. Women who plan to become pregnant should stop leflunomide and consult prescriber.

Breast-feeding patients
▶ Drug shouldn't be used by nursing mothers.

Pediatric patients
▶ Safety in children and adolescents hasn't been established. Not recommended for children under 18 years of age.

Patient teaching
▶ Explain the need for blood tests and monitoring, and the appropriate schedule for them.
▶ Instruct patient to use birth control during treatment and until drug is no longer active.
▶ Warn women to immediately notify prescriber about planned, suspected, or known pregnancy.

▶ levomethadyl acetate hydrochloride
Orlaam

Pharmacologic classification: *synthetic opiate agonist*

Therapeutic classification: *narcotic detoxification adjunct*

Controlled substance schedule II

Pregnancy risk category C

How supplied
Available by prescription only.
Oral solution: 10 mg/ml

Indications and dosages
Opiate addiction
Adults: dosage is highly individualized. Initially, 20 to 40 mg q 48 to 72 hours. Subsequent doses increased by 5 to 10 mg at 48- to 72-hour intervals until steady state occurs, usually in 1 to 2 weeks. Most patients are stable on 60 to 90 mg three times weekly.

Pharmacodynamics
Opiate agonist action: A synthetic opiate agonist structurally similar to methadone, drug suppresses withdrawal symptoms in opiate-tolerant people by cross-substituting for opiate agonists. Long-term use may produce sufficient tolerance to block the euphoric effects of opiate agonists.

Pharmacokinetics
Absorption: Drug is rapidly absorbed.
Distribution: Plasma levels are detectable within 30 minutes and peak within 2 hours.

Metabolism: Drug undergoes first-pass metabolism to demethylated metabolites.
Elimination: Duration of action is 48 to 72 hours.

Contraindications and precautions
Contraindicated in patients hypersensitive to drug.

    Use cautiously in patients with cardiac conduction defects or with hepatic or renal failure.

Interactions
Drug-drug
Carbamazepine, phenobarbital, phenytoin, rifampin: increased hepatic enzyme activity; may increase levomethadyl's peak activity or shorten its duration of action. Monitor patient closely for withdrawal symptoms.
Cimetidine, erythromycin, ketoconazole: decreased hepatic enzyme activity; may decrease levomethadyl's peak activity or prolong its duration of action. Monitor patient closely.
Naloxone, pentazocine, other opioid agonist-antagonists: may precipitate abstinence syndrome. Don't use together.

Drug-lifestyle
Alcohol use: increased CNS effects. Advise against concurrent use.

Effects on diagnostic tests
None reported.

Adverse reactions
CNS: asthenia, drowsiness, malaise, sedation.
CV: *bradycardia,* edema, prolonged QT interval.
EENT: blurred vision, rhinitis.
GI: *abdominal pain, constipation, diarrhea, dry mouth, nausea, vomiting.*
GU: *difficult ejaculation, impotence.*
Musculoskeletal: arthralgia, back pain.
Respiratory: *cough.*
Skin: *diaphoresis, rash.*
Other: abstinence syndrome with sudden withdrawal, chills, flulike syndrome, yawning.

Overdose and treatment
Overdose may cause extreme somnolence progressing to stupor or coma, respiratory depression, constricted pupils, muscle flaccidity, cold and clammy skin, bradycardia, and hypotension. Apnea, circulatory collapse, pulmonary edema, cardiac arrest, and death may occur in severe overdose.

    Treatment is symptomatic and supportive. Gastric emptying or activated charcoal may decrease drug absorption. Naloxone may be given. Peritoneal dialysis and hemodialysis aren't useful.

Special considerations
▶ Don't give drug on a daily basis because of risk of fatal overdose.
▶ Drug can be used only by certain clinics approved by the Food and Drug Administration, Drug Enforcement Agency, and designated state authority. It has no recognized clinical uses outside of addiction treatment programs. By law, take-home doses are forbidden.
▶ By law, oral solutions must be diluted before being given to patients. Diluent should be a different color than the one used to dilute methadone oral solution in the same clinic.

Most patients can tolerate the 72-hour interval between weekly regimens. If withdrawal is a problem during the 72-hour interval, increase the next dose or switch to an alternate-day schedule. Never give levomethadyl on 2 consecutive days; instead, give small supplemental doses of methadone. Consider the risk of drug diversion before giving patients take-home methadone.

When used to replace methadone, the suggested initial dose is 1.2 to 1.3 times the daily methadone dose three times weekly, not to exceed 120 mg. Adjust dosage according to patient response. The crossover to methadone should be done in a single dose rather than decreasing doses of methadone and increasing doses of levomethadyl.

Monitor patient's progress of overcoming addiction.

Withdrawal symptoms occur after discontinuing this drug.

Pregnant patients

If administering drug to women of childbearing age, ensure monthly pregnancy tests.

Patients who become pregnant should be switched to methadone.

Patient teaching

Explain how drug is administered, and review dose schedule.

Caution patient to avoid hazardous activities until full CNS effects of drug are known.

Advise patient to avoid alcohol while taking drug.

Stress the need for monthly pregnancy tests. Urge patient to use birth control and to notify prescriber immediately about planned, suspected, or known pregnancy.

▌levorphanol tartrate
Levo-Dromoran

Pharmacologic classification:
synthetic opioid

Therapeutic classification:
analgesic

Controlled substance schedule II

Pregnancy risk category C

How supplied
Available by prescription only
Injection: 2 mg/ml
Tablets: 2 mg

Indications and dosages
Moderate to severe pain
Adults: 1 mg I.V. every 3 to 6 hours p.r.n. or 1 to 2 mg I.M. or S.C. every 6 to 8 hours p.r.n. or 2 mg P.O. every 6 to 8 hours p.r.n. Initially, don't exceed 8 mg I.V. or I.M. or 12 mg P.O. in a 24-hour period.
Chronic pain in patients being converted from morphine
Adults: $\frac{1}{15}$ to $\frac{1}{12}$ of daily morphine dose P.O. Adjust dose according to clinical response.
Preoperative sedation
Adults: 1 to 2 mg I.M. or S.C. 60 to 90 minutes before surgery.
◩ DOSAGE ADJUSTMENT. Elderly or debilitated patients usually require less drug preoperatively. In patients with any condition affecting respiratory reserve, reduce dose by at least half. Reduce initial dosage in patients with severe hepatic or renal disease, hypothyroidism, Addison's disease, toxic psychosis, prostatic hypertrophy, urethral stricture, acute alcoholism or delirium tremens.

Pharmacodynamics

Analgesic action: Alters the transmission and perception of pain by acting at receptors in the gray matter of the brain and spinal cord.

Pharmacokinetics

Absorption: Action starts within 30 minutes after I.M. administration. Well absorbed after P.O. administration; plasma levels peak about 1 hour after dose. Peak analgesia occurs within 20 minutes after I.V. administration and 90 minutes after S.C. administration.
Distribution: About 40% bound to plasma proteins.
Metabolism: Extensively metabolized in the liver to inactive metabolites.
Excretion: Duration of effect is 6 to 8 hours. Eliminated primarily in urine as the glucuronide metabolite.

Contraindications and precautions

Contraindicated in patients hypersensitive to drug. Don't use in patients with acute or severe bronchial asthma because drug may cause respiratory depression, or in biliary surgery because it may increase pressure in the common bile duct.

Use cautiously in patients with impaired respiratory reserve or respiratory depression caused by uremia, severe infection, obstructive or restrictive respiratory conditions, intrapulmonary shunting, or chronic bronchial asthma and in patients with head injury or other intracranial lesions. Use cautiously in acute MI or in patients with myocardial dysfunction or coronary insufficiency because the effects on the cardiac workload are un-

known. Use cautiously in patients with severe hepatic or renal disease, hypothyroidism, Addison's disease, toxic psychosis, prostatic hypertrophy, urethral stricture, acute alcoholism, or delirium tremens.

Interactions
Drug-drug

CNS depressants, such as antihistamines, barbiturates, general anesthetics, hypnotics, other opioids, phenothiazines, sedatives, skeletal muscle relaxants, tranquilizers, tricyclic antidepressants: may cause severe respiratory depression, hypotension, or profound sedation or coma. Reduce dosage of one or both drugs.
MAO inhibitors: may interact. Avoid concomitant use.
Mixed agonist/antagonist opioid analgesics, such as buprenorphine, butorphanol, dezocine, nalbuphine, pentazocine: may precipitate withdrawal symptoms. Avoid concomitant use.

Drug-lifestyle

Alcohol: additive effects. Advise against concomitant use.

Effects on diagnostic tests

None reported.

Adverse reactions

CNS: abnormal dreams, abnormal thinking, *altered mood and mentation,* amnesia, CNS stimulation, **coma,** confusion, depression, dizziness, drug withdrawal, dyskinesia, hypokinesia, insomnia, lethargy, nervousness, personality disorder, *seizures.*
CV: *arrhythmias, bradycardia, cardiac arrest, flushing,* hypotension, palpitations, tachycardia.

EENT: abnormal vision, diplopia, pupillary disorder.
GI: abdominal pain, *biliary spasm, constipation,* dry mouth, dyspepsia, *nausea, vomiting.*
GU: *difficulty urinating,* **renal failure,** urine retention.
Respiratory: *apnea,* cyanosis, hypoventilation.
Skin: diaphoresis, *pruritus,* rash, urticaria.
Other: *shock,* injection site reaction.

Overdose and treatment

Overdose may cause decreased respiratory rate, periodic breathing, cyanosis, extreme somnolence progressing to stupor or coma, skeletal muscle flaccidity, cold and clammy skin, constricted pupils, bradycardia, and hypotension. Severe overdose may cause apnea, circulatory collapse, cardiac arrest and death.

Treatment is supportive and symptomatic. Naloxone will reverse the effects. Several doses may be necessary.

Special considerations

▶ Dosage must be individualized according to pain level and patient's age, weight, physical status, underlying disease, and use of other drugs.
▶ Excessive preoperative doses may delay the return of spontaneous respiration or prolong postoperative hypoventilation.
▶ Drug is 4 to 8 times more potent than morphine and has a longer half-life.
▶ Administer by slow I.V. injection.
▶ Monitor patient for orthostatic hypotension.
▶ Keep narcotic antagonist, such as naloxone, and resuscitation equipment available when giving drug by I.V. route.
▶ Neurologic exams may be complicated because of drug's effect on level of consciousness.
▶ Drug may obscure the diagnosis or clinical course of abdominal conditions.
▶ For patients on round-the-clock dosing, allow 72 hours between dosage changes.
▶ Withdrawal symptoms shouldn't occur in patients receiving the drug postoperatively or for less than one week, but they may occur after prolonged use. Reduce dose gradually.

Breast-feeding patients
▶ No data exist to demonstrate whether drug appears in breast milk. Because of serious potential reactions, drug shouldn't be used in nursing mothers.

Pediatric patients
▶ Safety and effectiveness in patients under age 18 haven't been established.

Geriatric patients
▶ Use drug cautiously and reduce initial dose by half because drug effects may be increased.

Patient teaching
▶ Advise patient that drug may be habit-forming.
▶ Warn ambulatory patient about getting out of bed or walking.
▶ Caution patient to avoid hazardous activities until full CNS effects of drug are known.
▶ Advise patient to avoid alcohol while taking drug.

▶ lidocaine 2.5% and prilocaine 2.5% cream
EMLA Anesthetic Disc, EMLA cream

Pharmacologic classification:
amide-type local anesthetic

Therapeutic classification:
analgesic, local anesthetic

Pregnancy risk category B

How supplied
Available by prescription only
Anesthetic disc: 1 g
Cream: 5 g, 30 g

Indications and dosages
To provide local analgesia on normal intact skin during minor dermal procedures, such as I.V. cannulation and venipuncture
Adults: apply 2.5 g of cream (half of 5-g tube) over 20 cm^2 of skin surface and cover with occlusive dressing. Or apply 1 anesthetic disc. Leave intact for at least 1 hour.
Infants up to 3 months or who weigh less than 5 kg (11 lb): apply 1 g of cream over 10 cm^2 of skin, cover with occlusive dressing, and leave intact for maximum of 1 hour.
Infants ages 4 to 12 months or who weigh 5 to 10 kg (11 to 22 lb): apply 2 g of cream over 20 cm^2 of skin, cover with occlusive dressing and leave intact for maximum of 4 hours.
Children ages 1 to 6 or who weigh 11 to 20 kg (22 to 44 lb): apply 10 g of cream over 100 cm^2 of skin, cover with occlusive dressing and leave intact for maximum of 4 hours.

Children ages 7 to 12 or who weigh more than 20 kg: apply 20 g of cream over 200 cm^2 of skin, cover with occlusive dressing and leave intact for maximum of 4 hours.
To provide local analgesia on normal intact skin during major dermal procedures such as split thickness skin graft harvesting
Adults: apply 2 g of cream per 10 cm^2 of skin, cover with occlusive dressing, and allow to remain in contact with skin for at least 2 hours.
Adjunct to infiltration of local anesthetic in male genital skin for treating genital warts
Adults: apply 1 g of cream over 10 cm^2 of skin surface and cover with occlusive dressing for 15 minutes. Perform local anesthetic infiltration immediately after removing cream.
▧ **DOSAGE ADJUSTMENT.** In patients older than 3 months who weigh less than 5 kg, use 1 g of cream over 10 cm^2 of skin. In neonates and children who weigh less than 20 kg, the area and duration of application should be limited. Smaller areas of treatment are recommended in debilitated patients or patients with impaired elimination.

Pharmacodynamics
Analgesic and anesthetic actions: Provides dermal analgesia by releasing lidocaine and prilocaine near dermal pain receptors and nerve endings. Lidocaine and prilocaine stabilize neuronal membranes by inhibiting ionic fluxes needed to start and conduct impulses, thereby causing local anesthetic action.

Pharmacokinetics

Absorption: Systemic absorption is directly related to duration and area of application. Application over broken or inflamed skin or to 2000 cm^2 or more of skin could yield more systemic absorption. Analgesia is achieved 1 hour after application, peaks at 2 to 3 hours under occlusive dressing, and persists for 1 to 2 hours after removal.

Distribution: Lidocaine is about 70% bound to plasma proteins; prilocaine is 55% bound to plasma proteins. Both lidocaine and prilocaine cross the placenta and blood-brain barrier.

Metabolism: Unknown whether lidocaine or prilocaine are metabolized in the skin. Lidocaine is metabolized by the liver to a number of metabolites; prilocaine is metabolized by the liver and kidneys to various metabolites.

Excretion: More than 98% of an absorbed dose of lidocaine can be recovered in the urine as metabolites or parent drug. Duration of action is 1 to 2 hours after removal of cream or disc.

Contraindications and precautions

Contraindicated in patients hypersensitive to local anesthetics of the amide type or to any other component of the product. Don't use on mucous membranes or in any area where penetration or migration beyond the tympanic membrane into the middle ear is possible. Don't use in patients with congenital or idiopathic methemoglobinemia or in infants under age 12 months who are receiving treatment with methemoglobin-inducing drugs. Don't use before circumcision in pediatric patients or in neonates with a gestational age less than 37 weeks.

Use cautiously in acutely ill, debilitated, or elderly patients because they may be more sensitive to the systemic effects of lidocaine and prilocaine. Also, use cautiously in patients with a history of drug sensitivities, in patients with severe hepatic disease, and in breast-feeding women.

Interactions
Drug-drug

Acetaminophen, acetanilid, aniline dyes, benzocaine, chloroquine, dapsone, naphthalene, nitrates, nitrites, nitrofurantoin, nitroglycerin, nitroprusside, pamaquine, para-aminosalicylic acid, phenacetin, phenobarbital, phenytoin, primaquine, quinine, sulfonamides: increased risk of drug-induced methemoglobinemia. Use cautiously.

Class I antiarrhythmics (mexiletine, tocainide): potential toxicity and synergistic effects. Use together cautiously.

Effects on diagnostic tests
None reported.

Adverse reactions

Skin: *abnormal sensation,* altered temperature sensations, *blanching,* edema, *erythema,* itching, *paleness, pallor.*

Other: *anaphylaxis (urticaria, angioedema, bronchospasm, shock).*

Overdose and treatment

Toxic levels of lidocaine, prilocaine, or both can decrease cardiac output, total peripheral resistance, and mean arterial pressure. Provide symptomatic and supportive treatment.

There have been reports of significant methemoglobinemia in infants and children following excessive applications of EMLA cream. Spontaneous recovery after removal of the cream is likely. I.V. methylene blue may be effective if needed.

Special considerations

▶ When using drug for I.V. cannulation or venipuncture, consider preparing two sites in case cannulation or venipuncture fail at the first site.

▶ Decreasing the duration of application is likely to decrease the analgesic effect.

▶ Avoid contact with eyes.

▶ Monitor patient closely for effectiveness of analgesia and anesthesia during procedure.

▶ Very young patients, patients with glucose-6-phosphate deficiencies, and patients taking oxidizing drugs such as antimalarials and sulfonamides are more susceptible to methemoglobinemia.

▶ Long duration of application, large treatment area, small patients, or impaired renal and hepatic function may result in high blood levels.

▶ Monitor patient for CNS excitation or depression, which may be a sign of a systemic reaction.

▶ Application of cream to larger areas or for longer times than those recommended could result in serious systemic adverse effects. Systemic reactions may include CNS excitation or depression, light-headedness, nervousness, apprehension, euphoria, confusion, dizziness, drowsiness, tinnitus, blurred or double vision, vomiting, sensations of heat, cold or numbness, twitching, tremors, convulsions, unconsciousness, respiratory depression and arrest. Cardiac effects may include bradycardia, hypotension, and CV collapse leading to cardiac arrest.

▶ When drug is used with other local anesthetics, the amount absorbed from all drugs must be considered.

Breast-feeding patients

▶ Lidocaine and probably prilocaine appear in human milk. Use cautiously in breast-feeding women.

Pediatric patients

▶ Drug is less effective in children under age 7 than in older children and adults.

▶ Provide emotional and psychological support for young children undergoing medical or surgical procedures.

▶ If patient over 3 months old doesn't meet minimum weight requirement, maximum dose should correspond to patient's weight, not age.

Patient teaching

▶ Advise patient to use cream only on intact skin and to avoid contact with mucous membranes and eyes.

▶ Urge patient to apply cream carefully and not to exceed the recommended area or duration of application.

▶ Tell patient to avoid spreading out the cream and to apply the occlusive dressing carefully to avoid leakage around the edges of the dressing. Application of a secondary protective covering at the application site may be helpful.

▶ Caution patient to avoid scratching, rubbing, or exposing treated area to extreme heat or cold until sensation has returned. Duration of anesthesia is at least 1 hour after removal of the occlusive dressing.

▶ Urge parent to carefully monitor child while drug is in use and to protect child from accidental ingestion of cream or dressing.

▶ Advise parent to remove cream and notify prescriber immediately if child becomes dizzy, sleepy, or develops duskiness of the face or lips after applying cream.

▶ If child will undergo a painful procedure, help parent prepare child for the procedure, and explain what to expect and what the child may feel.

▶ Tell parent to use distraction techniques and to calmly reassure child during the procedure.

▶ **lidocaine (lignocaine)**
Xylocaine

▶ **lidocaine hydrochloride**
Anestacon, Dilocaine, L-Caine, Lidoderm Patch, Lidoject, LidoPen Auto-Injector, Nervocaine, Xylocaine, Xylocaine Viscous, Zilactin-L

Pharmacologic classification:
amide derivative

Therapeutic classification:
ventricular antiarrhythmic, local anesthetic

Pregnancy risk category B

How supplied
Available without a prescription
Cream: 0.5%
Gel: 0.5%, 2.5%
Liquid: 2.5%
Ointment: 2.5%
Spray: 0.5%
Transdermal patch: 5%
Available by prescription only
Injection: 5 mg/ml, 10 mg/ml, 15 mg/ml, 20 mg/ml, 40 mg/ml, 100 mg/ml, 200 mg/ml
Jelly: 2%
Ointment: 5%
Premixed solutions: 2 mg/ml, 4 mg/ml, 8 mg/ml in D_5W
Spray: 10%
Topical solution: 2%, 4%

Indications and dosages
Local anesthesia of skin or mucous membranes, pain from dental extractions, stomatitis
Adults and children: 2% to 5% solution or ointment or 15 ml of Xylocaine Viscous applied q 3 to 4 hours to oral or nasal mucosa.
Local anesthesia in procedures involving the urethra
Adults: about 15 ml (male) or 3 to 5 ml (female) instilled into urethra.
Pain, burning, or itching caused by burns, sunburn, or skin irritation
Adults and children: liberal application.
Pain from postherpetic neuralgia
Adults: 1 to 3 patches applied to intact skin, covering most painful area, once daily for up to 12 hours. Smaller areas are recommended for debilitated patients or those with poor elimination. Applying patch to larger areas or for excessive times could increase lidocaine absorption and cause serious adverse effects.

Pharmacodynamics
Ventricular antiarrhythmic action:
One of the oldest antiarrhythmics, lidocaine remains among the most

widely used drugs for treating acute ventricular arrhythmias. A class IB antiarrhythmic, it suppresses automaticity and shortens the effective refractory period and action potential duration of His-Purkinje fibers and suppresses spontaneous ventricular depolarization during diastole. Therapeutic levels don't significantly affect conductive atrial tissue and AV conduction.

Unlike quinidine and procainamide, lidocaine doesn't significantly alter hemodynamics when given in usual doses. It seems to act preferentially on diseased or ischemic myocardial tissue; it inhibits reentry mechanisms and halts ventricular arrhythmias.

Local anesthetic action: As a local anesthetic, lidocaine blocks initiation and conduction of nerve impulses by decreasing the permeability of the nerve cell membrane to sodium ions.

Pharmacokinetics

Absorption: Drug is absorbed after oral administration; however, a significant first-pass effect occurs in the liver and only about 35% of drug reaches the systemic circulation. Oral doses high enough to achieve therapeutic blood levels result in an unacceptable toxicity.

Distribution: Drug is distributed widely throughout the body; it has a high affinity for adipose tissue. After I.V. bolus administration, an early, rapid decline in plasma levels occurs; this stems mainly from distribution into highly perfused tissues, such as the kidneys, lungs, liver, and heart, followed by a slower elimination phase in which metabolism and redistribution into

skeletal muscle and adipose tissue occur. The first (early) distribution phase occurs rapidly, creating a need for a constant infusion after the initial bolus dose. Distribution volume declines in patients with liver or hepatic disease, resulting in toxic levels with usual doses. About 60% to 80% of circulating drug is bound to plasma proteins. Usual therapeutic drug level is 1.5 to 5 mcg/ml. Although toxicity may occur within this range, levels above 5 mcg/ml are considered toxic and warrant dosage reduction.

Metabolism: Lidocaine is metabolized in the liver to two active metabolites. Less than 10% of a parenteral dose escapes metabolism and reaches the kidneys unchanged. Metabolism is affected by hepatic blood flow, which may decrease after MI and with heart failure. Liver disease also may limit metabolism.

Excretion: Half-life has a biphasic pattern, with an initial phase of 7 to 30 minutes followed by a terminal half-life of 1½ to 2 hours. Elimination half-life may be prolonged in patients with heart failure or liver disease. Continuous infusions longer than 24 hours also may cause an apparent half-life increase.

Contraindications and precautions

Contraindicated in patients with hypersensitivity to amide-type local anesthetics, Stokes-Adams syndrome, Wolff-Parkinson-White syndrome, and severe degrees of SA, AV, or intraventricular block if patient doesn't have an artificial pacemaker. Also contraindicated in

patients with inflammation or infection in puncture region, septicemia, severe hypertension,
spinal deformities, and neurologic
disorders.

Use cautiously in elderly patients, in patients who weigh less
than 50 kg (110 lb), and in patients
with renal or hepatic disease, complete or second-degree heart block,
sinus bradycardia, or heart failure.

Interactions
Drug-drug
*Antiarrhythmics, including pheny-
toin, procainamide, propranolol,
quinidine:* may cause additive or
antagonist effects and additive toxicity. Monitor patient closely.
Beta blockers, cimetidine: may
cause lidocaine toxicity from reduced hepatic clearance. Monitor
patient for toxicity.
Succinylcholine: use of high-dose
lidocaine with succinylcholine
may increase neuromuscular effects of succinylcholine. Monitor
patient closely.

Drug-herb
Pareira: may add to or potentiate
neuromuscular blockade. Advise
against use together.

Effects on diagnostic tests
Because I.M. lidocaine therapy
may increase CK levels, isoenzyme tests should be performed
for differential diagnosis of acute
MI.

Adverse reactions
CNS: anxiety, lethargy, muscle
twitching, nervousness, paresthesia, somnolence; *confusion,* hallucinations, *light-headedness, restlessness, seizures, stupor, tremor*
(systemic form); apprehension,
confusion, depression, euphoria,
light-headedness, restlessness,
seizures, slurred speech, stupor,
tremors, unconsciousness (topical
form).
CV: bradycardia, CARDIAC AR-
REST, edema; *hypotension, new or
worsened arrhythmias* (systemic
form); *arrhythmias,* hypotension,
myocardial depression (topical
form).
EENT: *blurred or double vision,
tinnitus* (systemic form); blurred
or double vision, tinnitus (topical
form).
GI: nausea, vomiting (topical
form).
Respiratory: *respiratory arrest,
status asthmaticus.*
Skin: dermatologic reactions, diaphoresis, rash, sensitization.
Other: *anaphylaxis,* sensation of
cold (systemic form), soreness at
injection site.

Overdose and treatment
Overdose may cause CNS toxicity,
such as seizures or respiratory depression, and CV toxicity (as indicated by hypotension).

Treatment includes stopping
drug and providing supportive
measures. Maintain a patent airway, and give other respiratory
support measures immediately as
needed. Give diazepam or thiopental for seizures. To treat significant
hypotension, consider a vasopressor (such as dopamine or norepinephrine).

Special considerations
▶ Drug may be helpful in treating
neuropathic pain because of its
sodium channel blockade. It also is
effective for topical mucositis pain
in conjunction with opiates. And
it's used to treat status epilepticus

and ventricular arrhythmias caused by MI, cardiac manipulation, or cardiac glycosides.

▶ Don't give lidocaine with epinephrine (for local anesthesia) to treat arrhythmias. Use caution when giving epinephrine solutions in CV disorders and in body areas with limited blood supply (ears, nose, fingers, toes).

▶ Don't use preservative-containing solutions for spinal, epidural, or caudal block.

▶ For epidural use, inject a 2- to 5-ml test dose at least 5 minutes before giving total dose to check for intravascular or subarachnoid injection. Motor paralysis and extensive sensory anesthesia indicate subarachnoid injection.

▶ Use infusion pump or microdrip system and timer to monitor infusion precisely. Never exceed infusion rate of 4 mg/minute, if possible. A faster rate greatly increases risk of toxicity.

▶ Therapeutic serum levels range from 2 to 5 mcg/ml.

▶ Monitor patient's vital signs and serum electrolyte, BUN, and creatinine levels.

▶ Monitor ECG constantly if giving drug by I.V. route, especially if patient has liver disease, heart failure, hypoxia, respiratory depression, hypovolemia, or shock, because these conditions may affect drug metabolism, excretion, or distribution volume, predisposing patient to drug toxicity.

▶ Discard partially used vials if solution contains no preservative.

▶ Doses of up to 400 mg I.M. have been advocated in prehospital phase of acute MI.

▶ A patient who receives lidocaine I.M. will show a sevenfold increase in serum CK level. Such CK originates in skeletal muscle, not the heart. Test isoenzyme levels to confirm MI if using the I.M. route.

▶ In many severely ill patients, seizures may be the first sign of toxicity. However, severe reactions are usually preceded by somnolence, confusion, and paresthesia. Regard all evidence of toxicity as serious, and promptly reduce dosage or stop drug. Continued infusion could lead to seizures and coma. Give oxygen via nasal cannula, if not contraindicated. Keep oxygen and resuscitation equipment nearby.

▶ Assess patient for signs of excessive depression of cardiac conductivity (such as sinus node dysfunction, PR-interval prolongation, QRS-interval widening, and appearance or exacerbation of arrhythmias). If they occur, reduce dosage or discontinue drug.

Pediatric patients

▶ Safety and effectiveness in children haven't been established.

▶ Use of an I.M. autoinjector device isn't recommended.

Geriatric patients

▶ Because elderly patients tend to have other disorders and declining organ function, use conservative lidocaine doses.

Patient teaching

▶ Tell patient to report adverse reactions promptly.

▶ **lithium carbonate**
Carbolith◇, **Duralith**◇, **Eskalith,**
Eskalith CR, Lithane, Lithizine◇,
Lithobid, Lithonate, Lithotabs

▶ **lithium citrate**
Cibalith-S

Pharmacologic classification:
alkali metal

Therapeutic classification:
antimanic, antipsychotic

Pregnancy risk category D

How supplied
Available by prescription only
lithium carbonate
Capsules: 150 mg, 300 mg, 600 mg
Tablets: 300 mg
Tablets (sustained-release): 300 mg,
450 mg
lithium citrate
Syrup (sugarless): 300 mg/5 ml
(with 0.3% alcohol)

Indications and dosages
Chronic cluster or migraine
headaches
Adults: Drug has been used in uncontrolled clinical trials. Dosage
recommendations are undetermined.

Pharmacodynamics
Analgesic action: Unknown.
Antimanic action: Lithium probably exerts antipsychotic and antimanic effects by competing with
other cations for exchange at the
sodium-potassium ion pump, thus
altering cation exchange at the tissue level. It also inhibits adenyl cyclase, reducing intracellular levels
of cAMP and to a lesser extent,
cyclic guanosine monophosphate.

Pharmacokinetics
Absorption: Rate and extent of absorption vary with dosage form;
absorption is complete within 6
hours of oral administration from
conventional tablets and capsules.
Distribution: Drug is distributed
widely into the body, including
breast milk; levels in thyroid gland,
bone, and brain tissue exceed
serum levels. Effects peak in 30
minutes to 3 hours; liquid peaks at
15 minutes to 1 hour. Steady state
serum level achieved in 12 hours.
Therapeutic effect begins in 5 to
10 days and peaks within 3 weeks.
Therapeutic and toxic serum levels
and therapeutic effects show good
correlation. Therapeutic range is
0.6 to 1.2 mEq/L. Adverse reactions increase as level reaches 1.5
to 2 mEq/L—such levels may be
necessary in acute mania. Toxicity
usually occurs at levels above
2 mEq/L.
Metabolism: Lithium isn't metabolized.
Excretion: Drug is excreted 95%
unchanged in urine. About 50% to
80% of a given dose is excreted
within 24 hours. Level of renal
function determines elimination
rate.

Contraindications and
precautions
Contraindicated if therapy can't be
closely monitored and during pregnancy.
   Use cautiously in elderly patients; in patients with thyroid disease, seizure disorders, renal or
CV disease, severe dehydration or
debilitation, or sodium depletion;
and in patients receiving neuroleptics, neuromuscular blockers, and
diuretics.

Interactions
Drug-drug
ACE inhibitors: increased lithium levels. Monitor serum lithium levels.

Aminophylline, antacids, calcium, sodium, theophylline: may increase lithium excretion and decrease its effects by renal competition for elimination. Monitor patient for clinical effect.

Carbamazepine, mazindol, methyldopa, phenytoin, tetracyclines: increased lithium toxicity. Monitor lithium levels.

Chlorpromazine: decreased chlorpromazine effects. Monitor patient for drug effects.

Fluoxetine: increased lithium serum levels. Monitor lithium levels.

Haloperidol: increased risk of severe encephalopathy characterized by confusion, tremors, extrapyramidal effects, and weakness. Use this combination with caution.

Neuromuscular blockers, such as atracurium, pancuronium, succinylcholine: potentiated neuromuscular blocking effects. Monitor patient closely.

NSAIDs, such as indomethacin, phenylbutazone, piroxicam: decreased renal excretion of lithium. May require a 30% reduction in lithium dosage.

Sympathomimetics, especially norepinephrine: lithium may interfere with pressor effects. Monitor vital signs closely.

Thiazide diuretics: may decrease renal excretion and enhance lithium toxicity. Diuretic dosage may need to be reduced by 30%.

Drug-herb
Parsley: may promote or produce serotonin syndrome. Advise patient to avoid use together.

Psyllium seed: inhibited GI absorption. Advise patient to avoid use together.

Drug-food
Caffeine: may increase lithium excretion and decrease its effects by renal competition for elimination. Monitor patient for clinical effect.

Dietary sodium: may alter renal elimination of lithium. Increased sodium intake may increase drug elimination; decreased intake may decrease elimination. Monitor lithium levels and sodium intake.

Effects on diagnostic tests
Drug causes false-positive results on thyroid function tests.

Adverse reactions
CNS: ataxia, blackouts, ***coma,*** confusion, dizziness, drowsiness, EEG changes, ***epileptiform seizures,*** headache, impaired speech, incoordination, lethargy, muscle weakness, psychomotor retardation, restlessness, tremors, worsened organic mental syndrome.

CV: ***arrhythmias, bradycardia,*** hypotension, peripheral edema, *reversible ECG changes.*

EENT: blurred vision, tinnitus.

GI: abdominal pain, anorexia, diarrhea, dry mouth, flatulence, indigestion, metallic taste, nausea, *thirst,* vomiting.

GU: albuminuria, decreased creatinine clearance, elevated BUN and creatinine, glycosuria, *polyuria,* ***renal toxicity*** with long-term use.

Hematologic: elevated neutrophil count, *leukocytosis with WBC count of 14,000 to 18,000/mm³* (reversible).

Metabolic: goiter, hyponatremia, hypothyroidism (lowered T_3, T_4, and protein-bound iodine, but elevated ^{131}I uptake), transient hyperglycemia, weight gain.

Skin: acne, alopecia, diminished or absent sensation, drying and thinning of hair, pruritus, psoriasis, rash.

Overdose and treatment

Vomiting and diarrhea occur within 1 hour of acute ingestion. Death has occurred in patients who ingest 10 to 60 g of lithium, although patients have ingested 6 g with little toxic effect. Serum lithium levels above 3.4 mEq/L may be fatal.

Overdose with chronic lithium ingestion may follow altered pharmacokinetics, drug interactions, or volume or sodium depletion. It may cause sedation, confusion, hand tremors, joint pain, ataxia, muscle stiffness, increased deep tendon reflexes, visual changes, and nystagmus. Symptoms may progress to coma, movement abnormalities, tremors, seizures, and CV collapse.

Treatment is symptomatic and supportive; closely monitor vital signs. Induce emesis if patient isn't comatose and hasn't already vomited. If emesis isn't feasible, perform gastric lavage. Monitor fluid and electrolyte balance, and correct sodium depletion with normal saline solution. Institute hemodialysis if serum level is above 3 mEq/L, if patient has severe symptoms unresponsive to fluid and electrolyte correction, or if urine output decreases significantly. Serum rebound of tissue lithium stores (from high volume distribution) commonly occurs after dialysis and may necessitate prolonged or repeated hemodialysis. Peritoneal dialysis may help but is less effective.

Special considerations

▶ Lithium is used experimentally to increase WBC count in patients undergoing cancer chemotherapy and to treat cluster headaches, aggression, organic brain syndrome, and tardive dyskinesia. Drug has been used to treat SIADH.
▶ Drug is also used to prevent or control mania, depression in patients with bipolar illness, major depression, schizoaffective disorder, schizophrenic disorder, alcohol dependence, apparent mixed bipolar disorder in children, and chemotherapy-induced neutropenia in children and in patients with AIDS who receive zidovudine.
▶ Shake syrup form before administration.
▶ Give drug with food or milk to reduce GI upset.
▶ Determination of serum drug levels is crucial to safe use of drug. Don't use drug in patients who can't have regular serum drug level checks. Make sure patient or responsible family member can comply with instructions.
▶ Expect a lag of 1 to 3 weeks before beneficial effects are noticed. Other psychotropic drugs (such as chlorpromazine) may be necessary during interim period.
▶ Adjust fluid and salt ingestion to compensate if excessive loss occurs through protracted sweating or diarrhea. Patient should have fluid intake of 2,500 to 3,000 ml

daily and a balanced diet with adequate salt intake.

▶ Monitor fluid intake and output, especially when surgery is scheduled.

▶ Lithane tablets contain tartrazine, a dye that may cause an allergic reaction in certain people, particularly people with asthma who are sensitive to aspirin.

▶ EEG changes include diffuse slowing, widening of frequency spectrum, potentiation, and disorganization of background rhythm.

▶ Monitor baseline ECG, thyroid and renal studies, and electrolyte levels. Monitor lithium blood levels 8 to 12 hours after first dose (usually before morning dose), two or three times weekly the first month, then weekly to monthly on maintenance therapy.

▶ When lithium blood levels are below 1.5 mEq/L, adverse reactions usually remain mild.

▶ Monitor patient for edema or sudden weight gain.

▶ Acute neurotoxicity with delirium has occurred in patients receiving lithium and electroconvulsive therapy (ECT). Lithium dosage should be reduced or withdrawn before ECT.

▶ Arrange for outpatient follow-up of thyroid and renal functions every 6 to 12 months. Thyroid should be palpated to check for enlargement.

▶ Check urine for specific gravity level below 1.015, which may indicate diabetes insipidus.

▶ Drug may alter glucose tolerance in diabetic patients. Monitor blood glucose levels closely.

▶ Monitor serum levels and signs of impending toxicity.

▶ Monitor dosage carefully when patient's manic symptoms begin to subside because the ability to tolerate high serum lithium levels decreases as symptoms resolve.

Breast-feeding patients
▶ Lithium level in breast milk is 33% to 50% that of maternal serum level. Avoid breast-feeding during treatment with lithium.

Pediatric patients
▶ Drug isn't recommended for children under age 12.

Geriatric patients
▶ Elderly patients are more susceptible to chronic overdose and toxic effects, especially dyskinesias. These patients usually respond to a lower dosage.

Patient teaching
▶ Tell patient to take drug with food or milk.

▶ Advise patient to maintain adequate water intake and adequate, but not excessive, salt in diet.

▶ Explain that lithium has a narrow margin of safety. A serum drug level that is even slightly high can be dangerous.

▶ Explain the importance of regular follow-up visits to measure lithium serum levels.

▶ Warn patient and family to watch for signs of toxicity (diarrhea, vomiting, dehydration, drowsiness, muscle weakness, tremor, fever, and ataxia) and to expect transient nausea, polyuria, thirst, and discomfort during the first few days. If toxic symptoms occur, tell patient to withhold one dose and call promptly.

▶ Tell patient to explain to close friends or family members the signs of lithium overdose, in case emergency aid is needed.

▶ Warn ambulatory patient to avoid hazardous activities until CNS response to drug is known.
▶ Tell patient to avoid large amounts of caffeine because it interferes with drug effectiveness.
▶ Advise patient to consult prescriber before starting a weight-loss program.
▶ Tell patient not to switch brands of lithium or take other prescription or OTC drugs without consulting prescriber. Different brands may not provide equivalent effect.
▶ Warn patient against stopping drug abruptly.
▶ Instruct patient to wear or carry medical identification and instruction card with toxicity and emergency information.

▶ lorazepam
Apo-Lorazepam◇, Ativan, Novo-Lorazem◇

Pharmacologic classification: *benzodiazepine*

Therapeutic classification: *antianxiety drug, sedative-hypnotic*

Controlled substance schedule IV

Pregnancy risk category D

How supplied
Available by prescription only
Injection: 2 mg/ml, 4 mg/ml
Tablets: 0.5 mg, 1 mg, 2 mg
Tablets (S.L.)◇: 1 mg, 2 mg

Indications and dosages
Anxiety, tension, agitation, irritability, especially in anxiety neuroses or organic (especially GI or CV) disorders
Adults: 2 to 6 mg/day P.O. in divided doses. Maximum, 10 mg/day.

Insomnia
Adults: 2 to 4 mg P.O. h.s.
Preoperatively
Adults: 0.05 mg/kg I.M. 2 hours before surgery (maximum, 4 mg). Alternatively, 0.044 mg/kg (maximum, 2 mg) I.V. 15 to 20 minutes before surgery. In adults under age 50, dosage may be increased to 0.05 mg/kg (maximum, 4 mg) when increased lack of recall of preoperative events is desired.
Nausea and vomiting from chemotherapy*
Adults: 2.5 mg P.O. the evening before chemotherapy and a second dose just after chemotherapy starts. Alternatively, 1.5 mg/m^2 (maximum, 3 mg) I.V. over 5 minutes, 45 minutes before chemotherapy starts.

Pharmacodynamics
Anxiolytic and sedative actions: Lorazepam depresses the CNS at the limbic and subcortical levels of the brain. It produces an antianxiety effect by influencing the effect of the neurotransmitter GABA on its receptor in the ascending reticular activating system, which increases inhibition and blocks cortical and limbic arousal after stimulation of the reticular formation.

Pharmacokinetics
Absorption: When given orally, drug is well absorbed through the GI tract. Levels peak in 2 hours.
Distribution: Drug is distributed widely throughout the body and is about 85% protein-bound.
Metabolism: Drug is metabolized in the liver to inactive metabolites.
Excretion: The metabolites of lorazepam are excreted in urine as glucuronide conjugates.

Contraindications and precautions

Contraindicated in patients with acute angle-closure glaucoma or hypersensitivity to drug, other benzodiazepines, or its vehicle (used in parenteral dosage form).

Use cautiously in patients with pulmonary, renal, or hepatic impairment and in elderly, acutely ill, or debilitated patients. Don't use in pregnant patients, especially during the first trimester of pregnancy.

Interactions

Drug-drug

Antidepressants, antihistamines, barbiturates, general anesthetics, MAO inhibitors, narcotics, phenothiazines: lorazepam potentiates CNS depressant effects of these drugs. Monitor patient closely.
Cimetidine, disulfiram: diminished hepatic metabolism of lorazepam, which increases its plasma level. Decrease dose as needed.
Scopolamine: combined use of parenteral lorazepam and scopolamine may increase the risk of hallucinations, irrational behavior, and sedation. Avoid concomitant use.

Drug-lifestyle

Alcohol use: lorazepam potentiates the CNS depressant effects of alcohol. Advise against concurrent use.
Heavy smoking: accelerates lorazepam's metabolism, thus lowering effectiveness. Advise against concurrent use.

Effects on diagnostic tests

None reported.

Adverse reactions

CNS: agitation, amnesia, confusion, depression, disorientation, dizziness, *drowsiness,* headache, insomnia, *sedation,* unsteadiness, weakness.
EENT: visual disturbances.
GI: abdominal discomfort, change in appetite, nausea.
Other: *acute withdrawal syndrome* after sudden discontinuation in physically dependent persons.

Overdose and treatment

Overdose may cause somnolence, confusion, coma, hypoactive reflexes, dyspnea, labored breathing, hypotension, bradycardia, slurred speech, and unsteady gait or impaired coordination.

Treatment requires support of blood pressure and respiration until drug effects subside; monitor vital signs. Mechanical ventilatory assistance via endotracheal tube may be needed to maintain a patent airway and support adequate oxygenation. Flumazenil, a specific benzodiazepine antagonist, may be useful. Use I.V. fluids and vasopressors such as dopamine and phenylephrine to treat hypotension, if necessary. If patient is conscious, induce emesis. Use gastric lavage if ingestion was recent, but only if an endotracheal tube is present to prevent aspiration. After emesis or lavage, administer activated charcoal with a cathartic as a single dose. Dialysis is of limited value.

Special considerations

▶ Lorazepam reduces emotional reactivity to pain. It also is used to help relax patients with chronic pain, which potentiates opioid effects. Also, drug is effective for treating postoperative muscle spasm.

▶ Lorazepam is one of the preferred benzodiazepines for patients with hepatic disease.

▶ Drug has a high risk of abuse.

▶ Give oral drug in divided doses, with the largest dose given before bedtime.

▶ For I.V. administration, dilute lorazepam with an equal volume of a compatible diluent, such as D₅W, sterile water for injection, or normal saline solution. Administer diluted lorazepam solutions immediately.

▶ Drug may be injected directly into a vein or into the tubing of a compatible I.V. infusion, such as normal saline solution or D₅W solution. Don't exceed 2 mg/minute, and keep emergency resuscitative equipment nearby.

▶ Give I.M. dose undiluted, deep into a large muscle mass.

▶ Don't use solution if it's discolored or contains a precipitate.

▶ Parenteral lorazepam appears to have potent amnestic effects.

▶ Give lowest effective dose to avoid oversedation.

▶ Periodically assess hepatic function studies to prevent cumulative effects and to ensure adequate drug metabolism.

▶ Adverse effects don't usually occur with short-term use.

▶ Intra-arterial injection may cause arteriospasm. Don't give drug by this route.

Breast-feeding patients

▶ Drug may appear in breast milk. Don't administer to breast-feeding women.

Pediatric patients

▶ Closely observe neonate for withdrawal symptoms if mother took lorazepam for a prolonged period during pregnancy.

▶ Safe use of oral lorazepam in children under age 12 hasn't been established.

▶ Safe use of S.L. or parenteral lorazepam in children under age 18 hasn't been established.

Geriatric patients

▶ Elderly patients are more sensitive to CNS depressant effects of lorazepam. They may need assistance with ambulation and activities of daily living, especially when therapy starts or dosage increases.

▶ Lower doses usually are effective in elderly patients because they have decreased elimination.

▶ Parenteral administration is more likely to cause apnea, hypotension, bradycardia, and cardiac arrest in elderly patients.

Patient teaching

▶ Advise patient of potential for physical and psychological dependence with chronic use.

▶ Caution patient not to alter drug regimen without specific instructions.

▶ Teach safety measures, as appropriate, to protect from injury, such as gradual position changes and assisted walking.

▶ Advise patient of possible retrograde amnesia after I.V. or I.M. use.

▶ Tell patient to avoid large amounts of caffeine because it may interfere with drug effectiveness.

▶ Tell patient to discontinue drug slowly over 8 to 12 weeks, as directed, after long-term therapy.

▶ **magnesium citrate (citrate of magnesia)**
Citroma, Citro-Mag◇, Citro-Nesia

▶ **magnesium hydroxide (milk of magnesia)**
Milk of Magnesia, Milk of Magnesia-Concentrated, Phillips' Milk of Magnesia

▶ **magnesium sulfate (epsom salts)**

Pharmacologic classification: *magnesium salt*

Therapeutic classification: *antacid, antiulcer drug, laxative*

Pregnancy risk category NR

How supplied
Available without a prescription
magnesium citrate
Oral solution: about 168 mg magnesium/240ml
magnesium hydroxide
Oral suspension: 7% to 8.5% (about 80 mg magnesium/30ml)
magnesium sulfate
Granules: about 40 mg magnesium/5 g

Indications and dosages
Constipation, bowel evacuation before surgery
Adults and children age 12 years and older: 11 to 25 g magnesium citrate P.O. daily as a single dose or divided; 2.4 to 4.8 g (30 to 60 ml) magnesium hydroxide P.O. daily as a single dose or divided; 10 to 30 g magnesium sulfate P.O. daily as a single dose or divided.
Children ages 6 to 12 years: 5.5 to 12.5 g magnesium citrate P.O. daily as a single dose or divided; 1.2 to 2.4 g (15 to 30 ml) magnesium hydroxide P.O. daily as a single dose or divided; 5 to 10 g magnesium sulfate P.O. daily as a single dose or divided.
Children 2 to 6 years: 2.7 to 6.25 g magnesium citrate P.O. daily as a single dose or divided; 0.4 to 1.2 g (5 to 15 ml) magnesium hydroxide P.O. daily as a single dose or divided; 2.5 to 5 g magnesium sulfate P.O. daily as a single dose or divided.
Heartburn
Adults: 5 to 15 ml milk of magnesia P.O. t.i.d. or q.i.d.

Pharmacodynamics
Antiulcer action: Magnesium hydroxide neutralizes gastric acid, decreasing the direct acid irritant effect. This increases pH, which, in turn, leads to pepsin inactivation. Magnesium hydroxide also enhances mucosal barrier integrity and improves gastric and esophageal sphincter tone.
Antacid action: Drug reacts rapidly with hydrochloric acid in the stomach to form magnesium chloride and water.
Laxative action: Drug increases the osmotic gradient in the gut and draws in water, causing distention that stimulates peristalsis and bowel evacuation.

Pharmacokinetics
Absorption: About 15% to 30% of magnesium may be absorbed systemically.
Distribution: None.
Metabolism: None.
Excretion: Unabsorbed drug is excreted in feces; absorbed drug is excreted rapidly in urine.

Reactions may be *common*, uncommon, *life-threatening*, or COMMON AND LIFE-THREATENING.

Contraindications

Contraindicated in patients with abdominal pain, nausea, vomiting, or other symptoms of appendicitis or acute surgical abdomen; in those with myocardial damage, heart block, fecal impaction, rectal fissures, intestinal obstruction or perforation, or renal disease; and in pregnant patients about to deliver.

Use cautiously in patients with rectal bleeding.

Interactions

Drug-drug

Oral drugs: absorption of these drugs may be impaired. Separate administration times.

Effects on diagnostic tests

None reported.

Adverse reactions

GI: *abdominal cramping, diarrhea;* laxative dependence with long-term or excessive use, *nausea.*
Metabolic: fluid and electrolyte disturbances with daily use.

Special considerations

▶ Before giving drug for constipation, determine if the patient has adequate fluid intake, exercise, and diet.
▶ Keep in mind that drug is for short-term therapy.
▶ Magnesium sulfate is more potent than other saline laxatives.
▶ Drug produces watery stools in 3 to 6 hours; time administration so drug doesn't interfere with scheduled activities or sleep.
▶ Chill magnesium citrate before use to make it more palatable.
▶ Shake suspension well; give with large amount of water when used as laxative. When administering

through a nasogastric tube, make sure tube is placed properly and is patent. After instilling, flush tube with water to ensure passage to stomach and maintain tube patency.
▶ Prolonged laxative use may result in dehydration and electrolyte and vitamin abnormalities.
▶ Monitor serum electrolytes as ordered during prolonged use. Magnesium may accumulate in patients with renal insufficiency.

Breast-feeding patients

▶ Some magnesium may appear in breast milk, but no problems have been reported with use by breast-feeding women.

Pediatric patients

▶ Use as an antacid in children under age 6 requires a firm diagnosis because children tend to give vague descriptions of symptoms.

Patient teaching

▶ Instruct patient on drug administration.
▶ Teach patient about dietary sources of bulk, which include bran and other cereals, fresh fruit, and vegetables.
▶ Tell patient to refrigerate magnesium citrate to retain potency and palatability.
▶ Tell patient to use only as a temporary measure.
▶ Tell patient not to use drug if cramping, gas, abdominal pain, or nausea and vomiting occur.
▶ Instruct patient to notify prescriber if bleeding or any adverse reactions occur.
▶ Warn patient that frequent or prolonged use as a laxative may cause dependence.

▶ **magnesium salicylate**
Doan's Backache Pills, Doan's Extra Strength Caplets, Doan's Regular Caplets, Doan's Regular Strength Tablets, Maximum Strength Doan's Analgesic Caplets

Pharmacologic classification: *salicylate*

Therapeutic classification: *nonnarcotic analgesic, anti-inflammatory, antipyretic*

Pregnancy risk category C

How supplied
Available by prescription only
Tablets: 545 mg, 600 mg
Available without a prescription
Tablets: 325 mg, 500 mg

Indications and dosages
Arthritis
Adults: 545 mg to 1.2 g t.i.d. or q.i.d.
Analgesia
Adults and children over age 11: 300 to 600 mg P.O. q 4 hours, p.r.n.
Analgesia (self-medicated)
Adults and children over age 11: 500 mg to 1 g P.O. initially, then 500 mg q 4 hours p.r.n., not to exceed 3.5 g in 24 hours. Absorption of buffered or enteric-coated aspirin is increased by simultaneous administration. Use with caution in children; may receive the following doses q 4 hours, p.r.n., not to exceed five doses in 24 hours.
Children age 11: 450 mg P.O. q 4 hours.
Children ages 9 to 10: 375 mg P.O. q 4 hours.
Children ages 6 to 8: 300 mg P.O. q 4 hours.

Children ages 4 to 5: 225 mg P.O. q 4 hours.
Children ages 2 to 3: 150 mg P.O. q 4 hours.
Children under age 2: must be individualized.

Pharmacodynamics
Analgesic action: Drug acts by an ill-defined effect on the hypothalamus (central action) and by blocking generation of pain impulses (peripheral action). The peripheral action may involve inhibition of prostaglandin synthesis.
Anti-inflammatory action: Drug exerts effect by inhibiting prostaglandin synthesis; it may also inhibit the synthesis or action of other mediators of inflammation.
Antipyretic action: Drug relieves fever by acting on the hypothalamic heat-regulating center to produce peripheral vasodilation. This increases peripheral blood supply and promotes sweating, which leads to loss of heat and to cooling by evaporation.

Pharmacokinetics
Absorption: Magnesium salicylate is absorbed rapidly and completely from the GI tract.
Distribution: Drug is highly protein-bound.
Metabolism: Drug is hydrolyzed in the liver.
Excretion: Metabolites are excreted in urine.

Contraindications and precautions
Contraindicated in patients with hypersensitivity to drug, salicylates, or NSAIDs or those with severe chronic renal insufficiency because of risk of magnesium toxici-

---

Reactions may be *common*, uncommon, *life-threatening*, or COMMON AND LIFE-THREATENING.

ty. Also contraindicated in patients with bleeding disorders.

Use cautiously in patients with hypoprothrombinemia or vitamin K deficiency.

Interactions
Drug-drug
Anticoagulants, thrombolytics: potentiated platelet-inhibiting effects of magnesium salicylate. Monitor therapy closely for both drugs.

Corticosteroids: enhanced magnesium salicylate elimination. Monitor patient for drug effect.

GI-irritant drugs, such as antibiotics, corticosteroids, NSAIDs: potentiated adverse GI effects of magnesium salicylate. Use together with caution.

Highly protein-bound drugs, such as phenytoin, sulfonylureas, warfarin: increased risk of adverse effects and displacement of either drug. Monitor patient closely.

Urine acidifiers, such as ammonium chloride: increased magnesium salicylate blood levels. Monitor patient for magnesium salicylate toxicity.

Urine alkalizers, such as antacids in high doses: decreased magnesium salicylate blood levels. Monitor patient for decreased salicylate effect.

Drug-food
Food: delayed and decreased absorption of magnesium salicylate. However, it's recommended to give drug with food or milk to reduce GI upset.

Effects on diagnostic tests
High doses of drug may cause false-positive urine glucose test results using copper sulfate method; it may cause false-negative urine glucose test results using glucose enzymatic method. False increases or decreases have been seen in urine vanillylmandelic acid tests; false increases in serum uric acid have been seen. Magnesium salicylate may interfere with the Gerhardt test for urine aceto-acetic acid.

Adverse reactions
EENT: *dizziness, hearing loss, tinnitus.*
GI: *GI bleeding, GI distress,* GI ulceration, *nausea, vomiting.*
Hepatic: abnormal liver function test results, **hepatitis.**
Skin: *rash,* bruising.
Other: *hypersensitivity reactions* (*anaphylaxis,* asthma), **Reye's syndrome.**

Overdose and treatment
Overdose may cause metabolic acidosis with respiratory alkalosis, hyperpnea, and tachypnea from increased carbon dioxide production and direct stimulation of the respiratory center.

To treat overdose of magnesium salicylate, empty stomach immediately by inducing emesis with ipecac syrup if patient is conscious, or by gastric lavage. Administer activated charcoal via nasogastric tube. Provide symptomatic and supportive measures, such as respiratory support and correction of fluid and electrolyte imbalances. Monitor laboratory parameters and vital signs closely. Alkaline diuresis may enhance renal excretion.

Special considerations
▶ Drug may reduce GI disturbances.

▶ Drug inhibits platelet aggregation less than other salicylates.
▶ Discontinue use if dizziness, tinnitus or hearing impairment occurs.
▶ Monitor serum salicylate levels when drug is used long-term. The therapeutic blood salicylate level in arthritis patients is 10 to 30 mg/ 100 ml. Tinnitus may occur at plasma levels of 30 mg/100 ml and above, but this isn't a reliable indicator of toxicity, especially in very young patients and those over 60 years. With chronic therapy, mild toxicity may occur at plasma levels of 20 mg/100 ml.
▶ Evaluate hemoglobin, PT, and INR periodically.
▶ Monitor serum magnesium levels to prevent magnesium toxicity, especially in patients with renal insufficiency.
▶ Drug is also used for antipyresis.

Breast-feeding patients
▶ Salicylates appear in breast milk; avoid use of magnesium salicylate in breast-feeding women.

Pediatric patients
▶ Safety of long-term magnesium salicylate use in children has not been established.
▶ Because of the connection between salicylates and Reye's syndrome, the Centers for Disease Control and Prevention recommends that children with chickenpox or flulike symptoms not receive salicylates.
▶ Febrile, dehydrated children can develop toxicity rapidly.

Geriatric patients
▶ Patients over age 60 may be more susceptible to the toxic effects of

magnesium salicylate. Use with caution.
▶ The effects of salicylates on renal prostaglandins may cause fluid retention and edema, a significant drawback for elderly patients and those with heart failure.

Patient teaching
▶ Instruct patient to follow prescribed regimen and to report problems.
▶ Advise patient not to take drug longer than 10 days without medical supervision.
▶ Caution patient to keep drug out of children's reach.
▶ Tell patient to take with food to avoid adverse GI effects.

▶ **meclofenamate**
meclofenamate

Pharmacologic classification:
NSAID

Therapeutic classification:
anti-inflammatory, antipyretic, nonnarcotic analgesic

Pregnancy risk category C (D in third trimester)

How supplied
Available by prescription only
Capsules: 50 mg, 100 mg

Indications and dosages
Rheumatoid arthritis, osteoarthritis
Adults: 200 to 400 mg/day P.O. in three or four equally divided doses.
Mild to moderate pain
Adults: 50 to 100 mg P.O. q 4 to 6 hours. Maximum, 400 mg/day.
Dysmenorrhea
Adults: 100 mg P.O. t.i.d.

Pharmacodynamics

Analgesic, antipyretic, and anti-inflammatory actions: Mechanisms of action are unknown; meclofenamate is thought to inhibit prostaglandin synthesis.

Pharmacokinetics

Absorption: Drug is absorbed rapidly and completely from the GI tract. Food decreases the rate and extent of absorption.
Distribution: Drug is more than 99% bound to plasma proteins.
Metabolism: Drug is oxidized in the liver to active and inactive metabolites.
Excretion: Drug is excreted in urine, with some biliary excretion; plasma half-life after repeated doses is about 3 hours.

Contraindications and precautions

Contraindicated in patients hypersensitive to drug or with a history of aspirin- or NSAID-induced bronchospasm, urticaria, or rhinitis. Avoid use in pregnant patients.

Use cautiously in elderly patients, smokers, alcoholics, and patients with a history of peptic ulcer disease, blood dyscrasia, and hepatic, CV, or renal disease.

Interactions
Drug-drug

ACE inhibitors, antihypertensives, beta blockers, diuretics: meclofenamate may decrease effectiveness of these drugs. Monitor patient closely.
Anticoagulants, thrombolytics: may potentiate anticoagulant effects. Monitor coagulation studies.
Anti-inflammatory drugs, corticosteroids, corticotropin, salicylates: may cause increased GI adverse

effects, including ulceration and hemorrhage. Monitor patient for abdominal pain.
Aspirin: may decrease meclofenamate bioavailability. Avoid using together.
Diuretics: may increase nephrotoxicity. Monitor renal function.
Drugs that inhibit platelet aggregation, such as aspirin, carbenicillin (parenteral), cefamandole, cefoperazone, dextran, dipyridamole, moxalocillin, piperacillin, plicamycin, salicylates, sulfinpyrazone, ticarcillin, valproic acid: may cause bleeding problems. Monitor patient for bleeding.
Highly protein-bound drugs (coumarin derivatives, nifedipine, phenytoin, verapamil): meclofenamate may displace these drugs from binding sites. Monitor patient for toxicity.
Insulin, oral antidiabetic drugs: may potentiate hypoglycemic effects. Monitor serum glucose.
Lithium, methotrexate: meclofenamate may decrease the renal clearance of these drugs. Monitor for toxicity.

Drug-lifestyle

Alcohol use: increased GI adverse effects. Advise against concurrent use.

Effects on diagnostic tests

Drug may cause false-positive test results of urine bilirubin in the diazo tablet test. Confirm suspected biliuria with other diagnostic tests, such as Harrison spot test.

Adverse reactions

CNS: confusion, dizziness, headache.
CV: edema.
EENT: tinnitus.

GI: abdominal pain, anorexia, constipation, diarrhea, flatulence, *GI bleeding,* nausea, peptic ulceration, stomatitis.
GU: impaired renal function, *renal failure.*
Hematologic: *agranulocytosis,* hemolytic anemia, *leukopenia, thrombocytopenia.*
Hepatic: altered liver function test results.
Skin: rash, urticaria.

Overdose and treatment

Overdose may cause CNS stimulation, irrational behavior, marked agitation, and generalized seizures. Renal toxicity may follow this phase of CNS stimulation.

To treat overdose, induce emesis with ipecac syrup or by gastric lavage. Administer activated charcoal via nasogastric tube. Provide symptomatic and supportive measures (respiratory support and correction of fluid and electrolyte imbalances). Appropriate therapy for seizure control with I.V. diazepam may be indicated. Monitor laboratory parameters and vital signs closely. Dialysis may prove beneficial in correcting azotemia or electrolyte abnormalities but not in removing the drug because of its protein-binding ability.

Special considerations

▶ For maximum analgesic effect, give drug before pain becomes severe.
▶ Adjust dose according to patient response.
▶ Institute safety measures to prevent injury if CNS effects occur.
▶ Check GI elimination patterns. Monitor for complaints of diarrhea.
▶ Check hydration status. Monitor for signs and symptoms of dehydration and electrolyte imbalance resulting from possible diarrhea.
▶ Meclofenamate contains sodium. Monitor patient for signs of fluid retention. Check weight and intake and output daily for significant changes. Restrict sodium intake as necessary.

Breast-feeding patients

▶ Meclofenamate is distributed in trace amounts into breast milk. Avoid use of meclofenamate in breast-feeding women.

Pediatric patients

▶ Safe long-term use of meclofenamate therapy in children under age 14 hasn't been established.

Geriatric patients

▶ Patients over age 60 may be more susceptible to the toxic effects of meclofenamate.
▶ The effects of this drug on renal prostaglandins may cause fluid retention and edema, a significant drawback for elderly patients, especially those with heart failure.

Patient teaching

▶ Instruct patient to avoid use of nonprescription medications, especially those containing aspirin and sodium. Tell patient to call before using any nonprescription medication.
▶ Reinforce signs and symptoms of possible adverse effects. Instruct patient to report them.
▶ Tell patient to record his weight two or three times weekly and to report any weight gain of 3 to 4 lb (1.4 to 1.8 kg) in 1 week.
▶ Instruct patient in diet therapy to assist with control of possible diarrhea. Reinforce need for fluids and

bland frequent meals if diarrhea occurs.

❯ Tell patient to take drug with food to avoid adverse GI side effects.

❯ Encourage patient to follow prescribed regimen and recommended schedule of follow-up. Warn women to call promptly if they become pregnant while taking meclofenamate.

❯ Caution patient that drowsiness may occur and to use care in activities requiring alertness, especially with initial exposure.

❯ Instruct patient in safety measures to prevent injury.

❯ mefenamic acid
Ponstan, Ponstel

Pharmacologic classification:
NSAID

Therapeutic classification:
anti-inflammatory, antipyretic, nonnarcotic analgesic

Pregnancy risk category C (D in third trimester)

How supplied
Available by prescription only
Capsules: 250 mg

Indications and dosages
Mild to moderate pain, dysmenor-rhea
Adults and children over age 14:
initially, 500 mg P.O. Then 250 mg q 4 hours, p.r.n. Don't exceed 1 week.

Pharmacodynamics
Analgesic, antipyretic, and anti-inflammatory actions: Unknown, although mefenamic acid is thought to inhibit prostaglandin synthesis.

Pharmacokinetics
Absorption: Drug is absorbed rapidly and completely from the GI tract.
Distribution: Mefenamic acid is highly protein-bound.
Metabolism: Drug is metabolized in the liver.
Excretion: Mefenamic acid is excreted mainly in urine, with some biliary excretion. Plasma half-life is about 2 hours.

Contraindications and precautions
Contraindicated in patients hypersensitive to drug and in patients with aspirin- or NSAID-induced asthma, urticaria, or rhinitis.

Give cautiously to patients with a history of GI disease, cardiac disease, hepatic or renal disease, blood dyscrasias, or diabetes mellitus, because it may worsen these conditions.

Interactions
Drug-drug
Acetaminophen, anti-inflammatory drugs, gold compounds: increased nephrotoxicity. Monitor renal function.
Anticoagulants, thrombolytics: may potentiate anticoagulant effects. Monitor coagulation studies.
Antihypertensives: decreased clinical effectiveness of these drugs. Monitor patient for clinical effectiveness.
Anti-inflammatory drugs, corticosteroids, corticotropin, salicylates: may cause increased GI adverse reactions, including ulceration and hemorrhage. Monitor patient for abdominal pain.
Aspirin: may decrease the bioavailability of mefenamic acid. Avoid concomitant use.

Diuretics: may increase nephrotoxicity and decrease clinical effectiveness of diuretics. Monitor renal function and patient for effectiveness.

Drugs that inhibit platelet aggregation, such as aspirin, azlocillin, carbenicillin (parenteral), cefamandole, cefoperazone, dextran, dipyridamole, mezlocillin, moxalactam, piperacillin, plicamycin, salicylates, sulfinpyrazone, ticarcillin, valproic acid: increased risk of bleeding problems. Monitor patient for bleeding tendencies.

Highly protein-bound drugs, such as coumarin derivatives, nifedipine, phenytoin, verapamil: mefenamic acid may displace these drugs from binding sites.Monitor patient for toxicity.

Insulin, oral antidiabetic drugs: potentiated hypoglycemic effects. Monitor serum glucose.

Lithium, methotrexate: mefenamic acid may decrease the renal clearance of these drugs. Monitor patient for toxic effects.

Drug-lifestyle
Alcohol use: increased risk of adverse GI reactions, including ulceration and hemorrhage. Advise against concurrent use.

Effects on diagnostic tests
Drug may cause false-positive results for urine bilirubin in the diazo tablet test. Confirm suspected biliuria with other diagnostic tests, such as Harrison spot test.

Adverse reactions
CNS: dizziness, drowsiness, headache, insomnia, nervousness, vertigo.
CV: edema.

EENT: blurred vision, eye irritation.
GI: anorexia, ***bleeding,*** *diarrhea*, flatulence, nausea, ***peptic ulceration***, vomiting.
GU: dysuria, hematuria, increased BUN, ***nephrotoxicity***.
Hematologic: ***agranulocytosis, aplastic anemia,*** decreased hematocrit, hemolytic anemia, increased PT, ***leukopenia, thrombocytopenia.***
Hepatic: elevated liver enzymes, ***hepatotoxicity***.
Metabolic: hyperkalemia.
Skin: rash, urticaria.

Overdose and treatment
Overdose may cause CNS stimulation, irrational behavior, marked agitation, and generalized seizures. Renal toxicity may follow this phase of CNS stimulation.

To treat overdose of mefenamic acid, empty stomach immediately by inducing emesis with ipecac syrup or by gastric lavage. Administer activated charcoal via nasogastric tube. Provide symptomatic and supportive measures (respiratory support and correction of fluid and electrolyte imbalances). Appropriate therapy for seizure control with I.V. diazepam may be indicated. Monitor laboratory parameters and vital signs closely. Mefenamic acid is not dialyzable.

Special considerations
▶ Patients with aspirin hypersensitivity, asthma, and rhinitis or nasal polyps have a high risk of bronchospasm.
▶ Stop drug if patient develops hypersensitivity, rash, or diarrhea.
▶ To maximize analgesic effect, give drug before pain is severe.

Reactions may be *common*, uncommon, *life-threatening*, or COMMON AND LIFE-THREATENING.

▌ Adjust dosage according to patient response.

▌ For acute pain, don't use drug longer than 1 week to avoid adverse effects of prolonged use.

▌ Serious GI toxicity, especially ulceration or hemorrhage, can occur at any time with NSAID use, especially in patients on long-term therapy.

▌ Institute safety measures to prevent injury that may occur because of CNS effects.

▌ Monitor GI elimination patterns for complaints of diarrhea.

▌ Assess patient for evidence of fluid retention, dehydration, or electrolyte imbalance. Check weight frequently for significant changes.

▌ NSAIDs may mask evidence of acute infection, such as fever, myalgia, erythema; carefully evaluate high-risk patients, such as diabetics.

▌ Insulin-dependent diabetic patients on mefenamic acid may have increased insulin requirements. Monitor serum glucose levels frequently.

Breast-feeding patients
▌ Mefenamic acid appears in breast milk; avoid use in breast-feeding women.

Pediatric patients
▌ Don't use mefenamic acid for long-term therapy in children under age 14; safety for this use hasn't been established.

Geriatric patients
▌ Patients over age 60 may be more susceptible to the toxic effects.
▌ The effects of this drug on renal prostaglandins may cause fluid retention and edema, a significant drawback for elderly patients and those with heart failure.

▌ Elderly patients are more likely to develop severe diarrhea than younger patients.

Patient teaching
▌ Tell patient to consult prescriber before taking any OTC medication.

▌ Review signs and symptoms of possible adverse effects. Instruct patient to call if any occur.

▌ Advise patient to record his weight two or three times weekly and to report any weight gain of 3 pounds or more within 1 week.

▌ Teach patient dietary measures to control possible diarrhea.

▌ Tell patient to take drug with food to avoid adverse GI effects.

▌ Advise patient of need for medical follow-up while taking mefenamic acid.

▌ Caution patient to avoid hazardous activities until full effects of drug are known.

▌ meperidine hydrochloride (pethidine hydrochloride)
Demerol

Pharmacologic classification:
opioid

Therapeutic classification:
analgesic, adjunct to anesthesia

Controlled substance schedule II

Pregnancy risk category C

How supplied
Available by prescription only
Injection: 10 mg/ml, 25 mg/ml, 50 mg/ml, 75 mg/ml, 100 mg/ml

Liquid: 50 mg/5 ml
Tablets: 50 mg, 100 mg

Indications and dosages
Moderate to severe pain
Adults: 50 to 150 mg P.O., I.M., I.V., or S.C. q 3 to 4 hours.
Children: 1 to 1.8 mg/kg P.O., I.M., I.V., or S.C. q 3 to 4 hours or 175 mg/m^2 daily in six divided doses. Maximum, 100 mg/dose.
Preoperative analgesia
Adults: 50 to 100 mg I.M., I.V., or S.C. 30 to 90 minutes before surgery.
Children: 1 to 2 mg/kg I.M., I.V., or S.C. 30 to 90 minutes before surgery. Don't exceed adult dose.
Support of anesthesia
Adults: Repeated slow I.V. injections of fractional doses (10 mg/ml) or continuous I.V. infusion of 1 mg/ml. Adjust dosage to meet patient's needs.
Obstetric analgesia
Adults: 50 to 100 mg I.M. or S.C. when pain becomes regular; may repeat q 1 to 3 hours.

Pharmacodynamics
Analgesic action: Drug is a narcotic agonist with actions and potency similar to those of morphine. Main action is at opiate receptors.

Pharmacokinetics
Absorption: Analgesia begins within 45 minutes and lasts 2 to 4 hours.
Distribution: Drug is distributed widely throughout the body and is 60% to 80% bound to plasma proteins.
Metabolism: Drug is metabolized primarily by hydrolysis in the liver to an active metabolite, normeperidine.

Excretion: About 30% of dose is excreted in urine as N-demethylated derivative; about 5% is excreted unchanged. Excretion is enhanced by acidifying the urine. Half-life of parent compound is 3 to 5 hours; half-life of metabolite is 8 to 21 hours.

Contraindications and precautions
Contraindicated in patients hypersensitive to drug and in patients who took an MAO inhibitor within 14 days.

Use cautiously in elderly or debilitated patients and in those with increased intracranial pressure, head injury, asthma, other respiratory conditions, supraventricular tachycardia, seizures, acute abdominal conditions, renal or hepatic disease, hypothyroidism, Addison's disease, urethral stricture, or prostatic hyperplasia.

Interactions
Drug-drug
Anticholinergics: may cause paralytic ileus. Monitor patient for abdominal pain.
Cimetidine: increased respiratory and CNS depression, causing confusion, disorientation, apnea, or seizures. Reduce meperidine dosage.
CNS depressants, such as antihistamines, barbiturates, benzodiazepines, general anesthetics, muscle relaxants, opioid analgesics, phenothiazines, sedative-hypnotics, tricyclic antidepressants: potentiated respiratory and CNS depression, sedation, and hypotensive effects. Use together with caution.

General anesthetics: severe CV depression. Use together cautiously.

Isoniazid: potentiated adverse effects of isoniazid. Monitor patient closely.

MAO inhibitors: may cause unpredictable and occasionally fatal reactions. Don't use together or within 14 days of each other.

Narcotic antagonists: acute withdrawal syndrome in patients physically dependent on drug. Avoid using together.

Drug-herb
Parsley: may promote or produce serotonin syndrome. Advise against concurrent use.

Drug-lifestyle
Alcohol use: potentiated respiratory and CNS depression, sedation, and hypotensive effects. Avoid concomitant use.

Effects on diagnostic tests
Drug increases plasma amylase or lipase levels through increased biliary tract pressure; levels may be unreliable for 24 hours after meperidine administration.

Adverse reactions
CNS: *clouded sensorium, dizziness, euphoria,* hallucinations, headache, *light-headedness,* paradoxical excitement, *sedation,* **seizures** with large doses, *somnolence,* syncope, tremor.
CV: **bradycardia, cardiac arrest,** *hypotension,* **shock,** tachycardia.
GI: biliary tract spasms, *constipation,* dry mouth, ileus, *nausea, vomiting.*
GU: *urine retention.*
Respiratory: *respiratory arrest, respiratory depression.*

Musculoskeletal: muscle twitching.
Skin: *diaphoresis,* pruritus, urticaria.
Other: induration after S.C. injection, local tissue irritation, pain at injection site, phlebitis after I.V. delivery, physical dependence.

Overdose and treatment
Overdose typically causes CNS depression, respiratory depression, skeletal muscle flaccidity, cold and clammy skin, mydriasis, bradycardia, and hypotension. Other acute toxic effects include hypothermia, shock, apnea, cardiopulmonary arrest, circulatory collapse, pulmonary edema, and seizures.

To treat acute overdose, first establish adequate respiration via a patent airway and ventilate as needed; administer a narcotic antagonist (naloxone) to reverse respiratory depression. (Because the duration of action of meperidine is longer than that of naloxone, repeated dosing is necessary.) Naloxone shouldn't be given unless the patient has clinically significant respiratory or CV depression. Monitor vital signs.

If patient presents within 2 hours of ingestion of an oral overdose, empty the stomach immediately by inducing emesis (ipecac syrup) or using gastric lavage. Use caution to avoid risk of aspiration. Administer activated charcoal via nasogastric tube for further removal of meperidine, and acidify urine to help remove drug.

Provide symptomatic and supportive treatment (continued respiratory support, correction of fluid and electrolyte imbalance). Monitor laboratory values, vital signs, and neurologic status close-ly.

Special considerations
▶ Oral dose is less than half as effective as parenteral dose. Give I.M. if possible. When changing from parenteral to oral route, dosage should be made based on conversion charts.
▶ Alternating meperidine with a peripherally active nonopioid analgesic (aspirin, acetaminophen, NSAIDs) may improve pain control while allowing lower opioid dosages.
▶ Because drug toxicity commonly appears after several days of treatment, this drug isn't recommended for treatment of chronic pain.
▶ High doses increase seizure potential due to excessive CNS stimulation.
▶ Drug may be administered to some patients who are allergic to morphine.
▶ Syrup has local anesthetic effect. Give with water.
▶ Question patient carefully regarding possible use of MAO inhibitors within the past 14 days.
▶ Monitor respiratory and CV function. Do not give if respirations are below 12 breaths/minute, if respiratory rate or depth is decreased, or if change in pupils is noted.
▶ Monitor bowel and bladder function.
▶ Meperidine and its active metabolite normeperidine accumulate. Monitor the patient for neurotoxic effects, especially in burn patients and those with poor renal function, sickle cell anemia, or cancer.

▶ During I.V. administration, tachycardia may occur, possibly as a result of drug's atropine-like effects.
▶ S.C. injection is very painful.
▶ Give slowly by direct I.V. injection; meperidine may also be given by slow continuous I.V. infusion, preferably as a diluted solution. Drug is compatible with most I.V. solutions, including D_5W, normal saline, and Ringer's or lactated Ringer's solutions.
▶ Keep narcotic antagonist (naloxone) available when giving this drug I.V.

Breast-feeding patients
▶ Drug appears in breast milk; use with caution in breast-feeding women.

Pediatric patients
▶ Drug shouldn't be administered to infants under age 6 months.

Geriatric patients
▶ Lower doses are usually indicated for elderly patients, because they may be more sensitive to the therapeutic and adverse effects of drug.

Patient teaching
▶ Caution patient to avoid hazardous activities until full CNS effects of drug are known.
▶ Tell patient to avoid alcohol during therapy.

▌ mepivacaine hydrochloride
Carbocaine, Polocaine, Polocaine MPF

Pharmacologic classification:
amide

Therapeutic classification:
local anesthetic

Pregnancy risk category C

How supplied:
Injection: 1%, 1.5%, 2%, 3%

Indications and dosages
Infiltration anesthesia
Adults: 40 ml of 1% solution or 80 ml of 0.5% solution (400 mg).
Cervical, brachial, intercostal or pudendal nerve block
Adults: 5 to 40 ml of 1% solution (50 to 400 mg) or 5 to 20 ml of 2% solution (100 to 400 mg). For pudendal block, inject half the total dose on each side.
Combined paracervical and pudendal block
Adults: up to 15 ml of 1% solution (150 mg) transvaginally injected on each side.
Paracervical block
Adults: up to 10 ml of 1% solution (100 mg) injected slowly on each side every 90 minutes. Wait 5 minutes between sides.
Therapeutic nerve block to manage pain
Adults: 1 to 5 ml of 1% or 2% solution (10 to 100 mg).
Caudal epidural block
Adults: initially, 5 ml as a test dose. After 5 minutes, give total dose: 15 to 30 ml of 1% solution (150 to 300 mg) or 10 to 25 ml of 1.5% solution (150 to 375 mg) or

10 to 20 ml of 2% solution (200 to 400 mg).
Dental infiltration, nerve block procedures
Adults: 1.8 ml (36 mg) of 2% solution that also contains levonordefrin or 1.8 ml (54 mg) of 3% solution injected slowly with frequent aspiration. Maximum, 3 mg/kg, up to 400 mg.
Children: maximum dose is child's weight in pounds divided by 150 and multiplied by 400 mg.
◼ DOSAGE ADJUSTMENT. Reduce dosage in children, elderly patients, and debilitated or acutely ill patients.

Pharmacodynamics
Nerve blocking action: Blocks nerve conduction near the site of injection by decreasing the permeability of nerve cell membranes to sodium ions, thus decreasing the rate of depolarization of the nerve membrane, increasing the threshold for electrical excitability, and preventing propagation of the action potential.

Pharmacokinetics
Absorption: In epidural block, onset of 2% solution is 7 to 15 minutes; for dental anesthesia, onset is ½ to 2 minutes in the upper jaw and 1 to 4 minutes in the lower jaw.
Distribution: 60% to 85% bound to plasma proteins; 50% of dose is distributed into bile.
Metabolism: Mainly metabolized in the liver; up to 5% of dose metabolized to carbon dioxide.
Excretion: In epidural block, duration of anesthesia for 2% solution is 115 to 150 minutes; in caudal block, duration of anesthesia for 1% to 2% solution is 105 to 170

minutes; for dental anesthesia, duration of anesthesia for 3% solution is 10 to 100 minutes. Drug is excreted via the lungs, urine, and feces.

Contraindications and precautions
Contraindicated in patients hypersensitive to mepivacaine or other drugs of the amide type. Don't use in patients with myasthenia gravis, severe shock, or impaired cardiac conduction. Epidural route is contraindicated in patients with meningitis, spinal fluid block, cranial or spinal hemorrhage, tumors, poliomyelitis, syphilis, tuberculosis, or metastatic spinal cord lesions.

Use cautiously in severely debilitated patients and in patients with cardiac disease, hyperthyroidism and other endocrine diseases, and liver disease. Use cautiously in patients with skin infections.

Interactions
None reported.

Effects on diagnostic tests
None reported.

Adverse reactions
CNS: anxiety, apprehension, confusion, disorientation, dizziness, drowsiness, nervousness, restlessness, *seizures,* shivering, tremors, twitching, unconsciousness.
CV: *arrhythmias, bradycardia, cardiac arrest, CV collapse,* hypotension.
EENT: blurred vision, miosis, tinnitus.
GI: nausea, vomiting.
Respiratory: *respiratory arrest.*

Other: chills, transient burning at injection site.

Overdose and treatment
Overdose may cause CNS and CV effects. Treatment is supportive and symptomatic.

Special considerations
▶ Adverse reactions usually occur from high plasma levels of drug.
▶ Drug should be used only by clinicians knowledgeable in diagnosing and managing dose-related toxicity and other emergencies that may result from local anesthetics. Keep resuscitative equipment and drugs readily available.
▶ Use smallest dose and concentration needed for desired effect.
▶ Watch closely for adverse reactions, which may indicate high plasma drug levels.
▶ Prepare 0.5% solution by diluting 1% solution with normal saline solution.
▶ Solutions of 1%, 1.5%, or 2% containing no preservatives may be used in epidural or caudal anesthesia.
▶ Inject slowly and with frequent aspiration to avoid intravascular injection.
▶ During epidural use, monitor patient closely for signs of inadvertent intravascular or subarachnoid injection, such as motor paralysis and extensive sensory anesthesia.
▶ Some forms of drug may contain sulfites, which may cause allergic reactions in susceptible patients.

Breast-feeding patients
▶ No data exist to demonstrate whether drug appears in breast milk. Safety hasn't been established.

Pediatric patients
▶ Reduce dosage in children.
▶ Use solutions under 2% concentration for children younger than age 3 or who weigh less than 14 kg (30 lb),

Geriatric patients
▶ Reduce dosage in elderly patients.

Patient teaching
▶ Advise patient that anesthetized part of body may temporarily lose sensation and motor activity.

▶ meprobamate
Apo-Meprobamate◇, Equanil, Meprospan, Miltown, Neuramate

Pharmacologic classification: *carbamate*

Therapeutic classification: *antianxiety drug*

Controlled substance schedule IV

Pregnancy risk category D

How supplied
Available by prescription only
Tablets: 200 mg, 400 mg, 600 mg
Capsules (sustained-release): 200 mg, 400 mg

Indications and dosages
Anxiety and tension
Adults: 1.2 to 1.6 g P.O. daily in three or four equally divided doses. Maximum, 2.4 g/day. For sustained-release capsules, 400 to 800 mg b.i.d.
Children ages 6 to 12: 100 to 200 mg P.O. b.i.d. or t.i.d. For sustained-release capsules, 200 mg b.i.d.

Pharmacodynamics
Anxiolytic action: Although cellular mechanism is unknown, drug causes nonselective CNS depression similar to that of barbiturates. It acts at multiple CNS sites, including the thalamus, hypothalamus, limbic system, and spinal cord, but not the medulla or reticular activating system.

Pharmacokinetics
Absorption: After oral administration, drug is well absorbed; serum levels peak in 1 to 3 hours. Sedation usually occurs within 1 hour.
Distribution: Meprobamate is distributed throughout the body; 20% is protein-bound. Drug is excreted in breast milk at two to four times the serum level; it also crosses the placenta.
Metabolism: Drug is metabolized rapidly in the liver to inactive glucuronide conjugates. Half-life is 6 to 17 hours.
Excretion: Metabolites of drug and 10% to 20% of a single dose as unchanged drug are excreted in urine.

Contraindications and precautions
Contraindicated in patients hypersensitive to meprobamate or related compounds (such as carbromal, carisoprodol, mebutamate, tybamate) and in those with porphyria. Avoid use of drug during first trimester of pregnancy.

Use cautiously in elderly or debilitated patients and in those with impaired renal or hepatic function, seizure disorders, or suicidal tendencies.

Interactions
Drug-drug
CNS depressants, such as antihistamines, barbiturates, narcotics, tranquilizers: potentiated CNS depressant effects. Monitor patient closely.

Drug-lifestyle
Alcohol use: potentiated effects of alcohol. Advise against concurrent use.

Effects on diagnostic tests
Drug therapy may falsely elevate urine 17-ketosteroids, 17-ketogenic steroids (as determined by the Zimmerman reaction), and 17-hydroxycorticosteroid levels (as determined by the Glenn-Nelson technique).

Adverse reactions
CNS: ataxia, dizziness, *drowsiness,* headache, **seizures,** slurred speech, syncope, vertigo.
CV: *arrhythmias,* hypotension, palpitations, tachycardia.
GI: diarrhea, nausea, vomiting.
Hematologic: *agranulocytosis, aplastic anemia, thrombocytopenia.*
Skin: erythematous maculopapular rash, *hypersensitivity reactions,* pruritus, urticaria.

Overdose and treatment
Overdose may cause drowsiness, lethargy, ataxia, coma, hypotension, shock, and respiratory depression.

Treatment of overdose is supportive and symptomatic, including maintaining adequate ventilation and a patent airway, with mechanical ventilation, if needed.

Treat hypotension with fluids and vasopressors as needed. Empty gastric contents by emesis or lavage if ingestion was recent, followed by activated charcoal and a cathartic. Treat seizures with parenteral diazepam. Peritoneal dialysis and hemodialysis may effectively remove drug. Serum levels above 100 mcg/ml may be fatal.

Special considerations
▶ Reduced anxiety allows pain medications to be more effective.
▶ Provide a calm environment for the patient, if possible.
▶ Take safety precautions, especially for elderly patients and especially when treatment starts or dosage increases. Raise side rails, as needed, and provide assistance with walking.
▶ Drug abuse and addiction may occur.
▶ Assess level of consciousness and vital signs frequently.
▶ Periodic evaluation of CBC is recommended during long-term therapy.
▶ Withdraw drug gradually. Abrupt withdrawal after long-term therapy may cause severe generalized tonic-clonic seizures.

Breast-feeding patients
▶ Drug appears in breast milk at two to four times the serum level. Do not use in breast-feeding women.

Pediatric patients
▶ Safety hasn't been established in children under age 6.

Geriatric patients
▶ Elderly patients may have more pronounced CNS effects. Use lowest dose possible.

Patient teaching
▶ Inform patient about risk of physical or psychological dependence with long-term use.
▶ Advise patient not to increase dose or frequency and not to abruptly discontinue drug or decrease dose unless prescribed.
▶ Tell patient to avoid alcohol and other CNS depressants, such as antihistamines, narcotics, and tranquilizers, while taking drug, unless prescribed.
▶ Caution patient to avoid hazardous activities until full CNS effects of drug are known.
▶ Recommend ice chips or sugarless candy or gum to relieve dry mouth.
▶ Urge patient to notify prescriber about sore throat, fever, or unusual bleeding or bruising.

▶ methadone hydrochloride
Dolophine, Methadose

Pharmacologic classification: *opioid*

Therapeutic classification: *analgesic, narcotic detoxification adjunct*

Controlled substance schedule II

Pregnancy risk category C

How supplied
Available by prescription only
Injection: 10 mg/ml
Oral solution: 5 mg/5 ml, 10 mg/5 ml, 10 mg/ml (concentrate)
Tablets: 5 mg, 10 mg, 40 mg for oral solution (for narcotic abstinence syndrome)

Indications and dosages
Severe pain
Adults: 2.5 to 10 mg P.O., I.M., or S.C. q 3 to 4 hours, p.r.n. or around-the-clock.
Narcotic abstinence syndrome
Adults: individualized at 15 to 20 mg/day P.O. Maintenance, 20 to 120 mg/day P.O. Adjust dosage as needed. Amounts above 120 mg/day require state and federal approval. If patient feels nauseated, give 25% of total P.O. dose in two injections, S.C. or I.M.

Pharmacodynamics
Analgesic action: Methadone is an opiate agonist; analgesic activity results from its affinity for opiate receptors—an action similar to that of morphine.

Pharmacokinetics
Absorption: Methadone is well absorbed from the GI tract. Oral administration delays onset and prolongs duration of action as compared to parenteral administration. Onset of action occurs within 30 to 60 minutes; peak effect is seen at 1½ to 2 hours.
Distribution: Drug is highly bound to tissue protein, which may explain its cumulative effects and slow elimination.
Metabolism: Methadone is metabolized primarily in the liver by N-demethylation.
Excretion: Duration of action is 4 to 6 hours after I.V. administration and 22 to 48 hours after repeated oral administration. Half-life is prolonged (7 to 11 hours) in patients with hepatic dysfunction. Urine excretion, the major route, is dose-dependent. Metabolites are also excreted in feces via bile.

Contraindications and precautions

Contraindicated in patients hypersensitive to drug.

Use cautiously in elderly or debilitated patients and in those with severe renal or hepatic impairment, acute abdominal conditions, hypothyroidism, Addison's disease, prostatic hyperplasia, urethral stricture, head injury, increased intracranial pressure, asthma, or other respiratory disorders.

Interactions

Drug-drug

Cimetidine: may increase respiratory and CNS depression, causing confusion, disorientation, apnea, or seizures. Reduce methadone dosage.

CNS depressants, such as antidepressants, antihistamines, barbiturates, benzodiazepines, general anesthetics, muscle relaxants, opioid analgesics, phenothiazines, sedative-hypnotics: potentiated respiratory and CNS depression, sedation, and hypotensive effects. Use together cautiously.

Opioid antagonists: acute withdrawal syndrome in patients physically dependent on drug. Use with caution. Monitor patient closely.

Rifampin: decreased methadone level. Monitor patient closely.

Drug-lifestyle

Alcohol use: potentiated respiratory and CNS depression, sedation, and hypotensive effects. Advise against concurrent use.

Effects on diagnostic tests

None reported.

Adverse reactions

CNS: agitation, *choreic movements, clouded sensorium, dizziness, euphoria,* headache, insomnia, *light-headedness, sedation, seizures* with large doses, *somnolence,* syncope.

CV: *bradycardia, cardiac arrest,* edema, *hypotension,* palpitations, ***shock.***

EENT: visual disturbances.

GI: *anorexia, biliary tract spasm, constipation, dry mouth, ileus,* increased serum amylase, *nausea, vomiting.*

GU: *decreased libido, urine retention.*

Respiratory: *respiratory arrest, respiratory depression.*

Skin: *diaphoresis,* pruritus, urticaria.

Other: pain at injection site, induration after S.C. injection, physical dependence, tissue irritation.

Overdose and treatment

Overdose typically causes CNS depression, respiratory depression, and miosis (pinpoint pupils). It also may cause hypotension, bradycardia, hypothermia, shock, apnea, cardiopulmonary arrest, circulatory collapse, pulmonary edema, and seizures. Toxicity may result from accumulation of drug over several weeks.

To treat acute overdose, establish adequate respiratory exchange. If patient has significant respiratory or CV depression, give an opioid antagonist (naloxone). Because methadone has a longer duration of action than naloxone, repeated naloxone doses will be needed. Monitor vital signs closely.

If oral ingestion occurred within 2 hours, induce emesis with ipecac syrup or perform gastric lavage.

Use caution to avoid risk of aspiration. Administer activated charcoal via nasogastric tube for further removal of drug in an oral overdose.

Provide symptomatic and supportive treatment, including continued respiratory support and correction of fluid or electrolyte imbalance. Monitor laboratory values, vital signs, and neurologic status closely.

Special considerations
▶ Drug is recommended for severe, chronic pain and for detoxification and maintenance of patients with opiate abstinence syndrome.
▶ Regimented, around-the-clock dosing is beneficial in severe, chronic pain. Tolerance may develop with long-term use, requiring a higher dose to achieve the same degree of analgesia.
▶ Dilute to a maximum of 10 mg/ml using normal saline solution. Give slowly by direct injection. Or dilute to 1 mg/ml and give as a slow I.V. infusion (15 to 35 mg/hour).
▶ Dispersible tablets may be dissolved in 4 oz (120 ml) of water or fruit juice; oral concentrate must be diluted to at least 3 oz (90 ml) with water before administration.
▶ Oral liquid form (not tablets) is legally required and is the only form available in drug maintenance programs.
▶ Oral dose is half as potent as injected dose.
▶ Patient treated for narcotic abstinence syndrome will usually require an additional analgesic if she needs pain control.
▶ Monitor patient closely because drug has a cumulative effect, and marked sedation can occur after repeated doses.
▶ Drug has a longer duration of action than morphine sulfate.
▶ Monitor circulatory and respiratory status and bowel and bladder function.
▶ Physical and psychological tolerance or dependence may occur. Be aware of potential for abuse. Do not abruptly discontinue use.
▶ Drug is effective for sickle cell crisis.
▶ Respiratory depression, hypotension, profound sedation, or coma may occur if drug is used with general anesthetics, tranquilizers, sedatives, hypnotics, alcohol, tricyclic antidepressants, or MAO inhibitors. Use together with extreme caution. Monitor patient's response.

Breast-feeding patients
▶ Methadone appears in breast milk; it may cause physical dependence in breast-feeding infants of women on methadone maintenance therapy.

Pediatric patients
▶ Drug isn't recommended for use in children.
▶ Safe use in adolescents hasn't been established.

Geriatric patients
▶ Elderly patients usually receive lower dosages because they may be more sensitive to drug effects.

Patient teaching
▶ If appropriate, tell patient that constipation is often severe during maintenance with methadone. Instruct her to use a stool softener or laxative.

▶ Caution patient to avoid hazardous activities because drug may cause drowsiness.

▶ methocarbamol
Robaxin

Pharmacologic classification:
carbamate derivative of guaifenesin

Therapeutic classification:
skeletal muscle relaxant

Pregnancy risk category C

How supplied
Available by prescription only
Tablets: 500 mg, 750 mg
Injection: 100 mg/ml parenteral in 10 ml vial

Indications and dosages
Adjunct in acute, painful musculoskeletal conditions
Adults: 1.5 g P.O. q.i.d. for 2 to 3 days. Maintenance, 4 to 4.5 g P.O. daily in three to six divided doses. Alternatively, 1 g I.M. or I.V. Maximum, 3 g daily I.M. or I.V. for 3 consecutive days.

Pharmacodynamics
Skeletal muscle relaxant action: Drug doesn't relax skeletal muscle directly. Its effects appear to be related to its sedative action; however, the exact mechanism of action is unknown.

Pharmacokinetics
Absorption: Drug is rapidly and completely absorbed from the GI tract. Action begins within 30 minutes after a single oral dose; it begins immediately after a single I.V. dose.

Distribution: Methocarbamol is widely distributed throughout the body.
Metabolism: Drug is extensively metabolized in the liver via dealkylation and hydroxylation. Half-life is 1 to 2 hours.
Excretion: Drug is rapidly and almost completely excreted in urine, mainly as its glucuronide and sulfate metabolites (40% to 50%), as unchanged drug (10% to 15%), and the remainder as unidentified metabolites.

Contraindications and precautions
Contraindicated in patients with hypersensitivity to drug, impaired renal function (injectable form), or seizure disorder (injectable form).

Interactions
Drug-drug
Anticholinesterase drugs: patients with myasthenia gravis may experience severe weakness if given methocarbamol. Monitor patient very closely.
CNS depressants, including anxiolytics, narcotics, psychotics, tricyclic antidepressants: may cause additive CNS depression. When used with other depressants, exercise care to avoid overdose.

Drug-lifestyle
Alcohol use: additive CNS depression. Advise against concurrent use.

Effects on diagnostic tests
Methocarbamol therapy causes false-positive results on tests for urine 5-hydroxyindoleacetic acid using quantitative method of Udenfriend. It also causes false-positive restuls for urine vanillyl-

mandelic acid in the Gitlow screening test. It causes no problem with the quantitative method of Sunderman.

Adverse reactions

CNS: confusion, dizziness, drowsiness, headache, light-headedness, mild muscular incoordination (I.M. or I.V.), *seizures* (I.V. only), syncope, vertigo.
CV: *bradycardia* (I.M. or I.V.), flushing, hypotension, thrombophlebitis.
EENT: blurred vision, conjunctivitis, diplopia, nystagmus.
GI: GI upset, metallic taste, nausea.
GU: discoloration of urine, hematuria (I.V. only).
Skin: pruritus, rash, urticaria.
Other: *anaphylactic reactions* (I.M. or I.V.), extravasation (I.V. only), fever.

Overdose and treatment

Overdose may cause extreme drowsiness, nausea and vomiting, and arrhythmias.

Treatment includes symptomatic and supportive measures. If ingestion was recent, induce emesis or perform gastric lavage. Maintain adequate airway, monitor urine output and vital signs, and give I.V. fluids if needed.

Special considerations

▶ Don't give drug by S.C. route.
▶ For I.M. use, don't give more than 500 mg in each gluteal region.
▶ For I.V. use, dilute 10 ml of drug in no more than 250 ml of solution. Use D_5W or normal saline solution for injection. Infuse slowly; maximum rate is 300 mg (3 ml)/minute.

▶ Patient should be supine during and for at least 15 minutes after I.V. injection.
▶ Drug may irritate veins, cause phlebitis, aggravate seizures, and cause fainting if injected rapidly.
▶ Drug is an irritant. Extravasation may cause thrombophlebitis and sloughing from hypertonic solution.
▶ Assist patient with walking after parenteral administration.
▶ Provide a safe environment; allow periods of rest.
▶ Monitor patient for orthostatic hypotension, especially with parenteral administration.
▶ Oral administration should replace parenteral use as soon as feasible.
▶ Adverse reactions after oral administration are usually mild and transient and subside with dosage reduction.
▶ To give drug via nasogastric tube, crush tablets and suspend in water or normal saline solution.
▶ If left standing, patient's urine may turn black, blue, brown, or green.
▶ Watch for sensitivity reactions, such as fever and skin eruptions.
▶ Drug is also used as supportive therapy in tetanus management. When used for tetanus, follow manufacturer's instructions.

Pregnant patients

▶ Safe use of methocarbamol hasn't been established during pregnancy. Drug shouldn't be used in women who are or may become pregnant, especially during early pregnancy, unless the benefits outweigh the possible hazards.

Breast-feeding patients
▶ Small amounts of drug appear in breast milk. Patient shouldn't breast-feed during treatment with methocarbamol.

Pediatric patients
▶ Use only for tetanus in children under age 12.

Geriatric patients
▶ Lower doses are indicated because elderly patients are more sensitive to drug effects.

Patient teaching
▶ Advise patient to change positions slowly, particularly from recumbent to upright, and to dangle legs before standing.
▶ Tell patient that urine may turn black, blue, green, or brown.
▶ Caution patient to avoid hazardous activities until full CNS effects of drug are known. Drug may cause drowsiness.
▶ Advise patient to avoid alcohol, including alcohol contained in OTC cold and cough preparations.
▶ Tell patient to store drug away from heat and light (not in bathroom medicine cabinet) and safely out of reach of children.
▶ Tell patient to take a missed dose as soon as she remembers it if within 1 hour of scheduled time. After 1 hour, patient should skip dose and resume regular schedule. Warn against doubling the dose.

▶ methotrexate, methotrexate sodium
Folex, Mexate, Mexate-AQ, Rheumatrex Dose Pack

Pharmacologic classification: *antimetabolite (specific to S phase of cell cycle)*

Therapeutic classification: *antineoplastic*

Pregnancy risk category X

How supplied
Available by prescription only
Injection: 20 mg, 25 mg, 50 mg, 100 mg, 250 mg, 1 g vials, lyophilized powder, preservative-free; 25 mg/ml vials, preservative-free solution; 2.5 mg/ml, 25 mg/ml vials, lyophilized powder, preserved
Tablets (scored): 2.5 mg

Indications and dosages
Severe, refractory rheumatoid arthritis
Adults: 7.5 to 15 mg weekly P.O. in single or divided doses.

Pharmacodynamics
Antineoplastic action: Methotrexate exerts cytotoxic effects by tightly binding with dihydrofolic acid reductase, an enzyme crucial to purine metabolism. As a result, it inhibits DNA, RNA, and protein synthesis.

Pharmacokinetics
Absorption: Absorption across the GI tract appears to be dose related. Lower doses are essentially completely absorbed, while absorption of larger doses is incomplete and variable. I.M. doses are absorbed

completely. Serum levels peak 30 minutes to 2 hours after an I.M. dose and 1 to 4 hours after an oral dose.

Distribution: Methotrexate is distributed widely throughout the body, with the highest levels found in the kidneys, gallbladder, spleen, liver, and skin. Drug crosses the blood-brain barrier but doesn't achieve therapeutic levels in the CSF. About 50% of the drug is bound to plasma protein.

Metabolism: Drug is metabolized only slightly in the liver.

Excretion: Drug is excreted primarily into urine as unchanged drug. Elimination has been described as biphasic, with a first phase half-life of 45 minutes and a terminal phase half-life of 4 hours.

Contraindications and precautions

Contraindicated in patients hypersensitive to drug and during pregnancy or breast-feeding. Also contraindicated in patients with psoriasis or rheumatoid arthritis who also have alcoholism, alcoholic liver, chronic liver disease, immunodeficiency syndrome, or blood dyscrasia.

Use cautiously in very young, elderly, or debilitated patients and in those with impaired renal or hepatic function, bone marrow suppression, aplasia, leukopenia, thrombocytopenia, anemia, folate deficiency, infection, peptic ulcer, or ulcerative colitis. Drug exits slowly from third space compartments, resulting in a prolonged terminal plasma half-life and risk of toxicity.

Interactions
Drug-drug

Folic acid: may decrease methotrexate effectiveness. Monitor patient for drug effects.

Immunizations: may not be effective when given during methotrexate therapy. Because of the risk of disseminated infections, live virus vaccines are generally not recommended during therapy.

NSAIDs, salicylates, sulfonamides, sulfonylureas: may increase therapeutic and toxic effects of methotrexate by displacing it from plasma proteins, increasing the levels of free methotrexate. Concurrent use of these drugs with methotrexate should be avoided if possible.

Oral antibiotics, such as chloramphenicol, nonabsorbable broad-spectrum antibiotics, tetracycline: may decrease methotrexate absorption. Monitor patient closely.

Phenytoin: serum phenytoin levels may be decreased by chemotherapeutic regimens that employ methotrexate, increasing the risk of seizures. Monitor phenytoin levels.

Probenecid, salicylates: increased therapeutic and toxic effects of methotrexate by inhibiting the renal tubular secretion of methotrexate. Combined use of these drugs requires a lower methotrexate dosage.

Pyrimethamine: drugs show similar pharmacologic action. Avoid concomitant use.

Drug-lifestyle

Sun exposure: increased risk of photosensitivity. Urge precautions.

Effects on diagnostic tests

Methotrexate may alter results of the laboratory assay for folate by inhibiting the organism used in the assay, thus interfering with the detection of folic acid deficiency.

Adverse reactions

CNS: *arachnoiditis* within hours of intrathecal use, dizziness, drowsiness, fatigue, headache, malaise, *necrotizing demyelinating leukoencephalopathy* (may occur a few years later), *seizures*, subacute *neurotoxicity* (may begin a few weeks later).

EENT: blurred vision, gingivitis, pharyngitis.

GI: abdominal distress, anorexia, diarrhea, enteritis, *GI ulceration and bleeding*, nausea, stomatitis, *vomiting.*

GU: cystitis, defective spermatogenesis, hematuria, menstrual dysfunction, nephropathy, *renal failure, tubular necrosis.*

Hematologic: anemia, *leukopenia, thrombocytopenia.*

Hepatic: *chronic hepatotoxicity, cirrhosis, hepatic fibrosis,* elevated transaminase levels.

Metabolic: diabetes, hyperuricemia.

Musculoskeletal: arthralgia, myalgia, osteoporosis in children with long-term use.

Respiratory: nonproductive cough, pneumonitis, *pulmonary fibrosis, pulmonary interstitial infiltrates.*

Skin: alopecia, *ecchymoses, erythematous rash, hyperpigmentation, photosensitivity, pruritus, psoriatic lesions (aggravated by exposure to sun), rash, urticaria.*

Other: chills, fever, reduced resistance to infection, *septicemia, sudden death.*

Overdose and treatment

Overdose may cause anemia, nausea, vomiting, myelosuppression, dermatitis, alopecia, and melena.

The antidote for hematopoietic toxicity (diagnosed or anticipated) is calcium leucovorin; it should begin as soon as possible, but within 1 hour after administration of methotrexate. The dosage of leucovorin should produce plasma levels higher than those of methotrexate. Since leucovorin blunts therapeutic response of methotrexate, consult specific disease protocol for details.

Special considerations

▶ Drug is used when NSAIDs or other antirheumatic drugs have proven ineffective.

▶ Drug is also used to treat trophoblastic tumors (choriocarcinoma, hydatidiform mole), acute lymphoblastic leukemia, meningeal leukemia, Burkitt's lymphoma (stage I or II), lymphosarcoma (stage III; malignant lymphoma), mycosis fungoides (advanced), psoriasis (severe), and as an adjunct treatment in osteosarcoma.

▶ Drug should be used as part of a comprehensive treatment program for rheumatoid arthritis that includes rest and physical therapy.

▶ Patients with active rheumatoid arthritis usually show the most improvement within the first 6 months of therapy.

▶ Dose modification may be needed in impaired hepatic or renal function, bone marrow depression, aplasia, leukopenia, thrombocytopenia, or anemia. Use cautiously in infection, peptic ulcer, ulcerative colitis, and in very young, old, or debilitated patients.

- GI adverse reactions may require drug discontinuation.
- Rash, redness, or ulcerations in mouth or pulmonary adverse reactions may signal serious complications.
- Avoid all I.M. injections in patients with thrombocytopenia.
- Leucovorin rescue is necessary with high-dose protocols (doses greater than 100 mg).
- Monitor uric acid levels.
- Monitor intake and output daily. Force fluids (2 to 3 L daily).
- Alkalinize urine by giving sodium bicarbonate tablets to prevent precipitation of drug, especially with high doses. Maintain urine pH at more than 6.5. Reduce dose if BUN level is 20 to 30 mg/dl or serum creatinine level is 1.2 to 2 mg/dl. Stop drug if BUN level exceeds 30 mg/dl or serum creatinine level exceeds 2 mg/dl.
- Watch for increases in AST, ALT, and alkaline phosphatase levels, which may signal hepatic dysfunction. Don't use methotrexate if patient has a risk of "third spacing."
- Watch for bleeding (especially GI) and infection.
- Monitor patient's temperature daily, and watch for cough, dyspnea, and cyanosis.
- Follow facility policy to reduce risks. Preparation and administration of parenteral drug form carries a risk of carcinogenic, mutagenic, and teratogenic effects.
- Dilution of drug depends on product, and infusion guidelines vary with dose.
- Methotrexate may be given undiluted by I.V. push.
- Drug can be diluted to a higher volume with normal saline solution for I.V. infusion.
- Reconstitute unpreserved solutions immediately before use, and discard any unused drug after 24 hours.
- For intrathecal administration, use only preservative-free form. Dilute with unpreserved normal saline solution.

Breast-feeding patients

- Drug appears in breast milk. To minimize the risk of serious adverse reactions, mutagenicity, and carcinogenicity in infant, stop breast-feeding during therapy.

Patient teaching

- Emphasize the importance of continuing drug despite nausea and vomiting. Tell patient to call immediately if she vomits shortly after taking a dose.
- Urge patient to maintain adequate fluid intake to increase urine output, prevent nephrotoxicity, and facilitate excretion of uric acid.
- To avoid potentially serious adverse effects, instruct patients also taking leucovorin to take exactly as prescribed.
- Warn patient to avoid alcoholic beverages during therapy.
- Tell patient to avoid prolonged exposure to sunlight and to use a highly protective sunscreen when exposed to sunlight.
- Teach patient good mouth care to prevent oral superinfection.
- Recommend salicylate-free analgesics for pain relief or fever reduction.
- Tell patient to avoid people with infections and to report signs of infection immediately.
- Advise patient to report unusual bruising or bleeding promptly.
- Explain that hair should grow back after treatment has ended.

▶ Caution patient to avoid conception during and immediately after therapy because of possible abortion or congenital anomalies.

▶ **methylcellulose**
Citrucel, Methylcellulose Tablets

Pharmacologic classification:
adsorbent

Therapeutic classification:
bulk-forming laxative

Pregnancy risk category C

How supplied
Available without a prescription
Powder: 105 mg/g, 364 mg/g
Tablets: 500 mg

Indications and dosages
Chronic constipation
Adults: maximum, 6 g/day, divided into 0.45- to 3-g/doses.
Children ages 6 to 12: maximum, 3 g/day divided into 0.45-g or 1.5-g doses.

Pharmacodynamics
Laxative action: Methylcellulose adsorbs intestinal fluid and serves as a source of indigestible fiber, stimulating peristaltic activity.

Pharmacokinetics
Absorption: Methylcellulose isn't absorbed. Action begins in 12 to 24 hours, but full effect may not occur for 2 to 3 days.
Distribution: Drug is distributed locally in the intestine.
Metabolism: None.
Excretion: Drug is excreted in feces.

Contraindications and precautions
Contraindicated in patients with abdominal pain, nausea, vomiting, or other symptoms of appendicitis or acute surgical abdomen and in those with intestinal obstruction or ulceration, disabling adhesions, or difficulty swallowing.

Interactions
Drug-drug
Oral drugs: methylcellulose may absorb oral drugs. Separate administration by at least 1 hour.

Effects on diagnostic tests
None reported.

Adverse reactions
GI: abdominal cramps, especially in severe constipation; *diarrhea* with excessive use; *esophageal, gastric, small intestinal, or colonic strictures* when drug is chewed or taken in dry form; laxative dependence with long-term or excessive use; *nausea; vomiting.*

Overdose and treatment
No information available.

Special considerations
▶ Drug may be effective in relieving constipation caused by analgesics.
▶ Drug is especially useful in patients with postpartum constipation, chronic laxative abuse, irritable bowel syndrome, diverticular disease, or colostomies; in debilitated patients; and in patients who need to empty colon before barium enema examinations.
▶ Bulk laxatives most closely mimic natural bowel function and don't promote laxative dependence.

▶ Give drug with at least 8 oz of water or juice.
▶ Drug may absorb oral drugs; schedule doses at least 1 hour away from all other drugs.
▶ Before giving drug for constipation, determine if patient has adequate fluid intake, exercise, and diet.

Breast-feeding patients
▶ Drug shows no risk to nursing infants.

Patient teaching
▶ Instruct patient to take other oral medications 1 hour before or after methylcellulose.
▶ Explain that full effect may not occur for 2 to 3 days.
▶ Instruct patient to drink plenty of fluids. Inadequate fluid intake while taking this medication may lead to fecal impaction.
▶ Tell patient to notify prescriber if abdominal pain doesn't resolve.

▶ methylergonovine maleate
Methergine

Pharmacologic classification: *ergot alkaloid*

Therapeutic classification: *oxytocic*

Pregnancy risk category C

How supplied
Available by prescription only
Injection: 0.2 mg/ml ampule
Tablets: 0.2 mg

Indications and dosages
Diagnosis of coronary artery spasm*
Adults: 0.1 to 0.4 mg I.V.

Pharmacodynamics
Oxytocic action: Drug stimulates contractions of uterine and vascular smooth muscle. The intense uterine contractions are followed by periods of relaxation. Drug produces vasoconstriction primarily of capacitance blood vessels, causing increased central venous pressure and elevated blood pressure. Drug increases the amplitude and frequency of uterine contractions and tone, which therefore impedes uterine blood flow.

Pharmacokinetics
Absorption: Absorption is rapid, with 60% of an oral dose appearing in the bloodstream. Plasma levels peak in about 3 hours. Onset of action is immediate after I.V. dose, 2 to 5 minutes after I.M. dose, and 5 to 15 minutes after oral dose.
Distribution: Drug appears to be rapidly distributed into tissues.
Metabolism: Extensive first-pass metabolism precedes hepatic metabolism.
Excretion: Drug is excreted primarily in feces, with a small amount in urine.

Contraindications and precautions
Contraindicated in pregnant patients and patients with hypertension, toxemia, or sensitivity to ergot preparations.
Use cautiously in patients with renal or hepatic disease, sepsis, or

obliterative vascular disease and during the first stage of labor.

Interactions
Drug-drug
Ergot alkaloids, local anesthetics with vasoconstrictors (such as lidocaine with epinephrine), sympathomimetic amines: enhanced vasoconstrictor potential. Use together with caution.

Drug-lifestyle
Smoking: enhances vasoconstriction. Urge patient to avoid concomitant use.

Effects on diagnostic tests
None reported.

Adverse reactions
CNS: *CVA* (with I.V. use), dizziness, hallucinations, headache, *seizures.*
CV: hypertension, hypotension, palpitations, thrombophlebitis, transient chest pain.
EENT: foul taste, nasal congestion, tinnitus.
GI: *diarrhea, nausea, vomiting.*
GU: hematuria.
Musculoskeletal: leg cramps.
Respiratory: dyspnea.
Skin: diaphoresis.

Overdose and treatment
Overdose may cause seizures and gangrene, with nausea, vomiting, diarrhea, dizziness, fluctuations in blood pressure, weak pulse, chest pain, tingling, and numbness and coldness in extremities.

Treatment of oral overdose requires that the patient drink tap water, milk, or vegetable oil to delay absorption. Follow with gastric lavage or emesis, and then activated charcoal and cathartics. Treat

seizures with anticonvulsants and hypercoagulability with heparin. Use vasodilators to improve blood flow as needed. Gangrene may require surgical amputation.

Special considerations
▶ Drug is also used to prevent and treat postpartum hemorrhage caused by uterine atony or subinvolution.
▶ Contractions begin 5 to 15 minutes after P.O. administration, 2 to 5 minutes after I.M. injection, and immediately following I.V. injection; they continue 3 hours or more after P.O. or I.M. administration, 45 minutes after I.V.
▶ Store tablets in tightly closed, light-resistant containers. Discard if discolored.
▶ Monitor blood pressure, pulse rate, and uterine response; watch for sudden change in vital signs or frequent periods of uterine relaxation, and character and amount of vaginal bleeding.
▶ Don't routinely administer drug by I.V. route because of the risk of inducing sudden hypertension and CVA.
▶ Administer I.V. solution only if it's clear and colorless.
▶ If I.V. administration is considered essential as a life-saving measure, give slowly over at least 60 seconds while monitoring blood pressure carefully. I.V. dose may be diluted to 5 ml with normal saline solution before use. Contractions begin immediately after I.V. use and continue for up to 45 minutes.
▶ Store I.V. solutions below 46.4° F (8° C).

Breast-feeding patients
▶ Ergot alkaloids inhibit lactation.

▶ Drug appears in breast milk, and ergotism has been reported in breast-fed infants.

Patient teaching
▶ Advise patient to avoid smoking while taking drug.
▶ Advise patient of adverse reactions.

▶ methylphenidate hydrochloride
Ritalin, Ritalin-SR

Pharmacologic classification:
piperidine CNS stimulant

Therapeutic classification:
CNS stimulant (analeptic)

Controlled substance schedule II

Pregnancy risk category NR

How supplied
Available by prescription only
Tablets: 5 mg, 10 mg, 20 mg
Tablets (sustained-release): 20 mg

Indications and dosages
Attention deficit hyperactivity disorder

Children age 6 and older: initially, 5 to 10 mg/day P.O. before breakfast and lunch, increased in 5- to 10-mg increments weekly, p.r.n., until optimum daily dose of 2 mg/kg is reached. Maximum, 60 mg/day.
Narcolepsy
Adults: 10 mg P.O. b.i.d. or t.i.d. 30 to 45 minutes before meals. Dosage varies with patient needs; average dose is 40 to 60 mg/day.

Pharmacodynamics
Analeptic action: The cerebral cortex and reticular activating system appear to be the primary sites of activity; methylphenidate releases nerve terminal stores of norepinephrine, promoting nerve impulse transmission. At high doses, effects are mediated by dopamine. It has a paradoxical calming effect in hyperactive children.

Pharmacokinetics
Absorption: Drug is absorbed rapidly and completely after oral administration; plasma levels peak in 1 to 2 hours. Duration of action is usually 4 to 6 hours (with considerable individual variation); sustained-release tablets may act for up to 8 hours.
Distribution: Unknown.
Metabolism: Methylphenidate is metabolized by the liver.
Excretion: Drug is excreted in urine.

Contraindications and precautions
Contraindicated in patients with hypersensitivity to drug, glaucoma, motor tics, family history of or diagnosis of Tourette syndrome, or history of marked anxiety, tension, or agitation.

Use cautiously in patients with history of seizures, drug abuse, hypertension, or EEG abnormalities.

Interactions
Drug-drug
Anticonvulsants (phenobarbital, phenytoin, primidone), coumarin anticoagulants, phenylbutazone, tricyclic antidepressants: methylphenidate may inhibit metabolism and increase serum levels of these drugs. Monitor patient for toxicity.

Bretylium, guanethidine: decreased hypotensive drug effects. Monitor patient.

MAO inhibitors or drugs that have MAO-inhibiting activity: may cause severe hypertension if methylphenidate taken within 14 days of such therapy. Avoid overlapping use.

Drug-food
Caffeine: may decrease drug efficacy in attention deficit hyperactivity disorder. Avoid use together.

Effects on diagnostic tests
None reported.

Adverse reactions
CNS: *akathisia, dizziness,* drowsiness, *dyskinesia, headache, insomnia, nervousness,* **seizures,** *Tourette syndrome.*
CV: *angina,* **arrhythmias,** *changes in blood pressure and pulse rate, palpitations, tachycardia.*
GI: abdominal pain, anorexia, nausea.
Hematologic: anemia, *leukopenia, thrombocytopenia, thrombocytopenic purpura.*
Metabolic: weight loss.
Skin: *erythema multiforme,* exfoliative dermatitis, rash, urticaria.

Overdose and treatment
Overdose may cause euphoria, confusion, delirium, coma, toxic psychosis, agitation, headache, vomiting, dry mouth, mydriasis, self-injury, fever, diaphoresis, tremors, hyperreflexia, hyperpyrexia, muscle twitching, seizures, flushing, hypertension, tachycardia, palpitations, and arrhythmias.

Treat overdose symptomatically and supportively: induce emesis if patient has intact gag reflex or perform gastric lavage. Maintain airway and circulation. Closely monitor vital signs and fluid and electrolyte balance. Keep patient in a cool room, monitor her temperature, minimize external stimulation, and protect her against self-injury. External cooling blankets may be needed.

Special considerations
▶ Drug is effective in treating sedative effects of long-acting opiates in cancer patients.
▶ Establish dosing schedule to help create normal morning waking pattern.
▶ Methylphenidate is the drug of choice for attention deficit hyperactivity disroder. Therapy usually stops after puberty.
▶ Drug has abuse potential; discourage use to combat fatigue. Some abusers dissolve tablets and inject drug.
▶ Monitor start of therapy closely; drug may precipitate Tourette syndrome.
▶ Make sure patient obtains adequate rest; fatigue may result as drug wears off.
▶ Intermittent drug-free periods during low-stress times (weekends, school holidays) may help prevent tolerance and allow decreased dosage when drug is resumed. Sustained-release form allows single, at-home dosing for school children.
▶ Monitor CBC, differential, and platelet counts if patient takes drug long-term.
▶ Drug impairs ability to perform tasks that require mental alertness.

Reactions may be *common,* uncommon, *life-threatening,* or **COMMON AND LIFE-THREATENING.**

▶ Monitor patient's height and weight; drug has been linked to growth suppression.

▶ If paradoxical aggravation of symptoms occurs during therapy, reduce dosage or discontinue drug.

▶ Check vital signs regularly for increased blood pressure or other signs of excessive stimulation; avoid late-day or evening dosing, especially of long-acting forms, to minimize insomnia.

▶ Drug may decrease seizure threshold in seizure disorders.

▶ Discourage methylphenidate use for analeptic effect; CNS stimulation superimposed on CNS depression may cause neuronal instability and seizures.

▶ After high-dose and long-term use, abrupt withdrawal may unmask severe depression. Reduce dosage gradually to prevent acute rebound depression.

Pregnant patients

▶ Don't give drug to women of childbearing age unless potential benefits outweigh the possible risks.

Pediatric patients

▶ Drug isn't recommended for attention deficit hyperactivity disorder in children under age 6.

▶ It has been linked to growth suppression; all patients should be monitored.

Patient teaching

▶ Explain rationale for therapy and the antitipcated risks and benefits.

▶ Tell patient to avoid caffeine to prevent added CNS stimulation.

▶ Patient shouldn't alter dosage unless prescribed.

▶ Advise narcoleptic patient to take first dose on awakening; patient

with attention deficit hyperactivity disorder should receive last dose several hours before bed to avoid insomnia.

▶ Warn against chewing or crushing sustained-release dosage forms.

▶ Warn patient not to use drug to mask fatigue. Urge adequate rest.

▶ Urge patient to notify prescriber about excessive CNS stimulation.

▶ Advise patient to avoid hazardous activities until full sedative effect of drug is known.

methylprednisolone (systemic)
Medrol

methylprednisolone acetate
depMedalone 40, depMedalone 80, Depoject-40, Depoject-80, Depo-Medrol, Depopred-40, Depopred-80, Duralone-40, Duralone-80, Medralone, Rep-Pred 40, Rep-Pred 80

methylprednisolone sodium succinate
A-Methapred, Solu-Medrol

Pharmacologic classification: *glucocorticoid*

Therapeutic classification: *anti-inflammatory, immunosuppressant*

Pregnancy risk category C

How supplied
Available by prescription only
methylprednisolone
Tablets: 2 mg, 4 mg, 8 mg, 16 mg, 24 mg, 32 mg

methylprednisolone acetate
Injection: 20 mg/ml, 40 mg/ml,
80 mg/ml suspension
methylprednisolone sodium succinate
Injection: 40 mg, 125 mg, 500 mg,
1,000 mg, 2,000 mg/vial

Indications and dosages
Inflammation
methylprednisolone
Adults: 2 to 60 mg P.O. daily in
four divided doses, depending on
disease being treated.
Children: 0.117 to 1.66 mg/kg daily or 3.3 to 50 mg/m^2 P.O. daily in
three to four divided doses.
methylprednisolone acetate
Adults: 10 to 80 mg I.M. daily; or
4 to 80 mg into joints and soft tissue, p.r.n., q 1 to 5 weeks; or 20 to
60 mg into lesion.
methylprednisolone sodium succinate
Adults: 10 to 250 mg I.M. or I.V. q
4 hours.
Children: 0.03 to 0.2 mg/kg or 1 to
6.25 mg/m^2 I.M. or I.V. daily in divided doses.
Treatment or minimization of motor and sensory defects caused by acute spinal cord injury*
Adults: initially, 30 mg/kg I.V. over
15 minutes followed in 45 minutes
by I.V. infusion of 5.4 mg/kg/hour
for 23 hours.

Pharmacodynamics
Anti-inflammatory action: Drug
stimulates synthesis of enzymes
needed to decrease inflammatory
response. It suppresses the immune system by reducing activity
and volume of the lymphatic system, producing lymphocytopenia
(primarily of T lymphocytes), decreasing immunoglobulin and
complement levels, decreasing

passage of immune complexes
through basement membranes, and
possibly depressing reactivity of
tissue to antigen-antibody interactions.

Drug is an intermediate-acting
glucocorticoid. It has no mineralocorticoid activity but is a potent
glucocorticoid, with five times the
potency of an equal weight of hydrocortisone. It's used primarily as
an anti-inflammatory and immunosuppressant.

Methylprednisolone may be administered orally. The sodium succinate form may be given I.M. or
by I.V. injection or infusion, usually at 4- to 6-hour intervals. The acetate suspension may be given by
intra-articular, intrasynovial, intrabursal, intralesional, or soft tissue
injection. It has a slow onset but a
long duration of action. Injectable
forms are usually used only when
the oral forms can't be used.

Pharmacokinetics
Absorption: Drug is absorbed
readily after oral administration.
After oral and I.V. administration,
effects peak in 1 to 2 hours. The
acetate suspension for injection
has a variable absorption over 24
to 48 hours, depending on whether
it is injected into an intra-articular
space or a muscle, and on the
blood supply to that muscle.
Distribution: Drug is distributed
rapidly to muscle, liver, skin, intestines, and kidneys. Adrenocorticoids are distributed into
breast milk and through the placenta.
Metabolism: Drug is metabolized
in the liver to inactive glucuronide
and sulfate metabolites.
Excretion: Inactive metabolites
and small amounts of unmetabo-

lized drug are excreted by the kidneys. Small amounts of drug are excreted in feces. Biological half-life of methylprednisolone is 18 to 36 hours.

Contraindications and precautions

Contraindicated in patients allergic to any component of the formulation, in those with systemic fungal infections, and in premature infants (acetate and succinate).

Use cautiously in patients with renal disease, GI ulceration, hypertension, osteoporosis, diabetes mellitus, hypothyroidism, cirrhosis, diverticulitis, nonspecific ulcerative colitis, recent intestinal anastomoses, thromboembolic disorders, seizures, myasthenia gravis, heart failure, tuberculosis, emotional instability, ocular herpes simplex, and psychotic tendencies.

Interactions
Drug-drug
Amphotericin B, diuretics: increased risk of hypokalemia, which may increase the risk of toxicity in patients concurrently receiving cardiac glycosides. Monitor serum potassium and digoxin levels.
Antacids, cholestyramine, colestipol: decreased corticosteroid effect by decreasing the amount absorbed. Separate administration times.
Anticholinesterase: creates profound weakness. Use together cautiously.
Barbiturates, phenytoin, rifampin: decreased corticosteroid effects because of increased hepatic metabolism. Monitor patient.

Cyclosporine: increased cyclosporine levels. Monitor serum drug levels.
Estrogens: may reduce corticosteroid metabolism by increasing the level of transcortin, thus prolonging corticosteroid half-life. Adjust dose as needed.
Insulin, oral antidiabetic drugs: increased risk of hyperglycemia. Adjust dosage as needed.
Isoniazid, salicylates: increased metabolism of these drugs. Adjust dosage as needed.
Oral anticoagulants: decreased anticoagulant effects. Monitor PT and INR.
Ulcer-causing drugs, such as NSAIDs: increased risk of GI ulceration. Assess patient for abdominal complaints.
Vaccines: drug may decrease effectiveness. Avoid concomitant use.

Effects on diagnostic tests

Drug suppresses reactions to skin tests, causes false-negative results in the nitroblue tetrazolium test for systemic bacterial infections, and decreases ^{131}I uptake and protein-bound iodine levels in thyroid function tests.

Adverse reactions

CNS: *euphoria,* headache, *insomnia,* paresthesia, pseudotumor cerebri, psychotic behavior, *seizures,* vertigo.
CV: *arrhythmias, fatal arrest or circulatory collapse* (following rapid administration of large I.V. doses), edema, *heart failure,* hypertension, *thromboembolism,* thrombophlebitis.
EENT: cataracts, glaucoma.

GI: GI irritation, increased appetite, nausea, *pancreatitis, peptic ulceration,* vomiting.

GU: increased urine glucose and calcium levels, menstrual irregularities.

Metabolic: decreased T_3 and T_4 levels, hypercholesterolemia, hyperglycemia, hypocalcemia, hypokalemia.

Musculoskeletal: muscle weakness, osteoporosis.

Skin: acne, delayed wound healing, various skin eruptions.

Other: *acute adrenal insufficiency* (may result from abrupt withdrawal after long-term therapy or from increased stress, as from infection, surgery, or trauma), carbohydrate intolerance, cushingoid state (moonface, buffalo hump, central obesity), growth suppression in children, hirsutism, susceptibility to infection.

Overdose and treatment

Acute ingestion, even in massive doses, rarely causes a problem. Toxic signs and symptoms rarely occur if drug is used for less than 3 weeks, even at large doses.

Special considerations

▶ Drug may be used as adjuvant therapy in chronic cancer pain. It's also used to treat multiple sclerosis, shock, and severe lupus nephritis (off label).

▶ Never use acetate form for I.V. delivery; use only sodium succinate form. Reconstitute according to manufacturer's directions using the supplied diluent or bacteriostatic water for injection with benzyl alcohol.

▶ When giving a direct injection, inject diluted drug into a vein or free-flowing compatible I.V. solution over at least 1 minute. When giving an intermittent or continuous infusion, dilute solution according to manufacturer's instructions, and give over the prescribed duration. If used for continuous infusion, change solution every 24 hours.

▶ Compatible solutions include D_5W, normal saline solution, and dextrose 5% in normal saline solution.

▶ Give oral dose with food when possible. Critically ill patients may require concomitant antacid or H_2-receptor antagonist therapy.

▶ For better results and less toxicity, give once daily in the morning.

▶ Always adjust to lowest effective dose.

▶ Monitor patient's weight, blood pressure, serum electrolyte levels, and sleep patterns. Euphoria may initially interfere with sleep, but most patients adjust in 1 to 3 weeks.

▶ Assess patient for infection.

▶ Watch for depression or psychotic tendencies, especially in high-dose therapy.

▶ Monitor serum glucose levels.

▶ Don't confuse Solu-Medrol with Solu-Cortef (hydrocortisone sodium succinate). Solu-Medrol shouldn't be given intrathecally.

▶ Most adverse reactions to corticosteroids are dose-dependent or duration-dependent.

▶ Long-term use of drug causes adverse physiologic effects, including suppression of the hypothalamus-pituitary-adrenal axis, cushingoid appearance, muscle weakness, and osteoporosis.

▶ Abrupt withdrawal can cause anorexia, arthralgia, depression, dizziness, dyspnea, fainting, fatigue, fever, lethargy, orthostatic hypotension, hypoglycemia, rebound inflammation, weakness. After prolonged use, it may be fatal.

Pediatric patients
▶ Long-term use of adrenocorticoids in children and adolescents may delay growth and maturation.

Geriatric patients
▶ In elderly patients, weigh the risks and benefits; lower doses are recommended.
▶ Check blood pressure, blood glucose and electrolytes at least every 6 months.

Patient teaching
▶ Tell patient not to stop drug abruptly.
▶ Instruct patient to take oral form of drug with milk or food.
▶ Teach patients the signs of early adrenal insufficiency: fatigue, muscle weakness, joint pain, fever, anorexia, nausea, dyspnea, dizziness, and fainting.
▶ Instruct patient to carry or wear medical identification that identifies her need for supplemental systemic glucocorticoids during stress. This card should contain health care provider's name, medication, and dose needed.
▶ Warn patient on long-term therapy about cushingoid symptoms and to notify prescriber about sudden weight gain or swelling.
▶ Advise patient on long-term therapy to consider exercise or physical therapy. Also, as appropriate, recommend a vitamin D or calcium supplement.

▶ Instruct patient to avoid exposure to infections (such as chickenpox or measles) and to contact prescriber if such exposure occurs.

▶ methysergide maleate
Sansert

Pharmacologic classification:
ergot alkaloid

Therapeutic classification:
vasoconstrictor

Pregnancy risk category X

How supplied
Available by prescription only
Tablets: 2 mg

Indications and dosages
Prevention of migraine and cluster headaches
Adults: 4 to 8 mg/day P.O. in divided doses with meals.

Pharmacodynamics
Vasoconstrictor action: Drug competitively blocks serotonin peripherally and may act as a serotonin agonist in the CNS (brain stem). Its antiserotonin effects inhibit the peripheral vasoconstrictor and pressor effects of serotonin, inhibit the inflammation induced by serotonin, and reduce the increased rate of platelet aggregation caused by serotonin.

The mechanism involved in prophylaxis of vascular headaches by methysergide is unknown; however, its effectiveness may result from humoral factors affecting the pain threshold and from its central serotonin-agonist effect.

Pharmacokinetics

Absorption: Drug is rapidly absorbed from the GI tract.
Distribution: Methysergide is widely distributed in body tissues.
Metabolism: Drug is metabolized in the liver to methylergonovine and glucuronide metabolites.
Excretion: 56% of a dose is excreted in urine as unchanged drug and its metabolites. Plasma elimination half-life is 10 hours.

Contraindications and precautions

Contraindicated in debilitated patients, pregnant patients, and patients with severe hypertension or arteriosclerosis, peripheral vascular insufficiency, renal or hepatic disease, coronary artery disease, phlebitis or cellulitis of lower limbs, collagen diseases, fibrotic processes, or valvular heart disease.

Use cautiously in patients with peptic ulcer or suspected coronary artery disease and in those with aspirin or tartrazine allergies.

Interactions
Drug-drug

Beta blockers: peripheral ischemia, resulting in cold limbs and increased risk of peripheral gangrene.
Narcotic analgesics: drug may reverse the analgesic activity of these drugs. Monitor patient for increased pain.

Effects on diagnostic tests

None reported.

Adverse reactions

CNS: *ataxia,* drowsiness, *euphoria,* hallucinations or feelings of dissociation, hyperesthesia, insomnia, light-headedness, lethargy, rapid speech, weakness, *vertigo.*
CV: bruits; cold, numb, painful limbs with or without paresthesia and diminished or absent pulses; *fibrotic thickening of cardiac valves and aorta, inferior vena cava, and common iliac branches (retroperitoneal fibrosis);* flushing; murmurs; orthostatic hypotension; peripheral edema; tachycardia; vasoconstriction, causing abdominal pain, chest pain, vascular insufficiency in legs.
GI: constipation, diarrhea, heartburn, nausea, vomiting.
Hematologic: eosinophilia, *neutropenia.*
Musculoskeletal: arthralgia, myalgia.
Respiratory: *pulmonary fibrosis* (causing dyspnea, tightness and pain in chest, pleural friction rubs, and effusion).
Skin: hair loss, rash.

Overdose and treatment

Overdose may cause hyperactivity, euphoria, dizziness, peripheral vasospasm with diminished or absent pulses, and coldness, mottling, and cyanosis of extremities.

Treatment requires supportive measures with prolonged and careful monitoring. If patient is conscious and ingestion recent, induce emesis; if he's unconscious, insert cuffed endotracheal tube and perform gastric lavage followed by sodium chloride (magnesium sulfate) cathartic. Administer I.V. fluids if needed. Monitor vital signs. Apply warmth (not direct heat) to ischemic limbs if vasospasm occurs. Administer vasodilators (nitroprusside, tolazoline, or prazosin) if needed.

Contact local or regional poison control center for more information.

Special considerations

▶ Don't use drug to treat acute episodes of migraine, vascular headache, or muscle contraction headache.
▶ If drug is given for cluster headaches, it's usually administered only during the cluster.
▶ Drug has also been used to control diarrhea in patients with cancer.
▶ Protective effect develops in 1 to 2 days and persists for 1 to 2 days after drug stops.
▶ Separate each 6-month course of therapy with 3- to 4-week drug-free intervals.
▶ Adverse reactions occur in up to half of patients.
▶ GI effects may be reduced by gradual introduction of drug and by giving it with food or milk.
▶ Reduce dosage gradually for 2 to 3 weeks before stopping drug.
▶ Monitor patient's cardiac and renal function, CBC, and erythrocyte sedimentation rate before and during therapy.

Breast-feeding patients

▶ Drug may appear in breast milk. Avoid breast-feeding during drug therapy.

Pediatric patients

▶ Drug isn't recommended for children because of risk of fibrosis.

Geriatric patients

▶ Use with caution.

Patient teaching

▶ Tell patient to take drug with food.

▶ Caution patient to avoid hazardous activities until full CNS effects of drug are known. Drug may cause drowsiness.
▶ Warn patient to avoid alcoholic beverages because alcohol may worsen headaches.
▶ Caution patient to avoid smoking because it may increase adverse drug effects.
▶ Tell patient to avoid prolonged exposure to very cold temperatures because cold may increase adverse drug effects.
▶ Caution patient regarding caloric intake to avoid excessive weight gain.
▶ Tell patient not to take drug for longer than 6 months at a time and to wait 3 to 4 weeks before starting another 6-month treatment period.
▶ Tell patient to immediately notify prescriber about numbness or tingling in hands or feet, red or violet blisters on hands and feet, flank or chest pain, shortness of breath, leg cramps when walking, or any other evidence of impaired circulation.
▶ Tell patient to report illness or infection, which may increase sensitivity to drug effects.
▶ Explain that after stopping drug, her body may need time to adjust depending on the amount used and the duration of time involved.
▶ Drug may contain tartrazine, which can cause an allergic reaction.

▶ metoclopramide hydrochloride
Apo-Metoclop◇, Clopra, Maxeran◇, Maxolon, Octamide PFS, Reclomide, Reglan

Pharmacologic classification:
para-aminobenzoic acid derivative

Therapeutic classification:
antiemetic, GI stimulant

Pregnancy risk category B

How supplied
Available by prescription only
Injection: 5 mg/ml
Solution: 10 mg/ml
Syrup: 5 mg/5 ml
Tablets: 5 mg, 10 mg

Indications and dosages
Prevention or reduction of chemotherapy-induced nausea and vomiting
Adults: 1 to 2 mg/kg I.V. q 2 hours for two doses, beginning 30 minutes before emetogenic chemotherapy. Then q 3 hours for three doses.
Gastroesophageal reflux
Adults: 10 to 15 mg P.O. q.i.d., p.r.n., 30 minutes before meals and h.s.
Postoperative nausea and vomiting
Adults: 10 to 20 mg I.M. near end of surgical procedure, repeated q 4 to 6 hours, p.r.n.
Vomiting
Adults: 10 mg P.O. taken 30 minutes before meals.

Pharmacodynamics
Antiemetic action: Drug inhibits dopamine receptors in the brain's chemoreceptor trigger zone to inhibit or reduce nausea and vomiting.
GI stimulant action: Drug relieves esophageal reflux by increasing lower esophageal sphincter tone and reduces gastric stasis by stimulating motility of the upper GI tract, thus reducing gastric emptying time.

Pharmacokinetics
Absorption: After oral administration, drug is absorbed rapidly and thoroughly from the GI tract; action begins in 30 to 60 minutes. After I.M. administration, about 74% to 96% of drug is bioavailable; action begins in 10 to 15 minutes. After I.V. administration, onset of action occurs in 1 to 3 minutes.
Distribution: Drug is distributed to most body tissues and fluids, including the brain. Drug crosses the placenta and is distributed in breast milk.
Metabolism: Drug isn't metabolized extensively; a small amount is metabolized in the liver.
Excretion: Drug is mostly excreted in urine and feces. Hemodialysis and peritoneal dialysis remove minimal amounts. Duration of effect is 1 to 2 hours.

Contraindications and precautions
Contraindicated in patients for whom stimulation of GI motility might be dangerous (in those with hemorrhage, obstruction, or perforation) and in patients with hypersensitivity to drug, pheochromocytoma, or seizure disorders.

Use cautiously in patients with history of depression, Parkinson's disease, and hypertension.

Interactions
Drug-drug
Acetaminophen, aspirin, diazepam, levodopa, lithium, tetracycline: increased absorption of these drugs. Monitor patient for effects and toxicity.

Anticholinergics, opiates: may antagonize metoclopramide's effect on GI motility. Monitor patient closely.

Antihypertensives, CNS depressants (sedatives, tricyclic antidepressants): may increase CNS depression. Monitor patient closely.

Butyrophenone antipsychotics, phenothiazine: may potentiate extrapyramidal reactions. Use together cautiously.

Cyclosporine: faster gastric emptying time may increase cyclosporine absorption. Monitor patient for increased immunosuppressive and toxic effects.

Digoxin: decreased digoxin absorption. Monitor serum digoxin level.

MAO inhibitors: metoclopramide releases catecholamines in patients with essential hypertension. Use with extreme caution.

Drug-lifestyle
Alcohol use: increased CNS depression. Advise against concurrent use.

Effects on diagnostic tests
None reported.

Adverse reactions
CNS: *akathisia, anxiety, confusion, depression,* dizziness, *drowsiness,* dystonic reactions, extrapyramidal symptoms, *fatigue,* hallucinations, headache, *insomnia, lassitude, restlessness,* **suicidal ideation, seizures,** tardive dyskinesia.

CV: **bradycardia,** hypotension, supraventricular tachycardia, transient hypertension.

GI: bowel disturbances, diarrhea, nausea.

GU: decreased libido, incontinence, urinary frequency.

Hematologic: *agranulocytosis, neutropenia.*

Metabolic: prolactin secretion.

Respiratory: *bronchospasm.*

Skin: rash, urticaria.

Other: fever, porphyria.

Overdose and treatment
Overdose is rare but may cause drowsiness, dystonia, seizures, and extrapyramidal effects.

Treatment includes administration of antimuscarinics, antiparkinsonians, or antihistamines with antimuscarinic activity (such as 50 mg diphenhydramine, given I.M.).

Special considerations
❯ Drug has been used experimentally to treat anorexia nervosa, dizziness, migraine, intractable hiccups. It also has been investigated for promoting postpartum lactation. Oral form is being used experimentally to treat nausea and vomiting.
❯ Drug is also used for delayed gastric emptying caused by diabetic gastroparesis and to facilitate small-bowel intubation and aid in radiologic examination.
❯ Drug may be used to facilitate nasoduodenal tube placement.
❯ Closely monitor blood pressure in patients receiving I.V. form of drug.
❯ Give lower doses (10 mg or less) by direct injection over 1 to 2 minutes. Dilute doses larger than 10 mg

in 50 ml of a compatible diluent, and infuse over at least 15 minutes. Protection from light is unnecessary if infusion mixture is administered within 24 hours. If infusion mixture is protected from light and refrigerated, stability is 48 hours.
▶ Drug is compatible with D_5W, normal saline solution for injection, dextrose 5% in half-normal saline injection, Ringer's injection, or lactated Ringer's injection.
▶ Administer by I.V. infusion 30 minutes before chemotherapy.
▶ Don't use drug for more than 12 weeks. It isn't recommended for long-term use.
▶ Diphenhydramine may be used to counteract extrapyramidal effects of high-dose metoclopramide.
▶ Monitor patient's bowel sounds.

Breast-feeding patients
▶ Because drug appears in breast milk, use caution when administering it to breast-feeding women.

Pediatric patients
▶ Children have an increased risk of adverse CNS effects.

Geriatric patients
▶ Use drug with caution, especially if patient has impaired renal function. Dosage may need to be decreased.
▶ Elderly patients have an increased risk of extrapyramidal symptoms and tardive dyskinesia.

Patient teaching
▶ Warn patient to avoid hazardous activities for 2 hours after each dose because drug may cause drowsiness. Until extent of CNS

effect is known, advise patient not to consume alcohol.
▶ Tell patient to report twitching or involuntary movements.
▶ Instruct patient to take medication 30 minutes before each meal.

▶ **metoprolol succinate**
Lopressor, Toprol XL

▶ **metoprolol tartrate**
Apo-Metoprolol◊, Apo-Metoprolol (Type L)◊, Betaloc◊, Betaloc Durules◊, Lopressor◊, Novometoprol◊, Nu-Metop◊

Pharmacologic classification:
beta blocker

Therapeutic classification:
adjunctive treatment of acute MI, antihypertensive

Pregnancy risk category C

How supplied
Available by prescription only
Injection: 1 mg/ml in 5-ml ampules or prefilled syringes
Tablets: 50 mg, 100 mg
Tablets (extended-release): 50 mg, 100 mg, 200 mg

Indications and dosages
Angina
Adults: 100 mg in two divided doses. Maintenance, 100 to 400 mg/day. Alternatively, 100 mg/day P.O. of extended-release tablets (maximum, 400 mg/day).
Migraine prophylaxis*
Adults: 50 to 100 mg b.i.d.

Pharmacodynamics
Action after acute MI: The exact mechanism by which drug decreas-

es mortality after MI is unknown. Metoprolol reduces heart rate, systolic blood pressure, and cardiac output. Drug also appears to decrease the occurrence of ventricular fibrillation in these patients.

Antihypertensive action: Metoprolol is a cardioselective beta$_1$-antagonist; exact mechanism of antihypertensive effect is unknown. Drug may reduce blood pressure by blocking adrenergic receptors (thus decreasing cardiac output), by decreasing sympathetic outflow from the CNS, or by suppressing renin release.

Migraine prophylaxis action: Mechanism isn't known.

Pharmacokinetics

Absorption: Orally administered metoprolol is absorbed rapidly and almost completely from GI tract; food enhances absorption. Following a single oral dose, drug appears in plasma in 10 minutes. Plasma levels peak in 90 minutes. After I.V. administration, maximum beta blockade occurs in 20 minutes. Maximum effect occurs after 1 week of treatment.

Distribution: Drug is distributed widely throughout the body; about 12% is protein-bound.

Metabolism: Drug is metabolized in the liver.

Excretion: About 95% of a given dose of metoprolol is excreted in urine within 72 hours, largely as metabolites.

Contraindications and precautions

Contraindicated in patients with hypersensitivity to drug or other beta blockers. Also contraindicated in patients with sinus bradycardia, heart block greater than first-degree, cardiogenic shock, overt cardiac failure, or right ventricular failure secondary to pulmonary hypertension when used to treat hypertension or angina. When used to treat MI, drug is contraindicated in patients with heart rate less than 45 beats/minute, second- or third-degree heart block, PR interval of 0.24 second or longer with first-degree heart block, systolic blood pressure less than 100 mm Hg, or moderate to severe cardiac failure.

Use cautiously in patients with impaired hepatic or respiratory function, diabetes, or heart failure.

Interactions

Drug-drug

Antihypertensives, including diuretics: metoprolol may potentiate antihypertensive effects. Monitor blood pressure.

Cardiac glycosides: enhanced bradycardia. Monitor heart rate.

Sympathomimetics: metoprolol may antagonize beta-adrenergic effects of these drugs. Monitor patient.

Thyroid hormones: metoprolol's action may be impaired when hypothyroid patient is converted to euthyroid state. Monitor patient.

Verapamil: may decrease metoprolol bioavailability when given with antiarrhythmics. Monitor patient.

Drug-food

Food: enhanced metoprolol absorption. Give drug with food.

Effects on diagnostic tests

None reported.

Adverse reactions

CNS: depression, *dizziness, fatigue.*

CV: *AV block, bradycardia, heart failure,* hypotension.
GI: diarrhea, nausea.
Hepatic: elevated liver enzymes.
Respiratory: *bronchospasm,* dyspnea.
Skin: rash.

Overdose and treatment

Overdose may cause severe hypotension, bradycardia, heart failure, and bronchospasm.

After acute ingestion, induce emesis or perform gastric lavage. Give activated charcoal to reduce absorption. Subsequent treatment is usually symptomatic and supportive.

Special considerations

▶ Drug is also used to treat mild to severe hypertension and as an early intervention in acute MI.
▶ For effective migraine prophylaxis, patient must take drug as prescribed.
▶ Avoid late-evening doses to minimize insomnia.
▶ Reduce dosage in patients with impaired hepatic function.
▶ Monitor blood pressure and pulse rate.
▶ Give undiluted by direct injection. Although mixing with other drugs should be avoided, metoprolol is compatible when mixed with meperidine hydrochloride or morphine sulfate or when administered with alteplase infusion at a Y-site connection.
▶ Signs of hypoglycemia may be masked in diabetic patients.

Breast-feeding patients

▶ Metoprolol appears in breast milk. An alternative feeding method is recommended during therapy.

Pediatric patients

▶ Safety and efficacy in children haven't been established. No dosage recommendation exists for children.

Geriatric patients

▶ Elderly patients may require lower maintenance dosages because of delayed metabolism.
▶ These patients may experience enhanced adverse effects. Use with caution.

Patient teaching

▶ Instruct patient to take the drug exactly as prescribed and to take with meals. Tell patient not to stop drug suddenly and to inform prescriber of any unpleasant adverse effects.
▶ Explain common adverse effects the patient may experience. Tell patient to notify prescriber if any of the following occur: shortness of breath, swelling of limbs, decrease in pulse rate, depression, or dizziness.
▶ Tell patient to talk to pharmacist or prescriber before taking any OTC medications that may contain stimulants (such as cough and cold preparations, decongestants).
▶ If patient misses a dose, tell her to skip it and resume therapy with the next scheduled dose.
▶ Explain to patient that when being used for migraine prophylaxis, the drug helps to prevent the recurrence and severity of migraines.

Reactions may be *common,* uncommon, *life-threatening*, or COMMON AND LIFE-THREATENING.

▶ mexiletine hydrochloride
Mexitil

Pharmacologic classification:
lidocaine analogue, sodium channel antagonist

Therapeutic classification:
ventricular antiarrhythmic

Pregnancy risk category C

How supplied
Available by prescription only
Capsules: 150 mg, 200 mg, 250 mg

Indications and dosages
Diabetic neuropathy*
Adults: 150 mg/day for first 3 days, 300 mg/day for next 3 days, and then 10 mg/kg/day.

Pharmacodynamics
Antiarrhythmic action: Mexiletine is structurally similar to lidocaine and exerts similar electrophysiologic and hemodynamic effects. A class IB antiarrhythmic, it suppresses automaticity and shortens the effective refractory period and action potential duration of His-Purkinje fibers and suppresses spontaneous ventricular depolarization during diastole. At therapeutic serum levels, the drug doesn't affect conductive atrial tissue or AV conduction.

Unlike quinidine and procainamide, mexiletine doesn't significantly alter hemodynamics when given in usual doses. Its effects on the conduction system inhibit reentry mechanisms and halt ventricular arrhythmias. Drug has no significant negative inotropic effect.

Pharmacokinetics
Absorption: About 90% of drug is absorbed from the GI tract; serum levels peak in 2 to 3 hours. Rate of absorption decreases with conditions that speed gastric emptying.
Distribution: Drug is widely distributed throughout the body. About 50% to 60% of circulating drug is bound to plasma proteins. Usual therapeutic level is 0.5 to 2 mcg/ml. Although toxicity may occur within this range, levels above 2 mcg/ml are considered toxic and are associated with an increased frequency of adverse CNS effects, warranting dosage reduction.
Metabolism: Drug is metabolized in the liver to relatively inactive metabolites. Less than 10% of a parenteral dose escapes metabolism and reaches the kidneys unchanged. Metabolism is affected by hepatic blood flow, which may be reduced in patients who are recovering from MI and in those with heart failure. Liver disease also limits metabolism.
Excretion: In healthy patients, drug's half-life is 10 to 12 hours. Elimination half-life may be prolonged in patients with heart failure or liver disease. Urine excretion increases with urine acidification and slows with urine alkalinization.

Contraindications and precautions
Contraindicated in patients with cardiogenic shock or second- or third-degree AV block who don't have an artificial pacemaker.

Use cautiously in patients with hypotension, heart failure, first-degree heart block, ventricular pacemaker, preexisting sinus node dysfunction, or seizure disorders.

◇ Available in Canada only   *Unlabeled use

Interactions
Drug-drug
Bicarbonate: decreased mexiletine excretion. Watch for toxicity.
Cimetidine: decreased mexiletine metabolism and increased serum levels. Monitor patient for toxicity.
Drugs that alter gastric emptying time (such as aluminum- and magnesium-containing antacids, atropine, narcotics), urine alkalinizers (such as high-dose antacids, carbonic anhydrase inhibitors, sodium): may delay mexiletine absorption. Monitor patient for drug effect.
Drugs that alter hepatic enzyme function, such as phenobarbital, phenytoin, rifampin: may induce hepatic metabolism of mexiletine and thus reduce serum drug levels. Monitor patient for effect.
Metoclopramide: increased mexiletine absorption. Monitor patient.
Theophylline: mexiletine may increase serum theophylline levels. Monitor theophylline levels.
Urine acidifiers, such as ammonium chloride: enhanced mexiletine excretion. Monitor patient.

Effects on diagnostic tests
None reported.

Adverse reactions
CNS: *blurred vision,* changes in sleep habits, *confusion,* depression, *diplopia, dizziness,* fatigue, *headache,* incoordination, light-headedness, *nervousness,* paresthesia, speech difficulties, tinnitus, *tremor,* weakness.
CV: angina, chest pain, ***new or worsened arrhythmias,*** nonspecific edema, palpitations.
GI: *abdominal pain, altered appetite, constipation, diarrhea, dry* mouth, heartburn, nausea, upper GI distress, vomiting.
Hepatic: transient elevation of liver enzymes.
Skin: rash.

Overdose and treatment
Overdose typically causes extensions of adverse CNS effects. Seizures are the most serious effect.

Treatment usually involves symptomatic and supportive measures. In acute overdose, emesis induction or gastric lavage should be performed. Urine acidification may accelerate drug elimination. If patient has bradycardia and hypotension, atropine may be given.

Special considerations
▶ Drug is used to treat life-threatening documented ventricular arrhythmias, including ventricular tachycardia.
▶ Drug is useful in treating neuropathic pain via sodium channel blockade.
▶ Dosage should be administered with meals, if possible.
▶ Monitor therapeutic levels as ordered. Levels range from 0.5 to 2 mcg/ml.
▶ Avoid administering drug within 1 hour of antacids that contain aluminum-magnesium hydroxide.
▶ Monitor blood pressure and heart rate and rhythm for significant change.
▶ Tremor, usually a fine hand tremor, is common in patients taking larger doses of mexiletine.
▶ Monitor patient for toxicity; one of the first signs is a fine hand tremor. This progresses to dizziness then ataxia and nystagmus.

▶ Because of proarrhythmic effects, drug isn't recommended for non-life-threatening arrhythmias.
▶ When changing from lidocaine to mexiletine, stop infusion when first mexiletine dose is given. Keep infusion line open, however, until arrhythmia appears to be satisfactorily controlled.
▶ Patients who aren't controlled by dosing every 8 hours may respond to dosing every 6 hours.
▶ Patients who respond well to mexiletine (300 mg or less every 8 hours) can be maintained on an every-12-hours schedule, with the same total daily dose, improving patient compliance.

Breast-feeding patients
▶ Drug appears in breast milk. Alternative feeding method should be used during therapy.

Geriatric patients
▶ Most elderly patients need reduced dosages because of reduced hepatic blood flow and therefore, decreased metabolism.
▶ Elderly patients may be more susceptible to adverse CNS effects.

Patient teaching
▶ Tell patient to take drug with food to reduce risk of nausea.
▶ Instruct patient to report unusual bleeding or bruising, signs of infection (such as fever, sore throat, stomatitis, or chills), or fatigue.

▶ midazolam hydrochloride
Versed

Pharmacologic classification:
benzodiazepine

Therapeutic classification:
adjunct for induction of general anesthesia, amnesic, drug for conscious sedation, preoperative sedative

Controlled substance schedule IV

Pregnancy risk category D

How supplied
Available by prescription only
Injection: 1 mg/ml in 2-ml, 5-ml, and 10-ml vials; 5 mg/ml in 1-ml, 2-ml, 5-ml, and 10-ml vials; 5 mg/ml in 2-ml disposable syringe
Syrup: 2 mg/ml in 118 ml bottle

Indications and dosages
Preoperative sedation to induce sleepiness or drowsiness and relieve apprehension
Adults under age 60: 0.07 to 0.08 mg/kg I.M. about 1 hour before surgery. May be administered with atropine or scopolamine and reduced doses of narcotics.
◪ Dosage adjustment. Reduce dosage in patients over age 60, patients with COPD, patients at high risk during surgery, and patients who have received concomitant narcotics or other depressants.
Conscious sedation
Adults under age 60: initially, 1 to 2.5 mg I.V. over at least 2 minutes; repeat after 2 minutes, if needed, up to a total dose of 5 mg. Added doses to maintain desired level of sedation may be given slowly in

---

increments of 25% of dose used to reach the sedation endpoint.

Adults age 60 and over: 1.5 mg or less over at least 2 minutes. If additional drug is needed, don't exceed 1 mg over 2 minutes. Total doses exceeding 3.5 mg aren't usually necessary.

Induction of general anesthesia
Unpremedicated adults under age 55: 0.3 to 0.35 mg/kg I.V. over 20 to 30 seconds if patient hasn't received preanesthesia medication. Give 0.2 to 0.25 mg/kg I.V. over 20 to 30 seconds if patient has received preanesthesia medication. Increments of 25% of the initial dose may be needed to complete induction.

Unpremedicated adults age 55 and over: initially, 0.3 mg/kg. For debilitated patients, initial dose is 0.2 to 0.25 mg/kg. For premedicated patients, 0.15 mg/kg may be sufficient.

Continuous infusion for sedation of intubated and mechanically ventilated patients as a component of anesthesia or during treatment in the critical care setting
Adults: If a loading dose is necessary to rapidly initiate sedation, give 0.01 to 0.05 mg/kg slowly or infused over several minutes, with dose repeated at 10- to 15-minute intervals until adequate sedation is achieved. For maintenance of sedation, usual infusion rate is 0.02 to 0.10 mg/kg/hour (1 to 7 mg/hour). Infusion rate should be titrated to the desired amount of sedation. Drug can be adjusted up or down by 25% to 50% of the initial infusion rate to achieve optimal sedation without oversedation.
Children: After a loading dose of 0.05 to 0.2 mg/kg over 2 to 3 min-

utes in intubated patients only, an infusion may be initiated at 0.06 to 0.12 mg/kg/hour (1 to 2 mcg/kg/minute). For optimal sedation, dose may be adjusted up or down by 25% of the initial or subsequent infusion rate.
Neonates: Use only on intubated neonates. No loading dose is used in neonates. Neonates less than 32 weeks old receive 0.03 mg/kg/hour (0.5 mcg/kg/minute). Neonates older than 32 weeks receive 0.06 mg/kg/hour (1 mcg/kg/minute). Infusion may be run more rapidly in the first few hours to obtain a therapeutic blood level. Rate of infusion should be frequently and carefully reassessed to administer the lowest possible amount of drug.

Sedation, anxiolysis, and amnesia before diagnostic, therapeutic or endoscopic procedures or before induction of anesthesia in children
Children (syrup only): Single dose 0.25 to 1 mg/kg P.O. Maximum, 20 mg/dose. Lower doses may provide adequate therapeutic effect for children ages 6 to 16 or cooperative patients.

Pharmacodynamics
Sedative and anesthetic actions: Like other benzodiazepines, midazolam probably facilitates the action of GABA in providing a short-acting CNS depressant action.
Amnesic action: Mechanism of action isn't known.

Pharmacokinetics
Absorption: Absorption after I.M. administration appears to be 80% to 100%; serum levels peak in 45 minutes and are about half of those

after I.V. administration. Sedation begins within 15 minutes after an I.M. dose and within 2 to 5 minutes after I.V. injection. After I.V. administration, induction of anesthesia occurs in 1½ to 2½ minutes. Following oral doses of syrup in children ages 6 months to 2 years, serum levels peak in 10 to 15 minutes; in children ages 2 to 12 years, level peaks in 45 to 60 minutes. Absorption is slower, and peak levels lower, after oral doses of syrup in children ages 12 to 16 years.

Distribution: Drug has a large volume of distribution and is about 97% protein-bound. It crosses the placenta and enters fetal circulation.

Metabolism: Midazolam is metabolized in the liver.

Excretion: Metabolites of midazolam are excreted in urine. Half-life of drug is 2 to 6 hours. Duration of sedation is usually 1 to 4 hours.

Contraindications and precautions

Contraindicated in patients hypersensitive to drug and those with acute angle-closure glaucoma, shock, coma, or acute alcohol intoxication.

Use cautiously in patients with uncompensated acute illnesses and in elderly or debilitated patients.

Interactions
Drug-drug
CNS and respiratory depressants, such as antidepressants, antihistamines, barbiturates, narcotics, tranquilizers: potentiated effects. Monitor patient closely.

Droperidol, fentanyl, narcotics used before surgery: potentiated hypnotic effects of midazolam. Monitor patient closely.

Erythromycin: may decrease plasma midazolam clearance. Monitor patient for increased effects.

Inhaled anesthetics: midazolam may decrease the needed dose of inhaled anesthetics by depressing respiratory drive. Monitor patient closely.

Isoniazid: may decrease midazolam metabolism. Monitor patient for increased effects.

Drug-lifestyle
Alcohol use: potentiated effects of alcohol. Avoid use together.

Effects on diagnostic tests
None reported.

Adverse reactions
CNS: amnesia, drowsiness, headache, oversedation.

CV: *cardiac arrest,* variations in blood pressure (hypotension) and pulse rate.

GI: *nausea,* vomiting.

Respiratory: *apnea, decreased respiratory rate,* hiccups, *respiratory arrest.*

Other: *pain, tenderness at injection site.*

Overdose and treatment
Overdose may cause confusion, stupor, coma, respiratory depression, and hypotension.

Treatment is supportive and includes maintaining patient's airway and ensuring adequate ventilation with mechanical support, if necessary. Monitor vital signs. Give I.V. fluids or ephedrine for hypotension. Flumazenil, a specific benzodiazepine-receptor antagonist, is indicated for complete or partial reversal of the sedative effects.

Special considerations

▶ Laryngospasm and broncho-spasm rarely occur; keep counter-measures readily available.
▶ Anyone who administers mida-zolam must be familiar with air-way management and be able to closely monitor cardiopulmonary function. Continuously monitor patients who have received mida-zolam to detect potentially life-threatening respiratory depression.
▶ When preparing infusion, use 5 mg/ml vial and dilute to 0.5 mg/ml with D_5W or normal saline solution.
▶ Don't use solution that's discolored or contains a precipitate.
▶ Before I.V. administration, ensure the immediate availability of oxygen and resuscitative equipment. Apnea and death have been reported with rapid I.V. administration. Avoid intra-arterial injection because the hazards of this route are unknown. Avoid extravasation.
▶ Administer I.V. dose slowly over at least 2 minutes; wait at least 2 minutes when adjusting doses to effect.
▶ Solutions of D_5W, normal saline solution, and lactated Ringer's solution are compatible with midazolam.
▶ Administer I.M. dose deep into a large muscle mass to prevent tissue injury.
▶ Individualize dosage; use smallest effective dose possible.
▶ Syrup form must be given only to patients visually monitored by a health care professional.
▶ Midazolam can be mixed in the same syringe with morphine, meperidine, atropine, and scopolamine.

▶ Hypotension occurs more frequently in patients premedicated with narcotics. Monitor vital signs.

Breast-feeding patients

▶ It isn't known whether drug passes into breast milk; use with caution in breast-feeding women.

Pediatric patients

▶ Safety and efficacy haven't been established in children for nonoral dose forms.
▶ Consider the amount of benzyl alcohol when giving high dose of drug to a neonate because of increased risk of hypotension, metabolic acidosis, and kernicterus.

Geriatric patients

▶ Elderly or debilitated patients, especially those with COPD, are at significantly increased risk for respiratory depression and hypotension. Use smallest dose possible Use with great caution. Oral forms aren't recommended.

Patient teaching

▶ Caution patient to avoid hazardous activities until drug's effects have worn off.
▶ Instruct patient as necessary in safety measures, such as assisted walking and gradual position changes, to prevent injury.
▶ Tell patient to consult prescriber before taking OTC medications.

Reactions may be *common*, uncommon, *life-threatening*, or COMMON AND LIFE-THREATENING.

▶ mineral oil
Fleet Mineral Oil, Fleet Mineral Oil Enema, Kondremul◇, Kondremul Plain, Lansoÿl◇, Milkinol, Neo-Cultol, Nujol◇, Petrogalar Plain

Pharmacologic classification: *lubricant oil*

Therapeutic classification: *laxative*

Pregnancy risk category C

How supplied
Available without a prescription
Emulsion: 2.5 ml/5 ml, 1.4 g/5 ml
Jelly: 180 ml
Rectal oil enema: 120 ml
Suspension: 1.4 ml/5 ml, 2.75 ml/5 ml, 4.75 ml/5 ml

Indications and dosages
Constipation, preparation for bowel studies or surgery
Adults and children age 12 and older: 5 to 45 ml P.O. as a single dose or in divided doses, or 120-ml enema.
Children ages 6 to 11: 5 to 15 ml P.O. daily as a single dose or in divided doses, or 30- to 60-ml enema.
Children ages 2 to 5: 30- to 60-ml enema.

Pharmacodynamics
Laxative action: Mineral oil acts mainly in the colon, lubricating the intestine and retarding colonic fluid absorption.

Pharmacokinetics
Absorption: Mineral oil normally is absorbed minimally; with emulsified drug form, significant absorption occurs. Action begins in 6 to 8 hours.
Distribution: Mineral oil is distributed locally, primarily in the colon.
Metabolism: None.
Excretion: Mineral oil is excreted in feces.

Contraindications and precautions
Contraindicated in patients with abdominal pain, nausea, vomiting, or other symptoms of appendicitis or acute surgical abdomen and in those with fecal impaction or intestinal obstruction or perforation. Also contraindicated in patients with colostomy, ileostomy, ulcerative colitis, and diverticulitis.

Use cautiously in elderly, debilitated, and young patients.

Interactions
Drug-drug
Anticoagulants, cardiac glycosides, fat-soluble vitamins (A, D, E, and K), oral contraceptives, sulfonamides: impaired absorption. Monitor patient for decreased drug effects.
Stool softeners, such as docusate: increased mineral oil absorption to potentially toxic levels. Avoid use together.

Effects on diagnostic tests
None reported.

Adverse reactions
GI: abdominal cramps (especially in severe constipation), anal irritation, anal pruritus, decreased absorption of nutrients and fat-soluble vitamins (resulting in deficiency), *diarrhea* (with excessive use), hemorrhoids, *nausea,* perianal discomfort, slowed healing after hemorrhoidectomy, *vomiting.*

Respiratory: *lipid pneumonia.*
Other: laxative dependence with long-term or excessive use.

Overdose and treatment
No information available.

Special considerations
▶ Before giving drug for constipation, determine whether patient has adequate fluid intake, exercise, and diet.
▶ Avoid administering drug to patients lying flat; drug may aspirate into the lungs, and pneumonitis may result.
▶ Don't give drug with food because doing so may delay gastric emptying, resulting in delayed drug action and increased aspiration risk. Separate by at least 2 hours.
▶ To improve taste, give emulsion and suspension with fruit juice or carbonated beverages.
▶ Administer cleansing enema 30 minutes to 1 hour after retention enema.
▶ Reduce or divide dose or use emulsified drug to avoid leakage through anal sphincter.

Pediatric patients
▶ Mineral oil isn't recommended for children under age 6 because of risk of aspiration.
▶ Enema form is contraindicated in children under age 2.

Geriatric patients
▶ Because of increased aspiration risk, use caution when administering drug to elderly patients.

Patient teaching
▶ Instruct patient not to take mineral oil with stool softeners.
▶ Warn patient that mineral oil may leak through anal sphincter, especially with repeated use or with enema form. Undergarment protection may be desired.

▶ **misoprostol**
Cytotec

Pharmacologic classification: *prostaglandin E analogue*

Therapeutic classification: *antiulcer drug, gastric mucosal protectant*

Pregnancy risk category X

How supplied
Available by prescription only
Tablets: 100 mcg, 200 mcg

Indications and dosages
Prevention of NSAID-induced gastric ulcer
Adults: 200 mcg P.O. q.i.d with meals and h.s. Reduce dosage to 100 mcg P.O. q.i.d. in patients who can't tolerate this dosage.
Duodenal or gastric ulcer
Adults: 100 to 200 mcg P.O. q.i.d. with meals and h.s.

Pharmacodynamics
Antiulcer action: Drug enhances the production of gastric mucus and bicarbonate, and it decreases basal, nocturnal, and stimulated gastric acid secretion.

Pharmacokinetics
Absorption: Drug is rapidly absorbed after oral administration.
Distribution: Drug is less than 90% bound to plasma proteins. Levels peak in about 12 minutes.
Metabolism: Drug is rapidly de-esterified to misoprostol acid, the biologically active metabolite. The de-

esterified metabolite undergoes further oxidation in several body tissues.
Excretion: About 15% of an oral dose appears in feces; the balance is excreted in urine. Terminal half-life is 20 to 40 minutes.

Contraindications and precautions
Contraindicated in pregnant and breast-feeding patients and in those allergic to prostaglandins.

Interactions
Drug-drug
Antacids: decreased misoprostol levels. Monitor patient.
Aspirin: decreased aspirin availability. Monitor patient.

Drug-food
Food: reduces drug levels, but probably has no significant effect.

Effects on diagnostic tests
Misoprostol modestly decreases basal pepsin secretion.

Adverse reactions
CNS: headache.
GI: *abdominal pain, constipation, diarrhea, dyspepsia, flatulence, nausea, vomiting.*
GU: cramps, dysmenorrhea, hypermenorrhea, menstrual disorders, spotting.

Overdose and treatment
There's been little clinical experience with overdose. Cumulative daily doses of 1,600 mcg have been administered, with only minor GI discomfort noted. Treatment should be supportive.

Special considerations
▶ Drug is also used to prevent acute graft rejection in renal transplantation.
▶ Drug has been used for treatment and prophylaxis of reflux esophagitis, alcohol-induced gastritis, hemorrhagic gastritis, and fat malabsorption in cystic fibrosis.
▶ Diarrhea is usually dose-related and develops within the first 2 weeks of therapy. It can be minimized by administering the drug after meals and at bedtime, by avoiding magnesium-containing antacids.
▶ Starting treatment at a lower dose may minimize adverse effects.
▶ Misoprostol shouldn't be prescribed for a woman of childbearing age unless she needs NSAID therapy, is at high risk of developing gastric ulcers, is capable of complying with effective contraception, has received both oral and written warnings regarding the hazards of misoprostol therapy, has had a negative serum pregnancy test within 2 weeks before beginning therapy, and will begin therapy on the second or third day of her next normal menstrual period.

Breast-feeding patients
▶ Breast-feeding isn't recommended because of potential for drug-induced diarrhea in infant.

Pediatric patients
▶ Safety hasn't been established in children under age 18.

Patient teaching
▶ Explain importance of not giving drug to anyone else.
▶ Make sure patient understands that a miscarriage could result if drug is taken by a pregnant woman.

▶ morphine sulfate
**Astramorph PF, Duramorph,
Epimorph◇, Infumorph, MS
Contin, MSIR, MS/L, MS/S, OMS
Concentrate, Oramorph SR, RMS
Uniserts, Roxanol, Statex◇**

Pharmacologic classification:
opioid

Therapeutic classification:
narcotic analgesic

Controlled substance schedule II

Pregnancy risk category C

How supplied
Available by prescription only
Injection (with preservative):
1 mg/ml, 2 mg/ml, 3 mg/ml, 4 mg/
ml, 5 mg/ml, 8 mg/ml, 10 mg/ml,
15 mg/ml, 25 mg/ml, 50 mg/ml
Injection (without preservative):
500 mcg/ml, 1 mg/ml, 10 mg/ml,
25 mg/ml
Oral solution: 4 mg/ml, 10 mg/
5 ml, 20 mg/5 ml, 20 mg/ml,
100 mg/5 ml
Suppositories: 5 mg, 10 mg, 20 mg,
30 mg
Tablets: 15 mg, 30 mg
Tablets (extended-release): 15 mg,
30 mg, 60 mg, 100 mg, 200 mg
Tablets (soluble): 10 mg, 15 mg,
30 mg

Indications and dosages
Severe pain
Adults: 10 mg q 4 hours S.C. or
I.M., or 10 to 30 mg P.O., or 10 to
20 mg P.R. q 4 hours, p.r.n., or
around the clock. May be injected
slow I.V. (over 4 to 5 minutes) 2.5
to 15 mg diluted in 4 to 5 ml water.
Administer controlled-release
tablets 30 mg q 8 to 12 hours or as

an epidural injection, 5 mg via an
epidural catheter q 24 hours.
Children: 0.1 to 0.2 mg/kg S.C. q
4 hours. Maximum dose is 15 mg.
Drug may be administered by con-
tinuous I.V. infusion or by intra-
spinal and intrathecal injection.
*Preoperative sedation and adjunct
to anesthesia*
Adults: 8 to 10 mg I.M., S.C., or
I.V.
Pain from acute MI
Adults: 8 to 15 mg I.M., S.C., or
I.V. Additional, smaller doses may
be given at 3- to 4-hour intervals,
p.r.n.
*Adjunctive treatment of acute pul-
monary edema*
Adults: 10 to 15 mg I.V. at no more
than 2 mg/minute.

Pharmacodynamics
Analgesic action: Morphine is the
principal opium alkaloid, the
standard for opiate agonist analgesic activity. Mechanism of action is thought to be via the opiate receptors, altering patient's
perception of pain. Drug is particularly useful in severe, acute
pain or severe, chronic pain and
also has a central depressant effect on respiration and on the
cough reflex center.

Pharmacokinetics
Absorption: Variable absorption
from the GI tract. Analgesia peaks
within 60 minutes.
Distribution: Morphine is distributed widely throughout the body.
Metabolism: Drug is metabolized
primarily in the liver. One metabolite, morphine 6-glucuromide, is
active.
Excretion: Duration of action is 3
to 7 hours. Morphine is excreted

in urine and bile. Morphine 6-glucuromide may accumulate after continuous dosing in patients with renal failure, leading to enhanced, prolonged opiate activity.

Contraindications and precautions
Contraindicated in patients with hypersensitivity to drug or conditions that would preclude administration of opioids by I.V. route (acute bronchial asthma or upper airway obstruction).

Use cautiously in elderly or debilitated patients and in those with head injury, increased intracranial pressure, seizures, pulmonary disease, prostatic hyperplasia, hepatic or renal disease, acute abdominal conditions, hypothyroidism, Addison's disease, or urethral strictures.

Interactions
Drug-drug
Anticholinergics: increased risk of paralytic ileus. Monitor patient for abdominal pain.
Cimetidine: increased respiratory and CNS depression, causing confusion, disorientation, apnea, or seizures. Reduced dosage of morphine is usually necessary.
CNS depressants, such as antihistamines, barbiturates, benzodiazepines, general anesthetics, MAO inhibitors, muscle relaxants, opioid analgesics, phenothiazines, sedative-hypnotics, tricyclic antidepressants: potentiated respiratory and CNS depression, sedation, and hypotensive effects. Monitor patient closely.
General anesthetics: increased risk of severe CV depression. Monitor patient closely.

Narcotic antagonists: patients who become physically dependent on this drug may experience acute withdrawal syndrome if given a narcotic antagonist. Avoid using together.

Drug-lifestyle
Alcohol use: potentiated respiratory and CNS depressive, sedative, and hypotensive effects. Advise against concurrent use.

Effects on diagnostic tests
None reported.

Adverse reactions
CNS: depression, *dizziness,* hallucinations, light-headedness, *sedation, somnolence, clouded sensorium, euphoria,* nervousness, *nightmares (with long-acting oral forms),* **seizures** (with large doses), syncope.
CV: *bradycardia, cardiac arrest,* hypertension, *hypotension,* **shock,** tachycardia.
GI: *anorexia, biliary tract spasms, constipation, dry mouth, ileus, nausea, vomiting.*
GU: *decreased libido, urine retention.*
Hematologic: *thrombocytopenia.*
Metabolic: increased plasma amylase levels.
Respiratory: *apnea, respiratory arrest, respiratory depression.*
Skin: *diaphoresis, edema,* pruritus, skin flushing (with epidural administration).
Other: *physical dependence.*

Overdose and treatment
Rapid I.V. administration may result in overdose because of the delay in maximum CNS effect (30 minutes). The most common signs

and symptoms of morphine overdose are miosis (pinpoint pupils) and respiratory depression with or without CNS depression. Other acute toxic effects include hypotension, bradycardia, hypothermia, shock, apnea, cardiopulmonary arrest, circulatory collapse, pulmonary edema, and seizures.

To treat acute overdose, establish adequate respiration via a patent airway and ventilate, as needed; administer a narcotic antagonist such as naloxone to reverse respiratory depression. Because duration of action of morphine is longer than that of naloxone, repeated naloxone doses are necessary. Give naloxone only if patient has clinically significant respiratory or CV depression. Monitor vital signs closely.

If patient presents within 2 hours of ingestion of an oral overdose, empty the stomach immediately by inducing emesis with ipecac syrup or using gastric lavage. Use caution to minimize risk of aspiration. Administer activated charcoal via nasogastric tube for further removal of drug in an oral overdose.

Provide symptomatic and supportive treatment, including continued respiratory support and correction of fluid or electrolyte imbalance. Monitor laboratory values, vital signs, and neurologic status closely.

Special considerations

▶ When administering drug, use a pain scale and assess patient after giving drug.
▶ Morphine is drug of choice in relieving pain of MI; it may cause transient decrease in blood pressure.
▶ Regimented (around-the-clock) scheduling or use of long-acting form is beneficial in severe, chronic pain.
▶ Use immediate-release form for breakthrough pain.
▶ Oral solutions of varied strengths are available, including an intensified oral solution.
▶ Note the disparity between oral and parenteral doses.
▶ When given by direct injection, 2.5 to 15 mg may be diluted in 4 or 5 ml of sterile water and given over 4 to 5 mintes. Alternatively, drug may be mixed with D_5W to 0.1 to 1 mg/ml and administered by continuous infusion device. Morphine sulfate is compatible with most common I.V. solutions.
▶ For S.L. administration, measure out oral solution with tuberculin syringe and administer dose a few drops at a time to allow maximal S.L. absorption and minimize swallowing.
▶ Use rectal form for confused or sedated patients.
▶ Refrigeration of rectal suppositories isn't necessary.
▶ In some patients, rectal and oral absorption may not be equivalent.
▶ Epidural morphine has proven to be an excellent analgesic for patients with postoperative pain.
▶ After epidural injection, monitor patient closely for respiratory depression for up to 24 hours. Check respiratory rate and depth according to protocol (for example, every 15 minutes for 2 hours, and then hourly for 18 hours). Some clinicians advocate a dilute naloxone infusion (5 to 10 mcg/kg/hour) during the first 12 hours to mini-

mize respiratory depression without altering pain relief.
▶ Monitor circulatory, respiratory, bladder and bowel functions carefully.
▶ Some morphine injections contain sulfites that may cause allergic-type reactions.
▶ Preservative-free preparations are now available for epidural and intrathecal administration. The use of the epidural route is increasing.
▶ Give antipruritic drugs to reduce adverse effects.
▶ Morphine may worsen or mask gallbladder pain.
▶ Long-term therapy in patients with advanced renal disease may lead to toxicity from accumulation of the active metabolite.

Breast-feeding patients
▶ Morphine appears in breast milk. To avoid sedating the infant, wait 2 to 3 hours after last dose before breast-feeding.

Geriatric patients
▶ Lower doses are usually indicated for elderly patients, who may be more sensitive to drug effects.

Patient teaching
▶ Tell patient that oral liquid form of morphine may be mixed with fruit juice immediately before taking it to improve taste.
▶ If patient takes long-acting morphine tablets, instruct her to swallow them whole. Tablets shouldn't be broken, crushed, or chewed before swallowing.

▶ **nabumetone**
Relafen

Pharmacologic classification:
NSAID

Therapeutic classification:
antiarthritic

Pregnancy risk category C

How supplied
Available by prescription only
Tablets: 500 mg, 750 mg

Indications and dosages
Acute or chronic rheumatoid arthritis or osteoarthritis
Adults: initially, 1,000 mg/day P.O. as a single dose or in divided doses b.i.d. Adjust dosage based on patient response. Maximum, 2,000 mg/day.

Pharmacodynamics
Anti-inflammatory action: Drug probably acts by inhibiting the synthesis of prostaglandins. Drug also has analgesic and antipyretic action.

Pharmacokinetics
Absorption: Drug is well absorbed from the GI tract. After absorption, about 35% is rapidly transformed to 6-methoxy-2-naphthylacetic acid (6MNA), the principal active metabolite; the balance is transformed to unidentified metabolites. Administration with food increases the absorption rate and peak levels of 6MNA but does not change total drug absorbed. Levels peak in 2 to 4 hours.
Distribution: 6MNA is more than 99% bound to plasma proteins.

Metabolism: 6MNA is metabolized to inactive metabolites in the liver.

Excretion: Drug's metabolites are excreted primarily in urine. About 9% appears in feces. Elimination half-life is about 24 hours. Half-life is increased in patients with renal failure.

Contraindications and precautions

Contraindicated in patients with hypersensitivity reactions, history of aspirin- or NSAID-induced asthma, urticaria, other allergic-type reactions, and during the third trimester of pregnancy.

Use cautiously in patients with impaired renal or hepatic function, heart failure, hypertension, conditions that predispose to fluid retention, and history of peptic ulcer disease.

Interactions
Drug-drug

Drugs that are highly bound to plasma proteins, such as warfarin: increased risk of adverse reactions because nabumetone may displace drug. Use together with caution.

Effects on diagnostic tests
None reported.

Adverse reactions

CNS: *dizziness,* fatigue, *headache,* insomnia, nervousness, somnolence.
CV: edema, vasculitis.
EENT: *tinnitus.*
GI: *abdominal pain,* anorexia, *bleeding, constipation, diarrhea,* dry mouth, *dyspepsia, flatulence,* gastritis, *nausea,* stomatitis, ulceration, vomiting.

Respiratory: dyspnea, pneumonitis.
Skin: increased diaphoresis, *pruritus, rash.*

Overdose and treatment
After an accidental overdose, induce emesis or perform gastric lavage. Activated charcoal may limit the amount of drug absorbed.

Special considerations
▶ Drug may be used for other types of mild to moderate pain.
▶ Adjust dosage according to patient response.
▶ Drug may be given with antacids to reduce adverse GI effects.
▶ Use the lowest effective dose for long-term treatment.
▶ During long-term therapy, periodically monitor renal and liver function, CBC, and hematocrit. Monitor patient carefully for signs and symptoms of NSAID-induced ulcers and GI bleeding.
▶ Because NSAIDs impair the synthesis of renal prostaglandins, they can decrease renal blood flow and lead to reversible renal function impairment, especially in patients with preexisting renal failure, liver dysfunction, and heart failure; in elderly patients; and in those taking diuretics. Monitor these patients closely during therapy.

Breast-feeding patients
▶ The active metabolite of nabumetone, 6MNA, has been found in the milk of laboratory rats. Because of risk of serious toxicity to the infant, use in breast-feeding women is not recommended.

Pediatric patients
▶ Safety and efficacy haven't been established.

Geriatric patients
▶ No differences in safety or efficacy have been noted in elderly patients.

Patient teaching
▶ Tell patient to take drug with food, milk, or antacids to enhance drug absorption and avoid adverse GI effects.
▶ Stress the importance of follow-up examinations to detect adverse GI effects.
▶ Teach patient the signs and symptoms of GI bleeding, and tell him to report them immediately.
▶ Advise patient to limit alcohol intake because of risk of additive GI toxicity.

▶ nadolol
Corgard

Pharmacologic classification: *beta blocker*

Therapeutic classification: *antianginal, antihypertensive*

Pregnancy risk category C

How supplied
Available by prescription only
Tablets: 20 mg, 40 mg, 80 mg, 120 mg, 160 mg

Indications and dosages
Long-term prophylaxis of chronic stable angina
Adults: initially, 40 mg P.O. once daily. Dosage may be increased in 40- to 80-mg increments daily at 3- to 7-day intervals until optimum response occurs. Usual maintenance dosage is 40 or 80 mg once daily. Doses of up to 160 or 240 mg daily may be needed.
Prophylaxis of vascular headache*
Adults: 20 to 40 mg once daily; may gradually increase to 120 mg daily if necessary.

◻ DOSAGE ADJUSTMENT. Adjust dosage for patients with renal impairment. If creatinine clearance is 31 to 50 ml/min, give usual dose q 24 to 36 hours. If it's 10 to 30 ml/min, give usual dose q 24 to 48 hours. If it's below 10 ml/min, give usual dose q 40 to 60 hours.

Pharmacodynamics
Antianginal action: Nadolol decreases myocardial oxygen consumption, thus relieving angina, by blocking catecholamine-induced increases in heart rate, myocardial contraction, and blood pressure.
Antihypertensive action: Unknown. Drug may reduce blood pressure by blocking adrenergic receptors, thus decreasing cardiac output, by decreasing sympathetic outflow from the CNS, or by suppressing renin release.

Pharmacokinetics
Absorption: 30% to 40% of a dose of nadolol is absorbed from the GI tract; peak plasma levels occur in 2 to 4 hours. Absorption is not affected by food.
Distribution: Nadolol is distributed throughout the body; drug is about 30% protein-bound.
Metabolism: Drug isn't metabolized.
Excretion: Most of a given dose is excreted unchanged in urine; the remainder is excreted in feces. Plasma half-life is about 20 hours.

Antihypertensive and antianginal effects persist for about 24 hours.

Contraindications and precautions

Contraindicated in patients with bronchial asthma, sinus bradycardia and greater than first-degree heart block, and cardiogenic shock.

Use cautiously in patients with hyperthyroidism, heart failure, diabetes, chronic bronchitis, emphysema, and impaired renal or hepatic function and in those receiving general anesthesia before undergoing surgery.

Interactions
Drug-drug

Antiarrhythmics: may have additive or antagonistic cardiac effects and additive toxic effects. Monitor patient closely.

Antihypertensives, including diuretics: nadolol may potentiate antihypertensive effects of these drugs. Monitor blood pressure.

Antimuscarinics, such as atropine: may antagonize nadolol-induced bradycardia. Monitor heart rate.

Epinephrine: may cause a decrease in pulse rate with first- and second-degree heart block and hypertension. Monitor patient closely if used together.

Sympathomimetics, such as isoproterenol: nadolol may antagonize beta-adrenergic stimulating effects of these drugs. Monitor patient closely.

Tubocurarine and related drugs: may potentiate the neuromuscular blocking effect of these drugs at high doses. Monitor patient closely.

Drug-lifestyle

Cocaine: may inhibit therapeutic effects of nadolol. Discourage concurrent use.

Effects on diagnostic tests

None reported.

Adverse reactions

CNS: dizziness, fatigue.
CV: ***bradycardia, heart failure, hypotension,*** peripheral vascular disease, rhythm and conduction disturbances.
GI: abdominal pain, anorexia, constipation, diarrhea, nausea, vomiting.
Respiratory: ***increased airway resistance.***
Skin: rash.
Other: fever.

Overdose and treatment

Overdose may cause severe hypotension, bradycardia, heart failure, and bronchospasm.

After acute ingestion, empty stomach by induced emesis or gastric lavage and give activated charcoal to reduce absorption. Magnesium sulfate may be given orally as a cathartic. Subsequent treatment is usually symptomatic and supportive.

Special considerations

▶ Drug is also used to treat hypertension and arrhythmias.
▶ Individual dose adjustment may be necessary for migraine prophylaxis.
▶ Monitor patient's blood pressure during dosage adjustments.
▶ Monitor renal function during long-term therapy.
▶ Dosage adjustments may be necessary in patients with renal impairment.

▶ After long-term therapy, gradually decrease dose over 1 to 2 weeks before discontinuing drug. Abrupt withdrawal can exacerbate angina and cause an MI.

▶ Drug may mask signs of hyperthyroidism and hypoglycemia.

Breast-feeding patients

▶ Drug appears in breast milk; an alternative feeding method is recommended during therapy.

Pediatric patients

▶ Safety and efficacy in children haven't been established; use only if potential benefit outweighs risk.

Geriatric patients

▶ Elderly patients may require lower maintenance dosages of nadolol because of increased bioavailability or delayed metabolism; they also may experience enhanced adverse effects.

Patient teaching

▶ Tell patient not to discontinue nadolol abruptly. Drug should be tapered.

▶ **nalbuphine hydrochloride**
Nubain

Pharmacologic classification:
narcotic agonist-antagonist, opioid partial agonist

Therapeutic classification:
adjunct to anesthesia, analgesic

Pregnancy risk category NR

How supplied

Available by prescription only
Injection: 10 mg/ml, 20 mg/ml

Indications and dosages

Moderate to severe pain
Adults: 10 to 20 mg S.C., I.M., or I.V. q 3 to 6 hours, p.r.n., or around the clock. Maximum, 160 mg/day.
Supplement to anesthesia
Adults: 0.3 mg/kg to 3 mg/kg I.V. over 10 to 15 minutes. Maintenance, 0.25 to 0.5 mg/kg I.V.

Pharmacodynamics

Analgesic action: Analgesia is believed to result from drug's action at opiate receptor sites in the CNS, relieving moderate to severe pain. The narcotic antagonist effect may result from competitive inhibition at opiate receptors. Like other opioids, nalbuphine causes respiratory depression, sedation, and miosis. In patients with coronary artery disease or MI, it appears to produce no substantial changes in heart rate, pulmonary artery or wedge pressure, left ventricular end-diastolic pressure, pulmonary vascular resistance, or cardiac index.

Pharmacokinetics

Absorption: When administered orally, drug is about one-fifth as effective as an analgesic as it is when given I.M., apparently because of first-pass metabolism in the GI tract and liver. Action starts within 15 minutes and peaks in 30 minutes.
Distribution: Drug isn't appreciably bound to plasma proteins.
Metabolism: Drug is metabolized in the liver.
Excretion: Drug is excreted in urine and to some degree in bile. Duration of action is 3 to 6 hours.

Contraindications and precautions

Contraindicated in patients hypersensitive to drug.

Use cautiously in patients with history of drug abuse, emotional instability, head injury, increased intracranial pressure, impaired ventilation, MI accompanied by nausea and vomiting, upcoming biliary surgery, and hepatic or renal disease.

Interactions
Drug-drug
Barbiturate anesthetics, such as thiopental: additive CNS and respiratory depressant effects and, possible apnea. Use together cautiously.
Cimetidine: may increase narcotic nalbuphine toxicity, causing disorientation, respiratory depression, apnea, and seizures. Be prepared to administer a narcotic antagonist if toxicity occurs.
CNS depressants, such as antihistamines, barbiturates, benzodiazepines, muscle relaxants, narcotic analgesics, phenothiazines, sedative-hypnotics, tricyclic antidepressants: potentiated respiratory and CNS depression, sedation, and hypotensive effects. Reduced doses of nalbuphine are usually necessary.
Drugs extensively metabolized in the liver, such as digitoxin, phenytoin, rifampin: drug accumulation and enhanced effects may result. Monitor for toxicity.
General anesthetics: may cause severe CV depression. Monitor patient closely.
Narcotic antagonists: acute withdrawal syndrome if physically dependent patient receives high doses of narcotic antagonist. Use with caution, and monitor patient closely.

Drug-lifestyle
Alcohol use: potentiated effects. Advise against concurrent use.

Effects on diagnostic tests
Drug may interfere with enzyme tests for detection of opioids.

Adverse reactions
CNS: confusion, crying, depression, delusions, *dizziness,* euphoria, hallucinations, *headache,* hostility, nervousness, restlessness, *sedation,* speech difficulty, *vertigo,* unusual dreams.
CV: *bradycardia,* hypertension, hypotension, tachycardia.
EENT: blurred vision, *dry mouth.*
GI: biliary tract spasms, bitter taste, constipation, cramps, dyspepsia, *nausea, vomiting.*
GU: urinary urgency.
Respiratory: *asthma,* dyspnea, ***pulmonary edema*, *respiratory depression.***
Skin: burning, *clamminess,* pruritus, urticaria.

Overdose and treatment
Overdose typically causes CNS depression, respiratory depression, and miosis. It also may cause hypotension, bradycardia, hypothermia, shock, apnea, cardiopulmonary arrest, circulatory collapse, pulmonary edema, and seizures.

To treat acute overdose, establish adequate respiratory exchange via a patent airway and ventilation as needed; administer a narcotic antagonist such as naloxone, to reverse respiratory depression. Because the duration of action of nalbuphine is longer than that of naloxone, repeated naloxone dosing is necessary. Naloxone shouldn't be given in the absence of clinically significant respiratory or CV depression. Monitor vital signs closely.

Provide symptomatic and supportive treatment, such as continued respiratory support and correction of fluid or electrolyte imbalance. Monitor laboratory values, vital signs, and neurologic status closely.

Special considerations
▶ Drug also acts as a narcotic antagonist; it may precipitate abstinence syndrome in narcotic-dependent patients.
▶ Parenteral administration provides better analgesia than oral administration. Give I.V. doses by slow I.V. injection over at least 2 minutes into a vein or free-flowing I.V. solution, such as D_5W, normal saline solution, or lactated Ringer's solution. Rapid I.V. injection increases the risk of adverse effects.
▶ Before administration, inspect parenteral products for particulate matter and discoloration.
▶ Drug causes respiratory depression, which at 10 mg is equal to the respiratory depression produced by 10 mg of morphine.
▶ Monitor circulatory and respiratory status and bladder and bowel function.
▶ Constipation is commonly severe in maintenance therapy. Make sure stool softener or other laxative is ordered.
▶ Drug may cause orthostatic hypotension in ambulatory patients.
▶ Respiratory depression can be reversed with naloxone. Keep resuscitation equipment available, particularly during I.V. administration.
▶ Nalbuphine may obscure evidence of acute abdominal conditions or may worsen gallbladder pain.

Pregnant patients
▶ When drug is used during labor and delivery, watch for signs of respiratory depression in neonate.

Breast-feeding patients
▶ No data exist to demonstrate whether drug appears in breast milk; it should be used with caution in breast-feeding women.

Pediatric patients
▶ Safety in children under age 18 hasn't been established.

Geriatric patients
▶ Lower doses are usually indicated for elderly patients, who may be more sensitive to drug effects.

Patient teaching
▶ Instruct patient to avoid hazardous activities because drug may cause dizziness and fatigue.

▶ nalmefene hydrochloride
Revex

Pharmacologic classification:
opioid antagonist

Therapeutic classification:
narcotic antagonist

Pregnancy risk category B

How supplied
Available by prescription only
Injection: 100 mcg/ml, 1 mg/ml

Indications and dosages
Reversal of postoperative opioid effects
Adults: 100 mcg/ml dosage strength started at 0.25 mcg/kg I.V. and followed by 0.25-mcg/kg incremental doses at 2- to 5-minute intervals as needed. A cumulative total dose above 1 mcg/kg doesn't provide additional therapeutic effect.

Opioid overdose
Adults: 1 mg/ml dosage strength started at 0.5 mg/70 kg I.V. and followed by 1 mg/70 kg in 2 to 5 minutes if needed.

Pharmacodynamics
Opioid antagonist action: Drug blocks opioid receptors and thereby prevents or reverses the effects of opioids, including respiratory depression, sedation, and hypotension.

Pharmacokinetics
Absorption: Nalmefene is completely absorbed after I.M. or S.C. administration.
Distribution: Nalmefene is widely distributed and is about 45% bound to plasma protein.
Metabolism: Nalmefene is metabolized in the liver.
Excretion: Nalmefene is excreted in urine.

Contraindications and precautions
Contraindicated in patients hypersensitive to drug. Use with extreme caution in patients with known physical dependence on opioids or following surgery involving high doses of opioids.

Use cautiously in patients with CV, hepatic, or renal disease and in those who are receiving potentially cardiotoxic drugs.

Interactions
None known.

Effects on diagnostic tests
None reported.

Adverse reactions
CNS: agitation, confusion, depression, dizziness, headache, myo-clonus, nervousness, tremor, somnolence, withdrawal syndrome.
CV: *arrhythmias*, *bradycardia*, hypertension, hypotension, tachycardia, vasodilation.
GI: diarrhea, dry mouth, nausea, vomiting.
GU: urine retention.
Skin: pruritus.
Other: chills, fever, postoperative pain.

Overdose and treatment
Overdose in the absence of opioid agonists produces no serious adverse reactions. Overdose in patients physically dependent on opioids can cause withdrawal reactions that require medical attention.

Treatment of such patients should be symptomatic and supportive. Administration of large amounts of opioids in patients receiving opioid antagonists in an attempt to overcome a full blockade has resulted in adverse respiratory and circulatory reactions.

Special considerations
▶ Excessive doses of opioid antagonists in the postoperative setting have been associated with hypertension, tachycardia, and excessive mortality in patients at high risk for CV complications.
▶ Nalmefene may not completely reverse buprenorphine-induced respiratory depression.
▶ In postoperative cases where the patient is known to be at increased CV risk, drug can be diluted 1:1 with saline solution or sterile water and smaller initial and incremental doses of 0.1 mcg/kg used.
▶ Patients with renal failure may require incremental doses to be given slowly (over 60 seconds) to

minimize the hypertension and dizziness reported following the abrupt administration of the drug to such patients.

▶ If drug can't be administered I.V., a single 1-mg dose may produce therapeutic results within 15 minutes if administered I.M. or S.C.

▶ Nalmefene may produce acute withdrawal symptoms in patients with known physical dependence on opioids. If opioid dependency is suspected, administer a test dose of 0.1 mg/70 kg I.V. If no evidence of withdrawal occurs in 2 minutes, the recommended dose may be administered.

▶ Monitor patient's respiratory depth and rate closely. Duration of action of the opioid may exceed that of nalmefene, causing the patient to relapse into respiratory depression. Keep patient under close surveillance until there is no reasonable risk of recurrent respiratory depression.

▶ Drug is supplied in two concentrations: an ampule with a blue label contains 1 ml at a concentration suitable for postoperative use (100 mcg/ml) and an ampule with a green label contains 2 ml at a concentration suitable for management of overdose (1 mg/ml). Check concentration carefully before administering drug.

▶ A cumulative total dose above 1.5 mg/70 kg is unlikely to have an effect.

Breast-feeding patients
▶ No data exist to demonstrate whether nalmefene appears in breast milk; use caution when administering drug to breast-feeding women.

Pediatric patients
▶ Safety and effectiveness in neonates and children haven't been established.

Patient teaching
▶ Reassure patient and provide emotional support when treating opiate overdose.

▶ **naloxone hydrochloride**
Narcan

Pharmacologic classification:
narcotic (opioid) antagonist

Therapeutic classification:
narcotic antagonist

Pregnancy risk category B

How supplied
Available by prescription only
Injection: 0.4 mg/ml with preservatives, and 0.02 mg/ml, 0.4 mg/ml paraben-free

Indications and dosages
Respiratory depression known or suspected to result from natural or synthetic narcotics, methadone, nalbuphine, pentazocine, or propoxyphene
Adults: 0.4 to 2 mg I.V., S.C., or I.M., repeated q 2 to 3 minutes, p.r.n. If no response occurs after 10 mg have been given, diagnosis of narcotic-induced toxicity should be questioned.
Children: 0.01 mg/kg I.V. Give another 0.1 mg/kg if needed. Dosage for continuous infusion is 0.024 to 0.16 mg/kg/hour. If I.V. route isn't available, dose may be given I.M. or S.C. in divided doses.

Postoperative narcotic depression
Adults: 0.1 to 0.2 mg I.V. q 2 to 3 minutes, p.r.n., until desired response is obtained.
Children: 0.005 to 0.01 mg/kg dose I.M., I.V., or S.C., repeated q 2 to 3 minutes, p.r.n., until desired degree of reversal is obtained.
Neonates (asphyxia neonatorum): 0.01 mg/kg I.V. into umbilical vein repeated q 2 to 3 minutes for three doses. Drug level for use in neonates and children is 0.02 mg/ml.
Naloxone challenge for diagnosing opiate dependence
Adults: 0.16 mg I.M. naloxone; if no signs of withdrawal after 20 to 30 minutes, give second dose of 0.24 mg I.V.

Pharmacodynamics
Narcotic (opioid) antagonist action: Naloxone is essentially a pure antagonist. In patients who have received an opioid agonist or other analgesic with narcotic-like effects, naloxone antagonizes most of the opioid effects, especially respiratory depression, sedation, and hypotension. Because the duration of action of naloxone in most cases is shorter than that of the opioid, opiate effects may return as those of naloxone dissipate. Naloxone does not produce tolerance or physical or psychological dependence. The precise mechanism of action is unknown, but is thought to involve competitive antagonism of more than one opiate receptor in the CNS.

Pharmacokinetics
Absorption: Naloxone is rapidly inactivated after oral administration; therefore, it is given parenterally. Its onset of action is 1 to 2 minutes after I.V. administration

and 2 to 5 minutes after I.M. or S.C. administration. The duration of action is longer after I.M. use and higher doses, when compared with I.V. use and lower doses.
Distribution: Drug is rapidly distributed into body tissues and fluids.
Metabolism: Naloxone is rapidly metabolized in the liver, primarily by conjugation.
Excretion: Drug is excreted in urine. Duration of action is about 45 minutes, depending on route and dose. Plasma half-life has been reported to be from 60 to 90 minutes in adults and 3 hours in neonates.

Contraindications and precautions
Contraindicated in patients hypersensitive to drug.
  Use cautiously in patients with cardiac irritability and opiate addiction. When given to a narcotic addict, naloxone may produce an acute abstinence syndrome. Use with caution, and monitor patient closely.

Interactions
Drug-drug
Cardiotoxic drugs: may cause serious CV effects. Avoid concomitant use.

Effects on diagnostic tests
None reported.

Adverse reactions
CNS: *seizures.*
CV: *cardiac arrest,* hypertension (with higher-than-recommended doses), hypotension, tachycardia, *ventricular fibrillation.*
GI: nausea, vomiting (with higher-than-recommended doses).
Respiratory: pulmonary edema.

Reactions may be *common,* uncommon, *life-threatening,* or COMMON AND LIFE-THREATENING.

Skin: diaphoresis.
Other: tremors, withdrawal symptoms (in narcotic-dependent patients with higher-than-recommended doses).

Overdose and treatment
No serious adverse reactions to naloxone overdose are known except those of acute abstinence syndrome in narcotic-dependent persons.

Special considerations
▶ Naloxone is the safest drug to use when the cause of respiratory depression is uncertain.
▶ Naloxone isn't effective in treating respiratory depression caused by nonopioid drugs.
▶ Because naloxone's duration of activity is shorter than that of most narcotics, vigilance and repeated doses are usually necessary to manage acute narcotic overdose in a nonaddicted patient.
▶ Avoid depending on drug too much; that is, don't neglect attention to airway, breathing, and circulation. Maintain adequate respiratory and CV status at all times. Respiratory overshoot may occur; monitor for respiratory rate higher than before respiratory depression. Respiratory rate increases in 1 to 2 minutes, and effect lasts 1 to 4 hours.
▶ Naloxone via I.V. or S.C. routes is effective for treating pruritus associated with epidural opiate administration; administer in small increments to avoid complete reversal of opiates.
▶ Oral naloxone may be used to treat constipation.
▶ Naloxone may be administered by continuous I.V. infusion, which is necessary in many cases to control the adverse effects of epidurally administered morphine. Usual dose is 2 mg in 500 ml of D_5W or normal saline solution.
▶ Take a careful drug history to rule out narcotic addiction and to avoid inducing withdrawal symptoms (apply the same cautions to the baby of an addicted woman).
▶ Monitor patient closely for resedation.
▶ Monitor respiratory and cardiac status at all times until risk of resedation is unlikely.
▶ Before administration, inspect all parenteral products for particulate matter and discoloration.
▶ Be prepared to administer continuous I.V. infusion (necessary in many instances to control adverse effects of epidurally administered morphine). If 0.02 mg/ml is not available, be aware that adult concentration of 0.4 mg may be diluted by mixing 0.5 ml with 9.5 ml of sterile water for injection to make neonatal concentration (0.02 mg/ml).
▶ Naloxone can be diluted in dextrose 5% or normal saline solution. Use within 24 hours after mixing.

Breast-feeding patients
▶ No data exist to demonstrate whether drug appears in breast milk.

Geriatric patients
▶ Lower doses are usually indicated for elderly patients because they may be more sensitive to drug effects.

Patient teaching
▶ Inform family of use and administration of drug.

▶ Reassure family that patient will be monitored closely until effects of narcotic subside.

▶ naltrexone hydrochloride
ReVia

Pharmacologic classification:
narcotic (opioid) antagonist

Therapeutic classification:
narcotic detoxification adjunct

Pregnancy risk category C

How supplied
Available by prescription only
Tablets: 50 mg

Indications and dosages
Adjunct for maintenance of opioid-free state in detoxified persons
Adults: if naloxone challenge is negative and patient has been opioid-free for 7 to 10 days, give 25 mg P.O. If no withdrawal symptoms occur within 1 hour, give another 25 mg. Average dosage is 50 mg/day, but flexible maintenance schedule of 50 to 150 mg/day may be used, depending on schedule.
Alcoholism
Adults: 50 mg/day P.O.

Pharmacodynamics
Opioid antagonist action: Drug is essentially a pure opiate (narcotic) antagonist. Like naloxone, it has little or no agonist activity. Its precise mechanism of action is unknown, but it probably involves competitive antagonism of more than one opiate receptor in the CNS. When given to patients who haven't recently received opiates, it exhibits little or no pharmacologic effect. At oral doses of 30 to 50 mg daily, it produces minimal analgesia, only slight drowsiness, and no respiratory depression. However, pharmacologic effects, including psychotomimetic effects, increased systolic or diastolic blood pressure, respiratory depression, and decreased oral temperature, which are suggestive of opiate agonist activity, have reportedly occurred in a few patients. In patients who have received single or repeated large doses of opiates, naltrexone attenuates or produces a complete but reversible block of the pharmacologic effects of the narcotic. Naltrexone doesn't produce physical or psychological dependence, and tolerance to its antagonist activity reportedly does not develop.

Pharmacokinetics
Absorption: Naltrexone is well absorbed after oral administration, reaching peak plasma levels after 1 hour, although it does undergo extensive first-pass hepatic metabolism. Only 5% to 20% of an oral dose reaches the systemic circulation unchanged. Effects peak within 1 hour.
Distribution: Drug is about 21% to 28% protein-bound. Extent and duration of drug's antagonist activity appear directly related to plasma and tissue levels of drug. It is widely distributed throughout the body, but considerable variation exists between patients.
Metabolism: Oral naltrexone undergoes extensive first-pass hepatic metabolism. Its major metabolite is believed to be a pure antagonist also, and may contribute to its efficacy. Drug and hepatic metabolites may undergo enterohepatic recirculation.

Excretion: Naltrexone is excreted primarily by the kidneys. Elimination half-life is about 4 hours; half-life of major active metabolite is about 13 hours.

Contraindications and precautions

Contraindicated in patients receiving opioid analgesics, in opioid-dependent patients, in patients in acute opioid withdrawal, in patients with positive urine screen for opioids, and in patients with acute hepatitis or liver failure. Also contraindicated in patients hypersensitive to drug.

Use cautiously in patients with mild hepatic disease or history of hepatic impairment.

Interactions
Drug-drug

Drugs that alter hepatic metabolism: may increase or decrease serum naltrexone levels. Monitor patient closely.
Opiates: potentially severe opiate withdrawal. Drug shouldn't be used in patients receiving opiates or in nondetoxified patients physically dependent on opiates.
Opioid-containing drugs, such as antidiarrheals, cough and cold preparations, opioid analgesics: reduced opioid activity. Avoid concomitant use.

Effects on diagnostic tests
None known.

Adverse reactions

CNS: *anxiety,* depression, dizziness, fatigue, *headache, insomnia, nervousness,* somnolence, ***suicidal ideation.***

GI: *abdominal pain,* anorexia, constipation, increased thirst, *nausea, vomiting.*
GU: delayed ejaculation, impotence.
Hematologic: lymphocytosis.
Hepatic: ***hepatotoxicity***.
Musculoskeletal: *muscle and joint pain.*
Skin: rash.
Other: chills.

Overdose and treatment

Naltrexone overdose hasn't been documented. In one study, subjects who received 800 mg/day (16 tablets) for up to 1 week showed no evidence of toxicity.

In case of overdose, provide symptomatic and supportive treatment in a closely supervised environment. Contact the local or regional poison control center for further information.

Special considerations

▶ Don't give naltrexone unless naloxone challenge is negative. To perform it, give 0.2 mg I.V. If no signs of opiate withdrawal appear after 30 seconds, give 0.6 mg I.V. (Or give 0.8 mg S.C. and observe patient for 20 minutes for signs of withdrawal.) If no withdrawal signs appear, test result is negative.
▶ Drug can cause hepatocellular injury if given at higher-than-recommended doses. Naltrexone can cause or worsen signs and symptoms of abstinence in anyone not completely opioid-free.
▶ If an emergency requiring opiate analgesia occurs, patient who has been receiving naltrexone may need a higher-than-usual dose; the resulting respiratory depression may be deeper and more prolonged.

▶ Before administering drug, take a careful drug history to rule out possible narcotic use. Do not attempt treatment until the patient has been opiate-free for 7 to 10 days. Verify self-reporting of abstinence from narcotics by urinalysis. No withdrawal signs or symptoms should be reported by patient or be evident.

▶ Perform liver function tests before naltrexone use to establish a baseline and to evaluate possible drug-induced hepatotoxicity.

Breast-feeding patients
▶ No data exist to demonstrate whether drug appears in breast milk. Use caution when giving drug to breast-feeding women, especially because of its known hepatotoxicity.

Pediatric patients
▶ Safe use of naltrexone in patients under age 18 hasn't been established.

Geriatric patients
▶ Use in elderly patients isn't documented, but they would probably require reduced dosage.

Patient teaching
▶ Inform patient that opioid medications, such as cough and cold preparations, antidiarrheal products, and narcotic analgesics, may not be effective; recommend nonnarcotic alternative if available.
▶ Warn patient not to self-administer narcotics while taking naltrexone because serious injury, coma, or death may result.
▶ Explain that drug has no tolerance or dependence liability.
▶ Tell patient to report withdrawal signs and symptoms (tremors,

vomiting, bone or muscle pains, sweating, abdominal cramps).
▶ Tell patient to wear or carry medical identification that documents his use of naltrexone.

▶ naproxen
Naprosyn, EC-Naprosyn

▶ naproxen sodium
Aleve, Anaprox, Naprelan

Pharmacologic classification:
NSAID

Therapeutic classification:
anti-inflammatory, antipyretic, nonnarcotic analgesic

Pregnancy risk category B

How supplied
Available by prescription only
naproxen
Oral suspension: 125 mg/5 ml
Tablets: 250 mg, 375 mg, 500 mg
Tablets (controlled-release):
375 mg, 500 mg
Tablets (delayed-release): 375 mg, 500 mg
naproxen sodium
Tablets (film-coated): 275 mg, 550 mg
Available without a prescription
naproxen sodium
Capsules or tablets: 220 mg

Indications and dosages
Mild to moderate musculoskeletal or soft tissue irritation
naproxen
Adults: 250 to 500 mg P.O. b.i.d. Alternatively, 250 mg in the morning and 500 mg in the evening, 375 to 500 mg P.O. b.i.d. (delayed release), or 750 to 1,000 mg P.O. daily (controlled-release).

Reactions may be *common*, uncommon, *life-threatening*, or **COMMON AND LIFE-THREATENING.**

naproxen sodium

Adults: 275 to 550 mg P.O. b.i.d. Alternatively, 275 mg in the morning and 550 mg in the evening.

Mild to moderate pain, primary dysmenorrhea

naproxen

Adults: initially, 500 mg P.O., followed by 250 mg P.O. q 6 to 8 hours, p.r.n. Maximum, 1,250 mg naproxen or 1,000 mg P.O. daily (controlled release). Use 1,500 mg for a limited period for patients requiring greater analgesia.

naproxen sodium

Adults: initially, 550 mg P.O., followed by 275 mg P.O. q 6 to 8 hours, p.r.n. Maximum, 1,375 mg daily.

Self-medication: 220 mg q 8 to 12 hours. Maximum, 660 mg/day for adults under age 65 and 440 mg/day for adults age 65 and older. Advise against self-medication that lasts more than 10 days.

Acute gout

naproxen

Adults: initially, 750 mg, and then 250 mg q 8 hours until episode subsides. Or, 1,000 mg to 1,500 mg (controlled-release) P.O. on day 1, and then 1,000 mg P.O. daily until attack subsides.

naproxen sodium

Adults: initially, 825 mg, and then 275 mg q 8 hours until attack has subsided.

Juvenile rheumatoid arthritis

naproxen

Children: 10 mg/kg/day in two divided doses.

Pharmacodynamics

Analgesic, antipyretic, and anti-inflammatory actions: Unknown, although naproxen probably inhibits prostaglandin synthesis.

Pharmacokinetics

Absorption: Naproxen is absorbed rapidly and completely from the GI tract. Effect peaks at 2 to 4 hours.

Distribution: Drug is highly protein-bound. It crosses the placenta and is distributed into the milk.

Metabolism: Drug is metabolized in the liver.

Excretion: Drug is excreted in urine. Half-life is 10 to 20 hours.

Contraindications and precautions

Contraindicated in patients hypersensitive to drug and in patients with asthma, rhinitis, or nasal polyps.

Use cautiously in elderly patients and in patients with a history of peptic ulcer disease or renal, CV, GI, or hepatic disease.

Interactions

Drug-drug

Acetaminophen, gold compounds: increased nephrotoxicity may occur. Monitor renal function.

Anticoagulants, thrombolytics: may potentiate anticoagulant effects. Monitor PT and INR.

Antihypertensives, including diuretics: naproxen may decrease the clinical effectiveness. Using together may increase risk of nephrotoxicity. Monitor patient closely.

Anti-inflammatory drugs (aspirin, salicylates): increased risk of nephrotoxicity, bleeding problems, and adverse GI reactions, including ulceration and hemorrhage. Use cautiously together, and monitor patient's renal function, PT, and INR.

Aspirin: may decrease the bioavailability of naproxen. Avoid using together.

Corticosteroids, corticotropin, salicylates: increased adverse GI reactions, including ulceration and hemorrhage. Monitor patient for abdominal pain.

Coumadin derivatives, nifedipine, phenytoin, verapamil: toxicity may occur. Monitor patient for evidence of toxicity.

Drugs that inhibit platelet aggregation, such as aspirin, parenteral carbenicillin, cefamandole, cefoperazone, dextran, dipyridamole, mezlocillin, piperacillin, plicamycin, salicylates, sulfinpyrazone, ticarcillin, valproic acid: increased risk of bleeding problems. Monitor for bleeding tendencies.

Highly protein-bound drugs: naproxen may displace highly protein-bound drugs from binding sites. Monitor patient for clinical effects and toxicity.

Insulin, oral antidiabetic drugs: potentiated hypoglycemic effects. Monitor serum glucose.

Lithium, methotrexate: decreased renal clearance. Monitor patient for toxic effects.

Drug-lifestyle
Alcohol use: increased adverse GI reactions, including ulceration and hemorrhage. Advise against concomitant use.

Effects on diagnostic tests
Naproxen and its metabolites may interfere with urine 5-hydroxyindoleacetic acid and 17-hydroxycorticosteroid determinations.

Adverse reactions
CNS: *dizziness, drowsiness, headache,* vertigo.
CV: *edema,* palpitations.
EENT: auditory disturbances, *tinnitus,* visual disturbances.
GI: constipation, diarrhea, dyspepsia, *epigastric distress,* heartburn, *nausea, occult blood loss, peptic ulceration,* stomatitis, thirst.
GU: *nephrotoxicity.*
Hematologic: *agranulocytosis,* eosinophilia, *neutropenia, thrombocytopenia.*
Hepatic: elevated liver enzymes.
Respiratory: dyspnea.
Skin: ecchymosis, diaphoresis, *pruritus* purpura, *rash,* urticaria.

Overdose and treatment
Overdose may cause drowsiness, heartburn, indigestion, nausea, and vomiting.

    To treat naproxen overdose, induce emesis with ipecac syrup or perform gastric lavage. Give activated charcoal by nasogastric tube. Provide symptomatic and supportive measures, including respiratory support and correction of fluid and electrolyte imbalances. Monitor patient's laboratory values and vital signs closely. Hemodialysis is ineffective.

Special considerations
▶ Keep in mind that 220 mg of naproxen sodium equals 200 mg of naproxen. Likewise, 275 mg of naproxen sodium equals 250 mg of naproxen and 550 mg equals 500 mg of naproxen.
▶ Use lowest effective dose.
▶ Drug is used in mild to moderate chronic pain.
▶ Drug shouldn't be used in combination with aspirin or in patients with aspirin allergy.
▶ Relief usually begins within 2 weeks after beginning therapy with naproxen.

Reactions may be *common,* uncommon, *life-threatening,* or **COMMON AND LIFE-THREATENING.**

▶ Institute safety measures to prevent injury resulting from possible CNS effects.
▶ Drug can precipitate asthma.
▶ Monitor fluid balance and for evidence of fluid retention, especially significant weight gain.

Breast-feeding patients
▶ Because they're distributed into breast milk, avoid using naproxen and naproxen sodium during breast-feeding.

Pediatric patients
▶ Safe use of naproxen in children under age 2 hasn't been established.

Geriatric patients
▶ Patients over age 60 are more sensitive to adverse effects of drug, especially GI toxicity.
▶ Naproxen's effect on renal prostaglandins may cause fluid retention and edema. This may be significant in elderly patients, especially those with heart failure.

Patient teaching
▶ Tell patient to take drug with food to avoid adverse GI side effects.
▶ Teach patient not to break or crush controlled- or delayed-release tablets.
▶ Instruct patient to check his weight every 2 to 3 days and to report any gain of 3 lb (1.4 kg) or more over 1 week.
▶ Instruct patient in safety measures; caution him to avoid hazardous activities until full CNS effects of drug are known.
▶ Caution patient to avoid taking naproxen with other OTC drugs.
▶ Warn patient against combining naproxen (Naprosyn) with naprox-en sodium (Anaprox) because both drugs circulate in the blood as naproxen anion.
▶ Teach patient signs and symptoms of possible adverse reactions and tell him to report them promptly.

▶ naratriptan hydrochloride
Amerge

Pharmacologic classification:
*selective 5-hydroxytryptamine₁
(5-HT₁) receptor subtype agonist*

Therapeutic classification:
antimigraine

Pregnancy risk category C

How supplied
Available by prescription only
Tablets: 1 mg, 2.5 mg

Indications and dosages
Acute migraine headaches with or without aura
Adults: 1 or 2.5 mg P.O. as a single dose. Dose should be individualized based on possible benefit of 2.5-mg strength and the greater risk of adverse events. If headache returns or if only partial response occurs, may repeat dose after 4 hours. Maximum, 5 mg/24 hours.
◨ DOSAGE ADJUSTMENT. In patients with mild to moderate renal or hepatic impairment, consider a lower initial dose; don't exceed 2.5 mg over a 24-hour period. Do not use in patients with severe renal or hepatic impairment.

Pharmacodynamics
Antimigraine action: Naratriptan binds with high affinity to 5-HT₁D and 5-HT₁B receptors. One theory

suggests that activation of 5-$HT_{1D/1B}$ receptors located on intracranial blood vessels leads to vasoconstriction, which is associated with the migraine relief. Others believe that activation of 5-$HT_{1D/1B}$ receptors on sensory nerve endings in the trigeminal system results in the inhibition of pro-inflammatory neuropeptide release.

Pharmacokinetics

Absorption: Drug is well absorbed with about 70% oral bioavailability. Plasma levels peak in 2 to 4 hours.
Distribution: Steady state volume of drug's distribution is 170 L. Plasma protein-binding is 28% to 31%.
Metabolism: In vitro, naratriptan is metabolized by many cytochrome P-450 isoenzymes to inactive metabolites.
Excretion: Naratriptan is predominantly eliminated in urine, with 50% of dose recovered unchanged and 30% as metabolites. Mean elimination half-life is 6 hours.

Contraindications and precautions

Contraindicated in patients hypersensitive to drug or its components and in those with history, symptoms, or signs of ischemic cardiac, cerebrovascular (such as CVA or transient ischemic attack), or peripheral vascular syndromes (such as ischemic bowel disease). Also contraindicated in patients with significant underlying CV diseases, including angina pectoris, MI, and silent myocardial ischemia. Drug shouldn't be given to patients with uncontrolled hypertension, due to potential increase in blood pressure.

Contraindicated in patients with creatinine clearance below 15 ml/minute or Child-Pugh grade C hepatic impairment and in those with hemiplegic or basilar migraine.

Drug or other 5-HT_1 agonists are also contraindicated in patients with potential risk factors for coronary artery disease, such as hypertension, hypercholesterolemia, obesity, diabetes, strong family history of coronary artery disease, females with surgical or physiologic menopause, males over age 40, or smoking.

Interactions

Drug-drug

Ergot-containing or ergot-type drugs or other 5-HT_1 agonists: prolonged vasospastic reactions because their actions may be additive. Use of these drugs within 24 hours of naratriptan is contraindicated.
Oral contraceptives: slightly higher levels of naratriptan. Monitor patient.
Selective serotonin reuptake inhibitors, such as fluoxetine, fluvoxamine, paroxetine, sertraline: weakness, hyperreflexia, and incoordination when coadministered with 5-HT_1 agonists. If dual therapy is needed, monitor patient.

Drug-lifestyle

Smoking: increases naratriptan clearance by 30%. Advise patient to avoid smoking.

Effects on diagnostic tests

None reported.

Adverse reactions

CNS: dizziness, drowsiness, fatigue, malaise, paresthesias, vertigo.
CV: *abnormal ECG changes (prolonged PR, QT interval, ST/T wave abnormalities, PVCs, atrial flutter or fibrillation),* increased blood pressure, palpitations, syncope, *tachyarrhythmias.*
EENT: ear, nose, and throat infections, photophobia.
GI: hyposalivation, nausea, vomiting.
Other: warm or cold temperature sensations; pressure, tightness, heaviness sensations.

Overdose and treatment

Overdose may cause blood pressure to rise markedly ¼ to 6 hours after ingestion of the drug. In some patients, it returns to normal in 8 hours; in others, antihypertensives are needed.

No specific antidote exists. Perform ECG monitoring for evidence of ischemia. Monitor patient for at least 24 hours after an overdose or while symptoms persist. The effect of hemodialysis or peritoneal dialysis is unknown.

Special considerations

▶ Use drug only when a clear diagnosis of migraine has been established. It isn't intended for prophylactic therapy or for management of hemiplegic or basilar migraine.
▶ Give first dose in a medically equipped facility for patients at risk for coronary artery disease but determined to have a satisfactory CV evaluation. Consider ECG monitoring.
▶ Safety and effectiveness haven't been established for cluster headaches.

▶ Periodically reevaluate cardiac status of patients who have or develop risk factors for coronary artery disease.

Pregnant patients

▶ Don't give drug to patient with suspected or confirmed pregnancy.

Breast-feeding patients

▶ Use with caution in breast-feeding patients.

Pediatric patients

▶ Safety and effectiveness in children under age 18 haven't been established.

Geriatric patients

▶ Don't give drug to elderly patients.

Patient teaching

▶ Tell patient that drug is intended to relieve, not prevent, migraine headaches.
▶ Teach patient to alert physician of risk factors for coronary artery disease.
▶ Instruct patient to take dose soon after headache starts. If there's no response to the first tablet, tell patient to seek medical approval before taking second tablet.
▶ Tell patient that if more relief is needed after the first tablet, such as when a partial response occurs or if the headache returns, he may take a second tablet but no sooner than 4 hours after the first tablet. Inform him not to exceed two tablets within 24 hours.
▶ Instruct women not to use drug if pregnancy is suspected or confirmed.

❱ nicardipine hydrochloride
Cardene, Cardene SR

Pharmacologic classification:
calcium channel blocker

Therapeutic classification:
antianginal, antihypertensive

Pregnancy risk category C

How supplied
Available by prescription only
Capsules: 20 mg, 30 mg
Capsules (extended-release): 30 mg, 45 mg, 60 mg
Injection: 2.5 mg/ml in 10-ml ampules

Indications and dosages
Chronic stable angina
Adults: initially, 20 mg P.O. t.i.d. Adjust dosage based on patient response. Dosage range, 20 to 40 mg t.i.d. Extended-release capsules (for hypertension only) can be initiated at 30 mg b.i.d.; dose, 30 to 60 mg b.i.d.
◻ DOSAGE ADJUSTMENT. Start with 20 mg P.O. b.i.d. if patient has hepatic dysfunction. Then carefully adjust subsequent dose based on patient response.

Pharmacodynamics
Antihypertensive and antianginal actions: Nicardipine inhibits movement of calcium ions into cardiac and smooth muscle cells. Drug appears to act specifically on vascular muscle, and may cause a smaller decrease in cardiac output than other calcium channel blockers because of its vasodilatory effect.

Pharmacokinetics
Absorption: Drug is completely absorbed after oral administration. Plasma levels are detectable within 20 minutes and peak in about 1 hour. Absorption may be decreased if drug is taken with food. Therapeutic serum levels are 28 to 50 ng/ml.
Distribution: Drug is extensively (more than 95%) bound to plasma proteins.
Metabolism: A substantial first-pass effect reduces absolute bioavailability to about 35%. Drug is extensively metabolized in the liver, and the process is saturable. Increasing dosage yields nonlinear increases in plasma levels.
Excretion: Elimination half-life is about 8.6 hours after steady state levels are reached.

Contraindications and precautions
Contraindicated in patients hypersensitive to drug and in those with advanced aortic stenosis.

Use cautiously in patients with impaired renal or hepatic function, cardiac conduction disturbances, hypotension, or heart failure.

Interactions
Drug-drug
Cimetidine: increased plasma nicardipine levels. Monitor patient for toxic effects.
Cyclosporine: increased plasma cyclosporine levels. Careful monitoring is recommended.
Digoxin: may increase plasma levels of cardiac glycosides. Carefully monitor serum digoxin levels.
Fentanyl anesthesia: increased risk of severe hypotension. Monitor patient closely.

Effects on diagnostic tests
None reported.

Reactions may be *common*, uncommon, *life-threatening*, or COMMON AND LIFE-THREATENING.

Adverse reactions
CNS: asthenia, dizziness, headache, light-headedness, paresthesia.
CV: angina, *flushing, palpitations, peripheral edema,* tachycardia.
GI: abdominal discomfort, dry mouth, nausea.
Skin: rash.

Overdose and treatment
Overdose may cause hypotension, bradycardia, drowsiness, confusion, and slurred speech.

Treatment is supportive, with vasopressors administered as needed. I.V. calcium gluconate may be useful to counteract the effects of drug.

Special considerations
▶ When treating patients with chronic stable angina, S.L. nitroglycerin, prophylactic nitrate therapy, and beta blockers may be continued.
▶ Patients may experience increased frequency, severity, or duration of chest pain when therapy starts or dosage changes.
▶ Allow at least 3 days between oral dosage changes to ensure steady state plasma levels.
▶ Drug is also used for management of hypertension.
▶ Measure blood pressure frequently during initial therapy. Assess patient for orthostatic hypotension.
▶ When treating hypertension, measure blood pressure during times of plasma level trough (about 8 hours after dose or immediately before next doses). Because prominent effects may occur during peak plasma levels, measure blood pressure 1 to 2 hours after dose.
▶ Dilute solution in ampule before I.V. infusion. Recommended dilution is 0.1 mg/ml in dextrose or saline solution.
▶ Monitor blood pressure during I.V. administration because nicardipine I.V. decreases peripheral resistance.
▶ Adjust infusion rate if hypotension or tachycardia occurs, as ordered.
▶ When switching to oral therapy other than nicardipine, start therapy when infusion stops. If oral nicardipine will be used, give first dose of t.i.d. regimen 1 hour before stopping infusion.

Breast-feeding patients
▶ Substantial amounts of drug have been found in the milk of animals given nicardipine; breast-feeding isn't recommended.

Pediatric patients
▶ Safe use in children under age 18 hasn't been established.

Patient teaching
▶ Tell patient to take oral form of drug exactly as prescribed.
▶ Advise patient to report chest pain immediately.

▶ **nifedipine**
Adalat, Adalat CC, Procardia, Procardia XL

Pharmacologic classification:
calcium channel blocker

Therapeutic classification:
antianginal

Pregnancy risk category C

How supplied
Available by prescription only
Capsules: 10 mg, 20 mg

Tablets (extended-release): 30 mg, 60 mg, 90 mg

Indications and dosages
Prinzmetal's (variant) angina, chronic stable angina
Adults: starting dose is 10 mg P.O. t.i.d. Usual effective dosage range is 10 to 20 mg t.i.d., with some patients requiring up to 30 mg q.i.d. Maximum, 180 mg/day for capsules or 120 mg for extended-release tablets.

Pharmacodynamics
Antianginal action: Nifedipine dilates systemic arteries, resulting in decreased total peripheral resistance and modestly decreased systemic blood pressure with a slightly increased heart rate, decreased afterload, and increased cardiac index. Reduced afterload and decreased myocardial oxygen consumption probably account for the drug's value in treating chronic stable angina. In Prinzmetal's angina, nifedipine inhibits coronary artery spasm, increasing myocardial oxygen delivery.

Pharmacokinetics
Absorption: About 90% of dose is absorbed rapidly from the GI tract after oral administration; however, only about 65% to 70% of drug reaches the systemic circulation because of a significant first-pass effect in the liver. Serum levels peak in 30 minutes to 2 hours. Hypotensive effects may occur 5 minutes after S.L. administration. Therapeutic serum levels are 25 to 100 ng/ml.
Distribution: About 92% to 98% of circulating nifedipine is bound to plasma proteins.

Metabolism: Drug is metabolized in the liver.
Excretion: Drug is excreted in the urine and feces as inactive metabolites. Elimination half-life is 2 to 5 hours. Duration of effect ranges from 4 to 12 hours.

Contraindications and precautions
Contraindicated in patients hypersensitive to drug.

Use cautiously in elderly patients and patients with heart failure or hypotension. Use extended-release form cautiously in patients with GI narrowing. Use with caution in patients with unstable angina who aren't currently taking a beta blocker because they may have an increased risk of MI.

Interactions
Drug-drug
Beta blockers: may worsen angina, heart failure, and hypotension. Use together cautiously.
Cimetidine: may decrease nifedipine metabolism and increase drug levels. Use together cautiously.
Digoxin: may cause increased serum digoxin levels. Monitor serum digoxin level.
Fentanyl, hypotensive drugs: may cause excessive hypotension. Monitor blood pressure closely.
Phenytoin: may increase phenytoin levels. Monitor phenytoin levels.

Effects on diagnostic tests
None reported.

Adverse reactions
CNS: *dizziness, headache, lightheadedness,* nervousness, syncope, *weakness.*

CV: *flushing,* hypotension, ***heart failure, MI,*** palpitations, *peripheral edema.*
EENT: nasal congestion.
GI: abdominal discomfort, constipation, diarrhea, *nausea.*
Hepatic: increase in serum levels of alkaline phosphate, LD, AST, and ALT.
Metabolic: hypokalemia.
Musculoskeletal: muscle cramps.
Respiratory: cough, dyspnea, ***pulmonary edema.***
Skin: pruritus, rash.
Other: fever.

Overdose and treatment
Overdose typically causes extension of drug effects, primarily peripheral vasodilation and hypotension.

Treatment includes basic support measures, such as hemodynamic and respiratory monitoring. If patient requires blood pressure support by a vasoconstrictor, norepinephrine may be administered. Limbs should be elevated and any fluid deficit corrected.

Special considerations
▶ Drug is also used to manage hypertension.
▶ Monitor blood pressure regularly, especially if patient is also taking beta blockers or antihypertensives.
▶ Initial doses or dosage increases may worsen angina briefly.
Reassure patient that this symptom is temporary.
▶ Nifedipine isn't available in S.L. form. No advantage has been found in S.L. or buccal use.
▶ Although rebound effect hasn't been observed when drug is stopped, reduce dose slowly.

Geriatric patients
▶ Elderly patients may be more sensitive to drug's effects, and duration of effect may be prolonged; use caution.

Patient teaching
▶ Instruct patient to swallow capsules whole without breaking, crushing, or chewing them.
▶ Tell patient that he may experience hypotensive effects during dose adjustment; urge compliance with therapy.

▶ nimodipine
Nimotop

Pharmacologic classification:
calcium channel blocker

Therapeutic classification:
cerebral vasodilator

Pregnancy risk category C

How supplied
Available by prescription only
Capsules: 30 mg

Indications and dosages
Migraine headaches*
Adults: 120 mg/day P.O., 1 hour before or within 2 hours after meals.
◨ Dosage adjustment. Use lower doses in patients with hepatic failure. Start with 30 mg P.O. every 4 hours, and closely monitor patient's blood pressure and heart rate.

Pharmacodynamics
Antimigraine action: Unknown.
Neuronal-sparing action: Drug inhibits calcium ion movement across cardiac and smooth muscle

cell membranes, thus decreasing myocardial contractility and oxygen demand. It also dilates coronary arteries and arterioles. Although action isn't fully known, drug may dilate small cerebral resistance vessels and increase collateral circulation.

Pharmacokinetics
Absorption: Drug is well absorbed after oral administration. However, because of extensive first-pass metabolism, bioavailability is only about 3% to 30%.
Distribution: Drug is more than 95% protein-bound.
Metabolism: Drug is extensively metabolized in the liver. Drug and metabolites undergo enterohepatic recycling.
Excretion: Less than 1% is excreted as parent drug. Elimination half-life is 1 to 9 hours.

Contraindications and precautions
No known contraindications. Use cautiously in patients with hepatic failure.

Interactions
Drug-drug
Antihypertensives: enhanced hypotensive effect. Monitor blood pressure closely.
Calcium channel blockers: may enhance these drugs' CV effects. Monitor patient closely.
Phenytoin: increased phenytoin levels. Monitor phenytoin levels.

Drug-food
Food: decreased absorption. Give drug 1 hour before or 2 hours after meals.

Effects on diagnostic tests
None reported.

Adverse reactions
CNS: headache, psychic disturbances.
CV: edema, decreased blood pressure, flushing, tachycardia.
GI: abdominal discomfort, diarrhea, nausea.
Musculoskeletal: muscle cramps.
Respiratory: dyspnea.
Skin: dermatitis, rash.

Overdose and treatment
Overdose may cause nausea, weakness, drowsiness, confusion, bradycardia, and decreased cardiac output.

Treatment should be supportive. Give pressor amines for hypotension and cardiac pacing, atropine, or sympathomimetics for bradycardia. Calcium gluconate I.V. has been used to treat calcium channel blocker overdose.

Special considerations
▶ Drug is also used for improvement of neurologic deficits after subarachnoid hemorrhage from ruptured congenital aneurysms.
▶ Unlike other calcium channel blockers, nimodipine isn't used for angina or hypertension.
▶ Monitor patient's blood pressure and heart rate, especially at the start of therapy.
▶ Expect migraines to decrease in frequency, severity, and duration with 1 to 2 months of therapy. Additional studies are needed to evaluate benefits of long-term prophylactic therapy.
▶ If patient has a nasogastric tube, puncture the ends of liquid-filled capsule with an 18G needle and draw the contents into a syringe.

Instill dose into the tube and then flush the tube with 30 ml of normal saline solution.

Breast-feeding patients
▶ Substantial amounts of drug appear in the milk of lactating animals. Avoid breast-feeding during therapy.

Pediatric patients
▶ Safety and efficacy in children haven't been established.

Patient teaching
▶ Food decreases absorption. Advise patient to take drug 1 hour before or 2 hours after meals.
▶ Advise patient to rise slowly from lying to sitting or sitting to standing positions to avoid dizziness and hypotension, especially at start of therapy.

▶ nizatidine
Axid, Axid AR

Pharmacologic classification:
H₂-receptor antagonist

Therapeutic classification:
antiulcer drug

Pregnancy risk category B

How supplied
Available by prescription only
Capsules: 150 mg, 300 mg
Available without a prescription
Capsules: 75 mg

Indications and dosages
Active duodenal ulcer
Adults: 300 mg P.O. once daily h.s. Alternatively, 150 mg P.O. b.i.d.

Maintenance therapy for duodenal ulcer
Adults: 150 mg P.O. once daily h.s.
Gastroesophageal reflux disease
Adults: 150 mg P.O. b.i.d.
Heartburn
Adults: One 75-mg capsule P.O. 30 to 60 minutes before meals; use up to b.i.d.
◩ Dosage adjustment Give 150 mg/day for treatment or 150 mg every other day for maintenance therapy if patient's creatinine clearance is 20 to 50 ml/minute. Give 150 mg every other day for treatment or 150 mg every third day for maintenance therapy if creatinine clearance is below 20 ml/minute.

Pharmacodynamics
Antiulcer action: Nizatidine is a competitive, reversible inhibitor of H_2 receptors, particularly those in gastric parietal cells.

Pharmacokinetics
Absorption: Nizatidine is well absorbed (more than 90%) after oral administration. Absorption may be slightly enhanced by food and slightly impaired by antacids.
Distribution: About 35% of nizatidine is bound to plasma protein. Plasma levels peak 30 minutes to 3 hours after the dose is given.
Metabolism: Nizatidine probably undergoes hepatic metabolism. About 40% of excreted drug is metabolized; the remainder is excreted unchanged.
Excretion: More than 90% of an oral dose of nizatidine is excreted in urine within 12 hours. Renal clearance is about 500 ml/minute, which indicates excretion by active tubular secretion. Less than 6% of a dose is eliminated in feces. Elimination half-life is 1 to 2

hours. Moderate to severe renal impairment significantly prolongs half-life and decreases clearance.

Contraindications and precautions

Contraindicated in patients hypersensitive to H_2-receptor antagonists.

Use cautiously in patients with impaired renal function.

Interactions
Drug-drug
Aspirin: high doses of aspirin (3,900 mg/day) with nizatidine (150 mg b.i.d.) increase serum salicylate levels.

Drug-food
Tomato-based, mixed-vegetable juices: may decrease drug potency. Advise against concurrent use.

Effects on diagnostic tests

False-positive tests for urobilinogen may occur during nizatidine therapy.

Adverse reactions

CNS: somnolence.
CV: *arrhythmias.*
Hematologic: eosinophilia.
Hepatic: elevated liver function test results, hepatocellular injury.
Metabolic: hyperuricemia.
Skin: *diaphoresis,* rash, urticaria.
Other: fever.

Overdose and treatment

Overdose may cause cholinergic effects, including lacrimation, salivation, emesis, miosis, and diarrhea.

Treatment may include use of activated charcoal, emesis, or lavage with monitoring and supportive therapy.

Special considerations

▶ Giving antiulcer drugs with NSAID therapy is beneficial.
▶ Because drug is excreted primarily by the kidneys, reduce dosage in patients with moderate to severe renal insufficiency.
▶ Nizatidine is partially metabolized in the liver. In patients with normal renal function and uncomplicated hepatic dysfunction, the disposition of nizatidine is similar to that in patients with normal hepatic function.
▶ Effects of continuous drug therapy for over 1 year aren't known.
▶ Assess patient for abdominal pain. Assess for blood in emesis, stool, or gastric aspirate.

Breast-feeding patients
▶ Use with caution in women who are breast-feeding. Nizatidine is concentrated in the milk of lactating rats.

Pediatric patients
▶ Safety and efficacy in children haven't been established.

Geriatric patients
▶ Safety and efficacy appear similar to those in younger patients. However, consider that elderly patients have reduced renal function.

Patient teaching
▶ Advise patient not to smoke because it may increase gastric acid secretion and worsen the disease.

▶ nortriptyline hydrochloride
Aventyl, Pamelor

Pharmacologic classification:
tricyclic antidepressant

Therapeutic classification:
antidepressant

Pregnancy risk category NR

How supplied
Available by prescription only
Capsules: 10 mg, 25 mg, 50 mg, 75 mg
Solution: 10 mg/5 ml (4% alcohol)

Indications and dosages
Analgesic adjunct for phantom limb pain, migraine or chronic tension headache, diabetic neuropathy, tic douloureux, cancer pain, peripheral neuropathy with pain, postherpetic neuralgia, arthritic pain*
Adults: 50 to 150 mg P.O. daily.

Pharmacodynamics
Analgesic action: Unknown.
Antidepressant action: Drug probably inhibits reuptake of norepinephrine and serotonin in CNS nerve terminals (presynaptic neurons), which results in increased levels and enhanced activity of these neurotransmitters in the synaptic cleft. Nortriptyline inhibits reuptake of serotonin more actively than norepinephrine; it's less likely than other tricyclic antidepressants to cause orthostatic hypotension.

Pharmacokinetics
Absorption: Drug is absorbed rapidly from the GI tract after oral administration.
Distribution: Drug is distributed widely into the body, including the CNS and breast milk. It is 95% protein-bound. Plasma levels peak within 8 hours after a dose; steady state serum levels are achieved in 2 to 4 weeks. Therapeutic serum level ranges from 50 to 150 ng/ml.
Metabolism: Drug is metabolized by the liver; a significant first-pass effect may account for variability of serum levels in different patients taking the same dosage.
Excretion: Drug is mostly excreted in urine, with some in feces, via the biliary tract.

Contraindications and precautions
Contraindicated during acute recovery phase of MI, in patients hypersensitive to drug, and in patients who have taken an MAO inhibitor within 14 days.

Use cautiously in patients with history of urine retention or seizures, glaucoma, suicidal tendencies, CV disease, or hyperthyroidism and in those receiving thyroid hormones.

Interactions
Drug-drug
Antiarrhythmics (disopyramide, procainamide, quinidine), pimozide, thyroid hormones: may increase risk of arrhythmias and conduction defects. Monitor patient closely.
Anticholinergic drugs, such as antihistamines, antiparkinsonians, atropine, meperidine, pheno-

---

◇ Available in Canada only   *Unlabeled use

thiazines: increased risk of oversedation, paralytic ileus, visual changes, and severe constipation. Monitor patient closely.

Barbiturates: induce nortriptyline metabolism and decrease efficacy. Monitor patient for drug effect.

Beta blockers, cimetidine, methylphenidate, oral contraceptives, propoxyphene: may inhibit nortriptyline metabolism, increasing plasma levels and toxicity. Monitor patient for evidence of toxicity.

Central-acting antihypertensives, such as clonidine, guanabenz, guanadrel, guanethidine, methyldopa, reserpine: decreased hypotensive effects. Monitor patient's blood pressure.

CNS depressants, including analgesics, anesthetics, barbiturates, opioids, tranquilizers: increased risk of oversedation. Monitor patient closely.

Disulfiram, ethchlorvynol: may cause delirium and tachycardia. Avoid using together.

Haloperidol, phenothiazines: decreased nortriptyline metabolism and therapeutic efficacy. Monitor patient for clinical effect.

Metrizamide: increased risk of seizures. Use together cautiously.

Sympathomimetics, including ephedrine, epinephrine, phenylephrine, phenylpropanolamine: may increase blood pressure. Monitor blood pressure.

Warfarin: may increase PT and risk of bleeding. Monitor PT and INR.

Drug-lifestyle

Alcohol use: additive effects. Discourage alcohol use.

Heavy smoking: induces nortriptyline metabolism and decreases efficacy. Discourage smoking.

Effects on diagnostic tests

None reported.

Adverse reactions

CNS: agitation, ataxia, confusion, *dizziness, drowsiness,* EEG changes, extrapyramidal reactions, hallucinations, headache, insomnia, nervousness, nightmares, paresthesia, *seizures,* tremor, weakness.

CV: *CVA, heart block,* hypertension, hypotension, *MI,* prolonged conduction time (elongation of QT and PR intervals, flattened T waves on ECG), *tachycardia.*

EENT: *blurred vision,* mydriasis, tinnitus.

GI: anorexia, *constipation,* dry mouth, nausea, paralytic ileus, vomiting.

GU: elevated liver function test results, *urine retention.*

Hematologic: *agranulocytosis, bone marrow depression*, eosinophilia, *thrombocytopenia.*

Metabolic: increased serum glucose levels.

Skin: *diaphoresis,* photosensitivity, rash, urticaria.

Other: *hypersensitivity reaction.*

Overdose and treatment

The first 12 hours after acute ingestion are a stimulatory phase characterized by excessive anticholinergic activity (agitation, irritation, confusion, hallucinations, hyperthermia, parkinsonian symptoms, seizures, urine retention, dry mucous membranes, pupillary dilation, constipation, and ileus). This is followed by CNS depressant effects, including hypothermia, decreased or absent reflexes, sedation, hypotension, cyanosis, and cardiac irregularities, including tachycardia, conduction disturbances, and quinidine-like effects on the ECG.

Severity of overdose is best indicated by QRS complex prolonged beyond 100 ms, which usually indicates a serum level above 1,000 ng/ml. Metabolic acidosis may follow hypotension, hypoventilation, and seizures.

Treatment includes maintaining a patent airway, stable body temperature, and fluid and electrolyte balance. Induce emesis with ipecac syrup if patient is conscious; follow with gastric lavage and activated charcoal to prevent further absorption. Dialysis is usually ineffective. Consider use of cardiac glycosides or physostigmine if serious CV abnormalities or cardiac failure occurs. Treat seizures with parenteral diazepam or phenytoin; arrhythmias with parenteral phenytoin or lidocaine; and acidosis with sodium bicarbonate. Don't use quinidine, procainamide, or disopyramide to treat arrhythmias, since these agents can further depress myocardial conduction and contractility. Don't give barbiturates, which may enhance CNS and respiratory depressant effects.

Special considerations

▶ Drug is an adjuvant to opiate administration. It also is used to treat cancer patients with neuropathic pain.
▶ Drug may be administered at bedtime to reduce daytime sedation. Tolerance to sedative effects usually develops over the initial weeks of therapy.
▶ Daytime dosing may prevent insomnia, which may result from bedtime dosing.
▶ Withdraw drug gradually over a few weeks. It should be discontin-

ued at least 48 hours before surgical procedures.
▶ Abrupt withdrawal of long-term therapy may cause nausea, headache, and malaise, which don't indicate addiction.
▶ Drug is available in liquid form.
▶ Drug is usually used to treat depression and panic disorder.
▶ In patients with bipolar disorders, drug may cause manic phase symptoms to emerge.
▶ Monitor patient for adverse CNS and CV effects.

Breast-feeding patients
▶ Low levels of nortriptyline appear in breast milk; potential benefit to mother should outweigh potential harm to infant.

Pediatric patients
▶ Drug isn't recommended for children.
▶ Reduced dosages may be indicated for adolescents.

Geriatric patients
▶ Lower dosages may be indicated. Elderly patients are at greater risk for adverse cardiac effects.
▶ Nortriptyline is less likely to cause hypotension than other tricyclic antidepressants.

Patient teaching
▶ Explain that patient may not see full effects of drug therapy for up to 4 weeks after start of therapy.
▶ Warn patient about sedative effects.
▶ Recommend taking full daily dose at bedtime to prevent daytime sedation.
▶ Instruct patient to avoid alcoholic beverages, doubling doses after

missing one, and discontinuing drug abruptly, unless instructed.
▶ Warn patient about possible dizziness. Tell him to lie down for about 30 minutes after each dose at start of therapy and to avoid sudden position changes. Orthostatic hypotension is usually less severe than with amitriptyline.
▶ Suggest relieving dry mouth with sugarless chewing gum or candy.
▶ Caution patient to avoid hazardous activities during therapy.
▶ Urge patient to report unusual reactions promptly, such as confusion, movement disorders, fainting, rapid heartbeat, or difficulty urinating.

▶ **octreotide acetate**
Sandostatin

Pharmacologic classification:
synthetic octapeptide

Therapeutic classification:
somatotropic hormone

Pregnancy risk category B

How supplied
Available by prescription only
Injection: 0.05 mg/ml, 0.1 mg/ml, and 0.5 mg/ml in 1 ml ampules; 0.2 mg/ml and 1 mg/ml in 5 ml multidose vials

Indications and dosages
Flushing and diarrhea from carcinoid tumors
Adults: 100 to 600 mcg daily S.C. in two to four divided doses for first 2 weeks of therapy (usually 300 mcg daily). Subsequent dosage based on individual response.

Watery diarrhea from vasoactive intestinal peptide-secreting tumors (VIPomas)
Adults: initially, 200 to 300 mcg daily S.C. in two to four divided doses for first 2 weeks of therapy. Subsequent dosage based on individual response, but usually will not exceed 450 mcg daily.
Diarrheal states*
Adults: 100 to 500 mcg S.C. t.i.d.
Irritable bowel syndrome*
Adults: 100 mcg S.C. as a single dose to 125 mcg S.C. b.i.d.

Pharmacodynamics
Antidiarrheal action: Octreotide mimics the action of naturally occurring somatostatin and decreases the secretion of gastroenterohepatic peptides that may contribute to the adverse signs and symptoms seen in patients with metastatic carcinoid tumors and VIPomas. It isn't known if drug affects the tumor directly.

Pharmacokinetics
Absorption: Octreotide is absorbed rapidly and completely after injection. Plasma levels peak in less than 30 minutes.
Distribution: Drug is distributed to the plasma, where it binds to serum lipoprotein and albumin.
Metabolism: Drug is eliminated from the plasma at a slower rate than the naturally occurring hormone. Apparent half-life is about 1½ hours, with a duration of effect of up to 12 hours.
Excretion: About 35% of drug appears unchanged in the urine.

Contraindications and precautions
Contraindicated in patients hypersensitive to drug or its components.

Interactions

Drug-drug

Cyclosporine: octreotide may decrease plasma cyclosporine levels. Monitor drug levels.

Insulin, oral antidiabetic drugs (sulfonylureas), oral diazoxide: increased risk of hypoglycemia. May require dosage adjustments.

Effects on diagnostic tests

None reported.

Adverse reactions

CNS: dizziness, fatigue, headache, light-headedness.
CV: *arrhythmias,* conduction abnormalities, flushing, *sinus bradycardia.*
EENT: blurred vision.
GI: *abdominal pain or discomfort,* constipation, *diarrhea,* fat malabsorption, gallstones or biliary sludge, flatulence, *loose stools, nausea,* vomiting.
GU: pollakiuria, urinary tract infection.
Metabolic: hyperglycemia, hypoglycemia, hypothyroidism, suppressed secretion of growth hormone and gastroenterohepatic peptides (gastrin, glucagon, insulin, motilin, pancreatic polypeptide, secretin, and VIP).
Musculoskeletal: backache, joint pain.
Skin: alopecia, edema, erythema or pain at injection site, wheals.
Other: flulike symptoms.

Overdose and treatment

Doses of 1,000 mcg have been administered as an I.V. bolus in volunteers without adverse effects. Drug may produce metabolic changes in certain patients.

Special considerations

▶ Drug is also used to treat acromegaly, to decrease output of rectal or pancreatic fistulas, and to treat variceal bleeding and dumping syndrome.
▶ Fluid and electrolyte balance may be altered after therapy starts.
▶ Mild, transient hypoglycemia or hyperglycemia may occur during therapy. Observe patient for signs of glucose imbalance and monitor closely.
▶ Monitor laboratory values during therapy, such as urinary 5-hydroxyindoleacetic acid, plasma serotonin, plasma substance P for carcinoid tumors, and plasma VIP for VIPomas.
▶ Drug may alter fat absorption and aggravate fat malabsorption. Perform periodic assessment of 72-hour fecal fat and serum carotene.
▶ Use with octreotide may require dosage adjustment of other drugs such as beta blockers, calcium channel blockers, and electrolyte-controlling drugs.
▶ Half-life may be altered in patients with end-stage renal failure who undergo dialysis. Dosage adjustment may be necessary.
▶ Obtain baseline and periodic tests of thyroid function because drug's long-term effects on hypothalamic-pituitary function aren't known.
▶ Drug may decrease vitamin B_{12} levels during long-term treatment. Monitor patient's levels.
▶ Patients with acromegaly are more likely to experience adverse GI effects and bradycardia. Monitor patient closely.

Breast-feeding patients
▶ No data exist to demonstrate whether drug appears in breast milk.

Pediatric patients
▶ Doses of 1 to 10 mcg/kg appear to be tolerated well by children.

Patient teaching
▶ Because drug may cause gallstones, tell patient to report abdominal discomfort promptly.

▶ omeprazole
Prilosec

Pharmacologic classification:
substituted benzimidazole

Therapeutic classification:
gastric acid suppressant

Pregnancy risk category C

How supplied
Available by prescription only
Capsules (delayed-release): 10 mg, 20 mg

Indications and dosages
Active duodenal ulcer
Adults: 20 mg P.O. daily for 4 to 8 weeks.
Helicobacter pylori eradication to reduce the risk of duodenal ulcer recurrence
Triple therapy (omeprazole/clarithromycin/amoxicillin)
Adults: 20 mg P.O. b.i.d. plus 500 mg clarithromycin P.O. b.i.d. plus 1,000 mg amoxicillin P.O. b.i.d. for 10 days. In patients with an ulcer present at the time of initiation of therapy, an additional 18 days of omeprazole 20 mg once daily is recommended for ulcer healing and symptom relief.
Dual therapy (omeprazole/clarithromycin)
Adults: 40 mg each morning plus 500 mg clarithromycin t.i.d. for 14 days followed by 14 days of omeprazole 20 mg daily.
Severe erosive esophagitis; symptomatic, poorly responsive gastroesophageal reflux disease
Adults: 20 mg P.O. daily for 4 to 8 weeks. Patients with GERD should have failed initial therapy with an H$_2$ antagonist.
Pathological hypersecretory conditions, such as Zollinger-Ellison syndrome
Adults: initially, 60 mg P.O. daily; adjust dosage based on patient response. If daily dose exceeding 80 mg, divide it. Doses up to 120 mg t.i.d. have been administered. Continue therapy as long as clinically indicated.
Gastric ulcer
Adults: 40 mg P.O. daily for 4 to 8 weeks.
◪ DOSAGE ADJUSTMENT. Dosage adjustments may be necessary in patients with hepatic impairment.

Pharmacodynamics
Antisecretory action: Omeprazole inhibits the acid (proton) pump, H$_2$/K$^+$ adenosine triphosphatase (ATPase), located at the secretory surface of the gastric parietal cell. This action blocks the formation of gastric acid.

Pharmacokinetics
Absorption: Omeprazole is acid-labile and the formulation contains enteric-coated granules that permit absorption after drug leaves the stomach. Absorption is rapid, with peak levels occurring in less than

3½ hours. Bioavailability is about 40% because of instability in gastric acid as well as a substantial first-pass effect. Bioavailability increases slightly with repeated dosing, possibly because of drug's effect on gastric acidity.
Distribution: Drug is about 95% protein-bound.
Metabolism: Drug is primarily metabolized in the liver.
Excretion: Drug is primarily excreted by the kidneys. Plasma half-life is 30 to 60 minutes, but drug effects may persist for days.

Contraindications and precautions
Contraindicated in patients hypersensitive to drug or its components.

Interactions
Drug-drug
Drugs metabolized by hepatic oxidation, such as diazepam, phenytoin, propranolol, theophylline, warfarin: elimination may be impaired by omeprazole. Monitor patient closely.
Drugs that depend on low gastric pH for absorption, such as ampicillin esters, iron derivatives, itraconazole, ketoconazole: may have poor bioavailability in patients taking omeprazole. Separate administration times and observe for drug effects.

Drug-herb
Male fern: inactivated in alkaline environments. Advise patient concerning this effect.
Pennyroyal: drug may change the rate of formation of toxic metabolites. Advise against concurrent use.

Effects on diagnostic tests
Serum gastrin levels rise in most patients during first 2 weeks of therapy.

Adverse reactions
CNS: asthenia, dizziness, headache.
GI: abdominal pain, constipation, diarrhea, flatulence, nausea, vomiting.
Musculoskeletal: back pain.
Respiratory: cough, upper respiratory infection.
Skin: rash.

Overdose and treatment
Reports of overdose are rare. Symptoms include confusion, drowsiness, blurred vision, tachycardia, nausea, vomiting, diaphoresis, dry mouth, and headache. Amounts up to 360 mg daily have been well-tolerated. Dialysis is believed to be of little value because of the extent of binding to plasma proteins. Treatment should be symptomatic and supportive.

Special considerations
▶ Drug increases its own bioavailability with repeated administration. It's labile in gastric acid; less is lost to hydrolysis because drug raises gastric pH.
▶ Don't crush capsules.
▶ Monitor patient for decreased abdominal pain and improvement of symptoms.

Breast-feeding patients
▶ No data exist to demonstrate whether drug appears in breast milk. Avoid breast-feeding during therapy.

Pediatric patients
▶ Safe use in children hasn't been established.

Patient teaching
▶ Tell patient to take drug before meals and not to crush capsules.
▶ Explain the importance of taking drug exactly as prescribed.

▶ **ondansetron hydrochloride**
Zofran

Pharmacologic classification: *serotonin (5-HT₃)-receptor antagonist*

Therapeutic classification: *antiemetic*

Pregnancy risk category B

How supplied
Available by prescription only
Injection: 2 mg/ml in 20-ml multi-dose vials, 2-ml single-dose vials
Injection, premixed: 32 mg/50 ml in 5% dextrose single-dose vial
Tablets: 4 mg, 8 mg

Indications and dosages
Prevention of nausea and vomiting from initial and repeat courses of chemotherapy, including high-dose cisplatin
I.V. route
Adults and children age 4 and older: three I.V. doses of 0.15 mg/kg, with first dose infused over 15 minutes starting 30 minutes before chemotherapy and next two doses 4 and 8 hours after first dose. Alternatively, infuse a single 32-mg dose over 15 minutes, 30 minutes before chemotherapy starts.

P.O. route
Adults and children age 12 and over: 8 mg P.O. b.i.d. starting 30 minutes before chemotherapy starts, with subsequent dose 8 hours after first dose, then 8 mg q 12 hours for 1 to 2 days after completion of chemotherapy.
Children ages 4 to 11: 4 mg P.O. t.i.d. dosed the same times as for adults.
Prevention of radiation-induced nausea and vomiting
Adults: 8 mg P.O. t.i.d.
Prevention of postoperative nausea and vomiting
Adults: 16 mg P.O. 1 hour before anesthesia or 4 mg I.V. immediately before anesthesia or shortly postoperatively.
⊠ Dosage adjustment. Don't exceed 8 mg in patients with hepatic impairment.

Pharmacodynamics
Antiemetic action: Mechanism of action isn't fully defined; however, ondansetron is not a dopamine-receptor antagonist. Because serotonin receptors of the 5-HT₃ type are present both peripherally on vagal nerve terminals and centrally in the chemoreceptor trigger zone, it isn't certain whether ondansetron's antiemetic action is mediated centrally, peripherally, or both.

Pharmacokinetics
Absorption: Drug absorption is variable with oral administration. Level peaks within 2 hours, and bioavailability is 50% to 60%.
Distribution: Drug is 70% to 76% bound to plasma protein.
Metabolism: Drug is extensively metabolized by hydroxylation on

---

the indole ring, followed by glucuronide or sulfate conjugation. *Excretion:* 5% of dose is recovered in urine as parent compound. Half-life in adults is 3 to 6 hours.

Contraindications and precautions
Contraindicated in patients hypersensitive to drug. Use cautiously in patients with hepatic failure and liver failure.

Interactions
Drug-drug
Inducers or inhibitors of cytochrome P-450 enzyme: may change ondansetron clearance and half-life. No dosage adjustment is needed.

Drug-herb
Horehound: may enhance serotonergic effects. Advise against concurrent use.

Effects on diagnostic tests
None reported.

Adverse reactions
CNS: *dizziness, fatigue, headache, malaise, sedation.*
CV: chest pain.
GI: abdominal pain, *constipation, diarrhea,* xerostomia.
GU: gynecologic disorders, urine retention.
Hepatic: transient elevations in AST and ALT levels.
Musculoskeletal: *musculoskeletal pain.*
Respiratory: hypoxia.
Skin: injection-site reaction, rash.
Other: chills, fever.

Overdose and treatment
Doses more than 10 times the recommended amount have been given without incident.
 No recommended antidote exists. If overdose is suspected, manage with supportive therapy.

Special considerations
▶ For postoperative nausea and vomiting, give drug intraoperatively or immediately postoperatively.
▶ Drug is effective for managing postoperative pain related to nausea and vomiting, especially with gynecologic surgeries.
▶ Monitor patient's liver function tests.
▶ Dilute drug in 50 ml of D_5W injection or normal saline solution for injection before administration.
▶ Ondansetron is stable at room temperature for 48 hours after dilution with normal saline solution, D_5W, 5% dextrose and normal saline solution, 5% dextrose and half-normal saline solution, or 3% saline solution.

Breast-feeding patients
▶ No data exist to demonstrate whether drug appears in breast milk; caution is recommended.

Pediatric patients
▶ Little information is available for use in children age 3 and under.

Geriatric patients
▶ No age-related problems have been reported.

Patient teaching
▶ Advise patient that drug may help to relieve postoperative pain caused by vomiting.

▶ **opium tincture, deodorized (laudanum)**

▶ **opium tincture, camphorated (paregoric)**

Pharmacologic classification: *opiate*

Therapeutic classification: *antidiarrheal*

Controlled substance schedule II or III (based on amount of opium in product)

Pregnancy risk category B (D for high doses or long-term use)

How supplied
Available by prescription only
opium tincture
Alcoholic solution: equivalent to morphine 10 mg/ml
opium tincture, camphorated
Alcoholic solution: 2 mg morphine, 0.2 ml anise oil, 20 mg benzoic acid, 20 mg camphor, 0.2 ml glycerin, and ethanol to make 5 ml

Indications and dosages
Acute, nonspecific diarrhea
Adults: 0.6 ml opium tincture (range, 0.3 to 1 ml) P.O. q.i.d. (maximum, 6 ml daily) or 5 to 10 ml camphorated opium tincture daily, b.i.d., t.i.d., or q.i.d. until diarrhea subsides.
Children: 0.25 to 0.5 ml/kg camphorated opium tincture daily, b.i.d., t.i.d., or q.i.d. until diarrhea subsides.
Severe opiate withdrawal symptoms in neonates
Neonates: 1:25 dilution of opium tincture in water, given as 0.2 ml

P.O. q 3 hours. Adjust dosage to control withdrawal symptoms. Increase by 0.05 ml q 3 hours until symptoms are controlled. Once symptoms are stabilized for 3 to 5 days, gradually decrease dosage over a 2-to 4-week period.

Pharmacodynamics
Antidiarrheal action: Morphine, derived from the opium poppy and the most active ingredient in opium, increases GI smooth-muscle tone, inhibits motility and propulsion, and diminishes secretions. By inhibiting peristalsis, the drug delays passage of intestinal contents, increasing water resorption and relieving diarrhea.

Pharmacokinetics
Absorption: Morphine is absorbed variably from the gut.
Distribution: Although opium alkaloids are distributed widely in the body, the low doses used to treat diarrhea act primarily in the GI tract. Camphor crosses the placenta.
Metabolism: Opium is metabolized rapidly in the liver.
Excretion: Opium is excreted in urine; opium alkaloids (especially morphine) enter breast milk. Drug effect persists 4 to 5 hours.

Contraindications and precautions
Contraindicated in patients with acute diarrhea caused by poisoning until toxic material is removed from GI tract or in those with diarrhea caused by organisms that penetrate intestinal mucosa.
Use cautiously in patients with asthma, prostatic hyperplasia, he-

patic disease, and history of opium dependence.

Interactions
Drug-drug
Metoclopramide: may antagonize the effects of metoclopramide. Avoid using together.
Other CNS depressants: additive effects. Use together cautiously.

Effects on diagnostic tests
Opium tincture and camphorated opium tincture may prevent delivery of technetium Tc-99m disofenin to the small intestine during hepatobiliary imaging tests; delay test until 24 hours after last dose.

Adverse reactions
CNS: dizziness, light-headedness.
GI: increased serum amylase and lipase levels, nausea, vomiting.
Other: physical dependence after long-term use.

Overdose and treatment
Overdose may cause drowsiness, hypotension, seizures, and apnea.

Empty stomach by induced emesis or gastric lavage; maintain patent airway. Use naloxone to treat respiratory depression. Monitor patient for signs and symptoms of CNS or respiratory depression.

Special considerations
▶ Mix drug with sufficient water to ensure passage to stomach.
▶ Deodorized opium tincture (laudanum) is 25 times more potent than camphorated opium tincture (paregoric); take care not to confuse these drugs.
▶ Risk of physical dependence on drug increases with long-term use.

▶ Don't refrigerate drug.
▶ Monitor patient's vital signs and bowel function.

Breast-feeding patients
▶ Because opium alkaloids (especially morphine) appear in breast milk, drug's possible risks must be weighed against benefits.

Pediatric patients
▶ Opium tincture has been used to treat withdrawal symptoms in infants whose mothers are narcotic addicts.

Patient teaching
▶ Warn patient that physical dependence may result from long-term use.
▶ Caution patient to avoid hazardous activities because drug may cause drowsiness, dizziness, and blurred vision.
▶ Because drug is indicated only for short-term use, instruct patient to report diarrhea that persists longer than 48 hours.
▶ Advise patient to take drug with food if it causes nausea, vomiting, or constipation.
▶ Instruct patient to call immediately if she has shortness of breath or trouble breathing.
▶ Tell patient to drink adequate fluids while diarrhea persists.

▶ oxaprozin
Daypro

Pharmacologic classification:
NSAID

Therapeutic classification:
anti-inflammatory, antipyretic, nonnarcotic analgesic

Pregnancy risk category C

How supplied
Available by prescription only
Caplets: 600 mg

Indications and dosages
Acute or chronic osteoarthritis or rheumatoid arthritis
Adults: initially, 1,200 mg P.O. daily. Individualize to smallest effective dosage to minimize adverse reactions. Smaller patients or those with mild symptoms may require only 600 mg daily. Maximum, 1,800 mg or 26 mg/kg daily, whichever is lower, in divided doses.
◻ DOSAGE ADJUSTMENT. Elderly patients may need a reduced dose because of low body weight or disorders of aging. In patients with renal impairment, start with 600 mg daily and increase cautiously as needed.

Pharmacodynamics
Analgesic, antipyretic, and anti-inflammatory actions: Exact mechanism of action isn't clearly defined. Drug inhibits several steps along the arachidonic acid pathway of prostaglandin synthesis. One mode of action is presumed to be a result of inhibited cyclooxygenase activity and prostaglandin synthesis at the site of inflammation.

Pharmacokinetics
Absorption: Drug demonstrates high oral bioavailability (95%). Plasma levels peak 3 to 5 hours after dosing. Food may reduce the rate of absorption, but extent of absorption is unchanged.
Distribution: Drug is about 99.9% bound to albumin in plasma.
Metabolism: Drug is primarily metabolized in the liver by microsomal oxidation (65%) and glucuronic acid conjugation (35%).
Excretion: Glucuronide metabolites are excreted in urine (65%) and feces (35%). Elimination half-life in adults is 42 to 50 hours.

Contraindications and precautions
Contraindicated in patients hypersensitive to drug and in patients with reaction syndrome to aspirin or other NSAIDs (nasal polyps, angioedema, and bronchospasm).
Use cautiously in patients with renal or hepatic dysfunction, history of peptic ulcer, hypertension, CV disease, or conditions predisposing to fluid retention.

Interactions
Drug-drug
Aspirin: oxaprozin displaces salicylates from plasma protein-binding, increasing the risk of salicylate toxicity. Use of oxaprozin and aspirin isn't recommended.
Beta blockers, such as metoprolol: may cause a transient increase in blood pressure after 14 days of therapy. Consider routine blood pressure monitoring when starting oxaprozin therapy.
Oral anticoagulants: may increase the risk of bleeding. Monitor PT and INR.

Reactions may be *common*, uncommon, **life-threatening**, or COMMON AND LIFE-THREATENING.

Drug-lifestyle
Sun exposure: may cause photo-sensitivity reactions. Urge precautions.

Effects on diagnostic tests
None reported.

Adverse reactions
CNS: confusion, depression, sedation, sleep disturbances, somnolence.
EENT: blurred vision, tinnitus.
GI: abdominal pain or distress, anorexia, *constipation, diarrhea, dyspepsia,* flatulence, ***hemorrhage,*** *nausea,* stomatitis, ulcer, vomiting.
GU: dysuria, urinary frequency.
Hematologic: prolonged bleeding time.
Hepatic: elevated liver function test results with chronic use.
Skin: photosensitivity, *rash.*

Overdose and treatment
No specific information is available. Common symptoms of acute overdose with other NSAIDs (lethargy, drowsiness, nausea, vomiting, and epigastric pain) are typically reversible with supportive care. GI bleeding and coma have occurred after NSAID overdose. Hypertension, acute renal failure, and respiratory depression are rare. Symptomatic patients seen within 4 hours of ingestion or after a large overdose (5 to 10 times the usual dose) may need induced emesis or activated charcoal with an osmotic cathartic.

Special considerations
❯ Drug may be used for other mild to moderate types of pain such as dysmenorrhea, shoulder pain, and gout.

❯ Full therapeutic effect may be delayed for 2 to 4 weeks.
❯ Serious GI toxicity, including peptic ulceration and bleeding, can occur in patients taking NSAIDs despite the absence of GI symptoms. Patients at risk for developing peptic ulceration and bleeding are those with history of serious GI events, alcoholism, smoking, or other factors associated with peptic ulcer disease.
❯ Doses above 1,200 mg/day should be used for patients who weigh more than 110 lb (50 kg), who have normal renal and hepatic function, who are at low risk of peptic ulceration, and whose severity of disease justifies maximal therapy.
❯ Most patients tolerate once-daily dosing. Divided doses may be tried in patients unable to tolerate single doses.
❯ Elevated liver function test results can occur after chronic use. These abnormal findings may persist, worsen, or resolve with continued therapy. Rarely, patients may progress to severe hepatic dysfunction.
❯ Periodically monitor liver function tests in patients receiving long-term therapy, and closely monitor patients with abnormal test results.
❯ Anemia may occur in patients receiving oxaprozin. Obtain hemoglobin level or hematocrit in patients with prolonged therapy at intervals appropriate for their clinical situation.

Breast-feeding patients
❯ No data exist to demonstrate whether drug appears in breast milk. Use caution when administering drug to a breast-feeding woman.

◇ Available in Canada only   *Unlabeled use

Pediatric patients
▶ Safety and effectiveness in children haven't been established.

Geriatric patients
▶ Elderly patients may need a reduced dosage because of low body weight or disorders of aging.
▶ Elderly patients are less likely than younger patients to tolerate adverse reactions associated with oxaprozin.

Patient teaching
▶ Tell patient to take drug with milk or meals if adverse GI reactions occur.
▶ Because photosensitivity reactions may occur, advise patient to use a sunblock, wear protective clothing, and avoid prolonged exposure to sunlight.
▶ Warn patient to call immediately if signs and symptoms of GI bleeding or visual or auditory adverse reactions occur.

▶ oxazepam
Apo-Oxazepam◇, Novoxapam◇, Serax

Pharmacologic classification: *benzodiazepine*

Therapeutic classification: *antianxiety drug, sedative-hypnotic*

Controlled substance schedule IV

Pregnancy risk category D

How supplied
Available by prescription only
Tablets: 15 mg
Capsules: 10 mg, 15 mg, 30 mg

Indications and dosages
Alcohol withdrawal, severe anxiety
Adults: 15 to 30 mg P.O. t.i.d. or q.i.d.
Tension, mild to moderate anxiety
Adults: 10 to 15 mg P.O. t.i.d. or q.i.d.
▧ **Dosage adjustment.** In older adults, give 10 mg P.O. t.i.d.; then increase to 15 mg t.i.d. or q.i.d., p.r.n.

Pharmacodynamics
Anxiolytic and sedative-hypnotic actions: Oxazepam depresses the CNS at the limbic and subcortical levels of the brain. It produces an antianxiety effect by enhancing the effect of the neurotransmitter GABA on its receptor in the ascending reticular activating system, which increases inhibition and blocks both cortical and limbic arousal.

Pharmacokinetics
Absorption: When administered orally, oxazepam is well absorbed through the GI tract. Levels peak 3 hours after dosing. Action starts in 1 to 2 hours.
Distribution: Drug is distributed widely throughout the body. Drug is 85% to 95% protein-bound.
Metabolism: Drug is metabolized in the liver to inactive metabolites.
Excretion: Metabolites of oxazepam are excreted in urine as glucuronide conjugates. Half-life of drug is 6 to 11 hours.

Contraindications and precautions
Contraindicated in patients with psychosis or hypersensitivity to drug.

Use cautiously in elderly or debilitated patients; in those with history of drug abuse; and in those in whom a decrease in blood pressure is associated with cardiac problems.

Interactions
Drug-drug
Antacids: decreased rate of oxazepam absorption. Separate administration times.

Antidepressants, antihistamines, barbiturates, general anesthetics, MAO inhibitors, narcotics, phenothiazines: potentiated CNS depressant effects. Use together cautiously.

Cimetidine, disulfiram: diminished hepatic metabolism of oxazepam, which increases its plasma level. Monitor patient for toxic effects, and adjust dose as needed.

Levodopa: oxazepam may inhibit levodopa effects. Monitor patient for drug effects.

Drug-lifestyle
Alcohol use: potentiated CNS depressant effects of alcohol. Advise against alcohol use.

Heavy smoking: accelerates oxazepam metabolism, thus lowering effectiveness. Advise patient to avoid smoking.

Effects on diagnostic tests
None reported.

Adverse reactions
CNS: changes in EEG patterns, confusion, dizziness, *drowsiness,* headache, *lethargy,* slurred speech, syncope, tremor, vertigo.
CV: edema.
GI: nausea.
GU: altered libido.

Hepatic: *hepatic dysfunction.*
Skin: rash.

Overdose and treatment
Overdose may cause somnolence, confusion, coma, hypoactive reflexes, dyspnea, labored breathing, hypotension, bradycardia, slurred speech, and unsteady gait or impaired coordination.

Support blood pressure and respiration until the drug effects have subsided; monitor vital signs. Mechanical ventilatory assistance via endotracheal tube may be needed to maintain a patent airway and support adequate oxygenation. Flumazenil, a specific benzodiazepine antagonist, may be useful. As needed, use I.V. fluids and vasopressors, such as dopamine and phenylephrine, to treat hypotension. If the patient is conscious, induce emesis. Use gastric lavage if ingestion was recent, but only if an endotracheal tube is present to prevent aspiration. After emesis or lavage, administer activated charcoal with a cathartic as a single dose. Dialysis is of limited value.

Special considerations
▶ By reducing anxiety, drug potentiates the effects of analgesics.
▶ Provide patient with calm, serene environment, if possible.
▶ To discontinue therapy, reduce dosage gradually over 8 to 12 weeks.
▶ Oxazepam tablets contain tartrazine dye; check patient's history for allergy to this substance.
▶ Store drug in a cool, dry place away from light.
▶ Monitor hepatic and renal function studies to ensure normal function.

Breast-feeding patients
▶ The breast-fed infant whose mother uses oxazepam may become sedated, have trouble feeding, or lose weight; avoid use in breast-feeding women.

Pediatric patients
▶ Safe use in children under age 12 hasn't been established.
▶ Closely observe neonate for withdrawal symptoms if mother took oxazepam for a prolonged period during pregnancy.

Geriatric patients
▶ Elderly patients are more susceptible to the CNS depressant effects of oxazepam. Some may require supervision with ambulation and activities of daily living during initiation of therapy or after an increase in dose.
▶ Lower doses are usually effective in elderly patients because of decreased elimination.

Patient teaching
▶ Advise patient not to change part of drug regimen without consulting prescriber.
▶ Instruct patient in safety measures, such as gradual position changes and assisted ambulation, to prevent injury.
▶ Caution patient that sleepiness may not occur for up to 2 hours after taking oxazepam.
▶ Advise patient about risk of physical and psychological dependence with chronic use of oxazepam.
▶ Tell patient not to stop drug suddenly if he's been taking it for prolonged periods.

▶ oxybutynin chloride
Ditropan, Ditropan XL

Pharmacologic classification: *synthetic tertiary amine*

Therapeutic classification: *antispasmodic*

Pregnancy risk category B

How supplied
Available by prescription only
Syrup: 5 mg/5 ml
Tablets: 5 mg
Tablets (extended release): 5 mg, 10 mg, 15 mg

Indications and dosages
Bladder instability during voiding in patients with uninhibited and reflex neurogenic bladder
Adults: 5 mg P.O. b.i.d. to t.i.d. Maximum, 5 mg q.i.d.
Children over age 5: 5 mg P.O. b.i.d. Maximum, 5 mg t.i.d.
Overactive bladder
Adults: 5 mg P.O. daily. Increase by 5 mg as needed at about 1-week intervals. Maximum, 30 mg/day.

Pharmacodynamics
Antispasmodic action: Oxybutynin reduces the urge to void, increases bladder capacity, and reduces the frequency of contractions to the detrusor muscle. Drug exerts a direct spasmolytic action and an antimuscarinic action on smooth muscle.

Pharmacokinetics
Absorption: Drug is absorbed rapidly; levels peak in 3 to 6 hours. Action begins in 30 to 60 minutes and persists for 6 to 10 hours.
Distribution: Unknown.

Metabolism: Drug is metabolized by the liver.
Excretion: Drug is excreted principally in urine.

Contraindications and precautions

Contraindicated in patients with hypersensitivity to drug, myasthenia gravis, GI obstruction, glaucoma, adynamic ileus, megacolon, severe colitis, ulcerative colitis when megacolon is present, or obstructive uropathy; in elderly or debilitated patients with intestinal atony; and in hemorrhaging patients with unstable CV status.

Use cautiously in elderly patients and those with impaired renal or hepatic function, autonomic neuropathy, or reflux esophagitis.

Interactions
Drug-drug

CNS depressants: additive sedative effect. Monitor patient closely.
Digoxin: increased digoxin levels. Monitor serum digoxin levels.
Haloperidol: worsening of schizophrenia, decreased serum levels of haloperidol, and development of tardive dyskinesia may occur. Monitor patient closely.
Phenothiazines: increased incidence of anticholinergic adverse effects. Monitor patient closely.

Drug-lifestyle

Alcohol use: increased CNS effects. Advise against concurrent use.
Exercise, hot weather: may precipitate heat stroke. Advise caution.

Effects on diagnostic tests
None reported.

Adverse reactions
CNS: asthenia, confusion, dizziness, hallucinations, insomnia, restlessness.
CV: *palpitations, tachycardia,* vasodilation.
EENT: amblyopia, cycloplegia, decreased lacrimation, mydriasis.
GI: *constipation,* decreased GI motility, *dry mouth,* nausea, vomiting.
GU: *urinary hesitancy, urine retention.*
Skin: decreased diaphoresis, rash.
Other: fever, suppressed lactation.

Overdose and treatment
Overdose may cause restlessness, excitement, psychotic behavior, flushing, hypotension, circulatory failure, and fever. In severe cases, paralysis, respiratory failure, and coma may occur.

Treatment requires gastric lavage. Activated charcoal may be administered as well as a cathartic. Physostigmine may be considered to reverse symptoms of anticholinergic intoxication. Treat hyperpyrexia symptomatically with ice bags or other cold applications and alcohol sponges. Maintain artificial respiration if paralysis of respiratory muscles occurs.

Special considerations
❿ Antispasmotic action of drug reduces patient's discomfort.
❿ Before giving oxybutynin, anticipate confirmation of neurogenic bladder by cystometry and rule out partial intestinal obstruction in patients with diarrhea, especially those with colostomy or ileostomy.
❿ Discontinue drug periodically to determine if patient still requires medication.

▶ Drug may aggravate symptoms of hyperthyroidism, coronary artery disease, heart failure, arrhythmias, tachycardia, hypertension, or prostatic hyperplasia.
▶ Periodically prepare patient for cystometry to evaluate response to therapy.

Breast-feeding patients
▶ No data exist to demonstrate whether drug appears in breast milk. Use caution when administering to a breast-feeding woman.

Pediatric patients
▶ Dosage guidelines haven't been established for children under age 5.

Geriatric patients
▶ Elderly patients may be more sensitive to antimuscarinic effects.
▶ Drug is contraindicated in elderly and debilitated patients with intestinal atony.

Patient teaching
▶ Instruct patient regarding drug and dosage schedule; tell him to take a missed dose as soon as possible and not to double the doses.
▶ Tell patient not to crush or chew extended-release tablets. They may be administered without regard to food.
▶ Warn patient about possibility of decreased mental alertness or visual changes.
▶ Remind patient to use drug cautiously when in warm climates to minimize risk of heatstroke that may occur because of decreased sweating.

▶ oxycodone hydrochloride
Oxycontin, OxyFAST, OxyIR, Roxicodone, Supeudol ◇

Pharmacologic classification:
opioid

Therapeutic classification:
analgesic

Controlled substance schedule II

Pregnancy risk category C

How supplied
Available by prescription only
Oral solution: 5 mg/ml, 20 mg/ml
Tablets: 5 mg
Tablets (sustained-release): 10 mg, 20 mg, 40 mg, 80 mg

Indications and dosages
Moderate to severe pain
Adults: 5 mg P.O. q 6 hours
Chronic pain
Adults: initially, 10-mg sustained-release tablet q 12 hours; may increase dose q 1 to 2 days. Dosing frequency shouldn't be increased.

Pharmacodynamics
Analgesic action: Oxycodone acts on opiate receptors, providing analgesia for moderate to moderately severe pain. Episodes of acute pain, rather than chronic pain, appear to be more responsive to treatment with oxycodone.

Pharmacokinetics
Absorption: After oral administration, onset of analgesic effect occurs within 15 to 30 minutes and peak effect is reached within 1 hour.
Distribution: Drug is rapidly distributed.

Metabolism: Drug is metabolized in the liver.
Excretion: Oxycodone is excreted principally by the kidneys. Duration of analgesia is 6 hours; for sustained-release tablets, 12 hours.

Contraindications and precautions

Contraindicated in patients hypersensitive to drug.

Use cautiously in elderly or debilitated patients and in those with head injury, increased intracranial pressure, seizures, asthma, COPD, prostatic hyperplasia, severe hepatic or renal disease, acute abdominal conditions, urethral stricture, hypothyroidism, Addison's disease, or arrhythmias.

Interactions
Drug-drug

Anticholinergics: paralytic ileus. Monitor for abdominal pain.
Cimetidine: may increase respiratory and CNS depression, causing confusion, disorientation, apnea, or seizures. Avoid using together.
CNS depressants such as antihistamines, barbiturates, benzodiazepines, general anesthetics, muscle relaxants, narcotic analgesics, phenothiazines, sedative-hypnotics, tricyclic antidepressants: potentiated respiratory and CNS depression, sedation, and hypotensive effects. Use together cautiously, and reduce dosage as needed.
Drugs extensively metabolized in the liver such as digitoxin, phenytoin, rifampin: drug accumulation and enhanced effects. Use together cautiously, and reduce dosage as needed.

General anesthetics: increased risk of severe CV depression. Use together cautiously.
Opioid agonist-antagonist or antagonist: patients who become physically dependent on this drug may experience acute withdrawal syndrome. Avoid concurrent use unless absolutely necessary.
Oxycodone products containing aspirin: may increase anticoagulant's effect. Monitor clotting times, and use together cautiously.

Drug-lifestyle

Alcohol use: potentiated respiratory and CNS depression, sedation, and hypotensive effects. Advise against concurrent use.

Effects on diagnostic tests
None reported.

Adverse reactions
CNS: *clouded sensorium, dizziness, euphoria, light-headedness, sedation,* **seizure,** *somnolence.*
CV: **bradycardia,** *hypotension.*
GI: *constipation,* ileus, increased plasma amylase and lipase, *nausea, vomiting.*
GU: *urine retention.*
Hepatic: increased liver enzyme levels.
Respiratory: *respiratory depression.*
Skin: *diaphoresis,* pruritus, rash.
Other: physical dependence.

Overdose and treatment
Severe overdose may cause CNS depression, respiratory depression, and miosis. Other acute toxic effects include hypotension, bradycardia, hypothermia, shock, apnea, cardiopulmonary arrest, circulatory collapse, pulmonary edema, and convulsions.

To treat acute overdose, first establish adequate respiratory exchange via a patent airway and ventilation as needed; administer a narcotic antagonist such as naloxone to reverse respiratory depression. Because the duration of action of oxycodone is longer than that of naloxone, repeated naloxone dosing is necessary. Naloxone should not be given unless patient has clinically significant respiratory or CV depression. Monitor vital signs closely.

If ingestion occurred within 2 hours, empty the stomach immediately by inducing emesis with ipecac syrup or using gastric lavage. Use caution to avoid any risk of aspiration. Administer activated charcoal via nasogastric tube for further removal of the drug in an oral overdose.

Provide symptomatic and supportive treatment such as continued respiratory support and correction of fluid or electrolyte imbalance. Monitor laboratory values, vital signs, and neurologic status closely.

Dialysis may be helpful if combination products with aspirin or acetaminophen are involved.

Special considerations
▶ Drug is effective for short-term, acute pain or postoperative pain.
▶ Have patient rate pain using a scale, and then reevaluate pain after dosing.
▶ For full analgesic effect, administer drug before patient has intense pain.
▶ Oral solutions are effective when given via nasogastric tube; don't use sustained-release form in nasogastric tube.

▶ When using sustained-release form, breakthrough pain may require additional pain medication.
▶ Single-agent oxycodone solution or tablets are ideal for patients who can't take aspirin or acetaminophen.
▶ Oxycodone has high abuse potential.
▶ With chronic opioid use, dose tolerance is likely. Increase dose as necesssary and as ordered. Don't discontinue drug abruptly in these patients.
▶ Drug may obscure signs and symptoms of an acute abdominal condition or worsen gallbladder pain.
▶ Consider a stool softener for patients on long-term therapy.
▶ The 80-mg sustained-release tablets are for opioid-tolerant patients only.
▶ Monitor circulatory and respiratory status. Withhold dose and notify health care provider if respirations are shallow or if respiratory rate falls below 12 breaths/minute.
▶ Monitor patient's bladder and bowel patterns.

Breast-feeding patients
▶ No data exist to demonstrate whether drug appears in breast milk; use with caution in breast-feeding women.

Pediatric patients
▶ Dosage may be individualized for children; however, safety and effectiveness in children haven't been established.

Geriatric patients
▶ Lower doses are usually indicated for elderly patients, who may be more sensitive to the therapeutic and adverse effects of the drug.

Patient teaching
▶ For full analgesic effect, teach patient to take drug before pain becomes intense.
▶ Warn patient about possibility of decreased alertness or visual changes.
▶ Tell patient not to discontinue drug abruptly.
▶ Caution patient to avoid hazardous activities when taking drug.

▶ oxymorphone hydrochloride
Numorphan

Pharmacologic classification:
opioid

Therapeutic classification:
analgesic

Controlled substance schedule II

Pregnancy risk category C

How supplied
Available by prescription only
Injection: 1 mg/ml, 1.5 mg/ml
Suppository: 5 mg

Indications and dosages
Moderate to severe pain
Adults: 1 to 1.5 mg I.M. or S.C. q 4 to 6 hours, p.r.n., or around the clock; 0.5 mg I.V. q 4 to 6 hours, p.r.n., or around the clock; or 1 suppository administered P.R. q 4 to 6 hours, p.r.n., or around the clock.

Pharmacodynamics
Analgesic action: Oxymorphone effectively relieves moderate to severe pain via agonist activity at the opiate receptors. It has little or no antitussive effect.

Pharmacokinetics
Absorption: Oxymorphone is well absorbed after P.R., S.C., I.M., or I.V. administration. Onset of action occurs within 5 to 10 minutes.
Distribution: Drug is widely distributed.
Metabolism: Drug is primarily metabolized in the liver.
Excretion: Duration of action is 3 to 6 hours. Drug is excreted primarily in the urine as oxymorphone conjugates.

Contraindications and precautions
Contraindicated in patients hypersensitive to drug.

Use cautiously in elderly or debilitated patients and in those with head injury, increased intracranial pressure, seizures, asthma, COPD, acute abdomen conditions, prostatic hyperplasia, severe renal or kidney disease, urethral stricture, respiratory depression, Addison's disease, arrhythmias, or hypothyroidism.

Interactions
Drug-drug
Anticholinergics: paralytic ileus. Monitor for abdominal pain.
Cimetidine: increased respiratory and CNS depression, causing confusion, disorientation, apnea, or seizures. Reduced dosage of oxymorphone is usually necessary.
CNS depressants such as antihistamines, barbiturates, benzodiazepines, general anesthetics, muscle relaxants, opiates, phenothiazines, sedative-hypnotics, tricyclic antidepressants: potentiated respiratory and CNS depression, sedation, and hypotensive effects. Use together cautiously and reduce dosage as needed.

Drugs extensively metabolized in the liver, such as digitoxin, phenytoin, rifampin: drug accumulation and enhanced effects. Use together cautiously and reduce dosage as needed.
General anesthetics: severe CV depression. Monitor patient closely.
Narcotic antagonist: patients who become physically dependent on drug may experience acute withdrawal syndrome. Avoid concomitant use if possible.

Drug-lifestyle
Alcohol use: potentiated respiratory and CNS depression, sedation, and hypotensive effects. Advise against concurrent use.

Effects on diagnostic tests
None reported.

Adverse reactions
CNS: *clouded sensorium,* dizziness, *euphoria,* headache, lightheadedness, *sedation,* **seizures** with large doses, *somnolence.*
CV: **bradycardia**, *hypotension.*
GI: *constipation,* ileus, increased plasma amylase levels, *nausea, vomiting.*
GU: *urine retention.*
Respiratory: ***respiratory depression***.
Skin: pruritus.
Other: physical dependence.

Overdose and treatment
Oxymorphone overdose may cause CNS depression, extreme somnolence progressing to stupor and coma, respiratory depression, and miosis. Other acute toxic effects include hypotension, bradycardia, hypothermia, shock, apnea, cardiopulmonary arrest, circulatory collapse, pulmonary edema, and seizures.

To treat acute overdose, first establish adequate respiration via a patent airway and ventilate as needed; administer a narcotic antagonist such as naloxone, to reverse respiratory depression. Because drug's duration of action is longer than that of naloxone, repeated naloxone dosing is necessary. Naloxone should not be given unless the patient has clinically significant respiratory or CV depression. Monitor vital signs closely.

Provide symptomatic and supportive treatment such as continued respiratory support, and correction of fluid or electrolyte imbalance. Monitor laboratory values, vital signs, and neurologic status closely.

Special considerations
▶ Parenteral administration of drug is also indicated for preoperative medication, for support of anesthesia, for obstetric analgesia, and for relief of anxiety in dyspnea associated with acute left-sided heart failure and pulmonary edema.
▶ Drug isn't for use for mild pain.
▶ For better effect, administer drug before patient has intense pain.
▶ Drug is well absorbed P.R. and is an alternative to opioids with more limited dosage forms.
▶ Keep resuscitation equipment and narcotic antagonist (naloxone) available.
▶ Drug may worsen gallbladder pain.
▶ Refrigerate oxymorphone suppositories.
▶ Monitor circulatory and respiratory status. Withhold dose and notify if respirations are shallow or if

---

Reactions may be *common*, uncommon, ***life-threatening***, or **COMMON AND LIFE-THREATENING**.

respiratory rate falls below 12
breaths/minute.
▶ Monitor patient's bladder and
bowel patterns.
▶ Give by direct I.V. injection. If
necessary, drug may be diluted in
normal saline solution.

Breast-feeding patients
▶ No data exist to demonstrate
whether drug appears in breast
milk; use with caution in breast-
feeding women.

Pediatric patients
▶ Don't give drug to children under
age 12.

Geriatric patients
▶ Lower doses are usually indicated for elderly patients, who may be
more sensitive to the therapeutic
and adverse effects of the drug.

Patient teaching
▶ Instruct patient to ask for drug
before pain is intense.
▶ When drug is used postoperatively, encourage patient to turn,
cough, and deep breathe and to use
incentive spirometer to avoid atelectasis.
▶ Caution ambulatory patient about
getting out of bed or walking.
Warn outpatient to avoid driving
and other potentially hazardous activities that require mental alertness until drug's CNS effects are
known.
▶ Advise patient to avoid alcohol.

▶ pamidronate disodium
Aredia

Pharmacologic classification:
*bisphosphonate, pyrophosphate
analogue*

Therapeutic classification:
antihypercalcemic

Pregnancy risk category C

How supplied
Available by prescription only
Injection: 30 mg/vial, 60 mg/vial,
90 mg/vial

Indications and dosages
Paget's disease
Adults: 30 mg I.V. daily over 4
hours for 3 consecutive days for
total dose of 90 mg.
*Osteolytic bone lesions of multiple
myeloma*
Adults: 90 mg I.V. daily over 4
hours once monthly.

Pharmacodynamics
Antihypercalcemic action: Drug inhibits the resorption of bone. Drug
adsorbs to hydroxyapatite crystals
in bone and may directly block the
dissolution of calcium phosphate.
Drug apparently doesn't inhibit
bone formation or mineralization.

Pharmacokinetics
Absorption: Onset is rapid; duration of action is up to 6 months in
bone.
Distribution: After I.V. administration in animals, about 50% to 60%
of a dose is rapidly absorbed by
bone. Drug is also taken up by the
kidneys, liver, spleen, teeth, and
tracheal cartilage.

Metabolism: None.
Excretion: Drug is excreted by the kidneys; an average of 51% of a dose is excreted in urine within 72 hours of administration.

Contraindications and precautions

Contraindicated in patients hypersensitive to drug or other bisphosphonates, such as etidronate.

Use with extreme caution in patients with impaired renal function.

Interactions
Drug-drug
Solutions that contain calcium: pamidronate may form a precipitate when mixed with these solutions. Avoid mixing together.

Effects on diagnostic tests
None reported.

Adverse reactions
CNS: fatigue, headache, *seizures,* somnolence, syncope.
CV: atrial fibrillation, *hypertension,* tachycardia.
GI: *abdominal pain, anorexia, constipation,* **GI hemorrhage,** *nausea, vomiting.*
Hematologic: *anemia, leukopenia, thrombocytopenia.*
Metabolic: *hypocalcemia, hypokalemia, hypomagnesemia, hypophosphatemia.*
Musculoskeletal: *bone pain.*
Other: *fever, generalized pain, infusion-site reaction.*

Overdose and treatment
Symptomatic hypocalcemia could result from overdose; treat with I.V. calcium. Fever and hypotension can be rapidly corrected with steroids.

Special considerations
❱ Drug is also used for moderate to severe hypercalcemia associated with malignancy (with or without metastases).
❱ Pamidronate is used in addition to antineoplastics and opiate analgesics in the treatment of multiple myeloma.
❱ Paget's disease results in bone pain and fractures.
❱ Osteolytic destruction results in bone pain and immobility.
❱ Reconstitute vial with 10 ml sterile water for injection. Once drug is completely dissolved, add to 1,000 ml of D_5W or half-normal or normal saline solution injection. Don't mix with infusion solutions that contain calcium, such as Ringer's injection or lactated Ringer's injection. Administer in a single I.V. solution using its own line. Visually inspect for precipitate before administering.
❱ Injection solution is stable for 24 hours when refrigerated. Give only by I.V. infusion. Animal studies have shown evidence of nephropathy when drug is given as a bolus.
❱ Because drug can cause electrolyte disturbances, careful monitoring of serum electrolytes especially calcium, phosphate, and magnesium, is essential. Short-term administration of calcium may be necessary in patients with severe hypocalcemia. Also monitor creatinine, CBC, differential, hematocrit, and hemoglobin levels.
❱ Carefully monitor patients with preexisting anemia, leukopenia, or thrombocytopenia during first 2 weeks after therapy.
❱ Monitor patient's temperature. In trials, 27% of patients experienced a slightly elevated temperature for 24 to 48 hours after therapy.

Reactions may be *common,* uncommon, *life-threatening,* or COMMON AND LIFE-THREATENING.

▶ Consider retreatment if hypercalcemia recurs; allow a minimum of 7 days to elapse before retreatment to allow for full response to the initial dose.

Breast-feeding patients
▶ No data exist to demonstrate whether drug appears in breast milk. Use with caution in breast-feeding women.

Pediatric patients
▶ Safety and efficacy in children haven't been established.

Patient teaching
▶ Explain use and administration of drug to patient and family.
▶ Instruct patient to report adverse reactions promptly.

▶ pancuronium bromide
Pavulon

Pharmacologic classification:
nondepolarizing neuromuscular blocker

Therapeutic classification:
skeletal muscle relaxant

Pregnancy risk category C

How supplied
Available by prescription only
Injection: 1 mg/ml, 2 mg/ml parenteral

Indications and dosages
Adjunct to anesthesia to induce skeletal muscle relaxation, facilitate intubation and ventilation, and weaken muscle contractions in induced seizures
Adults and children over age 1 month: initially, 0.04 to 0.1 mg/kg I.V.; then 0.01 mg/kg q 25 to 60 minutes if needed. Dosage depends on anesthetic used, individual needs, and response. Doses are representative and must be adjusted.

Pharmacodynamics
Skeletal muscle relaxant action: Pancuronium prevents acetylcholine (ACh) from binding to receptors on the motor end plate, thus blocking depolarization. It may increase heart rate through direct blocking effect on the ACh receptors of the heart; increase is dose-related. Pancuronium causes little or no histamine release and no ganglionic blockade.

Pharmacokinetics
Absorption: After I.V. administration, onset of action occurs in 30 to 45 seconds, and effects peak in 2 to 3 minutes. Onset and duration are dose-related. After 0.06 mg/kg dose, effects begin to subside in 35 to 45 minutes. Repeated doses may increase the magnitude and duration of action.
Distribution: Pancuronium is 87% bound to plasma proteins.
Metabolism: Drug's metabolism is unknown; small amounts may be metabolized by the liver.
Excretion: Drug is mainly excreted unchanged in urine; some through biliary excretion.

Contraindications and precautions
Contraindicated in patients with hypersensitivity to bromides or preexisting tachycardia and in those for whom even a minor increase in heart rate is undesirable.

Use cautiously in elderly or debilitated patients and in those with impaired renal, pulmonary, or hepatic function; respiratory depression; myasthenia gravis; myasthenic syndrome of lung or bronchogenic cancer; dehydration; thyroid disorders; collagen diseases; porphyria; electrolyte disturbances; hyperthermia; or toxemic states. Also, use large doses cautiously in patients undergoing cesarean section.

Interactions
Drug-drug
Aminoglycoside antibiotics, beta blockers, clindamycin, depolarizing neuromuscular blockers, furosemide, general anesthetics, lincomycin, lithium, magnesium salts (parenteral), nondepolarizing neuromuscular blockers, polymyxin antibiotics, potassium-depleting drugs, quinidine, quinine, thiazide diuretics: potentiated effects of pancuronium. Monitor patient closely.
Opioid analgesics: may increase respiratory depression. Monitor patient closely.
Succinylcholine: may enhance and prolong neuromuscular blocking effects of pancuronium. Monitor patient closely.

Effects on diagnostic tests
None reported.

Adverse reactions
CV: increased blood pressure, tachycardia.
GI: excessive salivation.
Musculoskeletal: residual muscle weakness.
Respiratory: *prolonged, dose-related respiratory insufficiency or apnea.*
Skin: transient rashes.
Other: allergic or idiosyncratic *hypersensitivity reactions.*

Overdose and treatment
Overdose may cause prolonged respiratory depression, apnea, and CV collapse.

Use a peripheral nerve stimulator to monitor response and to evaluate neuromuscular blockade. Maintain an adequate airway and manual or mechanical ventilation until patient can maintain adequate ventilation unassisted. As needed, use neostigmine, edrophonium, or pyridostigmine to reverse effects.

Special considerations
▶ Administration before intubation requires presence of personnel trained in airway management, with emergency respiratory support available.
▶ Drug doesn't relieve pain or affect consciousness; assess need for analgesic or sedative.
▶ Administer sedative or general anesthetic before neuromuscular blockers.
▶ Keep emergency respiratory support equipment (endotracheal equipment, ventilator, oxygen, atropine, edrophonium, epinephrine, and neostigmine) immediately available.
▶ Reduce dosage when ether or other inhaled, neuromuscular blockade-enhancing anesthetics are used.
▶ If using succinylcholine, allow its effects to subside before administering pancuronium.
▶ Large doses may increase frequency and severity of tachycardia.
▶ Monitor baseline electrolyte levels, intake and output, and vital signs, especially heart rate and respiration.
▶ Don't mix in same syringe or give through same needle with bar-

---

Reactions may be *common,* uncommon, *life-threatening,* or COMMON AND LIFE-THREATENING.

biturates or other alkaline solutions. Use only fresh solutions.
▶ Store drug in refrigerator and not in plastic container or syringes. Plastic syringes may be used to administer dose.

Breast-feeding patients
▶ No data exist to demonstrate whether pancuronium appears in breast milk. Use with caution in breast-feeding women.

Pediatric patients
▶ Dosage for neonates under age 1 month must be carefully individualized.
▶ For infants over age 1 month and children, see adult dosage.

Geriatric patients
▶ Individualize the usual adult dose depending on response.

Patient teaching
▶ Explain all events and procedures to patient under the influence of pancuronium as he is able to hear.

▶ paroxetine hydrochloride
Paxil

Pharmacologic classification:
selective serotonin reuptake inhibitor

Therapeutic classification:
antidepressant

Pregnancy risk category B

How supplied
Available by prescription only
Tablets: 10 mg, 20 mg, 30 mg, 40 mg
Suspension: 10 mg/5ml

Indications and dosages
Diabetic neuropathy*
Adults: 10 to 60 mg/day P.O.
Headache*
Adults: 10 to 50 mg/day P.O.
▨ DOSAGE ADJUSTMENT. Start with 10 mg in elderly patients, debilitated patients, and patients with severe renal or hepatic impairment. Increase as needed to a maximum of 40 mg daily.

Pharmacodynamics
Analgesic action: Unknown.
Antidepressant action: Action is presumed to be linked to potentiation of serotonergic activity in the CNS, resulting from inhibition of neuronal reuptake of serotonin.

Pharmacokinetics
Absorption: Paroxetine is completely absorbed after oral dose.
Distribution: Drug is distributed throughout the body, including the CNS, with only 1% remaining in the plasma. About 93% to 95% of drug is bound to plasma protein.
Metabolism: About 36% of drug is metabolized in the liver. The principal metabolites are polar and conjugated products of oxidation and methylation, which are readily cleared.
Excretion: About 64% is excreted in urine (2% as parent compound and 62% as metabolite).

Contraindications and precautions
Contraindicated in patients taking MAO inhibitors or within 14 days of stopping an MAO inhibitor.
    Use cautiously in patients with history of seizures or mania; in those with severe, concurrent systemic illness; in those at risk for volume depletion; and in those

---

with hypersensitivity to selective serotonin reuptake inhibitors.

Interactions
Drug-drug
Cimetidine: decreased hepatic metabolism of paroxetine, leading to risk of toxicity. Dosage adjustments may be necessary.
Digoxin: paroxetine may decrease digoxin levels. Monitor the patient closely.
MAO inhibitors: increased risk of serious, sometimes fatal, adverse reactions. Avoid using together.
Phenobarbital: induces paroxetine metabolism, thereby reducing plasma levels of drug. Monitor clinical effects.
Phenytoin: altered pharmacokinetics of phenytoin. Adjust dosage as needed.
Procyclidine: increased procyclidine levels. Monitor the patient for excessive anticholinergic effects.
Theophylline: increased theophylline levels. Monitor patient closely.
Tricyclic antidepressants: increased toxicity. Reduce dosage as needed.
Warfarin: Paroxetine may increase risk of bleeding when used with warfarin. Monitor INR.

Drug-herb
St. John's wort: may result in sedative-hypnotic intoxication. Advise against concurrent use.

Drug-food
Tryptophan: may increase adverse reactions, such as diaphoresis, headache, nausea, and dizziness. Inform patient of these effects.

Drug-lifestyle
Alcohol use: may increase risk of adverse CNS effects. Advise patient to avoid alcohol during treatment.

Effects on diagnostic tests
None reported.

Adverse reactions
CNS: abnormal dreams, agitation, anxiety, *asthenia,* confusion, decreased levels, *dizziness, headache, insomnia, nervousness,* paresthesia, *somnolence, tremor.*
CV: chest pain, orthostatic hypotension, palpitations, vasodilation.
EENT: double vision, dysgeusia, lump or tightness in throat, visual disturbances.
GI: abdominal pain, *constipation, diarrhea, dry mouth,* dyspepsia, flatulence, increased or decreased appetite, *nausea,* vomiting.
GU: ejaculatory disturbances; female genital disorders including anorgasmia; male genital disorders including anorgasmia, erectile difficulties, delayed ejaculation or orgasm, impotence, and sexual dysfunction; urinary frequency; other urinary disorders.
Musculoskeletal: myalgia, myasthenia, myopathy.
Skin: *diaphoresis,* pruritus, rash.
Other: decreased libido, yawning.

Overdose and treatment
Overdose may cause nausea, vomiting, dizziness, sweating, facial flushing, drowsiness, sinus tachycardia, and dilated pupils.

Treatment includes gastric evacuation by induced emesis, gastric lavage, or both. In most cases, 20 to 30 g of activated charcoal may then be given every 4 to 6 hours during the first 24 to 48 hours after ingestion. Supportive care, frequent monitoring of vital signs, and careful observation are indicated. ECG and cardiac function monitoring are warranted with evidence of any abnormality.

Special caution must be taken with a patient who currently receives or recently received paroxetine if the patient ingests an excessive quantity of a tricyclic antidepressant. In such cases, accumulation of the parent tricyclic and its active metabolite may increase the possibility of clinically significant sequelae and extend the time needed for close medical observation.

Special considerations
▶ Drug is also used to treat depression, obsessive-compulsive disorder, panic disorder, and premature ejaculation.
▶ Patients with chronic headaches typically have fewer headaches per month while taking paroxetine.
▶ For best results, drug should be adjusted to effective dose.
▶ At least 14 days should elapse between stopping an MAO inhibitor and starting paroxetine. Likewise, at least 14 days should elapse between stopping paroxetine and starting an MAO inhibitor.
▶ Hyponatremia may occur with paroxetine use, especially in elderly patients, those taking diuretics, and those who are otherwise volume depleted. Monitor serum sodium levels.
▶ If signs of psychosis occur or increase, reduce dosage. Monitor patients for suicidal tendencies and allow them only a minimum supply of drug.

Breast-feeding patients
▶ Paroxetine appears in breast milk. Use caution when drug is administered to breast-feeding women.

Pediatric patients
▶ Safety and effectiveness in children haven't been established.

Geriatric patients
▶ Use cautiously and in lower dosages in elderly patients.

Patient teaching
▶ Tell patient that he may notice improvement in 1 to 4 weeks but that he must continue with the prescribed regimen to obtain continued benefits.
▶ Tell patient to abstain from alcohol while taking paroxetine.
▶ Caution patient to avoid hazardous activities until full effects of drug are known.
▶ Instruct patient to consult prescriber before taking other prescribed drugs, OTC medications, and herbal remedies while receiving paroxetine therapy.
▶ Instruct patient not to abruptly discontinue drug.

▶ pemoline
Cylert

Pharmacologic classification:
CNS stimulant, oxazolidinone-derivative stimulant

Therapeutic classification:
analeptic

Controlled substance schedule IV

Pregnancy risk category B

How supplied
Available by prescription only
Tablets: 18.75 mg, 37.5 mg, 75 mg

Tablets (chewable and containing povidone): 37.5 mg

Indications and dosages
Narcolepsy*
Adults: 50 to 200 mg daily, divided and given after breakfast and lunch.

Pharmacodynamics
Analeptic action: Pemoline differs structurally from methylphenidate and amphetamines but, like those drugs, pemoline has a paradoxical calming effect in children with attention deficit hyperactivity disorder (ADHD). Mechanism of action is unknown, but it may be mediated through dopaminergic mechanisms. Its CNS stimulant effect has been studied in narcolepsy in adults, in fatigue, in depressed and schizophrenic states, and in elderly patients.

Pharmacokinetics
Absorption: Drug is well absorbed after oral administration. Therapeutic effects peak within 4 hours and persist for about 8 hours.
Distribution: Unknown. Drug is 50% protein-bound.
Metabolism: Pemoline is metabolized by the liver to active and inactive metabolites.
Excretion: Drug and its metabolites are excreted in urine; 75% of an oral dose is excreted within 24 hours.

Contraindications and precautions
Contraindicated in patients with hepatic dysfunction, in patients hypersensitive to drug, and in patients with idiosyncratic reactions to drug.

Use cautiously in patients with impaired renal function.

Interactions
Drug-drug
Anticonvulsants: may decrease the seizure threshold. Monitor patient closely.

Drug-food
Caffeine: may decrease efficacy of pemoline in ADHD. Advise against concurrent use.

Effects on diagnostic tests
None reported.

Adverse reactions
CNS: abdominal pain, abnormal oculomotor function, depression, dizziness, drowsiness, dyskinetic movements, fatigue, hallucinations, *insomnia,* irritability, mild headache, **seizures,** *Tourette syndrome.*
GI: anorexia, nausea.
Hematologic: *aplastic anemia.*
Hepatic: elevated liver enzymes, *hepatic failure.*
Skin: rash.

Overdose and treatment
Overdose may cause irregular respiration, hyperreflexia, restlessness, tachycardia, hallucinations, excitement, and agitation.

Provide supportive treatment for symptoms. Perform gastric lavage if symptoms aren't severe (hyperexcitability or coma). Monitor vital signs and fluid and electrolyte balances. Keep patient in a cool room, monitor temperature, and minimize external stimulation. Protect patient from self-injury. Chlorpromazine or haloperidol

---

Reactions may be *common,* uncommon, *life-threatening,* or COMMON AND LIFE-THREATENING.

usually can reverse CNS stimulation. Hemodialysis may help.

Special considerations
▶ Because of the increased risk of life-threatening hepatic failure, drug shouldn't be considered first-line therapy for ADHD.
▶ Investigational uses include treatment of fatigue, mental depression, and schizophrenia.
▶ Give drug in a single morning dose for maximum daytime benefit and to minimize insomnia.
▶ Make sure patient obtains adequate rest; fatigue may result as drug wears off.
▶ Discourage pemoline use for analeptic effect because drug has abuse potential; CNS stimulation with CNS depression may cause neuronal instability and seizures.
▶ Abrupt withdrawal after high-dose long-term use may unmask severe depression. Lower dosage gradually to prevent acute rebound depression.
▶ Drug impairs ability to perform tasks requiring mental alertness.
▶ Carefully follow manufacturer's directions for reconstitution, storage, and administration of all preparations.
▶ Monitor start of therapy closely; drug may precipitate Tourette syndrome.
▶ Check vital signs regularly for increased blood pressure or other signs of excessive stimulation.
▶ Monitor blood and urine glucose levels in diabetic patients; drug may alter insulin requirements.
▶ Monitor CBC, differential, and platelet counts while patient is on long-term therapy.
▶ Determine baseline and periodically assess liver function tests. If abnormalities occur, discontinue therapy.
▶ Monitor patient's height and weight; drug has been linked to growth suppression.

Pediatric patients
▶ Drug isn't recommended for ADHD in children under age 6.

Patient teaching
▶ Explain need for therapy and the anticipated risks and benefits.
▶ Explain that drug effects may not appear for 3 to 4 weeks and that intermittent drug-free periods during low-stress times (weekends, school holidays) may help assess patient's condition, prevent tolerance, and permit decreased dosage when drug is resumed.
▶ Caution against altering dosage without consulting prescriber.
▶ Explain adverse reactions and the need to report them, particularly excessive CNS stimulation.
▶ Tell patient to avoid caffeine to prevent added CNS stimulation.
▶ Warn patient not to use drug to mask fatigue. Urge adequate rest.
▶ Advise diabetic patient to monitor blood glucose levels because drug may alter insulin needs.
▶ Caution patient to avoid hazardous activities until full sedative effects of drug are known.

❱ pentazocine hydrochloride
Talwin◇, Talwin-Nx (with naloxone hydrochloride)

❱ pentazocine lactate
Talwin

Pharmacologic classification:
narcotic agonist-antagonist, opioid partial agonist

Therapeutic classification:
adjunct to anesthesia, analgesic

Controlled substance schedule IV

Pregnancy risk category NR (C for Talwin-Nx)

How supplied
Available by prescription only
Injection: 30 mg/ml
Tablets: 50 mg

Indications and dosages
Moderate to severe pain
Adults: 50 to 100 mg P.O. or 30 mg I.M., I.V., or S.C. q 3 to 4 hours, p.r.n., or around the clock. Maximum, 600 mg P.O. or 360 mg parenterally daily. Doses above 30 mg I.V. or 60 mg I.M. or S.C. aren't recommended. For patients in labor, give 30 mg I.M. or 20 mg I.V. in 2- to 3-hour intervals.

Pharmacodynamics
Analgesic action: Unknown, but drug may be a competitive antagonist at some receptors and an agonist at others, resulting in relief of moderate pain.

Pentazocine can produce respiratory depression, sedation, miosis, and antitussive effects. It also may cause psychotomimetic and dysphoric effects. In patients with coronary artery disease, it elevates mean aortic pressure, left ventricular end-diastolic pressure, and mean pulmonary artery pressure. In patients with acute MI, I.V. pentazocine increases systemic and pulmonary arterial pressures and systemic vascular resistance.

Pharmacokinetics
Absorption: Drug is well absorbed after oral or parenteral administration. However, orally administered drug undergoes first-pass metabolism in the liver and less than 20% of a dose reaches the systemic circulation unchanged. Bioavailability is increased in patients with hepatic dysfunction; patients with cirrhosis absorb 60% to 70% of drug. Onset of analgesia is 15 to 30 minutes, with peak effect at 15 to 60 minutes.
Distribution: Drug appears to be widely distributed in the body.
Metabolism: Drug is metabolized in the liver, mainly by oxidation, but also by glucuronidation. Metabolism may be prolonged in patients with impaired hepatic function.
Excretion: Drug's duration of effect is 3 hours. There is considerable interpatient variability in its urine excretion. Small amounts of drug are excreted in the feces after oral or parenteral administration.

Contraindications and precautions
Contraindicated in patients with hypersensitivity to drug or its components and in children under age 12. Use cautiously in patients with impaired renal or hepatic function, acute MI, head injury, increased intracranial pressure, or respiratory depression.

Interactions
Drug-drug
Barbiturates, such as thiopental: if administered within a few hours, pentazocine may produce additive CNS and respiratory depressant effects and possible apnea. Use together cautiously.

Cimetidine: may increase pentazocine toxicity, causing disorientation, respiratory depression, apnea, and seizures. Give naloxone if toxicity occurs.

CNS depressants, such as antihistamines, barbiturates, benzodiazepines, muscle relaxants, narcotic analgesics, phenothiazines, sedative-hypnotics, tricyclic antidepressants: potentiated respiratory and CNS depression, sedation, and hypotensive effects. Reduce pentazocine dosage as needed.

Drugs extensively metabolized in the liver, such as digitoxin, phenytoin, rifampin: drug accumulation and enhanced effects may result. Monitor patient for toxicity.

General anesthetics: may cause severe CV depression. Monitor patient closely.

Narcotic agonist-antagonist or a single dose of an antagonist: acute withdrawal syndrome in patient physically dependent on pentazocine. Use with caution, and monitor patient closely.

Drug-lifestyle
Alcohol use: potentiated respiratory and CNS depression, sedation, and hypotensive effects. Advise against concurrent use.

Effects on diagnostic tests
None reported.

Adverse reactions
CNS: confusion, drowsiness, *dizziness, euphoria,* hallucinations, headache, *light-headedness,* psychotomimetic effects, *sedation,* syncope, visual disturbances.
CV: circulatory depression, hypertension, hypotension, **shock.**
EENT: dry mouth, blurred vision, nystagmus.
GI: constipation, *nausea,* taste alteration, *vomiting.*
GU: urine retention.
Hematologic: WBC depression.
Respiratory: *apnea,* dyspnea, **respiratory depression.**
Skin: diaphoresis; induration, nodules, sloughing and sclerosis at injection site; pruritus.
Other: **anaphylaxis, hypersensitivity reactions,** physical and psychological dependence.

Overdose and treatment
Pentazocine hydrochloride overdose hasn't been defined because of a lack of clinical experience with it. If overdose should occur, provide supportive measures as needed, such as oxygen, I.V. fluids, and vasopressors. Mechanical ventilation should be considered. Parenteral naloxone is an effective antagonist for respiratory depression because of pentazocine.

Special considerations
▶ For best results, give drug before patient has severe pain.
▶ Tablets aren't well absorbed.
▶ Pentazocine may obscure evidence of an acute abdominal condition or worsen gallbladder pain.
▶ Drug may cause orthostatic hypotension in ambulatory patients.
▶ Drug possesses narcotic antagonist properties. May precipitate

abstinence syndrome in narcotic-dependent patients.

▶ Use S.C. route only when necessary. Severe tissue damage is possible at injection site.

▶ Monitor respiratory status, circulatory status, and bowel and bladder function.

▶ Give slowly by direct I.V. injection. Don't mix in syringe with aminophylline, barbiturates, or other alkaline substances.

▶ Talwin-Nx, the available oral pentazocine, contains the narcotic antagonist naloxone, which prevents illicit I.V. use.

Breast-feeding patients
▶ No data exist to demonstrate whether drug appears in breast milk; use with caution in breast-feeding women.

Pediatric patients
▶ Use of drug isn't recommended in children under age 12.

Geriatric patients
▶ Lower doses are usually indicated for elderly patients, who may be more sensitive to the therapeutic and adverse effects of drug.

Patient teaching
▶ Tell patient to report rash, confusion, disorientation, or other serious adverse effects.

▶ Warn patient that Talwin-Nx is for oral use only. Severe reactions may result if tablets are crushed, dissolved, and injected.

▶ Tell patient to avoid use of alcohol and other CNS depressants.

▶ pentobarbital sodium
Nembutal

Pharmacologic classification:
barbiturate

Therapeutic classification:
anticonvulsant, sedative-hypnotic

Controlled substance schedule: II (III for suppositories)

Pregnancy risk category D

How supplied
Available by prescription only
Capsules: 50 mg, 100 mg
Elixir: 18.2 mg/5 ml
Injection: 50 mg/ml, 1-ml and 2-ml disposable syringes; 2-ml, 20-ml, and 50-ml vials
Suppositories: 30 mg, 60 mg, 120 mg, 200 mg

Indications and dosages
To induce sedation
Adults: 20 to 40 mg P.O. b.i.d., t.i.d., or q.i.d.
Children: 2 to 6 mg/kg P.O. daily in divided doses, to maximum of 100 mg/dose.
To treat insomnia
Adults: 100 mg P.O. h.s. or 150 to 200 mg deep I.M.; 120 to 200 mg P.R.
Children: 2 to 6 mg/kg I.M. to maximum of 100 mg/dose. Or 30 mg P.R. (ages 2 months to 1 year), 30 to 60 mg P.R. (ages 1 to 4), 60 mg P.R. (ages 5 to 12), 60 to 120 mg P.R. (ages 12 to 14).
Preanesthesia
Adults: 150 to 200 mg I.M. or P.O. in two divided doses.

Pharmacodynamics
Anticonvulsant action: Drug suppresses the spread of seizure activ-

ity produced by epileptogenic foci in the cortex, thalamus, and limbic systems by enhancing the effect of GABA. Both presynaptic and postsynaptic excitability are decreased, and the seizure threshold is raised. *Sedative-hypnotic action:* Exact cellular site and mechanisms of action are unknown. Pentobarbital acts throughout the CNS as a non-selective depressant with a fast onset of action and short duration of action. Particularly sensitive to this drug is the reticular activating system, which controls CNS arousal. Pentobarbital decreases both presynaptic and postsynaptic membrane excitability by facilitating the action of GABA.

Pharmacokinetics

Absorption: Drug is absorbed rapidly after oral or rectal administration; onset of action, 10 to 15 minutes. Serum levels peak 30 to 60 minutes after oral administration. After I.M. injection, action starts in 10 to 15 minutes. After I.V. administration, action starts immediately. Serum levels needed for sedation and hypnosis are 1 to 5 mcg/ml and 5 to 15 mcg/ml, respectively. After oral or rectal administration, duration of hypnosis is 1 to 4 hours.
Distribution: Drug is distributed widely throughout the body. About 35% to 45% is protein-bound. Drug accumulates in fat with long-term use.
Metabolism: Drug is metabolized in the liver by penultimate oxidation.
Excretion: 99% of pentobarbital is eliminated as glucuronide conjugates and other metabolites in the urine. Terminal half-life ranges

from 35 to 50 hours. Duration of action is 3 to 4 hours.

Contraindications and precautions

Contraindicated in patients with hypersensitivity to barbiturates or porphyria or with severe respiratory disease when dyspnea or obstruction is evident.

Use cautiously in elderly or debilitated patients and in those with acute or chronic pain, mental depression, suicidal tendencies, history of drug abuse, or impaired hepatic function.

Interactions
Drug-drug

Antidepressants, antihistamines, narcotics, sedative-hypnotics, tranquilizers: potentiated CNS and respiratory depressant effects. Monitor patient closely.
Corticosteroids, digitoxin (not digoxin), doxycycline, estrogens (including oral contraceptives), xanthines (including theophylline): enhanced hepatic metabolism of these drugs. Monitor patient.
Disulfiram, MAO inhibitors, valproic acid: decreased pentobarbital metabolism. Monitor patient for toxicity.
Griseofulvin: impaired effectiveness of griseofulvin by decreasing absorption from the GI tract. Monitor patient.
Rifampin: may decrease pentobarbital levels by increasing hepatic metabolism. Monitor patient for drug effect.
Warfarin and other oral anticoagulants: pentobarbital enhances enzymatic degradation of these drugs. Patient may need increased anticoagulant dosage.

Drug-lifestyle

Alcohol use: pentobarbital may potentiate or add to CNS and respiratory depressant effects of alcohol. Advise against concurrent use.

Effects on diagnostic tests

Pentobarbital may cause a false-positive phentolamine test. Drug's physiologic effects may impair the absorption of cyanocobalamin Co57; it may decrease serum bilirubin levels in neonates, epileptic patients, and patients with congenital nonhemolytic unconjugated hyperbilirubinemia. EEG patterns show a change in low-voltage, fast activity; changes persist for a time after discontinuation of therapy.

Adverse reactions

CNS: *drowsiness,* hallucinations, *hangover, lethargy,* paradoxical excitement in elderly patients, somnolence, syncope.
CV: *bradycardia,* hypotension.
GI: nausea, vomiting.
Hematologic: exacerbation of porphyria.
Respiratory: *respiratory depression.*
Skin: rash, *Stevens-Johnson syndrome,* urticaria.
Other: *angioedema,* physical and psychological dependence.

Overdose and treatment

Overdose may cause unsteady gait, slurred speech, sustained nystagmus, somnolence, confusion, respiratory depression, pulmonary edema, areflexia, and coma. Typical shock syndrome with tachycardia and hypotension may occur. Jaundice, hypothermia followed by fever, and oliguria also may occur. Serum levels above 10 mcg/ml may produce profound coma; levels above 30 mcg/ml may be fatal.

Maintain and support ventilation and pulmonary function as necessary; support cardiac function and circulation with vasopressors and I.V. fluids, as needed. If patient is conscious and gag reflex is intact, induce emesis; if ingestion was recent, by administering ipecac syrup. If emesis is contraindicated, perform gastric lavage while a cuffed endotracheal tube is in place to prevent aspiration. Follow with administration of activated charcoal or sodium chloride cathartic. Measure intake and output, vital signs, and laboratory parameters. Maintain body temperature.

Alkalinization of urine may be helpful in removing drug from the body. Hemodialysis may be useful in severe overdose.

Special considerations

▶ Drug is used for sedation but has no analgesic effect and may cause restlessness or delirium in patients with pain.
▶ Drug is also used as an anticonvulsant.
▶ Assess patient's mental status before starting therapy.
▶ Administer I.M. dose deep into large muscle mass. Don't give more than 5 ml into any one site.
▶ Barbiturates given I.V. may cause severe respiratory depression, laryngospasm, or hypotension. Keep emergency resuscitation equipment available.
▶ To minimize deterioration, use I.V. injection solution within 30 minutes after opening container. Do not use cloudy, discolored, or precipitated solutions.

▶ Reserve I.V. injection for emergency treatment, which should be given under close supervision.

▶ Avoid I.V. administration at a rate exceeding 50 mg/minute to prevent hypotension and respiratory depression.

▶ Parenteral solution is alkaline. Local tissue reactions and injection site pain have followed I.V. use. Avoid extravasation. Assess patency of I.V. site before and during administration.

▶ To assure accuracy of rectal dose, don't divide suppositories.

▶ Long-term use isn't recommended; drug loses its sleep-promoting efficacy after 14 days of continued use. Long-term high dosage may cause drug dependence, and patient may experience withdrawal symptoms if drug suddenly stops. Withdraw barbiturates gradually.

▶ To prevent rebound of rapid-eye-movement sleep after prolonged therapy, discontinue gradually over 5 to 6 days.

▶ Administration of full loading doses over short periods of time to treat status epilepticus will require ventilatory support in adults.

▶ Nembutal tablets contain tartrazine dye, which may cause allergic reactions in susceptible persons.

▶ High-dose therapy for elevated intracranial pressure may require mechanically assisted ventilation.

▶ Watch for signs of barbiturate toxicity like coma, pupillary constriction, cyanosis, clammy skin, and hypotension. Overdose can be fatal.

▶ Skin eruptions may precede life-threatening reactions to barbiturate therapy. In some patients, high fever, stomatitis, headache, or rhinitis may precede skin reactions.

▶ Don't mix in syringe or in I.V. solutions or lines with other drugs.

Breast-feeding patients
▶ Pentobarbital appears in breast milk. Don't administer to breast-feeding women.

Pediatric patients
▶ Barbiturates may cause paradoxical excitement in children. Use with caution.

Geriatric patients
▶ Elderly patients usually require lower doses because of increased susceptibility to CNS depressant effects of pentobarbital.

▶ Confusion, disorientation, and excitability may occur in elderly patients. Use with caution.

Patient teaching
▶ Advise pregnant women of potential hazard to fetus or neonate when taking pentobarbital late in pregnancy. Withdrawal symptoms can occur.

▶ Tell patient not to take drug continuously for longer than 2 weeks.

▶ Emphasize the dangers of combining drug with alcohol. An excessive depressant effect is possible even if drug is taken the evening before ingestion of alcohol.

⏵ phenelzine sulfate
Nardil

Pharmacologic classification:
MAO inhibitor

Therapeutic classification:
antidepressant

Pregnancy risk category C

How supplied
Available by prescription only
Tablets: 15 mg

Indications and dosages
***Migraine headaches resistant to
other therapies****
Adults: 15 mg P.O. tid.

Pharmacodynamics
Antidepressant action: Depression
is thought to result from low CNS
levels of neurotransmitters, including norepinephrine and serotonin.
Phenelzine inhibits MAO, an enzyme that normally inactivates
amine-containing substances, thus
increasing the level and activity of
these substances.
Antimigraine action: Unknown.

Pharmacokinetics
Absorption: Drug is absorbed
rapidly and completely from the
GI tract.
Distribution: Unknown.
Metabolism: Drug is metabolized
in the liver.
Excretion: Drug is excreted mainly
in urine within 24 hours; some is
excreted in feces via the biliary
tract. Half-life is relatively short,
but enzyme inhibition is prolonged
and unrelated to half-life.

Contraindications and precautions
Contraindicated in patients with
hypersensitivity to drug, heart failure, pheochromocytoma, hypertension, liver disease, and CV disease.
Also contraindicated during therapy with other MAO inhibitors (iso-
carboxazid, tranylcypromine) or
within 10 days of such therapy or
within 10 days of elective surgery
requiring general anesthesia, cocaine use, or local anesthesia containing sympathomimetic vasoconstrictors. Contraindicated within 2
weeks of selective serotonin reuptake inhibitor use. Contraindicated
by some manufacturers in patients
over age 60 because of possibility
of existing cerebrosclerosis with
damaged vessels.

Use cautiously in patients at risk
for diabetes, suicide, or seizures
disorders and in those receiving
thiazide diuretics or spinal anes-
thesics.

Interactions
Drug-drug
*Amphetamines, ephedrine, OTC
cold medications, OTC hay fever
medications, OTC weight-reduction
products, phenylephrine, phenylpropanolamine:* serious CV toxicity. Avoid concomitant use.
*Barbiturates and other sedatives,
dextromethorphan, narcotics, tricyclic antidepressants:* increased
adverse reactions. Use cautiously
and in reduced dosages.
Disulfiram: tachycardia, flushing,
or palpitations. Avoid concomitant
use.
*General or spinal anesthetics nor-
mally metabolized by MAO:* severe
hypotension and excessive CNS
depression. Avoid concomitant
use, if possible.

Local anesthetics, including lidocaine, procaine: decreased effectiveness, resulting in poor nerve block. Discontinue phenelzine for at least 1 week before using these drugs.
Meperidine: circulatory collapse, coma, death. Never use together.
Serotonergic drugs such as fluoxetine, fluvoxamine, paroxetine, sertraline: serious adverse effects. Wait at least 2 weeks between drug use.

Drug-herb
Cacao: may potentiate vasopressor effects. Discourage concurrent use.
Ginseng: may cause adverse reactions including headache, tremors, mania. Discourage concurrent use.

Drug-food
Foods high in caffeine, tryptophan, or tyramine: may precipitate hypertensive crisis. Discourage concurrent use.

Drug-lifestyle
Alcohol use: may precipitate hypertensive crisis. Discourage concurrent use.

Effects on diagnostic tests
None reported.

Adverse reactions
CNS: *dizziness,* vertigo, headache, hyperreflexia, tremor, muscle twitching, *insomnia,* drowsiness, weakness, fatigue.
CV: edema, orthostatic hypotension.
GI: *anorexia,* dry mouth, constipation, nausea.
GU: elevated urinary catecholamine levels.
Hematologic: elevated WBC count.
Hepatic: elevated liver function test results.
Metabolic: weight gain.
Skin: diaphoresis.
Other: sexual disturbances.

Overdose and treatment
Overdose may worsen adverse reactions or cause exaggerated responses to normal pharmacologic activity; such symptoms become apparent slowly, within 24 to 48 hours, and may persist for up to 2 weeks. Agitation, flushing, tachycardia, hypotension, hypertension, palpitations, increased motor activity, twitching, increased deep tendon reflexes, seizures, hyperpyrexia, cardiorespiratory arrest, and coma may occur. Doses of 375 mg to 1.5 g have been ingested with fatal and nonfatal results.

Treat symptomatically and supportively. Give 5 to 10 mg of phentolamine by I.V. push for hypertensive crisis. Give I.V. diazepam for seizures, agitation, or tremors. Give beta blockers for tachycardia. Use cooling blankets for fever. Monitor vital signs and fluid and electrolyte balance. Use of sympathomimetics such as norepinephrine or phenylephrine is contraindicated in hypotension caused by MAO inhibitors.

Special considerations
▶ Drug is also used for severe depression.
▶ Exercise precautions for use of MAO inhibitors, given alone or with other drugs, for 14 days after stopping drug.
▶ At start of therapy, patient should lie down for 1 hour after taking phenelzine; to prevent dizziness from orthostatic blood pressure

changes, sudden changes to standing position should be avoided.

▶ In contrast to other MAO inhibitors, therapy with phenelzine and tricyclic antidepressants is generally well tolerated.

▶ Consider the inherent risk of suicide until significant improvement of depressive state occurs. High-risk patients should have close supervision during initial drug therapy. To reduce risk of suicidal overdose, prescribe the smallest quantity of tablets consistent with good management.

▶ Have phentolamine available to combat severe hypertension.

▶ Obtain baseline blood pressure, heart rate, CBC, and liver function test results before therapy, and continue to monitor throughout treatment.

Pediatric patients
▶ Drug isn't recommended for children under age 16.

Geriatric patients
▶ Drug isn't recommended for patients over age 60.

Patient teaching
▶ Warn patient not to take alcohol, other CNS depressants, or self-prescribed medications (such as cold, hay fever, or diet preparations) without consulting prescriber.

▶ Explain that many foods and beverages (such as wine, beer, cheeses, preserved fruits, meats, and vegetables) may interact with drug. A list of foods to avoid can usually be obtained from the dietary department or pharmacy at most hospitals.

▶ Tell patient to avoid hazardous activities that require alertness un-

til drug's full effect on the CNS is known. Suggest taking drug at bedtime to minimize daytime sedation.

▶ Instruct patient to take drug exactly as prescribed and not to double the dose if a dose is missed.

▶ Tell patient not to discontinue drug abruptly and to report any problems; dosage reduction can relieve most adverse reactions.

▶ phenobarbital
Barbita, Solfoton

▶ phenobarbital sodium
Luminal

Pharmacologic classification:
barbiturate

Therapeutic classification:
anticonvulsant, sedative-hypnotic

Controlled substance schedule IV

Pregnancy risk category D

How supplied
Available by prescription only
Capsules: 16 mg
Elixir: 15 mg/5 ml; 20 mg/5 ml
Injection: 30 mg/ml, 60 mg/ml, 65 mg/ml, 130 mg/ml
Tablets: 15 mg, 16 mg, 30 mg, 60 mg, 100 mg

Indications and dosages
To induce sedation
Adults: 30 to 120 mg P.O., I.M., or I.V. daily in two or three divided doses. Maximum, 400 mg/24 hours.
Children: 8 to 32 mg P.O. daily.
To treat insomnia
Adults: 100 to 200 mg P.O. or 100 to 320 mg I.M.

Reactions may be *common*, uncommon, *life-threatening*, or COMMON AND LIFE-THREATENING.

Preoperative sedation
Adults: 100 to 200 mg I.M. 60 to
90 minutes before surgery.
Children: 1 to 3 mg/kg I.V. or I.M.
60 to 90 minutes before surgery.

Pharmacodynamics
Anticonvulsant action: Phenobarbital suppresses the spread of
seizure activity produced by
epileptogenic foci in the cortex,
thalamus, and limbic systems by
enhancing the effect of GABA.
Both presynaptic and postsynaptic
excitability are decreased; also,
phenobarbital raises the seizure
threshold.
Sedative-hypnotic action: Exact
mechanism of action is unknown,
but phenobarbital acts throughout
the CNS as a nonselective depressant with a slow onset and a long
duration of action. Particularly
sensitive to this drug is the reticular activating system, which controls CNS arousal. Drug decreases
both presynaptic and postsynaptic
membrane excitability by facilitating the action of GABA.

Pharmacokinetics
Absorption: Drug is well absorbed
after oral and rectal administration,
with 70% to 90% reaching the
bloodstream. Absorption after I.M.
administration is 100%. After oral
administration, serum levels peak
in 1 to 2 hours; CNS levels peak in
1 to 3 hours. Action starts 20 to 60
minutes or more after oral dosing;
onset after I.V. administration is
about 5 minutes. A serum level of
10 mcg/ml is needed to produce sedation; 40 mcg/ml usually produces
sleep. Levels of 20 to 40 mcg/ml
are considered therapeutic for anticonvulsant therapy.

Distribution: Drug is distributed
widely throughout the body and is
about 25% to 30% protein-bound.
Metabolism: Drug is metabolized
by the hepatic microsomal enzyme
system.
Excretion: 25% to 50% of a phenobarbital dose is eliminated unchanged in urine; remainder is excreted as metabolites of glucuronic
acid. Drug's half-life is 5 to 7 days.

Contraindications and precautions
Contraindicated in patients with
barbiturate hypersensitivity, history of manifest or latent porphyria,
hepatic dysfunction, respiratory
disease with dyspnea or obstruction, and nephritis.
    Use cautiously in elderly or debilitated patients and in those with
acute or chronic pain, depression,
suicidal tendencies, history of drug
abuse, blood pressure alterations,
CV disease, shock, or uremia.

Interactions
Drug-drug
*Antidepressants, antihistamines,
narcotics, phenothiazines, sedative-
hypnotics, tranquilizers:* phenobarbital may add to or potentiate CNS
and respiratory depressant effects.
Monitor patient.
*Corticosteroids, digitoxin (not
digoxin), doxycycline, estrogens
(including oral contraceptives),
xanthines (including theophylline):*
enhanced hepatic metabolism of
these drugs. Monitor patient for
clinical effect.
Disulfiram, MAO inhibitors, valproic acid: decreased phenobarbital metabolism. Monitor patient for
toxicity.
Griseofulvin: impaired griseofulvin effectiveness by decreasing ab-

sorption from the GI tract. Monitor patient.

Rifampin: may decrease phenobarbital levels by increasing hepatic metabolism. Monitor patient.

Warfarin and other oral anticoagulants: phenobarbital enhances the enzymatic degradation of these agents. Patient may need increased anticoagulant dosage.

Drug-lifestyle
Alcohol use: phenobarbital may add to or potentiate CNS and respiratory depressant effects of alcohol. Advise against concurrent use.

Effects on diagnostic tests
Phenobarbital may cause a false-positive phentolamine test. The physiologic effects of drug may impair the absorption of cyanocobalamin Co57; it may decrease serum bilirubin levels in neonates, epileptics, and in patients with congenital nonhemolytic unconjugated hyperbilirubinemia. Barbiturates may increase sulfobromophthalein retention. EEG patterns show a change in low-voltage, fast activity; changes persist for a time after discontinuation of therapy.

Adverse reactions
CNS: depression, *drowsiness, hangover, lethargy,* paradoxical excitement in elderly patients, somnolence.
CV: *bradycardia,* hypotension.
GI: nausea, vomiting.
Hematologic: exacerbation of porphyria.
Respiratory: *apnea, respiratory depression.*
Skin: *erythema multiforme,* necrosis, nerve injury at injection site, pain, rash, *Stevens-Johnson*

syndrome, swelling, thrombophlebitis, urticaria.
Other: *angioedema,* physical and psychological dependence.

Overdose and treatment
Overdose may cause unsteady gait, slurred speech, sustained nystagmus, somnolence, confusion, respiratory depression, pulmonary edema, areflexia, and coma. Typical shock syndrome with tachycardia and hypotension along with jaundice, oliguria, and chills followed by fever may occur.

Treatment aims to maintain and support ventilation and pulmonary function as necessary; and to support cardiac function and circulation with vasopressors and I.V. fluids as needed. If patient is conscious and gag reflex is intact, induce emesis if ingestion was recent by administering ipecac syrup. If emesis is contraindicated, perform gastric lavage while a cuffed endotracheal tube is in place to prevent aspiration. Follow with administration of activated charcoal or sodium chloride cathartic. Measure intake and output, vital signs, and laboratory parameters. Maintain body temperature.

Alkalinization of urine may be helpful in removing drug from the body; hemodialysis may be useful in severe overdose. Oral activated charcoal may enhance phenobarbital elimination regardless of its route of administration.

Special considerations
▶ Drug is also used for treatment of all forms of epilepsy except absence seizures, febrile seizures in children and for status epilepticus.

▶ Drug may be used in combination with opiates to potentiate analgesic effects.

▶ Oral solution may be mixed with water or juice to improve taste.

▶ Don't crush or break extended-release form; this will impair drug action.

▶ Reconstitute powder for injection with 2.5 to 5 ml sterile water for injection. Roll vial in hands; don't shake.

▶ Administer parenteral dose within 30 minutes of reconstitution because phenobarbital hydrolyzes in solution and on exposure to air.

▶ Administer I.M. dose deep into a large muscle mass to prevent tissue injury.

▶ Don't use injectable solution if it contains a precipitate.

▶ Reserve I.V. injection for emergency treatment. Give slowly under close supervision. Monitor respirations closely.

▶ Use a relatively large vein for I.V. administration to prevent extravasation.

▶ Avoid I.V. administration at a rate exceeding 60 mg/minute to prevent hypotension and respiratory depression. Maximum effect may take up to 30 minutes after I.V. administration. Have emergency equipment available.

▶ Don't mix parenteral form with acidic solutions; precipitation may result.

▶ Administration of full loading doses over short periods of time to treat status epilepticus will require ventilatory support in adults.

▶ Full therapeutic effects aren't seen for 2 to 3 weeks, except when loading dose is used.

▶ Watch for barbiturate toxicity: coma, cyanosis, asthmatic breathing, clammy skin, and hypotension. Overdose can be fatal.

▶ Therapeutic blood levels are 15 to 40 mcg/ml.

Breast-feeding patients
▶ Phenobarbital passes into breast milk; avoid administering to breast-feeding women.

Pediatric patients
▶ Paradoxical hyperexcitability may occur in children; use with caution. Use of phenobarbital extended-release capsules isn't recommended in children under age 12.

Geriatric patients
▶ Elderly patients are more sensitive to drug's effects and usually need lower doses. Confusion, disorientation, and excitability may occur in elderly patients.

Patient teaching
▶ Advise patient of potential for physical and psychological dependence with prolonged use.

▶ Warn patient to avoid alcohol and other CNS depressants while taking drug. An excessive depressant effect is possible even if drug is taken the evening before ingestion of alcohol.

▶ Caution patient not to stop taking drug suddenly because this could cause a withdrawal reaction.

▶ Caution patient to avoid hazardous activities until full CNS effects of drug are known.

▶ phenytoin, phenytoin sodium, phenytoin sodium (extended)
Dilantin, Dilantin Kapseals, Dilantin Infatab, Dilantin-125

▶ phenytoin sodium (prompt)

Pharmacologic classification: *hydantoin derivative*

Therapeutic classification: *anticonvulsant*

Pregnancy risk category D

How supplied
Available by prescription only
phenytoin
Oral suspension: 30 mg/5 ml◊, 125 mg/5 ml
Tablets (chewable): 50 mg
phenytoin sodium
Injection: 50 mg/ml
phenytoin sodium (extended)
Capsules: 30 mg, 100 mg
phenytoin sodium (prompt)
Capsules: 30 mg, 100 mg

Indications and dosages
Neuritic pain, such as migraine, trigeminal neuralgia, and Bell's palsy
Adults: 200 to 600 mg P.O. daily in divided doses.
Skeletal muscle relaxation
Adults: 200 to 600 mg P.O. daily, p.r.n.

Pharmacodynamics
Analgesic action: Unknown.
Anticonvulsant action: Like other hydantoin derivatives, phenytoin stabilizes neuronal membranes and limits seizure activity by either increasing efflux or decreasing influx of sodium ions across cell membranes in the motor cortex during generation of nerve impulses. Phenytoin exerts its antiarrhythmic effects by normalizing sodium influx to Purkinje's fibers in patients with cardiac glycoside–induced arrhythmias. Drug is indicated for generalized tonic-clonic (grand mal) and partial seizures.
Other actions: Phenytoin inhibits excessive collagenase activity in patients with epidermolysis bullosa.

Pharmacokinetics
Absorption: Phenytoin is absorbed slowly from the small intestine; absorption is formulation-dependent and bioavailability may differ among products. Extended-release capsules give peak serum levels at 4 to 12 hours; prompt-release products peak at 1¼ to 3 hours. I.M. doses are absorbed erratically; about 50% to 75% of I.M. dose is absorbed in 24 hours.
Distribution: Drug is distributed widely throughout the body; therapeutic plasma levels are 10 to 20 mcg/ml, although in some patients they occur at 5 to 10 mcg/ml. Lateral nystagmus may occur at levels above 20 mcg/ml; ataxia usually occurs at levels above 30 mcg/ml; significantly decreased mental capacity occurs at 40 mcg/ml. Phenytoin is about 90% protein-bound, less so in uremic patients.
Metabolism: Drug is metabolized by the liver to inactive metabolites.
Excretion: Drug is excreted in urine and exhibits dose-dependent (zero-order) elimination kinetics; above a certain dosage level, small increases in dosage disproportionately increase serum levels.

Reactions may be *common*, uncommon, ***life-threatening***, or **COMMON AND LIFE-THREATENING**.

Contraindications and precautions
Contraindicated in patients with hydantoin hypersensitivity, sinus bradycardia, SA block, second- or third-degree AV block, or Adams-Stokes syndrome.

Use cautiously in elderly or debilitated patients; in those with hepatic dysfunction, hypotension, myocardial insufficiency, diabetes, or respiratory depression; and in those receiving hydantoin derivatives.

Interactions
Drug-drug
Acetaminophen, carbamazepine, corticosteroids, cyclosporine, dicumarol, digitoxin, disopyramide, dopamine, doxycycline, estrogens, furosemide, haloperidol, levodopa, mebendazole, meperidine, methadone, metyrapone, oral contraceptives, phenothiazines, quinidine, sulfonylureas: phenytoin may decrease the effects of these drugs by stimulating hepatic metabolism. Monitor patient for drug effects.
Allopurinol, benzodiazepines, chloramphenicol, chlorpheniramine, cimetidine, diazepam, disulfiram, fluconazole, ibuprofen, imipramine, isoniazid, metrodiazole, miconazole, omeprazole, phenacemide, phenylbutazone, salicylates, succinimides, trimethoprim, valproic acid: phenytoin's therapeutic effects may be increased. Monitor patient.
Amiodarone: phenytoin may decrease amiodarone effects by stimulating hepatic metabolism. Also, phenytoin's effects may increase. Monitor patient closely.
Antacids, antineoplastics, barbiturates, calcium, calcium gluconate, carbamazepine, charcoal, diazoxide, folic acid, loxapine, nitrofurantoin, pyridoxine, rifampin, sucralfate, or theophylline: phenytoin's therapeutic effects may be decreased. Monitor patient.
Drugs that lower the seizure threshold, such as antipsychotics: may attenuate phenytoin's therapeutic effects. Monitor patient.

Drug-lifestyle
Alcohol use: phenytoin's therapeutic effects may be decreased by alcohol. Advise against concurrent use

Effects on diagnostic tests
Drug may interfere with the 1-mg dexamethasone suppression test.

Adverse reactions
CNS: *ataxia, decreased coordination,* dizziness, headache, insomnia, *mental confusion,* nervousness, *slurred speech,* twitching.
CV: hypotension, periarteritis nodosa.
EENT: blurred vision, *diplopia, gingival hyperplasia* (especially in children), *nystagmus.*
GI: constipation, *nausea, vomiting.*
Hematologic: *agranulocytosis, leukopenia,* macrocythemia, megaloblastic anemia, *pancytopenia, thrombocytopenia.*
Hepatic: *toxic hepatitis.*
Metabolic: decreased serum levels of protein-bound iodine, hyperglycemia.
Musculoskeletal: osteomalacia.
Skin: bullous, discoloration of skin (purple glove syndrome) if given by I.V. push in back of hand, exfoliative or purpuric dermatitis, *hirsutism,* inflammation at injection site, lupus erythematosus, necrosis, pain, photosensitivity,

scarlatiniform or morbilliform rash, **Stevens-Johnson syndrome, toxic epidermal necrolysis**.
Other: hypertrichosis, lymphadenopathy.

Overdose and treatment

Early evidence of overdose may include drowsiness, nausea, vomiting, nystagmus, ataxia, dysarthria, tremor, and slurred speech; hypotension, arrhythmias, respiratory depression, and coma may follow. Death is caused by respiratory and circulatory depression. Estimated lethal dose in adults is 2 to 5 g.

Treat overdose with gastric lavage or emesis and follow with supportive treatment. Carefully monitor vital signs and fluid and electrolyte balances. Forced diuresis is of little or no value. Hemodialysis or peritoneal dialysis may be helpful.

Special considerations

▶ Drug is also used for treatment of generalized tonic-clonic seizures, status epilepticus, nonepileptic seizures (post-head trauma, Reye's syndrome); ventricular arrhythmias unresponsive to lidocaine or procainamide, and arrhythmias induced by cardiac glycosides; and prophylactic control of seizures during neurosurgery.

▶ Drug is effective in treating neurogenic pain caused by central or peripheral nerve damage. It also is useful in treating chronic neuralgias or neuropathy characterized by electric pain.

▶ Only extended-release capsules are approved for once-daily dosing; all other forms are given in divided doses every 8 to 12 hours.

▶ Oral or nasogastric feeding may interfere with absorption of oral suspension; separate doses as much as possible from feedings but no less than 1 hour. During continuous tube feeding, tube should be flushed before and after dose.

▶ If suspension is used, shake well.

▶ Avoid I.M. administration; it's painful and drug absorption is erratic.

▶ Abrupt withdrawal may precipitate status epilepticus.

▶ Phenytoin commonly is abbreviated as DPH (diphenylhydantoin), an older drug name.

▶ Monitoring of serum levels is essential because of dose-dependent excretion.

▶ Monitor CBC and serum calcium level every 6 months, and periodically monitor hepatic function as ordered. If megaloblastic anemia is evident, doctor may order folic acid and vitamin B_{12}.

▶ Mix I.V. doses in normal saline solution and infuse over 30 minutes to 1 hour; infusion must begin within 1 hour after preparation and an in-line filter is recommended. Mixtures with D_5W will precipitate. Never use cloudy solutions. Don't refrigerate solution or mix with other drugs. Discard 4 hours after preparation.

▶ Check patency of I.V. catheter before administering. Extravasation has caused severe local tissue damage.

▶ If using I.V. bolus, use slow (50 mg/minute) I.V. push or constant infusion; too-rapid I.V. injection may cause hypotension and circulatory collapse. Don't use I.V. push in veins on back of hand; larger veins are needed to prevent discoloration associated with purple glove syndrome.

▶ When giving I.V., continuous monitoring of ECG, blood pressure, and respiratory status is essential.

Breast-feeding patients
▶ Drug appears in breast milk; an alternative feeding method is recommended during therapy.

Pediatric patients
▶ Special pediatric-strength suspension (30 mg/5 ml) is available in Canada only. Take extreme care to use correct strength. Don't confuse with adult strength (125 mg/5 ml).

Geriatric patients
▶ Elderly patients metabolize and excrete phenytoin slowly; therefore, they may require lower doses.

Patient teaching
▶ Tell patient to use one brand of phenytoin. Changing brands may change therapeutic effect.
▶ Instruct patient to take drug with food or milk to reduce GI distress.
▶ Warn patient not to discontinue drug, except with medical supervision; to avoid hazardous activities that require alertness until CNS effect is determined; and to avoid alcoholic beverages, which can decrease effectiveness of drug and increase adverse reactions.
▶ Urge patient to wear or carry medical identification that shows need for phenytoin.
▶ Stress meticulous oral hygiene to minimize overgrowth and sensitivity of gums.

▶ pipecuronium bromide
Arduan

Pharmacologic classification:
nondepolarizing neuromuscular blocker

Therapeutic classification:
skeletal muscle relaxant

Pregnancy risk category C

How supplied
Available by prescription only
Injection: 10 mg/vial

Indications and dosages
To provide skeletal muscle relaxation during surgery as an adjunct to general anesthesia
Adults and children: Dosage is highly individualized. The following may serve as a guide, assuming that patient isn't obese and has normal renal function. Initial doses of 70 to 85 mcg/kg I.V. are used to provide conditions considered ideal for endotracheal intubation and will maintain paralysis for 1 to 2 hours. If succinylcholine is used for endotracheal intubation, initial doses of pipecuronium 50 mcg/kg will provide good relaxation for 45 minutes or more. Maintenance doses of 10 to 15 mcg/kg provide relaxation for about 50 minutes.
◩ DOSAGE ADJUSTMENT. Adjust dosage to ideal body weight in obese patients. Also, adjust dosage for patients with renal failure.

Pharmacodynamics
Muscle relaxant action: Like other nondepolarizing muscle relaxants, pipecuronium competes with acetylcholine for receptor sites at the motor end plate. Because this action may be antagonized by

cholinesterase inhibitors, it is considered a competitive antagonist.

Pharmacokinetics
Absorption: No information is available for any route other than I.V. Maximum onset of action occurs within 5 minutes.
Distribution: Volume of distribution (VD) is about 0.25 L/kg and increases in patients with renal failure. Other conditions associated with increased VD (including edema, old age, and CV disease) may delay onset.
Metabolism: Only about 20% to 40% of an administered dose is metabolized, probably in the liver. One metabolite (3-desacetyl pipecuronium) has about 50% of the neuromuscular blocking activity of the parent drug.
Excretion: Drug is primarily excreted by the kidneys. In preliminary studies, the half-life of drug has been estimated at 1.7 hours; it may increase to 4 hours or more in patients with severe renal disease.

Contraindications and precautions
Contraindicated in patients hypersensitive to drug. Use cautiously in patients with renal failure.

Interactions
Drug-drug
Aminoglycosides (gentamicin, kanamycin, neomycin, streptomycin), bacitracin, colistimethate sodium, colistin, polymyxin B, tetracyclines: potentiated neuromuscular blockade, leading to increased skeletal muscle relaxation and prolonged effects. Use together cautiously.
Magnesium salts: may enhance and prolong neuromuscular blockade. Monitor patient for increased muscle weakness.
Quinidine, volatile inhalation anesthetics: may intensify or prolong the action of nondepolarizing neuromuscular blocking agents. Monitor patient.

Effects on diagnostic tests
None reported.

Adverse reactions
CV: atrial fibrillation, ***bradycardia, CVA,*** hypertension, hypotension, myocardial ischemia, thrombosis, ***ventricular extrasystole.***
GU: anuria, increased creatinine levels.
Musculoskeletal: prolonged muscle weakness.
Respiratory: dyspnea, ***respiratory depression, respiratory insufficiency or apnea.***
Skin: rash, urticaria.

Overdose and treatment
No cases have been reported. Provide supportive treatment, and ventilate patient as necessary. Closely monitor vital signs.

Antagonists such as neostigmine shouldn't be used until there is some evidence of spontaneous recovery of neuromuscular function. A nerve stimulator is recommended to document antagonism of neuromuscular blockade.

Special considerations
▸ Use drug under direct medical supervision by personnel skilled in use of neuromuscular blockers and techniques for maintaining a patent airway. Don't use drug unless facilities and equipment for mechanical ventilation, oxygen therapy, and intubation and an antagonist are within reach.

Reactions may be *common,* uncommon, ***life-threatening,*** or COMMON AND LIFE-THREATENING.

▶ Because of its prolonged duration of action, drug is recommended only for procedures that take 90 minutes or longer.

▶ Use with other nondepolarizing neuromuscular blocking agents isn't recommended.

▶ Neuromuscular blockers don't obtund consciousness or alter pain threshold; administer sedatives or general anesthetics before pipecuronium, as ordered.

▶ Experimental evidence suggests that acid-base balance may influence the actions of pipecuronium.

▶ Alkalosis may counteract the paralysis, and acidosis may enhance it. Electrolyte disturbances may also influence response.

▶ Clinical trials have shown that edrophonium 0.5 mg/kg wasn't as effective as neostigmine 0.04 mg/kg in reversing the effects of pipecuronium. Higher doses of edrophonium and pyridostigmine have not been studied.

▶ Monitor respirations closely until patient recovers from neuromuscular blockade, as evidenced by tests of muscle strength (hand grip, head lift, and ability to cough).

▶ Monitor for bradycardia during anesthesia.

▶ Reconstitute with 10 ml of solution before use to yield 1 mg/ml. Large volumes of diluent or addition of drug to a hanging I.V. solution isn't recommended.

▶ When reconstituted with sterile water for injection or other compatible I.V. solution, such as normal saline injection, D_5W, lactated Ringer's injection, and dextrose 5% in saline, drug is stable for 24 hours if refrigerated.

▶ When reconstituted with bacteriostatic water for injection, drug is stable for 5 days at room temperature or in the refrigerator.

▶ If reconstituted with solution other than bacteriostatic water for injection, discard unused portions of drug.

▶ Pipecuronium may be administered after succinylcholine when the latter is used to facilitate intubation. There is no evidence to support the safe use of pipecuronium before succinylcholine to decrease adverse effects of the latter drug.

▶ Store powder at room temperature or in the refrigerator (36° to 86° F [2° to 30° C]).

Breast-feeding patients

▶ No data exist to demonstrate whether drug appears in breast milk. Use with caution in breast-feeding women.

Pediatric patients

▶ Drug isn't recommended for use in patients under age 3 months.

▶ Limited evidence suggests that children (age 1 to 14) under balanced anesthesia or halothane anesthesia may be less sensitive than adults.

▶ Bacteriostatic water contains benzyl alcohol and isn't intended for use in neonates.

Patient teaching

▶ Explain drug's purpose.

▶ Reassure patient and family that he will be monitored at all times.

▌ **piroxicam**
**Apo-Piroxicam◇, Feldene,
Novo-Pirocam◇**

Pharmacologic classification:
NSAID

Therapeutic classification:
*anti-inflammatory, antipyretic,
nonnarcotic analgesic*

**Pregnancy risk category B (D in
third trimester or near delivery)**

How supplied
Available by prescription only
Capsules: 10 mg, 20 mg

Indications and dosages
***Osteoarthritis and rheumatoid
arthritis***
Adults: 20 mg P.O. once daily. If
desired, the dose may be divided.
Juvenile rheumatoid arthritis*
*Children who weigh 15 to 30 kg
(33 to 67 lb)*: 5 mg P.O. daily.
*Children who weigh 31 to 45 kg
(68 to 100 lb):* 10 mg P.O. daily.
*Children who weigh 46 to 55 kg
(101 to 121 lb):* 15 mg P.O. daily.

Pharmacodynamics
*Analgesic, antipyretic, and anti-
inflammatory actions:* Unknown,
but piroxicam is thought to inhibit
prostaglandin synthesis.

Pharmacokinetics
Absorption: Drug is absorbed
rapidly from the GI tract. Effect
peaks 3 to 5 hours after dosing.
Food delays absorption.
Distribution: Piroxicam is highly
protein-bound.
Metabolism: Drug is metabolized
in the liver.

Excretion: Drug is excreted in
urine. Its long half-life (about 50
hours) allows for daily dosing.

Contraindications and
precautions
Contraindicated in patients hypersensitive to drug, in whom aspirin
or NSAIDs cause bronchospasm or
angioedema, and in patients who
are pregnant or breast-feeding.
   Use cautiously in the elderly and
in patients with GI disorders, history of renal, peptic ulcer, or cardiac disease, hypertension, or conditions that raise the risk of fluid
retention.

Interactions
Drug-drug
Acetaminophen, gold compounds:
increased nephrotoxicity. Monitor
renal function.
Anticoagulants, thrombolytics:
may potentiate anticoagulant effects. Monitor PT and INR.
Antihypertensives, diuretics: piroxicam may decrease effectiveness of
these drugs. Monitor patient for
clinical effect.
*Anti-inflammatory drugs (aspirin,
salicylates):* increased risk of
nephrotoxicity, bleeding problems,
and adverse GI reactions, including ulceration and hemorrhage.
Use cautiously together, and monitor patient's renal function, PT, and
INR.
Aspirin: may decrease the bioavailability of piroxicam. Avoid using together.
Corticosteroids, corticotropin:
may increase GI adverse effects,
including ulceration and hemorrhage. Monitor patient closely.
Diuretics: may increase nephrotoxicity. Monitor renal function.

Reactions may be *common*, uncommon, *life-threatening*, or COMMON AND LIFE-THREATENING.

Drugs that are highly protein-bound, such as coumarin derivatives, nifedipine, phenytoin, verapamil: piroxicam may displace highly protein-bound drugs from binding sites. Toxicity may occur.
Drugs that inhibit platelet aggregation, such as aspirin, carbenicillin (parenteral), cefamandole, cefoperazone, dextran, dipyridamole, mezlocillin, piperacillin, plicamycin, salicylates, sulfinpyrazone, ticarcillin, valproic acid: increased risk of bleeding problems. Monitor patient for bleeding tendencies and bruising.
Insulin, oral antidiabetic drugs: may potentiate hypoglycemic effects. Monitor serum glucose.
Lithium, methotrexate: decreased the renal clearance of these drugs. Monitor patient for toxicity.

Drug-lifestyle
Alcohol use: may increase GI adverse effects, including ulceration and hemorrhage. Advise against alcohol use.
Sun exposure: may cause photosensitivity reaction. Urge precautions.

Effects on diagnostic tests
None reported.

Adverse reactions
CNS: dizziness, drowsiness, headache, somnolence, vertigo.
CV: peripheral edema.
EENT: auditory disturbances.
GI: abdominal pain, anorexia, constipation, diarrhea, dyspepsia, *epigastric distress,* flatulence, *nausea, occult blood loss, peptic ulceration,* **severe GI bleeding,** stomatitis.

GU: elevated BUN level, ***nephrotoxicity.***
Hematologic: ***agranulocytosis,*** anemia, ***aplastic anemia,*** eosinophilia, ***leukopenia***, prolonged bleeding time, ***thrombocytopenia.***
Hepatic: elevated liver enzymes.
Skin: rash, *photosensitivity,* pruritus, urticaria.

Overdose and treatment
To treat piroxicam overdose, empty stomach immediately by inducing emesis with ipecac syrup or by gastric lavage. Administer activated charcoal via nasogastric tube. Provide symptomatic and supportive measures including respiratory support and correction of fluid and electrolyte imbalances. Monitor laboratory parameters and vital signs closely.

Special considerations
▶ Drug has been used to treat other types of mild to moderate pain.
▶ Effectiveness of piroxicam usually is not seen for at least 2 weeks after therapy begins. Evaluate response to drug as evidenced by reduced symptoms.
▶ Drug is usually administered as a single dose.
▶ Adverse skin reactions are more common with piroxicam than with other NSAIDs; photosensitivity reactions are the most common.
▶ Drug hasn't been proven safe to the fetus.

Breast-feeding patients
▶ Piroxicam may inhibit lactation.
▶ Because drug appears in breast milk at 1% of maternal serum levels, use an alternative feeding method during drug therapy.

Pediatric patients
▶ Safe use of long-term piroxicam in children hasn't been established.

Geriatric patients
▶ Patients over age 60 are more sensitive to the adverse effects of piroxicam. Use with caution.
▶ Through its effect on renal prostaglandins, piroxicam may cause fluid retention and edema. This may be significant in elderly patients and in those with heart failure.

Patient teaching
▶ Tell patient to take drug with food to avoid adverse GI effects.
▶ Caution patient to avoid hazardous activities requiring alertness until CNS effects are known. Instruct patient in safety measures to prevent injury.
▶ Tell patient to avoid aspirin and alcoholic beverages during therapy.
▶ Urge patient to consult prescriber before taking OTC medications.
▶ Instruct patient in signs and symptoms of adverse effects. Tell patient to report them immediately.
▶ Encourage patient to comply with recommended follow-up.

▶ **prednisolone (systemic)**
Delta-Cortef, Prelone

▶ **prednisolone acetate**
Key-Pred 25, Predalone 50, Predate-50, Predcor-50

▶ **prednisolone acetate and prednisolone sodium phosphate**
Predicort-RP

▶ **prednisolone sodium phosphate**
Hydeltrasol, Key-Pred-SP, Pediapred, Predate S

▶ **prednisolone tebutate**
Hydeltra T.B.A., Nor-Pred T.B.A., Predate TBA, Predcor-TBA

Pharmacologic classification: *glucocorticoid, mineralocorticoid*

Therapeutic classification: *anti-inflammatory, immunosuppressant*

Pregnancy risk category C

How supplied
Available by prescription only
prednisolone
Syrup: 15 mg/5 ml
Tablets: 5 mg
prednisolone acetate
Injection: 25 mg/ml, 50 mg/ml, 100 mg/ml suspension
prednisolone acetate and prednisolone sodium phosphate
Injection: 80 mg acetate and 20 mg sodium phosphate/ml suspension
prednisolone sodium phosphate
Injection: 20 mg/ml solution
Oral liquid: 6.7 mg (5 mg base)/5 ml

prednisolone tebutate
Injection: 20 mg/ml suspension

Indications and dosages
Severe inflammation, modification of immune response to disease
Adults: 2.5 to 15 mg P.O. b.i.d., t.i.d., or q.i.d.
Children: 0.14 to 2 mg/kg or 4 to 6 mg/m² daily in divided doses.
prednisolone acetate
Adults: 2 to 30 mg I.M. q 12 hours.
prednisolone sodium phosphate
Adults: 2 to 30 mg I.M. or I.V. q 12 hours, or into joints, lesions, and soft tissue, p.r.n.
prednisolone tebutate
Adults: 4 to 40 mg into joints and lesions, p.r.n.
prednisolone acetate and prednisolone sodium phosphate suspension
Adults: 0.25 to 1 ml into joints weekly, p.r.n.

Pharmacodynamics
Anti-inflammatory action: Prednisolone stimulates the synthesis of enzymes needed to decrease the inflammatory response. It suppresses the immune system by reducing activity and volume of the lymphatic system, thus producing lymphocytopenia primarily of T-lymphocytes, decreasing immunoglobulin and complement levels, decreasing passage of immune complexes through basement membranes, and possibly by depressing reactivity of tissue to antigen-antibody interactions.

The mineralocorticoids regulate electrolyte homeostasis by acting renally at the distal tubules to enhance the reabsorption of sodium ions and thus water from the tubular fluid into the plasma and enhance the excretion of both potassium and hydrogen ions.

Prednisolone is an adrenocorticoid with both glucocorticoid and mineralocorticoid properties. It's a weak mineralocorticoid with only half the potency of hydrocortisone but is a more potent glucocorticoid, having four times the potency of equal weight of hydrocortisone. It's used primarily as an anti-inflammatory agent and an immunosuppressant but isn't used for mineralocorticoid replacement therapy because of the availability of more specific and potent agents.

Prednisolone may be administered orally. Prednisolone sodium phosphate is highly soluble, has a rapid onset and a short duration of action, and may be given I.M. or I.V. Prednisolone acetate and tebutate are suspensions that may be administered by intra-articular, intrasynovial, intrabursal, intralesional, or soft-tissue injection. They have a slow onset but a long duration of action.

Prednisolone sodium phosphate and prednisolone acetate is a combination product of the rapid-acting phosphate salt and the slightly soluble, slowly released acetate salt. This product provides rapid anti-inflammatory effects with a sustained duration of action. It's a suspension and shouldn't be given I.V. It's particularly useful as an anti-inflammatory agent in intra-articular, I.D., and intralesional injections.

Pharmacokinetics
Absorption: Drug is absorbed readily after oral administration. After oral and I.V. administration, peak effects occur in about 1 to 2

hours. Acetate and tebutate suspensions for injection have a variable absorption rate over 24 to 48 hours, depending on whether they are injected into an intra-articular space or a muscle, and on the blood supply to that muscle. Systemic absorption occurs slowly after intra-articular injection.

Distribution: Drug is removed rapidly from the blood and distributed to muscle, liver, skin, intestines, and kidneys. Drug is extensively bound to plasma proteins transcortin and albumin. Only the unbound portion is active. Adrenocorticoids are distributed into breast milk and through the placenta.

Metabolism: Drug is metabolized in the liver to inactive glucuronide and sulfate metabolites.

Excretion: The inactive metabolites, and small amounts of unmetabolized drug, are excreted in urine. Insignificant quantities of drug are excreted in feces. Biological half-life of prednisolone is 18 to 36 hours.

Contraindications and precautions

Contraindicated in patients hypersensitive to drug or its ingredients and in patients with systemic fungal infections.

Use cautiously in patients with a recent MI, GI ulcer, renal disease, hypertension, osteoporosis, diabetes mellitus, hypothyroidism, cirrhosis, diverticulitis, nonspecific ulcerative colitis, recent intestinal anastamoses, thromboembolic disorders, seizures, myasthenia gravis, heart failure, tuberculosis, ocular herpes simplex, emotional instability, or psychotic tendencies.

Interactions
Drug-drug

Amphotericin B, diuretics: enhanced hypokalemia. The hypokalemia may increase the risk of toxicity in patients concurrently receiving cardiac glycosides. Monitor serum potassium and digoxin levels.

Antacids, colestipol, cholestyramine: decreased corticosteroid effect by decreasing the amount absorbed. Separate administration times.

Barbiturates, phenytoin, rifampin: decreased corticosteroid effects because of increased hepatic metabolism. Monitor patient.

Estrogens: may reduce the metabolism of corticosteroids by increasing the level of transcortin, thus prolonging the half-life. Adjust dose as needed.

Insulin, oral antidiabetic drugs: increased risk of hyperglycemia. Adjust dosage as needed.

Isoniazid, salicylates: increased metabolism of these drugs. Adjust dosage as needed.

Oral anticoagulants: decreased effects. Monitor PT and INR.

Ulcer-causing drugs, such as NSAIDs: increased risk of GI ulceration. Monitor patient for abdominal complaints.

Effects on diagnostic tests

Prednisolone suppresses reactions to skin tests and causes false-negative results in the nitroblue tetrazolium test for systemic bacterial infections.

Adverse reactions

CNS: cerebri, *euphoria, insomnia,* paresthesia, pseudotumor headache, psychotic behavior, ***seizures,*** vertigo.

CV: *arrhythmias,* edema, *heart failure,* hypertension, *thromboembolism,* thrombophlebitis.
EENT: cataracts, glaucoma.
GI: *peptic ulceration,* GI irritation, increased appetite, nausea, *pancreatitis,* vomiting.
GU: menstrual irregularities.
Metabolic: carbohydrate intolerance, hyperglycemia, hypokalemia.
Musculoskeletal: growth suppression in children, muscle weakness, osteoporosis.
Skin: acne, delayed wound healing, hirsutism, various skin eruptions.
Other: *acute adrenal insufficiency (with increased stress from infection, surgery, or trauma),* cushingoid state (moonface, buffalo hump, central obesity), susceptibility to infections.

Overdose and treatment

Acute ingestion, even in massive doses, is rarely a clinical problem. Toxic signs and symptoms rarely occur if drug is used for less than 3 weeks, even at large dosage ranges. However, chronic use causes adverse physiologic effects, including suppression of the hypothalamic-pituitary-adrenal axis, cushingoid appearance, muscle weakness, and osteoporosis.

Special considerations

▶ Drug may also be used as adjuvant therapy to cancer pain and to increase appetite in these patients.
▶ Always use lowest effective dose.
▶ Give oral dose with food when possible. Critically ill patients may require concomitant antacid or H_2-receptor antagonist therapy.
▶ Use only prednisolone sodium phosphate for I.V. route. When administering as direct injection, inject undiluted drug into a vein or

free-flowing compatible I.V. solution over at least 1 minute. When administering as an intermittant or continuous infusion, dilute solution according to manufacturer's instructions, and give over the prescribed duration. Compatible solutions include D_5W and normal saline.
▶ Monitor patient's weight, blood pressure, and serum electrolyte level.
▶ Monitor patient for infection.
▶ Watch for depression or psychotic tendencies, especially in high-dose therapy.
▶ Monitor serum glucose level.
▶ Don't confuse drug with prednisone.
▶ Most adverse reactions to corticosteroids are dose- or duration-dependent.
▶ Gradually reduce dosage after long-term therapy.
▶ Abrupt withdrawal of drug may cause rebound inflammation, fatigue, weakness, arthralgia, fever, dizziness, lethargy, depression, fainting, orthostatic hypotension, dyspnea, anorexia, and hypoglycemia. After prolonged use, sudden withdrawal may cause acute adrenal insufficiency and death.

Pediatric patients

▶ Long-term use of adrenocorticoids or corticotropin may suppress growth and maturation in children and adolescents.

Patient teaching

▶ Instruct patient to take oral form of drug with milk or food.
▶ Teach patient the signs of early adrenal insufficiency: fatigue, muscular weakness, joint pain, fever, anorexia, nausea, dyspnea, dizziness, and fainting.

▶ Warn patient on long-term therapy about cushingoid symptoms and the need to notify prescriber about sudden weight gain or swelling.

▶ Advise patient on long-term therapy to consider exercise or physical therapy. Also, patient should ask prescriber about vitamin D or calcium supplement.

▶ Instruct patient to avoid exposure to infections (such as chickenpox or measles) and to contact prescriber if exposure occurs.

▶ Tell patient not to discontinue drug abruptly without consulting prescriber.

▶ Instruct patient to wear or carry medical identification that shows his need for supplemental systemic glucocorticoids during stress, along with prescriber's name, medication, and dose taken.

▶ **prednisone**
Apo-Prednisone◇, Deltasone, Meticorten, Orasone, Prednicen-M, Sterapred, Winpred◇

Pharmacologic classification: *adrenocorticoid*

Therapeutic classification: *anti-inflammatory, immunosuppressant*

Pregnancy risk category C

How supplied
Available by prescription only
Oral solution: 5 mg/ml; 5 mg/5 ml
Syrup: 5 mg/5 ml
Tablets: 1 mg, 2.5 mg, 5 mg, 10 mg, 20 mg, 25 mg, 50 mg

Indications and dosages
Severe inflammation, modification of body's immune response to disease
Adults: 5 to 60 mg P.O. daily in single dose or divided doses. Must be individualized. Maximum, 250 mg/day. Maintenance dose given once daily or every other day.
Children: 0.14 mg/kg or 4 to 6 mg/m² P.O. daily in divided doses, or use the following schedule:
Ages 11 to 18: 20 mg P.O. q.i.d.
Ages 5 to 10: 15 mg P.O. q.i.d.
Ages 18 months to 4 years: 7.5 to 10 mg P.O. q.i.d.
Acute exacerbations of multiple sclerosis
Adults: 200 mg P.O. daily for 1 week, and then 80 mg every other day for 1 month.

Pharmacodynamics
Anti-inflammatory action: Prednisone is one of the intermediate-acting glucocorticoids, with greater glucocorticoid activity than cortisone and hydrocortisone, but less anti-inflammatory activity than betamethasone, dexamethasone, and paramethasone. Prednisone is about four to five times more potent as an anti-inflammatory agent than hydrocortisone, but it has only half the mineralocorticoid activity of an equal weight of hydrocortisone. Prednisone is the oral glucocorticoid of choice for anti-inflammatory or immunosuppressant effects.

Immunosuppressant action: Prednisone stimulates the synthesis of enzymes needed to decrease the inflammatory response. It reduces activity and volume of the lymphatic system, thus producing lymphocytopenia (primarily of T-lymphocytes), decreasing immuno-

---

globulin and complement levels, decreasing passage of immune complexes through basement membranes, and possibly by depressing reactivity of tissue to antigen-antibody interactions.

Pharmacokinetics

Absorption: Drug is absorbed readily after oral administration, with peak effects occurring in about 1 to 2 hours.
Distribution: Drug is distributed rapidly to muscle, liver, skin, intestines, and kidneys. Prednisone is extensively bound to plasma proteins transcortin and albumin. Only the unbound portion is active. Adrenocorticoids are distributed into breast milk and through the placenta.
Metabolism: Drug is metabolized in the liver to the active metabolite prednisolone, which in turn is then metabolized to inactive glucuronide and sulfate metabolites.
Excretion: The inactive metabolites and small amounts of unmetabolized drug are excreted by the kidneys. Insignificant quantities of drug are also excreted in feces. Biological half-life of prednisone is 18 to 36 hours.

Contraindications and precautions

Contraindicated in patients hypersensitive to drug and in patients with systemic fungal infections.

Use cautiously in patients with GI ulcer, renal disease, hypertension, osteoporosis, diabetes mellitus, hypothyroidism, cirrhosis, diverticulitis, nonspecific ulcerative colitis, recent intestinal anastamoses, thromboembolic disorders, seizures, myasthenia gravis, heart failure, tuberculosis, ocular herpes simplex, emotional instability, and psychotic tendencies.

Interactions
Drug-drug

Amphotericin B, diuretics: enhanced hypokalemia, which may increase the risk of toxicity in patients concurrently receiving cardiac glycosides. Monitor serum potassium and digoxin levels.
Antacids, cholestyramine, colestipol: decreased corticosteroid effect by decreasing the amount absorbed. Separate administration times.
Barbiturates, phenytoin, rifampin: decreased corticosteroid effects because of increased hepatic metabolism. Monitor patient.
Estrogens: may reduce the metabolism of corticosteroids by increasing the level of transcortin, thus prolonging the half-life. Adjust dosage as needed.
Insulin, oral antidiabetic drugs: hyperglycemia. Adjust dosage as needed.
Isoniazid, salicylates: increased metabolism of these drugs. Adjust dosage as needed.
Oral anticoagulants: decreased effects. Monitor PT and INR.
Ulcer-causing drugs, such as NSAIDs: increased risk of GI ulceration. Monitor patient for abdominal complaints.

Effects on diagnostic tests

Prednisone suppresses reactions to skin tests and causes false-negative results in the nitroblue tetrazolium test for systemic bacterial infections.

Adverse reactions

CNS: *euphoria,* headache, *insomnia,* paresthesia, pseudotumor

cerebri, psychotic behavior, *seizures,* vertigo.
CV: *arrhythmias,* edema, *heart failure,* hypertension, *thromboembolism,* thrombophlebitis.
EENT: cataracts, glaucoma.
GI: GI irritation, increased appetite, nausea, *pancreatitis, peptic ulceration,* vomiting.
GU: menstrual irregularities.
Metabolic: hyperglycemia, hypokalemia, and carbohydrate intolerance.
Musculoskeletal: growth suppression in children, muscle weakness, osteoporosis.
Skin: acne, delayed wound healing, hirsutism, various skin eruptions.
Other: *acute adrenal insufficiency* (with increased stress from infection, surgery, or trauma), cushingoid state (moonface, buffalo hump, central obesity), susceptibility to infections.

Overdose and treatment
Acute ingestion, even in massive doses, is rarely a clinical problem. Toxic signs and symptoms rarely occur if drug is used for less than 3 weeks, even at large dosage ranges. However, chronic use causes adverse physiologic effects, including suppression of the hypothalamic-pituitary-adrenal axis, cushingoid appearance, muscle weakness, and osteoporosis.

Special considerations
▶ Drug is also used as an adjunct to anti-infective therapy in the treatment of moderate to severe *Pneumocystis carinii* pneumonia.
▶ Drug may also be used as adjuvant therapy to cancer pain and to increase appetite in these patients.

▶ Use of corticosteroids in patient decreases pain; thus, decreasing need for opiate intake.
▶ If patient can't swallow tablets, liquid forms are available. The oral concentrate (5 mg/ml) may be diluted in juice or another flavored diluent or mixed in semisolid food such as applesauce before administration.
▶ Always use lowest effective dose.
▶ Most adverse reactions to corticosteroids are dose- or duration-dependent.
▶ For better results and less toxicity, give daily dose in the morning.
▶ Give oral dose with food when possible. Critically ill patients may require concomitant antacid or H_2-receptor antagonist therapy.
▶ Don't confuse with prednisolone.
▶ Gradually reduce dosage after long-term therapy.
▶ Abrupt withdrawal may cause anorexia, arthralgia, depression, dizziness, fainting, fatigue, fever, rebound hypoglycemia, hypotension, inflammation, lethargy, orthostatic dyspnea, weakness. After prolonged use, sudden withdrawal may cause acute adrenal insufficiency and death.
▶ Monitor patient's weight, blood pressure, and serum electrolyte levels.
▶ Monitor patient for infection.
▶ Watch for depression or psychotic tendencies, especially in high-dose therapy.
▶ Monitor patient's serum glucose levels.

Pediatric patients
▶ Long-term use of prednisone in children or adolescents may delay growth and maturation.

Patient teaching
▶ Tell patient not to discontinue drug abruptly without prescriber's consent.
▶ Instruct patient to take oral form of drug with milk or food.
▶ Teach patient the signs of early adrenal insufficiency: fatigue, muscular weakness, joint pain, fever, anorexia, nausea, dyspnea, dizziness, and fainting.
▶ Instruct patient to wear or carry medical identification that shows his need for supplemental systemic glucocorticoids during stress, his prescriber's name, and the drug and dose taken.
▶ Warn patient on long-term therapy about cushingoid symptoms and the need to notify prescriber about sudden weight gain or swelling.
▶ Advise patient on long-term therapy to consider exercise or physical therapy. Also, patient should ask prescriber about vitamin D or calcium supplement.
▶ Instruct patient to avoid exposure to infections (such as chickenpox or measles) and to contact prescriber if exposure occurs.

▶ procaine hydrochloride
Novocain

Pharmacologic classification:
ester-type local anesthetic

Therapeutic classification:
local anesthetic, injectable

Pregnancy risk category C

How supplied
Available by prescription only
Injection: 1% in 2-ml and 6-ml ampules and in 30-ml vials, 2% in 30-ml vials, 10% in 2-ml ampules

Indications and dosages
Infiltration anesthesia
Adults: 350 mg to 600 mg as a 0.25% or 0.5% solution
Peripheral nerve block
Adults: up to 200 ml of a 0.5% solution, up to 100 ml of a 1% solution or up to 50 ml of a 2% solution
Spinal anesthesia
Adults: For the perineum, 0.5 ml of 10% solution (50 mg) diluted with an equal volume of diluent; for perineum and legs, 1 ml of 10% solution (100 mg) diluted with an equal volume of diluent; up to costal margin, 2 ml of 10% solution (200 mg) and 1 ml of diluent. Maximum initial dose, 1 gram.
▧ Dosage adjustment. Give reduced doses to debilitated, obstetric, and acutely ill patients and to patients with increased abdominal pressure or cardiac or liver disease.

Pharmacodynamics
Local anesthetic action: Procaine blocks the generation and conduction of nerve impulses by increasing the threshold for electrical excitation in the nerve, by slowing propagation of the nerve impulse, and by reducing the rate of the action potential.

Pharmacokinetics
Absorption: Absorption depends on dose and concentration of drug, route of administration, and vascularity of site. Use of a vasoconstrictor decreases absorption rate.
Distribution: Depending on route of administration, procaine is distributed to some extent to all body tissues.
Metabolism: Drug is hydrolyzed by plasma cholinesterase to para-

aminobenzoic acid and diethyl-aminoethanol.

Excretion: Drug is excreted mainly in urine as metabolites; less than 2% recovered as unchanged drug.

Contraindications and precautions

Contraindicated in patients hypersensitive to procaine, to its components, or to para-aminobenzoic acid or its derivatives.

Use cautiously in patients with hepatic disease, severe hypotension, shock, heart block, disturbances of cardiac rhythm or impaired CV function and in those with inflammation or infection at puncture site.

Interactions
Drug-drug

CNS depressants: may cause additive CNS effects; reduce dosage of CNS depressants.

Succinylcholine: prolonged neuromuscular blockade. Use cautiously together.

Sulfonamides: procaine inhibits the action of sulfonamides. Don't use in conditions in which a sulfonamide drug is needed.

Effects on diagnostic tests

None reported

Adverse reactions

CNS: anxiety, nervousness, *seizures* followed by drowsiness.
CV: *arrhythmias, bradycardia, cardiac arrest,* edema, hypotension, myocardial depression.
EENT: blurred vision, tinnitus.
GI: nausea, vomiting.
Respiratory: *respiratory arrest, status asthmaticus.*
Skin: dermatological reactions.
Other: *anaphylaxis.*

Overdose and treatment

Overdose is usually from high plasma levels or an unintentional subarachnoid injection of the drug and can result in seizures as well as underventilation and apnea.

Treatment involves establishing a patent airway and administering oxygen. This may prevent seizures if they haven't already occurred. Administer medications to control seizures as appropriate.

Special considerations

▶ The dose will differ with the anesthetic procedure, the area to be anesthetized, the vascularity of the area, the number of neuronal segments to be blocked, the degree of block and the duration of anesthesia desired, as well as individual patient conditions and tolerance. Incremental doses should always be used.

▶ The smallest dose and concentration needed to produce the result should be administered to avoid serious adverse effects.

▶ Keep resuscitative equipment and drugs readily available when using a local anesthetic.

▶ For infiltration anesthesia or peripheral nerve block; if vasoconstrictive effect is desired, add 0.5 ml to 1 ml of epinephrine 1:1000 per 100 ml of anesthetic solution.

▶ Inspect product for particulate matter or discoloration.

▶ To prepare 60 ml of a 0.5% solution (5 mg/ml), dilute 30 ml of the 1% solution with 30 ml of normal saline solution for injection. To prepare 60 ml of a 0.25% solution (2.5 mg/ml), dilute 15 ml of the 1% solution with 45 ml of normal saline solution for injection.

▶ For spinal anesthesia, dilute 10% solution with normal saline solution injection, sterile water for injection, or CSF. For hyperbaric technique, use dextrose injection prior to administration. Rate of injection is 1 ml/5 seconds.

▶ Discard partially used bottles of unpreserved solution.

▶ Always inject slowly, with frequent aspirations to prevent intravascular injection.

▶ Observe patient carefully when giving anesthesia by monitoring CV and respiratory status and consciousness.

Breast-feeding patients
▶ No data exist to demonstrate whether drug appears in human breast milk. Use caution when administering to a breast-feeding woman.

Pediatric patients
▶ Reduce dosages in children.

Geriatric patients
▶ Reduce dosages in elderly patients.

Patient teaching
▶ Inform patient that he may experience temporary loss of sensation following proper administration of anesthesia.

▶ Explain to the patient that respiratory and CV systems will be monitored.

▶ ## prochlorperazine
Compazine, Stemetil ◇

▶ ## prochlorperazine edisylate
Compazine

▶ ## prochlorperazine maleate
Compazine, Compazine Spansule, Stemetil ◇

Pharmacologic classification:
phenothiazine (piperazine derivative)

Therapeutic classification:
antianxiety drug, antiemetic, antipsychotic

Pregnancy risk category C

How supplied
Available by prescription only
prochlorperazine edisylate
Injection: 5 mg/ml
Spansules (sustained-release): 10 mg, 15 mg, 30 mg
Suppositories: 2.5 mg, 5 mg, 25 mg
Syrup: 1 mg/ml
prochlorperazine maleate
Tablets: 5 mg, 10 mg, 25 mg

Indications and dosages
Preoperative nausea control
Adults: 5 to 10 mg I.M. 1 to 2 hours before induction of anesthesia, repeated once in 30 minutes if necessary; or 5 to 10 mg I.V. 15 to 30 minutes before induction of anesthesia, repeated once if necessary; or 20 mg/L D_5W and normal saline solution by I.V. infusion, added to infusion 15 to 30 minutes before induction. Maximum parenteral dosage is 40 mg daily.
Severe nausea, vomiting
Adults: 5 to 10 mg P.O. t.i.d. or q.i.d.; or 15 mg of sustained-

release form P.O. on arising; or 10 mg of sustained-release form P.O. q 12 hours; or 25 mg P.R. b.i.d.; or 5 to 10 mg I.M. injected deeply into upper outer quadrant of gluteal region. Repeat q 3 to 4 hours, p.r.n. May be given I.V. Maximum parenteral dose, 40 mg daily.

Children who weigh 18 to 39 kg (39 to 86 lb): 2.5 mg P.O. or rectally t.i.d.; or 5 mg P.O. or P.R. b.i.d.; or 0.132 mg/kg deep I.M. injection. Control usually obtained with one dose. Maximum, 15 mg daily.

Children who weigh 14 to 17 kg (31 to 38 lb): 2.5 mg P.O. or P.R. b.i.d. or t.i.d.; or 0.132 mg/kg deep I.M. injection. Control usually is obtained with one dose. Maximum, 10 mg daily.

Children who weigh 9 to 14 kg (20 to 30 lb): 2.5 mg P.O. or P.R. daily or b.i.d.; or 0.132 mg/kg deep I.M. injection. Control usually is obtained with one dose. Maximum, 7.5 mg daily.

Anxiety

Adults: 5 mg P.O. t.i.d. or q.i.d.

▷ Dosage adjustment. Elderly patients tend to require lower doses adjusted to individual effects.

Pharmacodynamics

Antiemetic action: Drug exibits this action due to dopamine receptor blockade in the medullary chemoreceptor trigger zone.

Antipsychotic action: Prochlorperazine is thought to exert these effects by postsynaptic blockade of CNS dopamine receptors, thus inhibiting dopamine-mediated effects.

Other actions: Prochlorperazine has many other central and peripheral effects: It produces alpha and ganglionic blockade and counter-acts histamine- and serotonin-mediated activity. Its most prevalent adverse reactions are extrapyramidal. It is used primarily as an antiemetic; it is ineffective against motion sickness.

Pharmacokinetics

Absorption: Rate and extent of absorption vary with administration route: oral tablet absorption is erratic and variable, with onset of action ranging from ¼ to 1 hour; oral concentrate absorption is more predictable. I.M. drug is absorbed rapidly.

Distribution: Drug is distributed widely into the body, including breast milk. Drug is 91% to 99% protein-bound. Peak effect occurs at 2 to 4 hours; steady state serum levels are achieved within 4 to 7 days.

Metabolism: Drug is metabolized extensively by the liver, but no active metabolites are formed; duration of action is about 3 to 4 hours and 10 to 12 hours for the extended-release form.

Excretion: Drug is mostly excreted in urine via the kidneys; some is excreted in feces via the biliary tract.

Contraindications and precautions

Contraindicated in patients hypersensitive to phenothiazines and in those with CNS depression including coma; during pediatric surgery; when using spinal or epidural anesthetic, adrenergic blockers, or ethanol; and in infants under age 2.

Use cautiously in patients with impaired CV function, glaucoma, seizure disorders; in those who have been exposed to extreme heat; and in children with acute illness.

Interactions
Drug-drug
Aluminum- and magnesium-containing antacids, antidiarrheals: decreased absorption. Separate administration times.

Antiarrhythmics, disopyramide, procainamide, quinidine: increased risk of arrhythmias and conduction defects. Use together with caution.

Anticholinergics, including antidepressants, antihistamines, antiparkinsonians, atropine, MAO inhibitors, meperidine, phenothiazines: increased risk of oversedation, paralytic ileus, visual changes, and severe constipation. Monitor patient.

Appetite suppressants, sympathomimetics (including ephedrine, epinephrine, phenylephrine, phenylpropanolamine): may decrease their stimulatory and pressor effects and may cause epinephrine reversal (hypotensive response to epinephrine). Use together cautiously.

Beta blockers: may inhibit prochlorperazine metabolism, increasing plasma levels and toxicity. Monitor patient for toxicity.

Bromocriptine: prochlorperazine may antagonize therapeutic effect on prolactin secretion. Monitor patient for clinical effects.

Central-acting antihypertensives, such as clonidine, guanabenz, guanadrel, guanethidine, methyldopa, reserpine: inhibited blood pressure response. Monitor blood pressure.

CNS depressants, including barbiturates, epidural anesthetics, general anesthetics, magnesium sulfate (parenteral), narcotics, spinal anesthetics, tranquilizers: in-creased risk of oversedation, respiratory depression, and hypotension. Monitor patient.

High-dose dopamine: decreased vasoconstricting effects. Monitor patient for clinical effects.

Levodopa: decreased effectiveness and increased toxicity (because of dopamine blockade). Monitor patient for drug effects.

Lithium: risk of severe neurologic toxicity with an encephalitis-like syndrome, and decreased therapeutic response to prochlorperazine. Use together cautiously.

Metrizamide: increased risk of seizures. Use together cautiously.

Nitrates: hypotension may occur. Monitor blood pressure.

Phenobarbital: enhanced renal excretion. Monitor patient for drug effects.

Phenytoin: inhibited metabolism and increased toxicity of phenytoin. Monitor phenytoin levels.

Propylthiouracil: increased risk of agranulocytosis. Monitor hematologic studies.

Drug-food
Caffeine: increased prochlorperazine metabolism. Discourage concurrent use.

Drug-lifestyle
Alcohol use: additive effects. Discourage alcohol use.

Heavy smoking: increased prochlorperazine metabolism. Discourage smoking during therapy.

Sun exposure: may cause photosensitivity. Urge precautions.

Effects on diagnostic tests
Prochlorperazine causes false-positive test results for urine porphyrins, urobilinogen, amylase, and 5-hydroxyindoleacetic acid be-

cause of darkening of urine by metabolites; it also causes false-positive urine pregnancy results in tests using human chorionic gonadotropin as the indicator.

Adverse reactions
CNS: confusion, dizziness, EEG changes, *extrapyramidal reactions,* pseudoparkinsonism, sedation.
CV: ECG changes, *orthostatic hypotension,* tachycardia.
EENT: *blurred vision, ocular changes.*
GI: *constipation, dry mouth,* ileus.
GU: dark urine, inhibited ejaculation, menstrual irregularities, *urine retention.*
Hematologic: *agranulocytosis, hemolytic anemia, **thrombocytopenia, transient leukopenia.***
Hepatic: *cholestatic jaundice.*
Metabolic: hyperglycemia, hyperprolactinemia, hypoglycemia, increased appetite, weight gain.
Skin: *allergic reactions*, exfoliative dermatitis, mild photosensitivity.
Other: gynecomastia.

Overdose and treatment
Overdose may cause CNS depression characterized by deep, unarousable sleep and possible coma, hypotension or hypertension, extrapyramidal symptoms, dystonia, abnormal involuntary muscle movements, agitation, seizures, arrhythmias, ECG changes, hypothermia or hyperthermia, and autonomic nervous system dysfunction.

Treatment is symptomatic and supportive and includes maintaining vital signs, airway, stable body temperature, and fluid and electrolyte balance. Don't induce vomiting: Drug inhibits cough reflex, and aspiration may occur. Use gastric lavage, then activated charcoal and saline cathartics. Dialysis doesn't help. Regulate body temperature as needed. Treat hypotension with I.V. fluids: Don't give epinephrine. Treat seizures with parenteral diazepam or barbiturates, arrhythmias with parenteral phenytoin (1 mg/kg with rate adjusted to blood pressure), and extrapyramidal reactions with benztropine or parenteral diphenhydramine 2 mg/kg/minute.

Special considerations
▶ Drug is also used to treat psychotic disorders.
▶ Drug is only used when vomiting can't be controlled by other measures or when only a few doses are needed. If more than 4 doses are needed in 24 hours, reevaluate patient.
▶ Reevaluate patient's analgesics; they may need adjustment if antiemetic gives no relief.
▶ Oral forms may cause stomach upset. Give with food or fluid.
▶ Liquid and injectable formulations may cause a rash after contact with skin.
▶ Drug may cause a pink to brown discoloration of urine.
▶ Drug causes high risk of extrapyramidal effects and, in institutionalized psychiatric patients, photosensitivity reactions; patient should avoid exposure to sunlight or heat lamps.
▶ Benadryl is effective in treating extrapyramidal effects.
▶ Drug is ineffective in treating motion sickness.
▶ Dilute the concentrate in 60 to 120 ml (2 to 4 oz) of water. Store the suppository form in a cool place.

▶ I.M. injection may cause skin necrosis. Don't mix with other medications in the syringe. Do not administer S.C.

▶ Administer I.M. injection deep into the upper outer quadrant of the buttock. Massaging the area after administration may prevent formation of abscesses.

▶ Solution for injection may be slightly discolored. Don't use if excessively discolored or if a precipitate is evident. Contact pharmacist.

▶ Don't give sustained-release form to children.

▶ Chewing gum, hard candy, or ice may help relieve dry mouth.

▶ Protect the liquid form from light.

▶ Monitor patient's blood pressure before and after parenteral administration.

▶ Give I.V. dose slowly (5 mg/minute). Take care to prevent extravasation.

▶ About 15 to 30 minutes before induction, add 20 mg of prochlorperazine per liter of D_5W and normal saline solution. Infusion rate shouldn't exceed 5 mg/minute. Maximum parenteral dosage is 40 mg daily. Infuse slowly, never as a bolus.

Breast-feeding patients
▶ Drug may enter breast milk and should be used with caution.

Pediatric patients
▶ Prochlorperazine isn't recommended for patients under age 2 or weighing less than 20 lb (9 kg).

Geriatric patients
▶ Elderly patients are at greater risk for adverse reactions, especially tardive dyskinesia, other extrapyramidal effects, and hypotension.

Patient teaching
▶ Explain risks of dystonic reactions and tardive dyskinesia. Tell patient to report abnormal body movements promptly.

▶ Tell patient to avoid sun exposure and to wear sunscreen when going outdoors to prevent photosensitivity reactions. (Note that heat lamps and tanning beds also may cause burning of the skin or skin discoloration.)

▶ Tell patient to avoid spilling the liquid form. Contact with skin may cause rash and irritation.

▶ Warn patient to avoid extremely hot or cold baths and exposure to temperature extremes, sunlamps, or tanning beds; drug may cause thermoregulatory changes.

▶ Advise patient to take drug exactly as prescribed, not to double doses after missing one, and not to share drug with others.

▶ Warn patient to avoid alcohol or taking other medications that may cause excessive sedation.

▶ Tell patient to dilute the concentrate in water; explain the dropper technique of measuring dose; teach correct use of suppository.

▶ Tell patient that hard candy, chewing gum, or ice chips can alleviate dry mouth.

▶ Urge patient to store drug safely away from children.

▶ Inform patient that interactions are possible with many drugs. Warn him to seek medical approval before taking self-prescribed medication.

▶ Warn patient not to stop taking drug suddenly and to promptly report difficulty urinating, sore throat, dizziness, or fainting.

Reassure patient that most reactions can be relieved by reducing dose.
▶ Caution patient to avoid hazardous activities until full effect of drug is known. Reassure patient that sedative effects subside and become tolerable in several weeks.

▶ **promethazine hydrochloride**
Anergan 25, Anergan 50, Histantil◇, Pentazine, Phencen-50, Phenergan, Phenergan Fortis, Phenergan Plain, Phenoject-50, Promet, Prorex-25, Prorex-50, Prothazine, Prothazine Plain, V-Gan-25, V-Gan-50

Pharmacologic classification:
phenothiazine derivative

Therapeutic classification:
antiemetic, antivertigo; antihistamine (H₂-receptor antagonist); preoperative, postoperative, or obstetric sedative and adjunct to analgesics

Pregnancy risk category NR

How supplied
Available by prescription only
Injection: 25 mg/ml, 50 mg/ml
Suppositories: 12.5 mg, 25 mg, 50 mg
Syrup: 6.25 mg/5 ml, 10 mg/5 ml, 25 mg/5 ml
Tablets: 12.5 mg, 25 mg, 50 mg

Indications and dosages
Motion sickness
Adults: 25 mg P.O. b.i.d.
Children: 12.5 to 25 mg P.O., I.M., or P.R. b.i.d.

Nausea
Adults: 12.5 to 25 mg P.O., I.M., or P.R. q 4 to 6 hours, p.r.n.
Children: 0.25 to 0.5 mg/kg I.M. or P.R. q 4 to 6 hours, p.r.n.
Sedation
Adults: 25 to 50 mg P.O. or I.M. h.s., or p.r.n.
Children: 12.5 to 25 mg P.O., I.M., or P.R. h.s.
Routine preoperative or postoperative sedation or as an adjunct to analgesics
Adults: 25 to 50 mg I.M., I.V., or P.O.
Children: 12.5 to 25 mg I.M., I.V., or P.O.
Obstetric sedation
25 to 50 mg I.M. or I.V. in early stages of labor, and 25 to 75 mg after labor is established; repeat q 2 to 4 hours, p.r.n. Maximum, 100 mg/day.

Pharmacodynamics
Antiemetic and antivertigo actions: The central antimuscarinic actions of antihistamines probably are responsible for their antivertigo and antiemetic effects; promethazine also is believed to inhibit the medullary chemoreceptor trigger zone.
Antihistamine action: Promethazine competes with histamine for the H₁-receptor, thereby suppressing allergic rhinitis and urticaria; drug does not prevent the release of histamine.
Sedative action: CNS depressant mechanism of promethazine is unknown; phenothiazines probably cause sedation by reducing stimuli to the brain-stem reticular system.

Pharmacokinetics
Absorption: Promethazine is well absorbed from the GI tract. Action begins 20 minutes after P.O., P.R.,

or I.M. administration and within 3 to 5 minutes after I.V. administration. Effects usually last 4 to 6 hours but may persist for 12 hours.
Distribution: Drug is distributed widely throughout the body; it crosses the placenta.
Metabolism: Drug is metabolized in the liver.
Excretion: Drug's metabolites are excreted in urine and feces.

Contraindications and precautions
Contraindicated in patients hypersensitive to drug; in those with intestinal obstruction, prostatic hyperplasia, bladder neck obstruction, seizure disorders, coma, CNS depression, and stenosing peptic ulcerations; in newborns, premature neonates, and breast-feeding patients; and in acutely ill or dehydrated children.

Use cautiously in patients with asthma or cardiac, pulmonary, or hepatic disease.

Interactions
Drug-drug
Antihistamines, CNS depressants (such as antianxiety drugs, barbiturates, sleeping aids, tranquilizers): additive CNS depression. Monitor patient closely.
Epinephrine: partial adrenergic blockade, producing further hypotension. Do not give together.
Levodopa: promethazine may block the antiparkinsonian action of levodopa.
MAO inhibitors: prolonged and intensified sedative and anticholinergic effects. Do not give together.

Drug-lifestyle
Alcohol use: additive CNS depression. Discourage alcohol use.

Sun exposure: may cause photosensitivity reactions. Urge precautions.

Effects on diagnostic tests
Discontinue drug 4 days before diagnostic skin tests to avoid preventing, reducing, or masking test response. Promethazine may cause either false-positive or false-negative pregnancy test results. It also may interfere with blood grouping in the ABO system.

Adverse reactions
CNS: confusion, disorientation, dizziness, *drowsiness,* extrapyramidal symptoms, *sedation,* sleepiness.
CV: hypertension, hypotension.
EENT: blurred vision.
GI: *dry mouth,* nausea, vomiting.
GU: urine retention.
Hematologic: *agranulocytosis, leukopenia, thrombocytopenia.*
Metabolic: hyperglycemia.
Skin: photosensitivity, rash.

Overdose and treatment
Overdose may cause either CNS depression (sedation, reduced mental alertness, apnea, and CV collapse) or CNS stimulation (insomnia, hallucinations, tremors, or seizures). Dry mouth, flushed skin, fixed and dilated pupils, and GI symptoms are common, especially in children.

Empty stomach by gastric lavage; don't induce vomiting. Treat hypotension with vasopressors, and control seizures with diazepam or phenytoin. Correct acidosis and electrolyte imbalance. Urine acidification promotes excretion of drug. Don't give stimulants.

Special considerations
▶ Drug is also used to treat rhinitis and allergy symptoms.
▶ Promethazine is used as an adjunct to analgesics, usually to increase sedation; it has no analgesic activity.
▶ Promethazine and meperidine may be mixed in the same syringe.
▶ The 50 mg/ml concentration is for I.M. use only; inject deep into large muscle mass. Don't administer drug S.C. because doing so could cause chemical irritation and necrosis.
▶ Give drug I.V., at no more than 25 mg/ml and 25 mg/minute; when using I.V. drip, wrap in aluminum foil to protect drug from light.
▶ Monitor patient for sedation.
▶ Monitor vital signs.
▶ Pronounced sedative effects may limit use in some ambulatory patients.

Breast-feeding patients
▶ Antihistamines such as promethazine shouldn't be used during breast-feeding. Many of these drugs appear in breast milk, exposing the infant to risks of unusual excitability, especially premature infants and other neonates, who may experience seizures.

Pediatric patients
▶ Use cautiously in children with respiratory dysfunction. Safety and efficacy in those younger than age 2 have not been established; do not give promethazine to infants under age 3 months.

Geriatric patients
▶ Elderly patients are usually more sensitive to adverse effects of antihistamines and are especially likely to experience a greater degree of dizziness, sedation, hyperexcitability, dry mouth, urine retention, and extrapyramidal symptoms than younger patients. Symptoms usually respond to a decrease in medication dosage.

Patient teaching
▶ Warn patient about possible photosensitivity and ways to avoid it.
▶ When treating motion sickness, tell patient to take first dose 30 to 60 minutes before travel; on succeeding days, he should take dose upon arising and with evening meal.

▶ proparacaine hydrochloride
Ak-Taine, Alcaine, Ophthaine, Ophthetic

Pharmacologic classification:
local anesthetic

Therapeutic classification:
local anesthetic

Pregnancy risk category C

How supplied
Available by prescription only
Ophthalmic solution: 0.5%

Indications and dosages
Anesthesia for tonometry
Adults and children: 1 or 2 drops of 0.5% solution instilled in eye just before procedure.
Anesthesia for removal of foreign bodies or sutures from the eye
Adults and children: 1 or 2 drops instilled 2 to 3 minutes before procedure or q 5 to 10 minutes for 1 to 3 doses.

Anesthesia for cataract extraction, glaucoma surgery
Adults and children: 1 drop of 0.5% solution instilled in eye q 5 to 10 minutes for 5 to 7 doses.
◩ Dosage adjustment. Dosage may need to be reduced in elderly, debilitated patients.

Pharmacodynamics
Anesthetic action: Produces anesthesia by preventing initiation and transmission of impulse at the nerve cell membrane.

Pharmacokinetics
Absorption: Action starts within 20 seconds of instillation and lasts 15 to 20 minutes.
Distribution: Unknown.
Metabolism: Unknown.
Excretion: Unknown.

Contraindications and precautions
Contraindicated in patients hypersensitive to ester-type local anesthetics, para-aminobenzoic acid or its derivatives, or any other ingredient in the preparation.

Use cautiously in patients with cardiac disease or hyperthyroidism.

Interactions
None reported.

Effects on diagnostic tests
None reported.

Adverse reactions
EENT: cycloplegic effect, hyperallergenic corneal reaction, occasional conjunctival congestion or hemorrhage, pupil dilation, softening and erosion of the corneal epithelium, transient pain.
Other: allergic contact dermatitis, *hypersensitivity.*

Overdose and treatment
Overdose is extremely rare with ophthalmic administration. Symptoms indicate CNS stimulation and may include alertness and agitation followed by depression.

Treat ocular overexposure with warm-water irrigation for at least 15 minutes.

Special considerations
▶ Proparacaine is the topical ophthalmic anesthetic of choice in diagnostic and minor surgical procedures.
▶ Drug is not for long-term use; may delay wound healing and may cause corneal opacification with accompanying loss of vision.
▶ Don't use discolored solution; store in tightly closed original container.
▶ Ophthaine brand packaging resembles that of Hemoccult in size and shape; check label carefully.
▶ Perform visual acuity in eye injuries.
▶ Discontinue drug if hypersensitivity occurs.

Patient teaching
▶ Warn patient not to rub or touch eye while cornea is anesthetized; this may cause corneal abrasion and greater discomfort when anesthesia wears off; advise use of a protective eye patch after procedures.
▶ Explain that corneal pain associated with an abrasion is relieved only temporarily by the application of proparacaine hydrochloride.
▶ Tell patient local irritation or stinging may occur several hours after instillation of proparacaine.
▶ Instruct patient to avoid contaminating the dropper and to replace cap after use.

❱ propoxyphene hydrochloride
Darvon

❱ propoxyphene napsylate
Darvon-N, Propacet 100 (with acetaminophen)

Pharmacologic classification:
opioid

Therapeutic classification:
analgesic

Controlled substance schedule IV

Pregnancy risk category NR

How supplied
Available by prescription only
propoxyphene hydrochloride
Capsules: 65 mg
Tablets: 65 mg
propoxyphene napsylate
Capsules: 50 mg, 100 mg
Suspension: 50 mg/5 ml
Tablets: 50 mg, 100 mg
propoxyphene napsylate and acetaminophen
Tablets: 100 mg propoxyphene napsylate, 650 mg acetaminophen

Indications and dosages
Mild to moderate pain
Adults: 65 mg (hydrochloride) P.O. q 4 hours, p.r.n., or 100 mg (napsylate) P.O. q 4 hours, p.r.n.
◺ DOSAGE ADJUSTMENT. Lower doses are usually indicated for elderly patients because they may be more sensitive to drug effects.

Pharmacodynamics
Analgesic action: Propoxyphene exerts its analgesic effect via opiate agonist activity and alters the patient's response to painful stimuli, particularly mild to moderate pain.

Pharmacokinetics
Absorption: After oral administration, drug is absorbed primarily in the upper small intestine. Equimolar doses of the hydrochloride and napsylate salts provide similar plasma levels. Onset of analgesia occurs in 20 to 60 minutes, and peak analgesic effects occur at 2 to 2½ hours.
Distribution: Drug enters the CSF and probably crosses the placental barrier; however, placental fluid and fetal blood levels haven't been determined.
Metabolism: Propoxyphene is degraded mainly in the liver; about one-quarter of a dose is metabolized to norpropoxyphene, an active metabolite.
Excretion: Drug is excreted in the urine. Duration of effect is 4 to 6 hours.

Contraindications and precautions
Contraindicated in patients hypersensitive to drug.
   Use cautiously in patients with impaired renal or hepatic function, emotional instability, or history of drug or alcohol abuse.

Interactions
Drug-drug
Antidepressants, such as doxepin: propoxyphene may inhibit metabolism of these drugs. Decrease antidepressant dosage.
Carbamazepine: increased carbamazepine effects. Monitor serum carbamazepine levels.
Cimetidine: enhanced respiratory and CNS depression, resulting in confusion, disorientation, apnea, or seizures. Use together cautiously.
CNS depressants, such as antidepressants, antihistamines, general

---

Reactions may be *common*, uncommon, *life-threatening*, or **COMMON AND LIFE-THREATENING**.

anesthetics, barbiturates, benzodiazepines, muscle relaxants, narcotic analgesics, phenothiazines, sedative-hypnotics: potentiation of adverse effects (respiratory depression, sedation, hypotension). Reduce propoxyphene dosage.

Drugs highly metabolized in the liver, such as digitoxin, phenytoin, rifampin: accumulation of either drug may occur. Withdrawal symptoms may result if used together. Monitor patient closely.

General anesthetics: severe CV depression. Monitor patient closely if used together.

Narcotic antagonists: acute withdrawal syndrome after a single dose in patients physically dependent on propoxyphene. Use with caution and monitor closely.

Drug-lifestyle
Alcohol use: potentiated CNS depressant effects of propoxyphene. Discourage concurrent use.

Effects on diagnostic tests
Drug may cause false decrease in test for urinary steroid excretion.

Adverse reactions
CNS: *dizziness,* euphoria, hallucinations, headache, light-headedness, *sedation,* weakness.
GI: abdominal pain, constipation, *nausea, vomiting.*
Hepatic: abnormal liver function tests.
Respiratory: *respiratory depression.*
Other: psychological and physical dependence.

Overdose and treatment
Overdose typically causes CNS depression, respiratory depression, and miosis. It also may cause hypotension, bradycardia, hypothermia, shock, apnea, cardiopulmonary arrest, circulatory collapse, pulmonary edema, and seizures.

Drug is known to cause ECG changes (prolonged QRS complex) and nephrogenic diabetes insipidus in acute toxic doses. Death from an acute overdose is most likely to occur within the first hour. Signs and symptoms of overdose with propoxyphene combination products may include salicylism from aspirin or acetaminophen toxicity.

To treat an acute overdose, first establish adequate respiration via a patent airway and ventilate as needed; administer a narcotic antagonist such as naloxone to reverse respiratory depression. Because the duration of action of drug is longer than naloxone, repeated dosing is necessary. Don't give naloxone if patient doesn't have clinically significant respiratory or CV depression. Monitor vital signs closely.

If patient shows symptoms within 2 hours of ingestion of an oral overdose, empty the stomach immediately by inducing emesis with ipecac syrup or gastric lavage. Use caution to avoid risk of aspiration. Administer activated charcoal via nasogastric tube for further removal of drug in an oral overdose.

Provide symptomatic and supportive treatment, including continued respiratory support and correction of fluid and electrolyte imbalances. Anticonvulsants may be needed; monitor laboratory parameters, vital signs, and neurologic status closely. Dialysis may be helpful in the treatment of overdose with propoxyphene combination products containing aspirin or acetaminophen.

Special considerations
▶ Propoxyphene can be considered a mild narcotic analgesic, but pain relief is equivalent to aspirin.
▶ Propoxyphene isn't an effective first-line drug.
▶ Drug isn't an appropriate choice for long-term pain management.
▶ Drug is toxic in high doses.
▶ Propoxyphene napsylate and acetaminophen combination contains 650 mg of Tylenol; patient should be made aware of Tylenol content of drug.
▶ Propoxyphene may obscure the signs and symptoms of an acute abdominal condition or worsen gallbladder pain.
▶ Don't prescribe drug maintenance purposes in narcotic addiction.
▶ Monitor patient for adequate and effective pain relief.
▶ Monitor liver function tests.

Breast-feeding patients
▶ Drug appears in breast milk; use with caution in breast-feeding women.

Patient teaching
▶ Warn patient not to exceed recommended dosage.
▶ Tell patient to take drug with food if GI upset occurs.
▶ Tell patient to avoid use of alcohol because it will cause additive CNS depressant effects.
▶ Warn patient of additive depressant effect that can occur if drug is prescribed for medical conditions requiring use of sedatives, tranquilizers, muscle relaxants, antidepressants, or other CNS-depressant drugs.

▶ **propranolol hydrochloride**
Inderal, Inderal LA

Pharmacologic classification:
beta blocker

Therapeutic classification:
adjunctive therapy in MI, adjunctive therapy in migraine, antianginal, antiarrhythmic, antihypertensive

Pregnancy risk category C

How supplied
Available by prescription only
Capsules (extended-release):
60 mg, 80 mg, 120 mg, 160 mg
Injection: 1 mg/ml
Solution: 4 mg/ml, 8 mg/ml, 20 mg/ 5 ml, 40 mg/5 ml, 80 mg/ml (concentrated)
Tablets: 10 mg, 20 mg, 40 mg, 60 mg, 80 mg, 90 mg

Indications and dosages
Management of angina
Adults: 10 to 20 mg t.i.d. or q.i.d., or one 80-mg sustained-release capsule daily. Dosage may be increased at 7- to 10-day intervals. Average optimum dose is 160 to 240 mg daily.
Prevention of frequent, severe, uncontrollable, or disabling migraine or vascular headache
Adults: initially, 80 mg daily in divided doses or one sustained-release capsule daily. Usual maintenance dosage is 160 to 240 mg daily, divided t.i.d. or q.i.d.
Adjunctive treatment of anxiety
Adults: 10 to 80 mg P.O. 1 hour before anxiety-provoking activity.

Pharmacodynamics
Antianginal action: Propranolol decreases myocardial oxygen consumption by blocking catechola-

mine access to beta-adrenergic receptors, thus relieving angina.
Antiarrhythmic action: Propranolol decreases heart rate and prevents exercise-induced increases in heart rate. It also decreases myocardial contractility, cardiac output, and SA and AV nodal conduction velocity.
Antihypertensive action: Exact mechanism of propranolol's antihypertensive effect is unknown; drug may reduce blood pressure by blocking adrenergic receptors (thus decreasing cardiac output), by decreasing sympathetic outflow from the CNS, and by suppressing renin release.
Migraine prophylactic action: Migraine-preventive effect of propranolol is thought to result from inhibition of vasodilation.
MI prophylactic action: Exact mechanism by which propranolol decreases mortality after MI is unknown.

Pharmacokinetics
Absorption: Drug is absorbed almost completely from the GI tract. Absorption is enhanced when given with food. Peak plasma levels occur 60 to 90 minutes after administration of regular-release tablets. After I.V. administration, peak levels occur in about 1 minute, with virtually immediate onset of action.
Distribution: Drug is distributed widely throughout the body; drug is more than 90% protein-bound.
Metabolism: Hepatic metabolism is almost total; oral dosage form undergoes extensive first-pass metabolism.
Excretion: About 96% to 99% of a given dose of propranolol is excreted in urine as metabolites; remainder is excreted in feces as un-

changed drug and metabolites. Biological half-life is about 4 hours.

Contraindications and precautions
Contraindicated in patients with bronchial asthma, sinus bradycardia and heart block greater than first-degree, cardiogenic shock, and heart failure unless failure is secondary to a tachyarrhythmia that can be treated with propranolol.

Use cautiously in elderly patients; in patients with impaired renal or hepatic function, nonallergic bronchospastic diseases, diabetes mellitus, or thyrotoxicosis; and in patients receiving other antihypertensives.

Interactions
Drug-drug
Aluminum hydroxide antacid: decreased GI absorption. Separate administration times.
Antihypertensives, especially such catecholamine-depleting drugs as reserpine: potentiated antihypertensive effects. Monitor blood pressure.
Atropine, tricyclic antidepressants, and other drugs with anticholinergic effects: may antagonize propranolol-induced bradycardia. Monitor heart rate.
Calcium channel blockers, especially I.V. verapamil: may depress myocardial contractility or AV conduction. On rare occasions, concurrent I.V. use of a beta blocker and verapamil has resulted in serious adverse reactions especially in patients with severe cardiomyopathy, heart failure, or recent MI. Use together cautiously.
Cimetidine: may decrease clearance of propranolol via inhibition

of hepatic metabolism, and thus also enhance its beta-blocking effects. Monitor patient closely.
Epinephrine: severe vasoconstriction. Monitor blood pressure and observe patient closely.
Insulin, oral antidiabetic drugs: alter dosage requirements in previously stable diabetic patients. Monitor serum glucose.
NSAIDs: may antagonize hypotensive effects of propranolol. Monitor blood pressure.
Phenytoin, rifampin: accelerated clearance of propranolol. Monitor patient.
Sympathomimetics, such as isoproterenol and MAO inhibitors: antagonized beta-adrenergic stimulating effects of these drugs. Monitor patient closely.
Tubocurarine and related compounds: high doses of propranolol may potentiate neuromuscular blocking effect of tubocurarine and related compounds. Monitor patient closely.

Drug-herb
Betel palm: may enhance CNS effects and reduce temperature elevating effects. Advise against concurrent use.

Drug-lifestyle
Alcohol use: slows the rate of absorption. Discourage alcohol use.

Effects on diagnostic tests
None reported.

Adverse reactions
CNS: *fatigue,* hallucinations, insomnia, *lethargy,* light-headedness, mental depression, vivid dreams.
CV: *bradycardia, heart failure, hypotension, intensification of AV block,* intermittent claudication.
GI: abdominal cramping, diarrhea, nausea, vomiting.
GU: elevated BUN levels.
Hematologic: *agranulocytosis.*
Hepatic: elevated serum transaminase, alkaline phosphatase, and LD levels.
Respiratory: *bronchospasm.*
Skin: rash.
Other: fever.

Overdose and treatment
Overdose may cause severe hypotension, bradycardia, heart failure, and bronchospasm.

After acute ingestion, induce emesis or empty stomach by gastric lavage; follow with activated charcoal to reduce absorption, and administer symptomatic and supportive care. Treat bradycardia with atropine (0.25 to 1 mg); if no response, administer isoproterenol cautiously. Treat cardiac failure with cardiac glycosides and diuretics, and hypotension with glucagon and/or vasopressors; epinephrine is preferred. Treat bronchospasm with isoproterenol and aminophylline.

Special considerations
▶ Drug is also used to treat hypertension; supraventricular, ventricular, and atrial arrhythmias; tachyarrhythmias caused by excessive catecholamine action during anesthesia, hyperthyroidism, and pheochromocytoma; to reduce mortality after MI; hypertrophic subaortic stenosis; preoperative pheochromocytoma; and essential, familial, or senile movement tremors.
▶ Propranolol has been used to treat aggression and rage, stage

---

fright, recurrent GI bleeding in cirrhotic patients, and menopausal symptoms.

▶ Drug is meant for prophylactic use against migraines; it isn't recommended to treat a migraine attack or to prevent or treat cluster headaches.

▶ Propranolol may reduce the frequency of anginal attacks and increase patient's activity tolerance.

▶ Give consistently with meals. Food may increase absorption of propranolol.

▶ Never administer propranolol as an adjunct in treatment of pheochromocytoma unless patient has been pretreated with alpha-adrenergic blocking agents.

▶ Drug may mask signs of hypoglycemia.

▶ Monitor blood pressure, ECG, and heart rate and rhythm frequently, especially I.V. administration. If the patient develops severe hypotension, notify the prescriber; a vasopressor may be prescribed.

▶ Give by direct injection into a large vessel or into the tubing of a free-flowing, compatible I.V. solution; continuous I.V. infusion is generally not recommended. Alternatively, dilute drug with normal saline and give by intermittant infusion over 10 to 15 minutes in 0.1 to 0.2 mg increments. Drug is compatible with D_5W and with half-normal saline, normal saline, and lactated Ringer's solutions.

▶ Double-check dose and route. I.V. doses are much smaller than oral doses.

Breast-feeding patients

▶ Drug appears in breast milk; an alternative feeding method is recommended during therapy.

Pediatric patients

▶ Safety and efficacy of propranolol in children haven't been established; use only if potential benefit outweighs risk.

Geriatric patients

▶ Elderly patients may require lower maintenance doses of propranolol because of increased bioavailability or delayed metabolism; they also may experience enhanced adverse effects.

Patient teaching

▶ Warn patient not to abruptly stop taking propranolol.

▶ Instruct patient on proper use, dosage, and potential adverse effects of propranolol.

▶ Tell patient to call before taking OTC drugs that may interact with propranolol, such as nasal decongestants or cold preparations.

▶ psyllium
Cillium, Fiberall, Hydrocil Instant, Konsyl, Konsyl-D, Metamucil, Naturacil, Reguloid, Serutan, Syllact, V-Lax

Pharmacologic classification:
adsorbent

Therapeutic classification:
bulk laxative

Pregnancy risk category C

How supplied
Available without a prescription
Chewable pieces: 1.7 g/piece
Granules: 2.5 g/teaspoon, 4.03 g/teaspoon
Powder: 3.3 g/teaspoon, 3.4 g/teaspoon, 3.5 g/teaspoon, 4.94 g/teaspoon

Powder (effervescent): 3.4 g/packet, 3.7 g/packet
Wafers: 1.7 g/wafer, 3.4 g/wafer

Indications and dosages
Constipation, bowel management, irritable bowel syndrome
Adults: 1 to 2 rounded tsp P.O. in full glass of liquid daily, b.i.d. or t.i.d., followed by second glass of liquid; or 1 packet P.O. dissolved in water daily; or 2 wafers b.i.d., or t.i.d.
Children over age 6: 1 level tsp P.O. in ¼ glass of liquid h.s.

Pharmacodynamics
Laxative action: Psyllium adsorbs water in the gut; it also serves as a source of indigestible fiber, increasing stool bulk and moisture, thus stimulating peristaltic activity and bowel evacuation.

Pharmacokinetics
Absorption: None; onset of action varies from 12 hours to 3 days.
Distribution: Psyllium is distributed locally in the gut.
Metabolism: Psyllium isn't metabolized.
Excretion: Psyllium is excreted in feces.

Contraindications and precautions
Contraindicated in patients hypersensitive to drug; patients with abdominal pain, nausea, vomiting, or other symptoms of appendicitis; and patients with intestinal obstruction or ulceration, disabling adhesions, or trouble swallowing.

Interactions
Drug-drug
Oral drugs: psyllium may adsorb oral drugs, such as anticoagulants, cardiac glycosides, and salicylates. Monitor patient for drug effects.

Effects on diagnostic tests
None reported.

Adverse reactions
GI: abdominal cramps, especially in severe constipation; diarrhea with excessive use; esophageal, gastric, small intestinal, and rectal obstruction when drug is taken in dry form; nausea; vomiting.

Overdose and treatment
No cases of overdose have been reported; probable clinical effects include abdominal pain and diarrhea.

Special considerations
▶ Psyllium and other bulk laxatives most closely mimic natural bowel function and do not cause laxative dependence; they are especially useful for patients with postpartum constipation or diverticular disease, for debilitated patients, for irritable bowel syndrome, and for chronic laxative users.
▶ Multiple approaches may be needed to treat constipation.
▶ Before administering drug, add at least 240 ml (8 oz) of water or juice and stir for a few seconds (improves drug's taste). Have patient drink mixture immediately to prevent it from congealing; then have him drink another glass of fluid.
▶ Separate administration of psyllium and oral anticoagulants, cardiac glycosides, and salicylates by at least 2 hours.
▶ Drug may reduce appetite if administered before meals.
▶ Give diabetic patients a sugar- and sodium-free psyllium product.

▶ Before giving for constipation, determine if the patient has adequate fluid intake, exercise, and diet.
▶ Monitor patient's bowel activity.

Breast-feeding patients
▶ Because drug isn't absorbed, it presumably is safe for use in breast-feeding women.

Patient teaching
▶ Warn patient not to swallow drug in dry form; he should mix it with at least 240 ml (8 oz) of fluid, stir briefly, drink immediately (to prevent mixture from congealing), and follow it with another 8 oz of fluid.
▶ Explain that drug may reduce appetite if taken before meals; recommend taking drug 2 hours after meals and any other oral medication.
▶ Advise diabetic patients and those with restricted sodium or sugar intake to avoid psyllium products containing salt or sugar. Advise patients who must restrict phenylalanine intake to avoid psyllium products containing aspartame.

▶ **ranitidine hydrochloride**
Zantac, Zantac 75, Zantac EFFERdose, Zantac GELdose

Pharmacologic classification:
H_2-receptor antagonist

Therapeutic classification:
antiulcer drug

Pregnancy risk category B

How supplied
Available by prescription only
Capsules: 150 mg, 300 mg
Granules (effervescent): 150 mg

Injection: 25 mg/ml
Injection (premixed): 50 mg/50 ml, 50 mg/100 ml
Syrup: 15 mg/ml
Tablets: 150 mg, 300 mg
Tablets (effervescent): 150 mg
Available without a prescription
Tablets: 75 mg

Indications and dosages
Duodenal and gastric ulcer (short-term treatment), pathologic hypersecretory conditions (such as Zollinger-Ellison syndrome)
Adults: 150 mg P.O. b.i.d. or 300 mg P.O. h.s. Alternatively, 50 mg I.V. or I.M. q 6 to 8 hours. Patients with Zollinger-Ellison syndrome may receive up to 6 g/day in divided doses.
Maintenance therapy in duodenal ulcer
Adults: 150 mg P.O. h.s.
Prevention of stress ulcer
Adults: Continuous I.V. infusion of 150 mg in 250 ml of compatible solution at 6.25 mg/hour using an infusion pump.
Gastroesophageal reflux disease
Adults: 150 mg P.O. b.i.d.
Erosive esophagitis
Adults: 150 mg or 10 ml (2 teaspoonfuls provides 150 mg of ranitidine) P.O. q.i.d. for up to 12 weeks. Maintenance dosage after healing, 150 mg b.i.d.
Occasional heartburn, acid indigestion, sour stomach
Adults and adolescents age 12 and older: 75 mg once or twice daily. Maximum, 150 mg in 24 hours.
◣ DOSAGE ADJUSTMENT. If patient's creatinine clearance is less than 50 ml/minute, reduce recommended dosage by half.

Pharmacodynamics
Antiulcer action: Ranitidine competitively inhibits the action of histamine at H_2 receptors in gastric parietal cells. This inhibition reduces basal and nocturnal gastric acid secretion as well as that caused by histamine, food, amino acids, insulin, and pentagastrin.

Pharmacokinetics
Absorption: About 50% to 60% of an oral dose is absorbed. Food doesn't significantly affect absorption. After I.M. injection, drug is absorbed rapidly from parenteral sites.
Distribution: Drug is distributed to many body tissues and appears in CSF and breast milk. It's about 10% to 19% protein-bound.
Metabolism: Ranitidine is metabolized in the liver.
Excretion: Drug is excreted in urine and feces. Half-life is 2 to 3 hours.

Contraindications and precautions
Contraindicated in patients hypersensitive to drug and in those with a history of acute porphyria.

Use cautiously in patients with impaired renal or hepatic function.

Interactions
Drug-drug
Antacids: decrease ranitidine absorption. Separate drugs by at least 1 hour.
Aspirin, NSAIDs: may cause GI irritation. Avoid concurrent use.
Diazepam: decreases diazepam absorption. Monitor patient closely.
Glipizide: may increase hypoglycemic effect. Adjust glipizide dosage if needed.

Ketoconazole: decreased ketoconazole bioavailability. Substitute fluconazole if concurrent use is necessary.
Procainamide: decreased renal clearance of procainamide. Adjust dosage as needed.
Warfarin: interference with warfarin clearance. Adjust dosage as needed.

Drug-lifestyle
Smoking: interference with drug action. Discourage concurrent use.

Effects on diagnostic tests
Drug may cause false-positive results in urine protein tests using Multistix.

Adverse reactions
CNS: malaise, vertigo.
EENT: blurred vision.
GU: increased serum creatinine.
Hematologic: *agranulocytopenia, pancytopenia, reversible leukopenia, thrombocytopenia*.
Hepatic: elevated liver enzymes, jaundice.
Skin: burning and itching at injection site.
Other: *anaphylaxis, angioedema.*

Overdose and treatment
No overdoses have been reported. If overdose occurs, treatment would involve induced emesis or gastric lavage and supportive measures as needed. Drug is removed by hemodialysis.

Special considerations
▶ When administering premixed I.V. infusion, give by slow I.V. drip over 15 to 20 minutes. Don't add other drugs to the solution. If given with a primary fluid system,

---

Reactions may be *common,* uncommon, *life-threatening,* or **COMMON AND LIFE-THREATENING.**

stop the primary solution during the infusion.

▶ To give drug by I.V. push, dilute to a total volume of 20 ml and inject over 5 minutes. No dilution necessary for I.M. delivery.

▶ To give drug by intermittent I.V. infusion, dilute 50 mg (2 ml) in 100 ml of a compatible solution (such as D_5W, normal saline solution for injection, $D_{10}W$ injection, 5% sodium bicarbonate injections, or lactated Ringer's injection) and infuse over 15 to 20 minutes.

▶ To give drug by continuous I.V. infusion, dilute 150 mg in 250 ml of compatible solution. Infuse at 6.25 mg/hour using an infusion pump.

▶ Debilitated patients may develop reversible confusion, agitation, depression, and hallucinations. Assess patient for these changes.

▶ If patient receives dialysis, give ranitidine afterward because procedure removes the drug.

Breast-feeding patients

▶ Drug appears in breast milk; use cautiously in breast-feeding women.

Geriatric patients

▶ Elderly patients may have more adverse reactions because of reduced renal clearance.

Patient teaching

▶ Instruct patient to take drug as directed, even after pain subsides, to ensure proper healing.

▶ If patient is taking a single daily dose, tell her to take it at bedtime.

▶ Tell patient to swallow oral drug whole with water. Warn against chewing it.

▶ Caution patient not to take OTC medications continuously for more than 2 weeks without consulting prescriber.

▶ Inform patient that smoking interferes with drug action.

▶ remifentanil hydrochloride
Ultiva

Pharmacologic classification:
μ-opioid agonist

Therapeutic classification:
analgesic, anesthetic

Controlled substance schedule II

Pregnancy risk category C

How supplied
Available by prescription only
Injection: 1 mg/3 ml, 2 mg/5 ml, 5 mg/10 ml vials

Indications and dosages
Induction of anesthesia through intubation
Adults: 0.5 to 1 mcg/kg/minute with hypnotic or volatile drug; may load with 1 mcg/kg over 30 to 60 seconds if endotracheal intubation will take place less than 8 minutes after remifentanil infusion starts.
Maintenance of anesthesia
Adults: 0.25 to 0.4 mcg/kg/minute based on concurrent anesthetics (nitrous oxide, isoflurane, propofol). Increase doses by 25% to 100% and decrease by 25% to 50% q 2 to 5 minutes, p.r.n. If rate exceeds 1 mcg/kg/minute, consider increases in concurrent anesthetics. May supplement with 1-mcg/kg boluses over 30 to 60 seconds q 2 to 5 minutes, p.r.n.

Continuation as analgesic in immediate postoperative period
Adults: 0.1 mcg/kg/minute, followed by infusion of 0.025 to 0.2 mcg/kg/minute. Adjust rate by 0.025-mcg/kg/minute increments q 5 minutes. Rates above 0.2 mcg/kg/minute may cause respiratory depression (less than 8 breaths/minute).

Monitored anesthesia care
Adults: for a single I.V. dose, give 0.5 to 1 mcg/kg over 30 to 60 seconds starting 90 seconds before placement of local or regional anesthetic. Decrease dose by 50% if given with 2 mg midazolam. For continuous I.V. infusion, give 0.1 mcg/kg/minute starting 5 minutes before giving local anesthetic; afterward, adjust infusion rate to 0.05 mcg/kg/minute. Adjust by 0.025 mcg/kg/minute q 5 minutes, p.r.n. Rates above 0.2 mcg/kg/minute may cause respiratory depression (less than 8 breaths/minute). Decrease dose by 50% if given with 2 mg midazolam. Avoid giving bolus doses to spontaneously breathing patient during continuous remifentanil infusion.

◨ DOSAGE ADJUSTMENT. Decrease initial dose by half in elderly patients, and adjust to desired effect. In obese patients (more than 30% over ideal body weight), base starting dose on ideal body weight. In patients over age 65, decrease starting dose by 50%. Cautiously adjust to effect.

Pharmacodynamics
Analgesic action: Drug binds to μ-opiate receptors throughout the CNS, resulting in analgesia.

Pharmacokinetics
Absorption: After I.V. administration, drug is rapidly absorbed. Blood level decreases 50% in 3 to 6 minutes after a 1-minute infusion because of rapid distribution and elimination processes, which are independent of drug administration.

Distribution: Initially, drug is distributed throughout the blood and rapidly perfused tissues; then it moves into peripheral tissues. Drug is about 70% bound to plasma proteins, of which two-thirds is bound to alpha₁-acid-glycoprotein.

Metabolism: Drug is rapidly metabolized by hydrolysis via blood and tissue esterases, resulting in an inactive carboxylic acid metabolite. Drug isn't metabolized by plasma cholinesterase and isn't appreciably metabolized by the liver or lungs.

Excretion: After hydrolysis, inactive metabolite is excreted by the kidneys with an elimination half-life of about 90 minutes. Clearance of active drug is high; elimination half-life is 3 to 10 minutes.

Contraindications and precautions
Contraindicated in patients hypersensitive to fentanyl analogues. Also, contraindicated by epidural and intrathecal routes because preparation contains glycine.

Interactions
Drug-drug
Barbiturate anesthetics, benzodiazepines, hypnotics, inhaled anesthetics: synergistic effect. Monitor patient closely.

Effects on diagnostic tests
None reported.

Reactions may be *common,* uncommon, *life-threatening,* or COMMON AND LIFE-THREATENING.

Adverse reactions
CNS: agitation, chills, dizziness, *headache.*
CV: ***bradycardia,*** flushing, hypertension, *hypotension,* tachycardia.
EENT: visual disturbances.
GI: *nausea, vomiting.*
Musculoskeletal: *muscle rigidity.*
Respiratory: ***apnea,*** *hypoxia,* ***respiratory depression.***
Skin: diaphoresis, pain at injection site, *pruritus.*
Other: chills, fever, postoperative pain, shivering, warm sensation.

Overdose and treatment
Overdose may cause apnea, chest wall rigidity, hypoxemia, hypotension, seizures, or bradycardia.

If these signs occur, stop drug, maintain patent airway, start assisted or controlled ventilation with oxygen, and maintain CV function. Give a neuromuscular blocker or opioid antagonist if decreased respiration is linked to muscle rigidity. Give I.V. fluids and vasopressors for hypotension and glycopyrrolate or atropine for bradycardia. Naloxone may be used to manage severe respiratory depression. Provide other supportive measures as needed.

Special considerations
▶ Before use, ask patient about previous personal or family adverse reactions to anesthesia.
▶ Don't use drug by itself for general anesthesia.
▶ Avoid using drug outside a monitored anesthesia care setting.
▶ Give continuous infusion via infusion device; give I.V. bolus only during maintenance of general anesthesia. In nonintubated patients, single doses should be administered over 30 to 60 seconds.

▶ Monitor vital signs and oxygenation continually throughout drug administration.
▶ If hypotension occurs, decrease administration rate or give I.V. fluids or catecholamines.
▶ If respiratory depression or skeletal muscle rigidity occurs in a spontaneously breathing patient, decrease infusion rate by half or temporarily discontinue infusion.
▶ Bradycardia has been reported and is responsive to ephedrine, atropine, and glycopyrrolate.
▶ When administration stops, clear I.V. tubing to avoid inadvertent administration of drug at a later time.
▶ Interruption of infusion causes rapid reversal of effects (no residual opioid effects after 5 to 10 minutes). Establish adequate postoperative analgesia before stopping drug.
▶ Effects of long-term use (more than 16 hours) in intensive care settings isn't known.
▶ Drug is incompatible with blood products; don't mix it with lactated Ringer's solution or dextrose 5% in lactated Ringer's solution. You can coadminister drug with these two diluents into a running I.V. administration set.

Breast-feeding patients
▶ Because fentanyl analogues appear in breast milk, use with caution in breast-feeding women.

Pediatric patients
▶ Use in children under age 2 hasn't been studied.

Patient teaching
▶ Reassure patient that she'll be monitored constantly during anesthesia.

▶ rizatriptan benzoate
Maxalt, Maxalt-MLT

Pharmacologic classification:
*selective 5-hydroxytryptamine
(5-HT$_{1B/1D}$) receptor agonist*

Therapeutic classification:
antimigraine

Pregnancy risk category C

How supplied
Tablets: 5 mg, 10 mg
Tablets (orally disintegrating):
5 mg, 10 mg

Indications and dosages
**Acute migraine headaches with or
without aura**
Adults: initially, 5 or 10 mg P.O. If
first dose is ineffective, another
dose may be given at least 2 hours
after the first. Maximum, 30 mg
over 24 hours.
◩ DOSAGE ADJUSTMENT. If patient receives propranolol, start with 5 mg
P.O. of rizatriptan. Maximum,
three doses (15 mg) over 24 hours.

Pharmacodynamics
Antimigraine action: Rizatriptan
probably acts as an agonist at serotonin receptors on extracerebral intracranial blood vessels, which
constricts the affected vessels, inhibits neuropeptide release, and reduces pain transmission in the
trigeminal pathways.

Pharmacokinetics
Absorption: Bioavailablity after
oral administration is 45%. Plasma
levels peak in 1 to 1½ hours.
Distribution: Rizatriptan is minimally plasma bound.
Metabolism: Primary metabolism
takes place via oxidative deamina-

tion by MAO-A to the indoleacetic
acid metabolite.
Excretion: Drug is excreted in
urine and feces after oral administration.

Contraindications and
precautions
Contraindicated in patients hypersensitive to drug or its inactive ingredients, in patients who took an
MAO inhibitor within 14 days, and
in patients with ischemic heart disease (angina, history of MI, or
documented silent ischemia), coronary artery vasospasm (Prinzmetal's variant angina), other significant underlying CV disease,
and uncontrolled hypertension.
Also, contraindicated within 24
hours of treatment with another
5-HT agonist or an ergotamine-
containing or ergot-type drug, such
as dihydroergotamine or methysergide.
   Use cautiously in patients with
hepatic or renal impairment and in
patients with risk factors for coronary artery disease (hypertension,
hypercholesterolemia, smoking,
obesity, diabetes, strong family
history of coronary artery disease,
surgical or physiologic menopause,
or male over age 40), unless a cardiac evaluation suggests that patient has no cardiac disease.

Interactions
Drug-drug
*Ergot-containing or ergot-type
drugs (such as dihydroergotamine,
methysergide), other 5-HT$_1$ agonists:* may cause prolonged vasospastic reactions. Don't use within
24 hours of rizatriptan.
MAO inhibitors: may increase
plasma rizatriptan levels. Allow at
least 14 days after stopping an

MAO inhibitor before starting rizatriptan.

Propranolol: may increase rizatriptan levels. Reduce rizatriptan dose to 5 mg.

Selective serotonin reuptake inhibitors: may cause weakness, hyperreflexia, and incoordination. Monitor patient.

Effects on diagnostic tests

None reported.

Adverse reactions

CNS: asthenia, decreased mental acuity, dizziness, euphoria, fatigue, headache, hypoesthesia, paresthesia, somnolence, tremor.
CV: chest pain, flushing, palpitations, pressure or heaviness.
EENT: neck, throat and jaw pain.
GI: diarrhea, dry mouth, nausea, vomiting.
Respiratory: dyspnea.
Other: hot flashes, pain, warm or cold sensations.

Special considerations

▶ Give drug only after a definite diagnosis of migraine has been made.
▶ Don't use drug for prophylactic therapy or for patients with hemiplegic migraine, basilar migraine, or cluster headaches.
▶ The safety of treating more than four headaches per month hasn't been established.
▶ Orally disintegrating tablets contain phenylalanine.
▶ If patient has risk factors for cardiac disease but a satisfactory CV evaluation, monitor her closely after the first dose.
▶ Assess CV status in patients who develop risk factors for coronary artery disease during treatment.

Breast-feeding patients

▶ Instruct patient not to breast-feed during therapy because effects on infant are unknown.

Pediatric patients

▶ Safety and effectiveness in children under age 18 haven't been established.

Patient teaching

▶ Tell patient that drug doesn't prevent migraine headaches.
▶ Advise patient to consult prescriber if headache returns after initial dose. With permission, a second dose may be taken at least 2 hours after the first. Warn against taking more than 30 mg over 24 hours.
▶ Caution patient to avoid hazardous activities until full effects of drug are known. It may cause somnolence and dizziness.
▶ Tell patient that food may delay drug's onset of action.
▶ If patient takes Maxalt-MLT, tell her to remove drug from blister pack immediately before use. Caution against popping the drug from the blister pack; instead, tell patient to carefully peel away the backing with dry hands and then place the tablet on her tongue and let it dissolve. Tell her to then swallow it with saliva. No water is needed or recommended.
▶ Explain the dissolving tablets don't relieve headache more rapidly than standard tablets.
▶ Advise patient to notify prescriber about planned, suspected, or known pregnancy.

▌ **rocuronium bromide**
Zemuron

Pharmacologic classification:
nondepolarizing neuromuscular blocker

Therapeutic classification:
skeletal muscle relaxant

Pregnancy risk category B

How supplied
Available by prescription only
Injection: 10 mg/ml

Indications and dosages
Adjunct to general anesthesia, facilitation of endotracheal intubation, skeletal muscle relaxation during surgery or mechanical ventilation
Dosage depends on anesthetic used, individual needs, and response. Dosages are representative and must be adjusted.
Adults and children age 3 months or older: initially, 0.6 to 1.2 mg/kg by I.V. bolus. In most patients, endotracheal intubation may take place within 2 minutes. Muscle paralysis should last about 31 minutes. Maintenance dosage of 0.1 mg/kg provides about another 12 minutes of muscle relaxation (0.15 mg/kg adds 17 minutes; 0.2 mg/kg adds 24 minutes).
◩ Dosage adjustment. In obese patients, initial dose should be based on patient's actual body weight.

Pharmacodynamics
Skeletal muscle relaxant action:
Rocuronium competes for cholinergic receptors at the motor end plate. This action is antagonized by acetylcholinesterase inhibitors, such as neostigmine and edrophonium.

Pharmacokinetics
Absorption: Drug is given I.V.
Distribution: Distribution half-life is 1 to 18 minutes. Drug is about 30% bound to plasma proteins.
Metabolism: No information available, but hepatic clearance could be significant. The rocuronium analogue 17-desacetyl-rocuronium, a metabolite, has rarely been observed in plasma or urine.
Excretion: About 33% of a dose is recovered in urine within 24 hours.

Contraindications and precautions
Contraindicated in patients hypersensitive to bromides.
    Use cautiously in patients with hepatic disease, severe obesity, bronchogenic carcinoma, electrolyte disturbances, neuromuscular disease, or altered circulation time caused by CV disease, age, or edematous states.

Interactions
Drug-drug
Aminoglycosides, bacitracin, colistimethate sodium, colistin, polymyxins, tetracylines, vancomycin: may enhance neuromuscular blocking action. Monitor patient closely.
Anticonvulsants, such as carbamazepine, phenytoin: may reduce magnitude of neuromuscular block or shorten duration. Monitor patient closely.
Enflurane, isoflurane: may prolong action of initial and maintenance rocuronium doses. As needed, decrease average infusion requirement of rocuronium by 40% com-

pared with opioid, nitrous oxide, oxygen anesthesia.

Quinidine: may cause recurrent paralysis. Monitor patient closely.

Effects on diagnostic tests
None reported.

Adverse reactions
CV: abnormal ECG, edema, tachycardia, transient hypotension and hypertension.
GI: nausea, vomiting.
Respiratory: asthma, ***bronchospasm***, hiccups.
Skin: pruritus, rash.

Overdose and treatment
No overdoses have been reported, but a neuromuscular blocker overdose may cause neuromuscular block beyond the time needed for surgery and anesthesia.

Primary treatment is maintenance of a patent airway and controlled ventilation until patient recovers normal neuromuscular function. After evidence of such recovery appears, further recovery may be facilitated by an anticholinesterase drug (such as neostigmine or edrophonium) and an anticholinergic.

Special considerations
▶ Drug should be administered only by staff experienced in airway management.
▶ Ensure a patent airway, and keep emergency resuscitation equipment (endotracheal supplies, ventilator, oxygen, atropine, edrophonium, epinephrine, neostigmine) readily available.
▶ Neuromuscular blockers don't obtund consciousness or alter the pain threshold. Patient needs a sedative or general anesthetic be-

fore receiving a neuromuscular blocker.
▶ Administer drug by rapid I.V. injection or by continuous I.V. infusion. Infusion rates are highly individualized.
▶ Compatible solutions include D_5W, normal saline solution for injection, dextrose 5% in normal saline solution for injection, sterile water for injection, and lactated Ringer's injection.
▶ Refrigerate reconstituted solution. Discard after 24 hours.
▶ Monitor the infusion site closely; drug is an irritant if it extravasates.
▶ Drug has an acid pH and shouldn't be mixed in the same syringe or infused simultaneously through the same needle with alkaline solutions (such as barbiturate solutions).
▶ Drug is well tolerated in patients with renal failure.
▶ Use a peripheral nerve stimulator to measure neuromuscular function during drug administration to monitor drug effect, determine the need for additional doses, and confirm recovery from neuromuscular block. Once spontaneous recovery starts, drug-induced neuromuscular blockade may be reversed with an anticholinesterase drug.

Pediatric patients
▶ Use of rocuronium in children under age 3 months hasn't been studied.

Patient teaching
▶ Teach patient about procedures to be performed.
▶ Talk to patient during procedures because she can still hear.
▶ Reassure patient and family that patient will be continuously monitored.

▶ ropivacaine hydrochloride
Naropin

Pharmacologic classification:
aminoamide

Therapeutic classification:
local anesthetic

Pregnancy risk category B

How supplied
Available by prescription only
E-Z off single-dose vials: 7.5 mg/
ml, 10 mg/ml in 10-ml vials
Infusion bottles: 2 mg/ml in 100-
ml and 200-ml bottles
Single-dose ampules: 2 mg/ml,
7.5 mg/ml, 10 mg/ml in 20-ml ampules; 5 mg/ml in 30-ml ampules
Single-dose vials: 2 mg/ml, 7.5 mg/
ml, 10 mg/ml in 20-ml vials; 5 mg/
ml in 30-ml vials
Sterile-pak single-dose vials: 2 mg/
ml, 7.5 mg/ml, 10 mg/ml in 20-ml
vials; 5 mg/ml in 30-ml vials

Indications and dosages
Lumbar epidural administration
for labor pain
Adults: initially, 20 to 40 mg (duration, ½ to 1½ hours), then 12 to
28 mg/hour as continuous infusion
or 20 to 30 mg/hour as incremental
"top-up" injections.
Lumbar epidural administration
for surgery
Adults: 75 to 200 mg (duration, 2
to 6 hours).
Lumbar epidural administration
for cesarean section
Adults: 100 to 150 mg (duration, 2
to 4 hours).
Lumbar epidural administration
for postoperative pain
Adults: 12 to 20 mg/hour as continuous infusion.

Thoracic epidural administration
to establish block for postopera-
tive pain relief
Adults: 25- to 75-mg doses.
Thoracic epidural administration
for postoperative pain
Adults: 8 to 16 mg/hour as continuous infusion.
Major nerve block (for example,
brachial plexus block)
Adults: 175 to 250 mg (duration, 5
to 8 hours).
Field block (such as minor nerve
blocks and infiltration)
Adults: 5 to 200 mg (duration, 2 to
6 hours).

Pharmacodynamics
Anesthetic action: Drug blocks the
generation and conduction of
nerve impulses, probably by increasing the threshold for electrical
excitation in the nerve by slowing
propagation of the nerve impulse
and reducing the rate of the action
potential. In general, progression
of anesthesia is related to the diameter, myelination, and conduction velocity of affected nerve
fibers. Clinically, loss of nerve
function follows this pattern: pain,
temperature, touch, proprioception, and skeletal muscle tone.

Pharmacokinetics
Absorption: Absorption depends
on dose and concentration of administered drug, on route of administration, on patient's hemodynamic or circulatory condition, and
on vascularity of administration
site. From the epidural space, drug
shows complete and biphasic absorption; mean half-lives of two
phases are 14 minutes and 4.2
hours, respectively. The slow absorption is a rate-limiting factor in
elimination of drug. Terminal half-

life is longer after epidural than after I.V. administration.

Distribution: After intravascular infusion, drug has steady state volume of distribution of 41 ± 7 L. Drug is 94% protein-bound, mainly to alpha$_1$ acid glycoprotein. An increase in total plasma levels during continuous epidural infusion has been observed secondary to a postoperative increase in alpha$_1$ acid glycoprotein.

Metabolism: Drug is extensively metabolized in the liver via cytochrome P-450$_{1A}$ to 3-hydroxy ropivacaine. About 37% of dose is excreted in urine as free drug and as conjugated metabolites.

Excretion: Drug is excreted mainly by the kidneys; 86% of the dose appears in urine after I.V. administration, only 1% of which relates to unchanged drug.

Contraindications and precautions

Contraindicated in patients hypersensitive to drug or to local anesthetics of the amide type.

Use cautiously in debilitated, elderly, and acutely ill patients because accumulation may result. Also use cautiously in patients with hepatic disease (especially repeat doses) and in patients with hypotension, hypovolemia, impaired CV function, or heart block.

Interactions
Drug-drug
Amide-type anesthetics: additive effects. Use together cautiously.
Fluvoxamine, imipramine, theophylline, verapamil: may competitively inhibit ropivacaine. Use together cautiously.

Effects on diagnostic tests
None reported.

Adverse reactions
CNS: anxiety, dizziness, headache, hypoesthesia, pain, paresthesia.
CV: ***bradycardia,*** chest pain, **FETAL BRADYCARDIA,** *fetal tachycardia,* hypertension, *hypotension,* tachycardia.
GI: *nausea,* neonatal vomiting, vomiting.
GU: oliguria, urine retention.
Hematologic: anemia.
Hepatic: neonatal jaundice.
Musculoskeletal: back pain.
Respiratory: *neonatal tachypnea,* ***respiratory distress.***
Skin: pruritus.
Other: **FETAL DISTRESS,** fever, neonatal fever, postoperative complications, rigors.

Overdose and treatment
Overdose may cause seizures followed by hypoxia, hypercarbia, and acidosis.

Treatment should be supportive and symptomatic. Discontinue drug. After unintentional subarachnoid injection, establish a patent airway and administer 100% oxygen. Doing so may prevent seizures if they haven't already occurred. Give drugs to control seizures as appropriate.

Special considerations
▶ Drug should only be used by persons familiar with its use. Keep resuscitation equipment immediately available.
▶ Use an adequate test dose (3 to 5 ml of short-acting local anesthetic solution containing epinephrine) before induction of complete block.

▶ Don't inject drug rapidly. Increase by incremental steps.

▶ Monitor patient for early signs of CNS toxicity: restlessness, anxiety, incoherent speech, light-headedness, numbness and tingling of mouth and lips, metallic taste, tinnitus, dizziness, blurred vision, tremors, twitching, depression, or drowsiness.

▶ To reduce the risk of serious adverse reactions, try to optimize the condition of patients who may be at risk, such as those with complete heart block, hepatic impairment, or renal impairment.

▶ Don't use drug in emergencies that demand a rapid onset of surgical anesthesia. Also, don't use drug for obstetric paracervical block, retrobulbar block, or spinal anesthesia (subarachnoid block) because insufficient data are available to support these uses.

▶ Don't use drug for I.V. regional anesthesia (bier block) because of a lack of clinical experience and a risk of toxic blood levels of ropivacaine.

▶ Don't use drug in ophthalmic surgery.

Breast-feeding patients

▶ No data exist to demonstrate whether drug appears in breast milk; use cautiously in breast-feeding patients.

Pediatric patients

▶ Don't use drug in children under age 12.

Patient teaching

▶ Tell patient that she may experience a temporary loss of sensation and motor activity in the anesthetized body part following proper administration of lumbar epidural anesthesia. Also explain adverse reactions that may occur.

▶ **salsalate**
Amigesic, Argesic-SA, Arthra-G, Disalcid, Marthritic, Mono-Gesic, Salflex, Salsitab

Pharmacologic classification:
NSAID

Therapeutic classification:
analgesic, anti-inflammatory

Pregnancy risk category C

How supplied

Available by prescription only
Capsules: 500 mg
Tablets: 500 mg, 750 mg

Indication and dosages

Rheumatoid arthritis, osteoarthritis, related rheumatic disorders
Adults: 3,000 mg P.O. daily in 2 or 3 divided doses.

Pharmacodynamics

Anti-inflammatory action: Although not fully defined, salsalate appears to selectively inhibit prostaglandin synthesis, providing anti-inflammatory action equivalent to aspirin or indomethacin. It doesn't inhibit platelet aggregation.

Pharmacokinetics

Absorption: Completely absorbed from the GI tract, principally in the small intestine.
Distribution: Widely and rapidly distributed into most body tissues and fluids.
Metabolism: Hydrolyzed to 2 molecules of salicylate.
Excretion: Almost completely excreted in urine.

Contraindications and precautions

Contraindicated in patients hypersensitive to salsalate and in patients with chickenpox, influenza, or flulike symptoms.

Use cautiously in patients with renal insufficiency or peptic ulcer disease.

Interactions
Drug-drug

Aspirin, salicylates: additive effects and possible increased salicylic acid levels. Avoid use together.

Drugs that are highly protein-bound: either drug may be displaced. Use together cautiously.

Drugs used to treat gout: antagonized uricosuric effects. Use together cautiously.

Drug-lifestyle

Alcohol use: may increase risk of GI bleeding and adverse effects. Advise against concurrent use.

Effects on diagnostic tests

May cause false-negative results in urine glucose tests that use glucose oxidase reagent, such as Clinistix or Tes-Tape. May cause false-positive results in tests using cupric sulfate method, such as Clinitest.

Adverse reactions

CNS: vertigo.
EENT: hearing impairment, tinnitus.
GI: abdominal pain, dyspepsia, nausea.
Hepatic: abnormal hepatic function.
Skin: rash.

Other: *Reye's syndrome, hypersensitivity reactions.*

Overdose and treatment

Salicylism may cause tinnitus, vertigo, headache, confusion, drowsiness, diaphoresis, hyperventilation, vomiting, and diarrhea. More severe intoxication will lead to disruption of electrolyte balance, dehydration, and hyperthermia.

Induce emesis with syrup of ipecac to prevent further absorption. If necessary, perform gastric lavage. Correct fluid and electrolyte imbalances with appropriate I.V. therapy. Maintain adequate renal function. In extreme cases, hemodialysis or peritoneal dialysis may be needed.

Special considerations

▶ Salicylates typically aren't useful for severe, acute visceral pain. They're most effective for low-intensity pain of nonvisceral origin, such as headache, neuralgia, myalgia, and arthralgia. They also may relieve mild to moderate postoperative pain, postpartum pain, oral surgery pain, dysmenorrhea, or other visceral pain, such as cancer pain and pain caused by trauma.
▶ In patients with arthritis, drug may relieve pain and stiffness; reduce swelling, tenderness, and the duration of morning stiffness; and decrease the number of joints involved.
▶ Although salicylates can be used to relieve pain in rheumatic conditions, they don't treat the underlying disease. Drug may be used with second-line antirheumatic drugs, such as antimalarials, gold compounds, or penicillamine.

▶ Salsalate may cause less GI irritation than aspirin.

▶ Drug may be used in patients who can't take aspirin or other NSAIDs that may interfere with normal platelet function.

▶ Assess patient for drug effects, evidence of GI bleeding, and the need for additional therapy.

Breast-feeding patients

▶ No data exist to demonstrate whether salsalate appears in breast milk, although salicylic acid (a primary metabolite of salsalate) does appear. Use cautiously in nursing women.

Pediatric patients

▶ Safety and effectiveness haven't been established.

Geriatric patients

▶ Elderly patients may attain therapeutic levels at lower dosages, which also reduces the risk of adverse effects.

Patient teaching

▶ Tell patient to take drug with food or milk to minimize gastric irritation.

▶ Caution patient not to use other OTC products without consulting prescriber because they may contain salicylates.

▶ Inform patient that it may take 3 to 4 days to achieve full benefit of the drug.

▶ scopolamine hydrobromide
Isopto Hyoscine, Scopace, Transderm-Scop

Pharmacologic classification: *anticholinergic*

Therapeutic classification: *antimuscarinic, cycloplegic mydriatic*

Pregnancy risk category C

How supplied
Available by prescription only
Injection: 0.3 and 1 mg/ml in 1-ml vials and ampules; 0.4 mg/ml and 0.86 mg/ml in 0.5-ml ampules
Ophthalmic solution: 0.25%
Tablets: 0.4 mg
Transdermal: 1.5 mg/72 hours

Indications and dosages
Antimuscarinic, adjunct to anesthesia, prevention of nausea and vomiting
Adults: 0.3 to 0.6 mg I.M., S.C., or I.V. (after dilution with sterile water for injection) as a single dose.
Children: 0.006 mg/kg I.M., S.C., or I.V. (after dilution with sterile water for injection) as a single daily dose. Maximum, 0.3 mg.
Prevention of nausea and vomiting from motion sickness
Adults: 1 transdermal patch applied behind the ear 4 hours before anticipated exposure to motion.
Iritis, uveitis
Adults: 1 to 2 drops of 0.25% solution daily or up to t.i.d.
Children: 1 drop of 0.25% solution up to t.i.d.

Pharmacodynamics
Antimuscarinic action: Scopolamine inhibits the muscarinic ac-

tions of acetylcholine on autonomic effectors, which decreases secretions and GI motility. It also blocks vagal inhibition of the SA node.
Mydriatic action: Scopolamine competitively blocks acetylcholine at cholinergic neuroeffector sites, antagonizing the effects of acetylcholine on the sphincter muscle and ciliary body, thereby producing mydriasis and cycloplegia. These effects are used to produce cycloplegic refraction and pupil dilation to treat preoperative and postoperative iridocyclitis.

Pharmacokinetics
Absorption: Drug is rapidly absorbed when given I.M. or S.C. Effects occur in 15 to 30 minutes. Systemic absorption of ophthalmic solution may result from drug passage through the nasolacrimal duct. Ophthalmic mydriatic effect peaks 20 to 30 minutes after administration. Cycloplegic effects peak 30 to 60 minutes after administration.
Distribution: Drug is distributed widely throughout body tissues. It crosses the placenta and probably the blood-brain barrier.
Metabolism: Drug is probably metabolized completely in the liver; however, its exact metabolic fate is unknown. Mydriatic and cycloplegic effects persist 3 to 7 days.
Excretion: Drug is probably excreted in urine as metabolites.

Contraindications and precautions
Systemic form is contraindicated in patients with angle-closure glaucoma, obstructive uropathy, obstructive disease of the GI tract, asthma, chronic pulmonary disease, myasthenia gravis, paralytic ileus, intestinal atony, unstable CV status in acute hemorrhage, or toxic megacolon. Ophthalmic form is contraindicated in patients with shallow anterior chamber, angle-closure glaucoma, or hypersensitivity to drug.

Use systemic form cautiously in children under age 6, in hot or humid environments, and in patients with autonomic neuropathy, hyperthyroidism, coronary artery disease, arrhythmias, heart failure, hypertension, hiatal hernia with reflux esophagitis, hepatic or renal disease, or ulcerative colitis. Use ophthalmic form cautiously in elderly patients, infants, children, and people with cardiac disease.

Interactions
Drug-drug
Anticholinergics: may cause additive toxicity. Avoid concomitant use.
CNS depressants (sedative-hypnotics, tranquilizers): may increase CNS depression. Monitor patient closely.
Oral potassium supplements (especially wax-matrix formulations): potassium-induced GI ulcerations may increase. Use together cautiously.
Slow-dissolving digoxin tablets: serum digoxin levels may rise with concurrent use. Monitor digoxin levels.

Drug-herb
Squaw vine: tannic acid may decrease metabolic breakdown of scopolamine. Monitor patient closely.
Jaborandi tree, pill-bearing spurge: effects of scopolamine may decrease. Monitor patient closely.

Drug-lifestyle
Alcohol use: may increase CNS depression. Discourage concurrent use.

Effects on diagnostic tests
None reported.

Adverse reactions
CNS: confusion, delirium, disorientation, dizziness, drowsiness, headache, hallucinations, irritability, restlessness.
CV: flushing, palpitations, ***paradoxical bradycardia,*** tachycardia.
EENT: blurred vision, conjunctivitis, dilated pupils, difficulty swallowing, edema, eye dryness, increased intraocular pressure, ocular congestion, photophobia, transient stinging and burning.
GI: *constipation,* dry mouth, *epigastric distress, nausea, vomiting.*
GU: urinary hesitancy, urine retention.
Respiratory: bronchial plugging, depressed respirations.
Skin: rash, dryness or contact dermatitis.
Other: fever.

Overdose and treatment
Overdose may cause excitability, seizures, CNS stimulation followed by depression, and such psychotic symptoms as disorientation, confusion, hallucinations, delusions, anxiety, agitation, and restlessness. Peripheral effects include dilated, nonreactive pupils; blurred vision; flushed, hot, dry skin; dry mucous membranes; dysphagia; decreased or absent bowel sounds; urine retention; hyperthermia; tachycardia; hypertension; and increased respirations.
    Treatment is mainly symptomatic and supportive, as needed.
Maintain a patent airway. If patient is awake and alert, induce emesis or perform gastric lavage and follow with a sodium chloride cathartic and activated charcoal to prevent further absorption. In life-threatening cases, give physostigmine to block the antimuscarinic effects of scopolamine. Give fluids, as needed, to treat shock. Give diazepam to control psychotic symptoms. Instill pilocarpine into the eyes to relieve mydriasis. If urine retention develops, catheterization may be necessary.

Special considerations
▶ Assess patient for pain before giving drug. Scopolamine may act as a stimulant if patient has pain, producing delirium if used without morphine or meperidine.
▶ Intermittent and continuous infusions aren't recommended. For direct injection, dilute with sterile water and inject diluted drug through patent line.
▶ Protect I.V. solutions from freezing and light; store at room temperature.
▶ Therapeutic doses may produce amnesia, drowsiness, and euphoria (desired effects for use as an adjunct to anesthesia). As necessary, reorient patient.
▶ Monitor patient, especially elderly patient, for transient excitement or disorientation.
▶ Transdermal patch delivers about 1.5 mg in 72 hours.
▶ Ophthalmic form is also used for cyclopegic refraction.
▶ Have patient lie down, tilt head back, or look at ceiling to aid instillation.
▶ Apply pressure to the lacrimal sac for 1 minute after instillation to

---

Reactions may be common, uncommon, *life-threatening,* or **COMMON AND LIFE-THREATENING.**

reduce the risk of systemic drug absorption.
▶ Decreased GI absorption of many drugs has been reported after the use of anticholinergics.
▶ Adverse reactions may be caused by atropine-like toxicity and are dose-related. Individual tolerance varies greatly.
▶ Many adverse reactions (such as dry mouth, constipation) are an expected extension of drug's pharmacologic activity.

Breast-feeding patients
▶ Avoid giving drug to breast-feeding women because it may appear in breast milk, raising the risk of toxicity in the infant. It also may decrease milk production.

Pediatric patients
▶ Use ophthalmic form cautiously, if at all, in infants and small children.

Geriatric patients
▶ Use caution and reduced dosages when giving drug to elderly patients.

Patient teaching
▶ Instruct patient to apply pressure to inner corner of eye for about 1 minute after instillation.
▶ Urge patient not to close his eyes tightly or blink for about 1 minute after instillation.
▶ Tell patient to wash his hands after applying a transdermal patch.
▶ Instruct patient to use only one patch at a time, and to remove it when he no longer needs the antiemetic effect.

▶ secobarbital sodium
Novosecobarb ◇ **, Seconal**

Pharmacologic classification:
barbiturate

Therapeutic classification:
anticonvulsant, sedative-hypnotic

Controlled substance schedule II

Pregnancy risk category D

How supplied
Available by prescription only
Capsules: 50 mg, 100 mg
Injection: 50 mg/ml in 2-ml disposable syringe

Indications and dosages
To induce preoperative sedation
Adults: 200 to 300 mg P.O. 1 to 2 hours before surgery or 1 mg/kg I.M. 15 minutes before surgery.
Children: 2 to 6 mg/kg P.O. (maximum, 100 mg) or 3 to 5 mg/kg I.M.
To treat insomnia
Adults: 100 mg/day P.O. or 100 to 200 mg/day I.M. for up to 2 weeks.

Pharmacodynamics
Sedative-hypnotic action: Drug acts throughout the CNS as a nonselective depressant with a rapid onset and short duration of action. Particularly sensitive to this drug is the reticular activating system, which controls CNS arousal. Secobarbital decreases both presynaptic and postsynaptic membrane excitability by facilitating the action of GABA. The exact cellular site and mechanisms of action are unknown.

Pharmacokinetics

Absorption: After oral administration, 90% of secobarbital is absorbed rapidly. After rectal administration, nearly 100% is absorbed. After oral or rectal administration, serum levels peak in 2 to 4 hours. Action starts within 15 minutes after an oral dose. It peaks within 30 minutes after an oral or rectal dose, 7 to 10 minutes after an I.M. dose, and 1 to 3 minutes after an I.V. dose. Levels of 1 to 5 mcg/ml are needed to produce sedation; 5 to 15 mcg/ml are needed for hypnosis. Hypnosis lasts 1 to 4 hours after oral doses of 100 to 150 mg.

Distribution: Drug is distributed rapidly throughout body tissues and fluids; about 30% to 45% is protein-bound.

Metabolism: Drug is oxidized in the liver to inactive metabolites. Duration of action is 3 to 4 hours.

Excretion: 95% of a dose is eliminated as glucuronide conjugates and other metabolites in urine. Drug has an elimination half-life of about 30 hours.

Contraindications and precautions

Contraindicated in patients hypersensitive to barbiturates and in patients with porphyria or respiratory disease involving dyspnea or obstruction.

Use cautiously in patients with acute or chronic pain (because drug can cause pain and paradoxical excitement), depression, suicidal tendencies, a history of drug abuse, or impaired hepatic or renal function.

Interactions
Drug-drug

Antidepressants, antihistamines, narcotics, sedative-hypnotics, tranquilizers: secobarbital may add to or potentiate CNS and respiratory depressant effects. Monitor CNS and respiratory status closely.

Beta blockers, corticosteroids, digitoxin (not digoxin), doxycycline, estrogens (including oral contraceptives), xanthines (including theophylline): secobarbital enhances hepatic metabolism of these drugs. Monitor patient for desired drug effects, and adjust dosages as needed.

Disulfiram, MAO inhibitors, valproic acid: decreased secobarbital metabolism and increased risk of toxicity. Use together with caution.

Griseofulvin: impaired griseofulvin effectiveness via decreased absorption from the GI tract. Monitor patient for desired drug effects; adjust dosage if needed.

Rifampin: may decrease secobarbital levels by increasing metabolism. Dosage adjustments may be needed.

Warfarin and other oral anticoagulants: secobarbital enhances enzymatic degradation of these drugs. Monitor patient's PT, PTT and INR closely. Increase anticoagulant dosage as needed.

Drug-lifestyle

Alcohol use: may potentiate CNS and respiratory depressant effects when combined with secobarbital. Discourage concurrent use.

Effects on diagnostic tests

Secobarbital may cause a false-positive phentolamine test. The physiologic effects of the drug may

---

impair absorption of cyanocobal-amin ^{57}Co.

Adverse reactions
CNS: altered EEG patterns, *drowsiness, hangover, lethargy,* paradoxical excitement in elderly patients, somnolence.
CV: hypotension with I.V. use.
GI: nausea, vomiting.
Hematologic: worsening of porphyria.
Hepatic: decreased serum bilirubin levels.
Respiratory: *respiratory depression.*
Skin: injection-site pain, rash, *Stevens-Johnson syndrome,* tissue reactions, urticaria.
Other: *angioedema,* physical and psychological dependence.

Overdose and treatment
Overdose may cause an unsteady gait, slurred speech, sustained nystagmus, somnolence, confusion, respiratory depression, pulmonary edema, areflexia, and coma. Typical shock syndrome with tachycardia and hypotension, jaundice, hypothermia followed by fever, and oliguria may occur.

Maintain and support ventilation and pulmonary function as needed. Support cardiac function and circulation with vasopressors and I.V. fluids as needed. If patient is conscious, gag reflex is intact, and ingestion was recent, induce emesis with ipecac syrup. If emesis is contraindicated, perform gastric lavage with a cuffed endotracheal tube in place. Follow with activated charcoal or a sodium chloride cathartic.

Measure patient's intake and output, vital signs, and laboratory values. Maintain body tempera-ture. Roll patient from side to side every 30 minutes to avoid pulmonary congestion. Alkalinization of urine may help to remove drug from the body. Hemodialysis may be useful in severe overdose.

Special considerations
▶ Drug is also used to treat status epilepticus.
▶ Drug may cause increased pain or paradoxical excitement in patients with acute or chronic pain.
▶ Give I.M. dose deep into large muscle mass to prevent tissue injury. Inject no more than 250 mg (5 ml) at any one site.
▶ Use I.V. route only in emergencies or when other routes are unavailable. Keep resuscitation equipment readily available.
▶ Dilute secobarbital injection with sterile water for injection, normal saline solution for injection, or Ringer's injection solution. Don't use solution that's discolored or precipitated.
▶ To prevent hypotension and respiratory depression, avoid I.V. administration at more than 50 mg/15 seconds. Total I.V. dose shouldn't exceed 500 mg.
▶ Monitor hepatic and renal studies often to prevent possible toxicity.

Breast-feeding patients
▶ Because drug enters breast milk, it shouldn't be given to breast-feeding women.

Pediatric patients
▶ Secobarbital sodium injection, diluted with lukewarm tap water to 10 to 15 mg/ml, may be given rectally to children. Give a cleansing enema before the drug enema.
▶ Drug may cause paradoxical excitement in children; use caution.

Geriatric patients
▶ Elderly patients are more susceptible to drug effects and usually need lower dosages.
▶ Confusion, disorientation, and excitability are more likely in elderly patients.

Patient teaching
▶ Emphasize the danger of combining drug with alcohol. An excessive depressant effect is possible even if drug is taken the evening before alcohol ingestion.

▶ senna

Black-Draught, Fletcher's Castoria, Gentlax S, Nytilax, Senexon, Senokot, Senolax, X-Prep

Pharmacologic classification:
anthra-quinone derivative

Therapeutic classification:
stimulant laxative

Pregnancy risk category C

How supplied
Available without a prescription
Dosages expressed as sennosides (active principal)
Granules: 15 mg/5 ml, 20 mg/5 ml
Liquid: 3 mg/ml
Suppositories: 30 mg
Syrup: 8.8 mg/5 ml
Tablets: 6 mg, 8.6 mg, 17 mg

Indications and dosages
Acute constipation, preparation for bowel examination
Black-Draught
Adults: 2 tablets or ¼ to ½ level tsp of granules mixed with water. Not recommended for children.

Other preparations
Adults and children age 12 and over: Usual dose is 2 tablets, 1 tsp of granules dissolved in water, 1 suppository, or 10 to 15 ml syrup h.s. Maximum dose varies with preparation used.
Children ages 6 to 11: 1 tablet, ½ tsp of granules dissolved in water, ½ suppository h.s., or 5 to 10 ml syrup. Maximum, 2 tablets b.i.d. or 1 tsp of granules b.i.d.
Children ages 2 to 5: 2.5 to 5 ml syrup h.s., ½ tablet, or ¼ tsp of granules dissolved in water. Maximum, 1 tablet b.i.d. or ½ tsp of granules b.i.d.

Pharmacodynamics
Laxative action: Senna has a local irritant effect on the colon, which promotes peristalsis and bowel evacuation. It also enhances intestinal fluid accumulation, thereby increasing moisture in stool.

Pharmacokinetics
Absorption: Senna is absorbed minimally. With oral administration, laxative effect occurs in 6 to 10 hours; with suppository, laxative effect occurs in 30 minutes to 2 hours.
Distribution: Senna may be distributed in bile, saliva, the colonic mucosa, and breast milk.
Metabolism: Absorbed portion of drug is metabolized in the liver.
Excretion: Unabsorbed senna is excreted mainly in feces; absorbed drug is excreted in urine and feces.

Contraindications and precautions
Contraindicated in patients with ulcerative bowel lesions; nausea, vomiting, abdominal pain, or other symptoms of appendicitis or acute

---

surgical abdomen; fecal impaction; or intestinal obstruction or perforation.

Interactions
None reported.

Effects on diagnostic tests
In the phenolsulfonphthalein excretion test, senna may turn urine pink to red, red to violet, or red to brown.

Adverse reactions
GI: *abdominal cramps* (especially in severe constipation), cathartic colon (which resembles ulcerative colitis radiologically) with long-term misuse, darkened pigmentation of rectal mucosa with long-term use (usually reversible 4 to 12 months after stopping drug), diarrhea, diarrhea in breast-feeding infants of mothers receiving senna, laxative dependence with excessive use, loss of normal bowel function with excessive use, malabsorption of nutrients, *nausea,* possible constipation after catharsis, vomiting, yellow or yellow-green cast to feces.
GU: red-pink discoloration in alkaline urine, yellow-brown color in acidic urine.
Metabolic: electrolyte imbalance (such as hypokalemia), protein-losing enteropathy.

Overdose and treatment
No information available.

Special considerations
▶ Long-term use may cause electrolyte imbalance.
▶ Protect drug from excessive heat and light.

Breast-feeding patients
▶ Senna enters breast milk, and diarrhea has been reported in nursing infants.

Pediatric patients
▶ Senna and other stimulant laxatives are used infrequently in children.

Geriatric patients
▶ Elderly persons commonly overuse laxatives and may be more prone to laxative dependence.

Patient teaching
▶ Instruct patient to take drug with a full glass of water, at bedtime, on an empty stomach.
▶ Warn patient that drug may turn urine pink, red, violet, or brown.
▶ Tell patient that stool may have a yellow or yellow-green cast.
▶ Caution patient not to use laxatives for more than 1 week because excessive use may cause dependence or electrolyte imbalance.

▶ sertraline hydrochloride
Zoloft

Pharmacologic classification:
selective serotonin reuptake inhibitor

Therapeutic classification:
antidepressant

Pregnancy risk category C

How supplied
Available by prescription only
Tablets: 25 mg, 50 mg, 100 mg

Indications and dosages

Depression, obsessive-compulsive disorder
Adults: 50 mg/day P.O. Adjust dosage as needed and tolerated; clinical trials used dosages of 50 to 200 mg/day. Make adjustments at intervals of no less than 1 week.

Panic disorder
Adults: 25 mg/day P.O. for one week, then increase to 50 mg/day.
◻ DOSAGE ADJUSTMENT. A lower or less frequent dosage should be used in patients with hepatic impairment. Particular care should be used in patients with renal failure.

Pharmacodynamics
Antidepressant action: Sertraline probably acts by blocking the reuptake of serotonin (5-hydroxytryptamine [5-HT]) into presynaptic neurons in the CNS, prolonging the action of 5-HT.

Pharmacokinetics
Absorption: Drug is well absorbed after oral administration; rate and extent are enhanced by food. Serum levels peak 4½ to 8¼ hours after a dose.
Distribution: In vitro studies indicate that drug is highly protein-bound (more than 98%).
Metabolism: Metabolism is probably hepatic; drug undergoes significant first-pass metabolism. N-desmethylsertraline is substantially less active than the parent compound.
Excretion: Drug is excreted mostly as metabolites in urine and feces. Mean elimination half-life is 26 hours. Steady state levels occur within 1 week of daily use in young, healthy patients.

Contraindications and precautions
Contraindicated in patients receiving MAO inhibitors.

Use cautiously in patients at risk for suicide and in those with seizure disorders, major affective disorder, or diseases or conditions that affect metabolism or hemodynamic responses.

Interactions
Drug-drug
Calcium-channel blockers, diazepam, haloperidol, methadone, phenothiazines, thiothixene, tolbutamide: clearance decreased by sertraline. Clinical significance is unknown, but monitor patient for increased drug effects.
Cimetidine: increased sertraline bioavailability, peak plasma levels, and half-life. Clinical significance is unknown.
Drugs highly bound to protein, such as warfarin: may cause interactions, increasing plasma levels of sertraline or the other highly bound drug. Small increases in PT have occurred with warfarin. Monitor patient closely.
MAO inhibitors: may cause serious changes in mental status, hyperthermia, autonomic instability, rapid fluctuations of vital signs, delirium, coma, and death. Don't administer within 14 days after stopping an MAO inhibitor. Similarly, allow 14 days after stopping sertraline before starting an MAO inhibitor.

Effects on diagnostic tests
None reported.

Adverse reactions
CNS: agitation, anxiety, confusion, *dizziness, fatigue, headache,*

hypertonia, hypoesthesia, *insomnia,* nervousness, paresthesia, *somnolence, tremor,* twitching.
CV: chest pain, hot flashes, palpitations.
GI: abdominal pain, anorexia, constipation, *diarrhea, dyspepsia, dry mouth,* flatulence, increased appetite, *loose stools, nausea,* thirst, vomiting.
GU: dysuria, *male sexual dysfunction,* nocturia, polyuria.
Hepatic: elevated liver enzymes.
Metabolic: decreased uric acid, minor increases in serum cholesterol and triglycerides.
Musculoskeletal: myalgia.
Skin: *diaphoresis,* pruritus, rash.

Overdose and treatment

Experience with sertraline overdose is limited. Treatment is supportive. Establish an airway, and maintain adequate ventilation. Because recent studies question the value of induced emesis or lavage, consider using activated charcoal in sorbitol to bind drug in the GI tract. No antidote exists. Monitor vital signs closely. Because drug has a large volume of distribution, hemodialysis, peritoneal dialysis, and forced diuresis probably aren't useful.

Special considerations

▶ Sertraline may be used to treat various types of headaches.
▶ Depressed patients who respond during the first 8 weeks of therapy will probably continue to respond to drug, although studies lasting more than 16 weeks are limited.
▶ If patient continues taking drug for prolonged therapy, periodically monitor effectiveness. No data exist to demonstrate whether periodic

dosage adjustments are needed to maintain effectiveness.
▶ Drug may activate mania or hypomania in patients with cyclic disorders.
▶ Assess patient for suicidal ideations.
▶ Weight loss may occur; adjust nutritional needs as necessary.

Breast-feeding patients

▶ No data exist to demonstrate whether drug appears in breast milk. Use with caution in breast-feeding women.

Pediatric patients

▶ Safety and efficacy in children haven't been established.

Geriatric patients

▶ Plasma clearance of drug is slower in elderly patients. Monitor patient closely for dose-related side effects.
▶ Drug may take 2 to 3 weeks of daily use before reaching steady state levels in elderly patients.

Patient teaching

▶ Tell patient to take drug once daily, either in the morning or evening, with or without food.
▶ Urge patient to avoid alcohol while taking drug and to consult prescriber before taking OTC medications or herbal remedies.
▶ Although problems have not been reported to date, caution patient to avoid hazardous tasks until full CNS effects of drug are known.

▶ sodium phosphates (sodium phosphate and sodium biphosphate)
Fleet Phospho-soda

Pharmacologic classification:
acid salt

Therapeutic classification:
sodium chloride laxative

Pregnancy risk category C

How supplied
Available without a prescription
Solution: 18 g sodium phosphate and 48 g sodium biphosphate/ 100 ml

Indications and dosages
Constipation
Adults: 20 to 30 ml of solution mixed with 120 ml (4 oz) of cold water.
Children ages 10 to 12: 10 ml of solution mixed with 120 ml of cold water.
Children ages 5 to 10: 5 ml of solution mixed with 120 ml of cold water.
Purgative action
Adults: 45 ml of solution mixed with 120 ml of cold water.

Pharmacodynamics
Laxative action: Sodium phosphate and sodium biphosphate exert an osmotic effect in the small intestine by drawing water into the intestinal lumen, producing distention that promotes peristalsis and bowel evacuation.

Pharmacokinetics
Absorption: About 1% to 20% of an oral dose of sodium and phosphate is absorbed. Action begins in 3 to 6 hours.
Distribution: Unknown.
Metabolism: Unknown.
Excretion: Unknown; probably excreted in feces and urine.

Contraindications and precautions
Contraindicated in patients on sodium-restricted diets and in patients with intestinal obstruction or perforation, edema, heart failure, megacolon, impaired renal function, and symptoms of appendicitis or acute surgical abdomen (pain, nausea, and vomiting).

Use cautiously in patients with large hemorrhoids or anal excoriations.

Interactions
Drug-drug
Antacids: may inactivate both drugs. Watch for drug effect.

Effects on diagnostic tests
None reported.

Adverse reactions
GI: *abdominal cramping.*
Metabolic: fluid and electrolyte disturbances, such as hypernatremia or hyperphosphatemia, with daily use.
Other: laxative dependence with long-term or excessive use.

Overdose and treatment
No information available; probable clinical effects include abdominal pain and diarrhea.

Special considerations
▶ Dilute drug with water before oral use. Follow dose with a full glass of water.

▶ Drug isn't routinely used for constipation but is commonly used to evacuate the bowel.

▶ Monitor serum electrolyte levels; when drug is given as sodium chloride laxative, up to 10% of sodium content may be absorbed.

Patient teaching
▶ Teach patient how to mix the drug and when to take it.
▶ Warn patient that frequent or prolonged use of drug may lead to laxative dependence.

▶ strontium-89 chloride
Metastron

Pharmacologic classification:
radioisotope

Therapeutic classification:
radioisotope for metastatic bone pain

Pregnancy risk category D

How supplied
Available by prescription only
Injection: 148 mBq (10.9 to 22.6 mg/ml) in 10-ml vial

Indications and dosages
Metastatic bone pain
Adults: 148 MBq, 4 millicuries (mCi) by slow I.V. injection over 1 to 2 minutes. Alternatively, give 1.5 to 2.2 MBq/kg or 40-60 mCi/kg. Don't repeat dose for at least 90 days.

Pharmacodynamics
Analgesic action: Drug selectively irradiates sites of primary metastatic bone involvement with minimal irradiation of soft tissues distant from the bone lesions.

Pharmacokinetics
Absorption: Rapidly cleared from the blood and selectively localized in bone mineral.
Distribution: Uptake of strontium-89 by bone occurs preferentially in sites of active osteogenesis; thus, primary bone tumors and areas of metastatic involvement (blastic lesions) can accumulate significantly greater concentrations of strontium-89 than surrounding normal bone.
Metabolism: Drug decays by beta emission and has a physical half-life of 50½ days.
Excretion: Excretion pathways are two-thirds urinary and one-third fecal in patients with bone metastases. Urine excretion, which is higher in people without bone lesions, is greatest in the first 2 days after injection.

Contraindications and precautions
Contraindicated in pregnant patients.

Use cautiously in patients with platelet counts below $60,000/mm^3$ or WBC counts below $2,400/mm^3$.

Interactions
None reported

Effects on diagnostic tests
None reported

Adverse reactions
CV: cutaneous flushing with rapid injection.
Hematologic: *bone marrow suppression*.
Other: transient increase in pain (flare reaction).

Overdose and treatment
No information available.

Special considerations

▶ Strontium-89 is a potential carcinogen; give it only to patients with well-documented metastatic bone disease.

▶ Like other radioactive drugs, strontium-89 requires careful handling and appropriate safety measures to minimize radiation to clinical staff.

▶ Verify dose and patient before administration because drug delivers a relatively high dose of radioactivity.

▶ Measure dose immediately before administration by using a suitable radioactivity calibration system.

▶ Don't give drug too rapidly. Patient may develop a calcium-like flushing sensation if the injection takes less than 30 seconds.

▶ Take special precautions to minimize risk of radioactive contamination of clothing, bed linens, and patient's environment. For example, catheterize patient with urinary incontinence.

▶ Expect bone marrow toxicity of variable intensity after administration, particularly involving WBCs and platelets.

▶ Monitor patient's peripheral blood cell counts at least once every other week. Typically, platelet count is depressed by about 30% compared with preadministration levels. The nadir of platelet depression in most patients is 12 to 16 weeks after drug administration. WBCs are usually depressed to a varying extent compared with preadministration levels. Recovery occurs slowly; counts typically reach preadministration levels 6 months after treatment unless patient's disease or additional therapy intervenes.

▶ When considering repeat dose, carefully evaluate patient's hematologic response to initial dose, current platelet level, and other evidence of marrow depletion. Repeat doses typically aren't recommended in less than 90 days.

▶ Because of delayed onset of pain relief (typically 7 to 20 days after injection), use of drug isn't recommended in patients with very short life expectancy.

Breast-feeding patients

▶ No data exist to demonstrate whether drug appears in breast milk. Breast-feeding should be discontinued just before drug administration.

Pediatric patients

▶ Safety and effectiveness in children under age 18 haven't been established.

Patient teaching

▶ Instruct patient to take radiation precautions for 1 week after injection because drug will be present in blood and urine.

▶ Explain that pain normally increases slightly 2 to 3 days after injection. As needed, recommend a temporary increase in pain medication until the pain subsides.

▶ Inform patient that pain relief usually begins 7 to 20 days after injection and lasts several months.

▶ Tell patient that routine blood tests may be needed periodically.

▶ Advise women of childbearing age to avoid pregnancy because drug may cause fetal harm.

▶ Urge patient to notify all health care providers about receiving strontium-89.

▶ sucralfate
Carafate

Pharmacologic classification:
pepsin inhibitor

Therapeutic classification:
antiulcer drug

Pregnancy risk category B

How supplied
Available by prescription only
Suspension: 1 g/10 ml
Tablets: 1 g

Indications and dosages
Short-term (up to 8 weeks) treatment of duodenal ulcer
Aspirin-induced gastric erosion*
Adults: 1 g P.O. q.i.d. 1 hour before meals and h.s.
Maintenance therapy for duodenal ulcer
Adults: 1 g P.O. b.i.d.

Pharmacodynamics
Antiulcer action: Sucralfate has a unique mechanism of action. It adheres to proteins at the ulcer site, forming a protective coating against gastric acid, pepsin, and bile salts. It also inhibits pepsin, exhibits a cytoprotective effect, and forms a viscous, adhesive barrier on the surface of the intact intestinal mucosa and stomach.

Pharmacokinetics
Absorption: Only about 3% to 5% of a dose is absorbed. Drug activity isn't related to the amount absorbed.
Distribution: Sucralfate acts locally at the ulcer site. Absorbed drug is distributed to many body tissues, including the liver and kidneys.

Metabolism: None.
Excretion: About 90% of a dose is excreted in feces; absorbed drug is excreted unchanged in urine. Duration of effect is 6 hours.

Contraindications and precautions
No known contraindications. Use cautiously in patients with chronic renal failure because of possible aluminum accumulation.

Interactions
Drug-drug
Antacids: may decrease binding of drug to gastroduodenal mucosa, impairing effectiveness. Give antacid 30 minutes before or 2 hours after sucralfate.
Cimetidine, digoxin, fat-soluble vitamins (A, D, E, and K), phenytoin, quinidine, quinolones, ranitidine, tetracycline, theophylline: sucralfate decreases absorption of these drugs. Avoid concomitant use.

Effects on diagnostic tests
None reported.

Adverse reactions
CNS: dizziness, headache, sleepiness, vertigo.
GI: bezoar formation, *constipation,* diarrhea, dry mouth, flatulence, gastric discomfort, indigestion, nausea, vomiting.
Musculoskeletal: back pain.
Skin: pruritus, rash.

Overdose and treatment
No information available.

Special considerations
▶ Drug treats ulcers as effectively as H_2-receptor antagonists.
▶ Drug is poorly water-soluble. For administration by nasogastric tube,

have pharmacist prepare a water-sorbitol suspension. Alternatively, place tablet in 60-ml syringe, add 20 ml of water, and let stand with tip facing upward for about 5 minutes, occasionally shaking gently. Resulting suspension may be administered from the syringe. After administration, flush tube several times to make sure patient received the entire dose.

▶ Assess patient's stool for frank or occult blood. Also, monitor patient for constipation.

▶ Therapy exceeding 8 weeks isn't recommended.

▶ Some experts believe that 2 g given b.i.d. is as effective as the standard regimen.

▶ Sucralfate may inhibit absorption of other drugs; schedule them 2 hours before or after sucralfate.

Breast-feeding patients
▶ The risks to breast-feeding infants must be weighed against benefits to mother.

Patient teaching
▶ Advise patient to continue taking drug as directed, even after pain begins to subside, to ensure adequate healing.

▶ Remind patient to take drug on an empty stomach and at least 1 hour before meals.

▶ If patient has trouble swallowing tablet, teach him to place it in 15 to 30 ml of water at room temperature, allow it to disintegrate, and then swallow the resulting suspension. This method is particularly useful for patients with esophagitis and painful swallowing.

▶ Tell patient that he may take an antacid 30 minutes before or 2 hours after sucralfate.

▶ Warn patient not to take drug for more than 8 weeks.

▶ Tell patient not to crush tablet.

▶ **sufentanil citrate**
Sufenta

Pharmacologic classification:
opioid

Therapeutic classification:
adjunct to anesthesia, analgesic, anesthetic

Controlled substance schedule II

Pregnancy risk category C

How supplied
Available by prescription only
Injection: 50 mcg/ml

Indications and dosages
Adjunct to general anesthesia
Adults: 1 to 8 mcg/kg I.V. with nitrous oxide and oxygen. Maintenance, 10 to 50 mcg.
Primary anesthetic
Adults: 8 to 30 mcg/kg I.V. with 100% oxygen and a muscle relaxant. Maintenance, 25 to 50 mcg.
Children: 10 to 25 mcg/kg I.V. with 100% oxygen and a muscle relaxant. Maintenance, up to 50 mcg.
◩ DOSAGE ADJUSTMENT. If patient weighs more than 20% over ideal body weight, determine dose based on ideal body weight.

Pharmacodynamics
Analgesic action: Sufentanil has a high affinity for opiate receptors with an agonist effect to provide analgesia. It's also used as an adjunct to anesthesia or as a primary anesthetic because of its potent CNS depressant effects.

Pharmacokinetics

Absorption: After I.V. administration, sufentanil has a more rapid onset of action (1½ to 3 minutes) than either morphine or fentanyl.

Distribution: Drug is highly lipophilic and is rapidly and extensively distributed in animals. It is highly protein-bound (more than 90%) and redistributed rapidly.

Metabolism: Drug appears to be metabolized mainly in the liver and small intestine. Relatively little accumulation occurs. Drug has an elimination half-life of about 2½ hours.

Excretion: Drug and its metabolites are excreted primarily in urine.

Contraindications and precautions

Contraindicated in patients hypersensitive to drug. Use cautiously in elderly or debilitated patients and in those with decreased respiratory reserve, head injuries, or renal, pulmonary, or hepatic disease.

Interactions

Drug-drug

Anticholinergics: may cause paralytic ileus. Monitor patient closely.

Beta blockers: enhanced sufentanil effects. Decrease sufentanil dosage as needed.

Cimetidine: may increase respiratory and CNS depression, causing confusion, disorientation, apnea, or seizures. Decreased sufentanil dosage is usually needed.

CNS depressants, such as antihistamines, barbiturates, benzodiazepines, general anesthetics, muscle relaxants, opioid analgesics, phenothiazines, sedative-hypnotics, tricyclic antidepressants: potentiated respiratory and CNS depression, sedation, and hypotensive effects. Use together cautiously.

General anesthetics: increased risk of severe CV depression. Use together cautiously.

Nitrous oxide: increased risk of CV depression with high sufentanil doses. Use together cautiously.

Opioid agonist-antagonist: acute withdrawal syndrome in patients physically dependent on sufentanil. Administer cautiously.

Pancuronium: may produce a dose-dependent elevation in heart rate during sufentanil and oxygen anesthesia. Use moderate doses of pancuronium or a less vagolytic neuromuscular blocker.

Drug-lifestyle

Alcohol use: may cause additive effects. Discourage concomitant use.

Effects on diagnostic tests

None reported.

Adverse reactions

CNS: somnolence.

CV: *arrhythmias, bradycardia,* hypertension, *hypotension,* tachycardia.

GI: nausea, vomiting.

Metabolic: increased plasma amylase and lipase levels, increased serum prolactin levels.

Musculoskeletal: intraoperative muscle movement.

Respiratory: *apnea, bronchospasm, chest wall rigidity.*

Skin: erythema, *pruritus.*

Other: chills.

Overdose and treatment

Although there's no clinical experience with acute sufentanil overdose, signs and symptoms probably would be similar to those of other opioids, with less CV toxicity. Acute opiate overdose typically causes CNS depression, respiratory depression, and miosis (pinpoint pupils). Other acute toxic effects include hypotension, bradycardia, hypothermia, shock, apnea, cardiopulmonary arrest, circulatory collapse, pulmonary edema, and seizures.

To treat acute overdose, establish adequate respiratory exchange via a patent airway and ventilation, as needed. Give a narcotic antagonist (naloxone) if patient has significant respiratory or CV depression. Because sufentanil has a longer duration of action than naloxone, repeated naloxone doses are needed. Monitor patient's vital signs closely. Provide symptomatic and supportive treatment as needed, such as continued respiratory support and correction of fluid or electrolyte imbalance. Monitor laboratory values, vital signs, and neurologic status closely.

Special considerations
▶ Sufentanil may produce dose-related rigidity of all skeletal muscles. Give a neuromuscular blocker appropriate to patient's CV status.
▶ Drug should be administered only by persons specifically trained to use I.V. anesthetics.
▶ Give drug by direct I.V. injection. It has been given by intermittent I.V. infusion, but drug compatibility and stability in I.V. solutions haven't been fully investigated.
▶ Sufentanil has a more rapid onset and shorter duration of action than fentanyl.
▶ When doses exceed 8 mcg/kg, postoperative mechanical ventilation and observation are essential because of extended postoperative respiratory depression.

Pediatric patients
▶ Safety and efficacy in children under age 2 have been documented in a limited number of patients, who were undergoing CV surgery.

Geriatric patients
▶ Lower dosages are usually indicated for elderly patients, who may be more sensitive to drug effects.

Patient teaching
▶ Explain patient's need for drug to patient and family.

▶ sulindac
Clinoril

Pharmacologic classification:
NSAID

Therapeutic classification:
anti-inflammatory, antipyretic, nonnarcotic analgesic

Pregnancy risk category NR

How supplied
Available by prescription only
Tablets: 150 mg, 200 mg

Indications and dosages
Osteoarthritis, rheumatoid arthritis, ankylosing spondylitis
Adults: initially, 150 mg P.O. b.i.d. May increase to 200 mg P.O. b.i.d.
Acute subacromial bursitis or supraspinatus tendinitis, acute gouty arthritis
Adults: 200 mg P.O. b.i.d. for 7 to 14 days. Dosage may be reduced as symptoms subside.

Pharmacodynamics
Analgesic, anti-inflammatory, and antipyretic actions: Mechanisms of action are unknown but proba-

bly stem from inhibited prostaglandin synthesis.

Pharmacokinetics

Absorption: Drug is rapidly and completely absorbed from the GI tract.

Distribution: Drug is highly protein-bound.

Metabolism: Sulindac is metabolized hepatically to the active sulfide metabolite and the inactive sulfone metabolite.

Excretion: Drug is excreted in urine. Half-life of parent drug is about 8 hours; half-life of active metabolite is about 16 hours.

Contraindications and precautions

Contraindicated in patients hypersensitive to drug and in patients for whom aspirin or NSAIDs raise the risk of acute asthma attack, urticaria, or rhinitis. Avoid use during pregnancy.

Use cautiously in patients with history of ulcer or GI bleeding, renal dysfunction, compromised cardiac function, hypertension, or conditions that predispose them to fluid retention.

Interactions
Drug-drug

Antacids: delayed and decreased sulindac absorption. Avoid concurrent use.

Anticoagulants, thrombolytics: may be potentiated by platelet-inhibiting effect of sulindac. Monitor patient for bleeding.

Aspirin, diflunisal: decreased plasma levels of the active sulfide metabolite. Monitor patient closely.

Dimethyl sulfoxide: may interact with sulindac, decreasing plasma levels of the active sulfide metabolite. Peripheral neuropathies have been reported with this combination. Monitor patient closely.

Drugs highly bound to protein (phenytoin, sulfonylureas, warfarin): either drug may be displaced, raising the risk of adverse effects. Monitor therapy closely for both drugs.

GI-irritating drugs, such as antibiotics, corticosteroids, NSAIDs: may potentiate the adverse GI effects of sulindac. Use together cautiously.

Lithium carbonate: NSAIDs decrease renal lithium clearance, increasing serum lithium levels and the risk of adverse effects. Monitor lithium levels frequently.

Probenecid: increases plasma levels of sulindac and its inactive sulfone metabolite. Sulindac may decrease the uricosuric effect of probenecid. Avoid concurrent use.

Drug-food

Any food: delayed and decreased sulindac absorption. Give drug on an empty stomach.

Effects on diagnostic tests
None reported.

Adverse reactions

CNS: dizziness, headache, nervousness, psychosis.

CV: edema, ***heart failure,*** hypertension, palpitations.

EENT: tinnitus, transient visual disturbances.

GI: anorexia, constipation, diarrhea, dyspepsia, *epigastric distress,* flatulence, *GI bleeding,* nausea, occult blood loss, ***pancreatitis, peptic ulceration,*** vomiting.

GU: increased BUN and serum creatinine, interstitial nephritis, ***nephrotic syndrome, renal failure.***

Hematologic: *agranulocytosis,* *aplastic anemia,* hemolytic anemia, *neutropenia,* prolonged bleeding time, *thrombocytopenia.*
Hepatic: elevated liver enzymes.
Metabolic: hyperkalemia.
Skin: pruritus, *rash.*
Other: *anaphylaxis, angioedema,* drug fever, *hypersensitivity syndrome.*

Overdose and treatment

Overdose may cause dizziness, drowsiness, mental confusion, disorientation, lethargy, paresthesias, numbness, vomiting, gastric irritation, nausea, abdominal pain, headache, stupor, coma, and hypotension.

To treat overdose, immediately induce emesis with ipecac syrup or perform gastric lavage. Give activated charcoal via nasogastric tube. Provide symptomatic and supportive measures, such as respiratory support and correction of fluid and electrolyte imbalances. Dialysis probably has little value because sulindac is highly protein-bound. Monitor laboratory values and vital signs closely.

Special considerations

▶ Symptoms may take 7 days or longer to improve. Evaluate patient's response in terms of symptom reduction.
▶ Take steps to prevent injury, such as raising side rails and assisting with ambulation.
▶ Assess cardiopulmonary status frequently. Monitor patient's vital signs, especially heart rate and blood pressure, to detect abnormalities.
▶ Assess patient's fluid balance. Monitor intake, output, and daily weight. Observe for presence and amount of edema.
▶ Sulindac may be the safest NSAID for patients with mild renal impairment. It may also be less likely to cause further renal toxicity.

Breast-feeding patients

▶ Safe use of sulindac during breast-feeding hasn't been established. Avoid use of drug in breast-feeding women.

Pediatric patients

▶ Safety of long-term drug use in children hasn't been established.

Geriatric patients

▶ Patients over age 60 are more sensitive to the adverse effects of sulindac. Use with caution.
▶ Because of its effect on renal prostaglandins, drug may cause fluid retention and edema. This may be significant in elderly patients and those with heart failure.

Patient teaching

▶ Instruct patient to check his weight two or three times weekly and to report a gain of 3 lb (1.4 kg) if it occurs in 1 week.
▶ Because drug causes sodium retention, advise patient to report edema and to have blood pressure checked routinely.
▶ Instruct patient in safety measures.
▶ Caution patient to avoid hazardous activities until full CNS effects of drug are known.
▶ Tell patient to avoid taking OTC medications and herbal remedies without consulting prescriber.
▶ Teach patient how to recognize possible adverse reactions, and explain when to notify prescriber about such reactions.

▶ sumatriptan succinate
Imitrex

Pharmacologic classification:
*selective 5-hydroxytryptamine
(5HT₁)-receptor agonist*

Therapeutic classification:
antimigraine

Pregnancy risk category C

How supplied
Available by prescription only
Injection: 12 mg/ml (0.5 ml in 1-
ml prefilled syringe), 6-mg single-
dose (0.5 ml in 2 ml) vial, and self-
dose system kit
Nasal spray: 5 mg, 20 mg unit
dose nasal spray device
Tablets: 25 mg, 50 mg

Indications and dosages
*Acute migraine headache with or
without aura*
Adults: 6 mg S.C. Maximum, two
6-mg injections in 24 hours, sepa-
rated by at least 1 hour. Or give
25 to 100 mg P.O. If response
doesn't occur in 2 hours, may give
a second dose of 25 to 100 mg.
Additional doses may be given in
2-hour or longer intervals. Maximum, 300 mg/day.
  For nasal spray, give single 5-
mg, 10-mg, or 20-mg dose in one
nostril; may repeat once after 2
hours for maximum of 40 mg/day.
To deliver a 10-mg dose, administer a 5-mg dose into each nostril.

Pharmacodynamics
Antimigraine action: Sumatriptan
selectively binds to a 5-HT₁ receptor subtype found in the basilar
artery and vasculature of the dura
mater. Here, sumatriptan activates
the receptor to cause vasoconstric-

tion, an action that probably relieves migraine pain.

Pharmacokinetics
Absorption: Bioavailability via
S.C. injection is 97% of that obtained via I.V. injection. After S.C.
injection, levels peak in about 12
minutes.
Distribution: Drug has a low
protein-binding capacity of about
14% to 21%.
Metabolism: About 80% of drug is
metabolized in the liver, primarily
to an inactive indoleacetic acid
metabolite.
Excretion: Drug is excreted primarily in urine, partly (20%) as
unchanged drug and partly as the
indoleacetic acid metabolite.
Elimination half-life is about 2
hours.

Contraindications and
precautions
Contraindicated in patients hypersensitive to drug, in patients who
took an MAO inhibitor within 14
days, in patients who take ergotamine, and in patients with uncontrolled hypertension, ischemic
heart disease (angina, Prinzmetal's
angina, history of MI, or documented silent ischemia), or hemiplegic or basilar migraine.
  Use cautiously in women of
childbearing age, pregnant women,
and patients who have risk factors
for coronary artery disease, such
as hypertension, hypercholesterolemia, obesity, diabetes, smoking,
family history, postmenopausal
status, or men over age 40.

Interactions
Drug-drug
Ergot and ergot derivatives: pro-
longed vasospastic effects when

---

given with sumatriptan. Don't give these drugs within 24 hours of sumatriptan therapy.

MAO inhibitors: sumatriptan appears to be metabolized by MAO inhibitors. Allow 2 weeks between use of oral sumatriptan and MAO inhibitors. Sumatriptan S.C. may be used with MAO inhibitors with careful patient monitoring.

Selective serotonin reuptake inhibitors: possible loss of migraine control and increased risk of serotonin syndrome. Monitor patient for weakness, progressive agitation, tingling, incoordination, chest pain, and dyspnea.

Drug-herb
Horehound: may enhance serotonergic effects. Discourage concurrent use.

Effects on diagnostic tests
None reported.

Adverse reactions
CNS: anxiety, *dizziness,* drowsiness, fatigue, headache, malaise, *vertigo,*
CV: *atrial fibrillation,* flushing, *MI,* pressure or tightness in chest, *ventricular fibrillation, ventricular tachycardia.*
EENT: altered vision, discomfort in throat, nasal cavity, sinus, mouth, jaw, or tongue.
GI: abdominal discomfort, dysphagia.
Musculoskeletal: muscle cramps, myalgia, neck pain.
Skin: diaphoresis.
Other: cold sensation, *burning sensation, heaviness, pressure, tightness, injection site reaction,* tight feeling in head, *tingling, warm or hot sensation.*

Overdose and treatment
No specific information available. However, overdose probably would cause seizures, tremor, inactivity, erythema of the limbs, reduced respiratory rate, cyanosis, ataxia, mydriasis, injection site reactions, and paralysis. Monitor patient carefully while evidence of overdose continues and for at least 10 hours afterward. Effect of hemodialysis or peritoneal dialysis on serum levels of sumatriptan is unknown.

Special considerations
▶ Don't use drug to manage hemiplegic or basilar migraine. Safety and effectiveness also haven't been established for cluster headache, which occurs in an older, predominantly male population.
▶ Don't give drug by I.V. route because coronary vasospasm may result.
▶ Nasal spray is usually well tolerated; however, adverse reactions seen with other forms of drug can still occur. Patient response to nasal spray may be varied.
▶ Clinical data on sumatriptan injection include rare reports of serious or life-threatening arrhythmias, such as atrial and ventricular fibrillation, ventricular tachycardia, MI, and marked ischemic ST elevations. Data also include rare but more frequent reports of chest and arm discomfort thought to be angina. Because such coronary events can occur, consider administering first dose in a supervised setting to patients in whom unrecognized coronary artery disease is relatively likely.
▶ Monitor patient for drug effect. The choice of dose should be made individually, weighing the possible

---

Reactions may be *common,* uncommon, *life-threatening,* or COMMON AND LIFE-THREATENING.

benefit of the 20-mg dose with the potential for a greater risk of adverse events.

Breast-feeding patients
▶ Drug appears in breast milk. Use caution when administering to breast-feeding women.

Pediatric patients
▶ Safety and effectiveness in children haven't been established.

Patient teaching
▶ Explain that drug is intended to relieve migraines, not to prevent or reduce the number of attacks.
▶ Tell patient that drug may be taken at any time during a migraine attack, but it works best when taken as soon as symptoms begin. If response is inadequate, oral dose may be repeated after 2 hours. Tell patient not to exceed maximum recommended amounts.
▶ Explain that additional injections are unlikely to provide relief if the first dose produces an inadequate response. However, a second dose may be given after 1 hour if symptoms recur.
▶ Urge patient not to use a second dose of nasal spray without consulting prescriber.
▶ Explain that drug is available in a spring-loaded injector system that facilitates self-administration. Review detailed information with patient. Make sure he understands how to load the injector, give the injection, and dispose of used syringes.
▶ Tell patient that redness and pain at injection site typically subside within 1 hour.
▶ Urge patient to immediately notify prescriber about persistent or severe chest pain, pain or tightness in the throat, wheezing, heart throbbing, rash, lumps, hives, or swollen eyelids, face, or lips.
▶ Tell women of childbearing age to immediately notify prescriber about planned, suspected, or known pregnancy.

▶ temazepam
Restoril

Pharmacologic classification: *benzodiazepine*

Therapeutic classification: *sedative-hypnotic*

Controlled substance schedule IV

Pregnancy risk category X

How supplied
Available by prescription only
Capsules: 7.5 mg, 15 mg, 30 mg

Indications and dosages
Insomnia
Adults: 7.5 to 30 mg P.O. 30 minutes before bedtime.
▧ DOSAGE ADJUSTMENT. In debilitated or elderly patients, start with 7.5 mg P.O. h.s. until individual response is determined. Also, give reduced dosages to patients with hepatic dysfunction.

Pharmacodynamics
Sedative-hypnotic action: Drug depresses the CNS at the limbic and subcortical levels of the brain. It causes a sedative-hypnotic effect by potentiating the effect of GABA on its receptor in the ascending reticular activating system, which increases inhibition and blocks cortical and limbic arousal.

Pharmacokinetics

Absorption: When given orally, drug is well absorbed through the GI tract. Action starts in 30 to 60 minutes. Levels peak in about 1½ hours.

Distribution: Drug is widely distributed throughout the body and is 96% protein-bound.

Metabolism: Drug is metabolized in the liver, primarily to inactive metabolites.

Excretion: Metabolites are excreted in urine as glucuronide conjugates. Half-life of drug is 4 to 20 hours.

Contraindications and precautions

Contraindicated in pregnant patients and in patients hypersensitive to drug or other benzodiazepines.

Use cautiously in patients with impaired renal or hepatic function, chronic pulmonary insufficiency, severe or latent mental depression, suicidal tendencies, or history of drug abuse.

Interactions

Drug-drug

CNS depressants, such as antihistamines, barbiturates, general anesthetics, MAO inhibitors, opioids, phenothiazines: potentiated CNS depressant effects. Use together with caution.

Haloperidol: decreased haloperidol levels. Dosage adjustment may be necessary.

Levodopa: benzodiazepines block levodopa's effects. Don't use together.

Drug-lifestyle

Alcohol use: increased risk of CNS depression. Discourage concurrent use.

Heavy smoking: accelerated temazepam metabolism and reduced effectiveness. Dosage adjustment may be necessary.

Effects on diagnostic tests

None reported.

Adverse reactions

CNS: anxiety, confusion, daytime sedation, depression, *drowsiness,* disturbed coordination, *dizziness,* euphoria, fatigue, headache, *lethargy,* minor changes in EEG patterns, nervousness, nightmares, weakness, vertigo.

EENT: blurred vision.

GI: diarrhea, dry mouth, nausea.

Hepatic: elevated liver enzymes.

Other: physical and psychological dependence.

Overdose and treatment

Overdose may cause somnolence, confusion, hypoactive or absent reflexes, dyspnea, labored breathing, hypotension, bradycardia, slurred speech, unsteady gait or impaired coordination and, ultimately, coma.

Support blood pressure and respiration until drug effects subside; monitor vital signs. As needed, provide mechanical ventilatory assistance via endotracheal tube to maintain a patent airway and support adequate oxygenation. Flumazenil, a specific benzodiazepine antagonist, may be useful. Give I.V. fluids and vasopressors, such as dopamine and phenylephrine, to treat hypotension as needed. If patient is conscious, induce emesis. If an endotracheal tube is in place and ingestion was recent, consider gastric lavage. After emesis or lavage, give activated charcoal with a cathartic as a single dose. Don't give barbiturates if excitation occurs. Dialysis is of limited value.

Special considerations
▶ Drug is useful for patients who have difficulty falling asleep or who awaken often at night.
▶ Assess the reason for the patient's insomnia; it may result from depression or another disorder.
▶ Drug has proven effective for up to 4 weeks of continuous use, but prolonged use isn't recommended.
▶ Remove all safety hazards, such as cigarettes, from patient's reach after giving drug.
▶ Impose safety measures, such as placing the call bell within each reach and raising the side rails, to prevent possible injury.
▶ Avoid abrupt withdrawal after long-term use; instead, taper the dosage gradually.
▶ Store drug in a cool, dry place away from light.
▶ Monitor hepatic function studies to detect toxicity.

Breast-feeding patients
▶ Temazepam appears in breast milk. A breast-fed infant may become sedated, have trouble feeding, or lose weight. Avoid use in breast-feeding women.

Pediatric patients
▶ Safe use in patients under age 18 hasn't been established.

Geriatric patients
▶ Elderly patients are more susceptible to the CNS depressant effects of temazepam. Use with caution.

▶ Lower doses are usually effective in elderly patients because of decreased elimination.
▶ Assist elderly patients with ambulation and activities of daily living, especially when therapy starts or dosage increases.

Patient teaching
▶ Inform patient that long-term use raises the risk of physical and psychological dependence.
▶ Instruct patient to consult prescriber before changing drug regimen.
▶ As needed, encourage safety measures to prevent injury, such as gradual position changes and assisted ambulation.
▶ Stress the risk of excessive CNS depression if drug is taken with alcohol.
▶ Tell patient that rebound insomnia may occur after stopping drug.
▶ Caution women to immediately notify prescriber about planned, suspected, or known pregnancy.

▶ tetracaine hydrochloride
Pontocaine, Pontocaine HCl

Pharmacologic classification:
ester local anesthetic

Therapeutic classification:
local anesthetic

Pregnancy risk category C

How supplied
Available by prescription only
Injection: 0.2%, 0.3%, 1%
Ophthalmic solution: 0.5%
Topical solution: 2%

Indications and dosages
Dosage for adults varies according to extent of block needed.

Low spinal (saddle) block in vaginal delivery
Adults: 2 to 5 mg (0.2 to 0.5 ml) as a 1% solution to be diluted with 10% dextrose.

Block of perineum
Adults: 5 mg (0.5 ml) as a 1% solution.

Block of perineum and legs
Adults: 10 mg (1 ml) as a 1% solution.

Block up to the costal margin
Adults: 15 to 20 mg (1.5 to 2 ml) as a 1% solution.

Anesthesia of the eye
Adults: 1 or 2 drops of a 0.5% solution.

Anesthesia of the larynx, trachea, or esophagus
Adults: Total dose shouldn't exceed 20 mg (8 ml of a 0.25% solution or 4 ml of a 0.5% solution).

◊ **Dosage adjustment.** Debilitated, geriatric, acutely ill, and obstetric patients should receive reduced dosages, along with patients who have increased abdominal pressure.

Pharmacodynamics
Local anesthetic action: Tetracaine blocks the generation and conduction of nerve impulses by increasing the threshold for electrical excitation in the nerve, by slowing propagation of the nerve impulse, and by reducing the rate of the action potential.

Pharmacokinetics
Absorption: Depends on dose, concentration, route of administration, and vascularity of tissue.

Distribution: Depending on the route, anesthetics are distributed to some extent to all tissues.

Metabolism: Metabolized by plasma esterase.

Excretion: Excreted mainly by the kidneys.

Contraindications and precautions
Contraindicated in patients hypersensitive to tetracaine hydrochloride, other local anesthetics of the ester type, p-aminobenzoic acid or its derivatives, and any ingredient in the formulation.

Use cautiously in patients with abnormal or low plasma esterase concentrations.

Interactions
Drug-drug
Cholinesterase inhibitors: prolonged ocular anesthesia and increased risk of toxicity. Use together cautiously.

CNS depressants: may cause additive CNS effects. Reduce dosage of CNS depressant.

Sulfonamides: tetracaine inhibits sulfonamide action. Don't use tetracaine in patients who need a sulfonamide.

Effects on diagnostic tests
None reported.

Adverse reactions
CNS: anxiety, nervousness, *seizures* followed by drowsiness.
CV: *arrhythmias, bradycardia, cardiac arrest,* edema, hypotension, myocardial depression.
EENT: blurred vision, burning or red eyes, tinnitus, transient stinging.
GI: nausea, vomiting.

Reactions may be *common,* uncommon, *life-threatening,* or COMMON AND LIFE-THREATENING.

Respiratory: *respiratory arrest, status asthmaticus.*
Skin: dermatologic reactions.
Other: *anaphylactoid reactions.*

Overdose and treatment
Acute emergencies typically stem from high plasma levels. Toxic reactions usually involve the CNS and CV systems.

To treat toxic reactions, immediately establish and maintain a patent airway or administer controlled ventilation with oxygen. If necessary, give drugs to control seizures. Give I.V. fluids, vasopressors, or both as needed to treat circulatory depression. Consider endotracheal intubation if you can't sustain a patent airway or if patient needs prolonged ventilatory support.

Special considerations
▶ Keep resuscitative equipment readily available when administering tetracaine.
▶ Use the smallest dose and lowest concentration needed to produce the desired effect.
▶ Monitor patient's blood pressure during spinal anesthesia.
▶ Protect drug from light, and store at 36° to 46° F (2° to 8° C).

Breast-feeding patients
▶ No data exist to demonstrate whether tetracaine appears in breast milk. Use cautiously in breast-feeding women.

Pediatric patients
▶ Safety and effectiveness haven't been established.

Geriatric patients
▶ Give reduced dosages to elderly patients.

Patient teaching
▶ After using ophthalmic product, caution patient not to rub or touch the affected eye until anesthesia has worn off.
▶ After using anesthetic in the mouth or throat, tell patient not to eat for 1 hour.
▶ Instruct patient not to chew food or gum while numbness persists to prevent biting the tongue or mucosa.
▶ Tell patient that anesthetized part of the body may temporarily lose feeling and motor activity.

▶ thiethylperazine maleate
Norzine, Torecan

Pharmacologic classification:
phenothiazine

Therapeutic classification:
antiemetic

Pregnancy risk category X

How supplied
Injection: 5 mg/ml
Tablets: 10 mg

Indications and dosages
Nausea and vomiting
Adults: 10 mg P.O. or I.M., once daily, b.i.d., or t.i.d.

Pharmacodynamics
Antiemetic action: Unknown. Probably acts on the chemoreceptor trigger zone to inhibit nausea and vomiting.

Pharmacokinetics
Absorption: Effects occur within 30 minutes after oral delivery.
Distribution: Unknown.
Metabolism: Unknown.

Excretion: Effects persist for 4 hours.

Contraindications and precautions

Contraindicated in pregnant patients, comatose patients, patients hypersensitive to phenothiazines, and patients with severe CNS depression or hepatic disease.

Use cautiously in patients hypersensitive to aspirin or tartrazine.

Interactions
Drug-drug

Antacids: inhibited absorption of oral phenothiazines. Separate antacid and phenothiazine doses by at least 2 hours.
Anticholinergics, including antidepressants, antiparkinsonians: increased anticholinergic activity and increased risk of pseudoparkinsonian symptoms. Use together cautiously.
Barbiturates: may decrease phenothiazine effect. Monitor patient for decreased antiemetic effect.

Effects on diagnostic tests

Drug may alter immunologic urine pregnancy test results.

Adverse reactions

CNS: confusion (especially in elderly patients), dizziness, EEG changes, *extrapyramidal symptoms,* pseudoparkinsonism, sedation.
CV: ECG changes, *orthostatic hypotension,* tachycardia.
EENT: *blurred vision, ocular changes.*
GI: *constipation, dry mouth,* increased appetite.
GU: dark urine, gynecomastia, inhibited ejaculation, menstrual irregularities, *urine retention.*

Hematologic: *agranulocytosis, transient leukopenia.*
Hepatic: cholestatic jaundice.
Metabolic: hyperprolactinemia, weight gain.
Skin: allergic reactions, *mild photosensitivity.*

Overdose and treatment

Overdose may cause severe extrapyramidal symptoms, hypotension, and sedation. CNS depression may lead to coma.

Treatment is symptomatic and supportive. Anticholinergic antiparkinsonians may be useful in controlling extrapyramidal symptoms. Avoid epinephrine and CNS stimulants that may cause seizures. Exchange transfusions may be useful, but hemodialysis isn't.

Special considerations

▶ Don't give drug by I.V. route because it may cause severe hypotension.
▶ Use drug only when vomiting can't be controlled by other measures or when only a few doses are needed.
▶ For nausea and vomiting from anesthesia and surgery, give deep I.M. injection shortly before or when terminating anesthesia.
▶ Monitor patient closely for adverse effects. If extrapyramidal symptoms occur, decrease dosage.
▶ If drug gets on skin, wash it off at once to prevent contact dermatitis.
▶ Torecan may contain tartrazine, to which some people are allergic.

Breast-feeding patients

▶ No data exist to demonstrate whether drug appears in breast milk. Breast-feeding isn't recommended during therapy.

Reactions may be *common,* uncommon, *life-threatening,* or COMMON AND LIFE-THREATENING.

Pediatric patients
▶ Safety and efficacy haven't been established in children under age 12.

Patient teaching
▶ Warn patient about possible hypotension, suggest that she stay in bed for 1 hour after receiving drug.
▶ Caution patient to avoid hazardous tasks until full CNS effects of drug are known.
▶ Instruct patient to immediately notify prescriber about decreased urine output, visual changes, and CNS effects.

▶ thiopental sodium
Pentothal

Pharmacologic classification:
barbiturate

Therapeutic classification:
anesthetic

Controlled substance schedule III

Pregnancy risk category C

How supplied
Available by prescription only
Injection: 250-mg (2.5%), 400-mg (2% or 2.5%), 500-mg (2.5%) syringes; 500-mg (2.5%), 1-g (2.5%), 2.5-g (2.5%), 5-g (2.5%), 1-g (2%), 2.5-g (2%), 5-g (2%) kits
Rectal suspension: 2-g disposable syringe (400 mg/g of suspension)

Indications and dosages
Reduction of intraoperative increase in intracranial pressure
Adults: 1.5 to 3.5 mg/kg intermittent I.V. bolus.

General anesthetic for short-term procedures
Adults and children: 2 to 4 ml 2.5% solution (50 to 100 mg) given I.V. for induction and repeated as a maintenance dose. Dosage must be individualized.
Seizures after anesthesia
Adults: 50 to 125 mg (2 to 5 ml 2.5% solution) I.V.
Basal anesthesia by rectal administration
Adults and children: 30 mg/kg P.R.

Pharmacodynamics
Anesthetic action: Thiopental produces anesthesia by direct depression of the polysynaptic midbrain reticular activating system. It decreases presynaptic (via decreased neurotransmitter release) and postsynaptic excitation. These effects may result from increased GABA levels, enhanced GABA effects, or a direct effect on GABA receptor sites.

Pharmacokinetics
Absorption: Thiopental I.V. produces peak brain levels in 10 to 20 seconds. Depth of anesthesia may increase for up to 40 seconds. Consciousness returns in 20 to 30 minutes.
Distribution: Drug is distributed throughout the body; highest initial level occurs in vascular areas of the brain, primarily gray matter; drug is 80% protein-bound. Redistribution of drug is primarily responsible for its short duration of action.
Metabolism: Drug is metabolized extensively but slowly in the liver.
Excretion: Unchanged thiopental isn't excreted in significant amounts; duration of action depends on tissue redistribution.

◇ Available in Canada only   *Unlabeled use

Contraindications and precautions
Contraindicated in patients hypersensitive to drug, in patients who can't have general anesthesia, and in patients with acute intermittent or variegate porphyria but not in other porphyrias. Don't use rectal form in patients with ulcerative, bleeding rectal lesions or tumors of the lower bowel or in those undergoing rectal surgery.

Use cautiously in patients with respiratory, cardiac, circulatory, renal, or hepatic dysfunction; severe anemia; shock; myxedema; or status asthmaticus (use extreme caution) because drug may worsen these conditions. Also use cautiously in breast-feeding patients and in patients with hypotension, Addison's disease, myasthenia gravis, or increased intracranial pressure.

Interactions
Drug-drug
Antihistamines, benzodiazepines, hypnotics, local anesthetics, opioids, phenothiazines, sedatives: potentiated or additive CNS depressant effects. Monitor patient closely.
Antihypertensives: increased risk of hypotension. Monitor blood pressure closely.

Drug-lifestyle
Alcohol use: increased CNS depressant effects. Discourage concurrent use.

Effects on diagnostic tests
None reported.

Adverse reactions
CNS: anxiety, dose-dependent alteration in EEG patterns, prolonged somnolence, restlessness, retrograde amnesia.
CV: *arrhythmias,* hypotension, *myocardial depression,* peripheral vascular collapse, tachycardia, thrombophlebitis.
GI: abdominal pain, cramping, diarrhea, nausea, rectal bleeding (rectal form), vomiting.
Respiratory: *apnea, bronchospasm,* coughing, hiccups, *laryngospasm, respiratory depression,* sneezing.
Skin: local irritation, necrosis from extravasation (unlikely at levels less than 2.5%), pain, swelling, ulceration.
Other: *allergic reactions,* gangrene after intra-arterial injection, shivering.

Overdose and treatment
Overdose may cause respiratory depression, respiratory arrest, hypotension, and shock.

Treat supportively, using mechanical ventilation if needed. Give I.V. fluids or vasopressors (dopamine, phenylephrine) for hypotension. Monitor vital signs closely.

Special considerations
▶ Keep resuscitation equipment readily available.
▶ Give a small test dose (25 to 75 mg) before I.V. use to assess tolerance or unusual sensitivity.
▶ During I.V. use, don't mix thiopental with solutions of succinylcholine, tubocurarine, or atropine. However, they can be given concomitantly.
▶ Monitor patient closely for signs of respiratory depression.
▶ Discontinue drug if patient develops peripheral vascular col-

lapse, respiratory arrest, or hypersensitivity.

Pediatric patients
▶ Use drug cautiously in children.

Geriatric patients
▶ Lower dosages may be indicated for elderly patients.

Patient teaching
▶ Caution patient to avoid alcohol and other CNS depressants after drug administration.
▶ Advise patient to avoid hazardous tasks until full CNS effects of drug are known.
▶ Tell patient to report adverse reactions.

▶ tiludronate disodium
Skelid

Pharmacologic classification:
bisphosphonate analogue

Therapeutic classification:
antihypercalcemic

Pregnancy risk category C

How supplied
Available by prescription only
Tablets: 200 mg

Indications and dosages
Paget's disease
Adults: 400 mg P.O. with 6 to 8 oz (180 to 240 ml) of water taken once daily, 2 hours before or after meals, for 3 months.

Pharmacodynamics
Antihypercalcemic action: Tiludronate is thought to suppress bone resorption by reducing osteoclastic activity. It appears to inhibit osteo-

clasts by inhibiting the osteoclastic proton pump and by disrupting the cytoskeletal ring structure, possibly by inhibiting protein-tyrosine-phosphatase, thus leading to detachment of osteoclasts from the bone surface.

Pharmacokinetics
Absorption: Bioavailability on an empty stomach is 8%. Food and beverages other than water can reduce bioavailability by up to 90%.
Distribution: Drug is widely distributed in bone and soft tissue. Protein-binding is about 90%, mainly to albumin.
Metabolism: Tiludronate doesn't appear to be metabolized.
Excretion: Drug is excreted mainly in urine. Mean plasma half-life is 150 hours.

Contraindications and precautions
Contraindicated in patients hypersensitive to any component of drug and in patients with creatinine clearance below 30 ml/minute.

Use cautiously in patients with upper GI disease, such as dysphagia, esophagitis, esophageal ulcer, hiatal hernia, or gastric ulcer.

Interactions
Drug-drug
Aluminum antacids, calcium supplements, magnesium antacids: may dramatically reduce tiludronate bioavailability when given 1 hour before tiludronate. Don't give these drugs within 2 hours of tiludronate.
Aspirin: may decrease tiludronate bioavailability by up to half when taken within 2 hours after dose. Don't give aspirin within 2 hours of drug.

Indomethacin: may increase tiludronate bioavailability. Dosage adjustment may be needed.

Drug-food
Any food: delays drug absorption. Don't give drug within 2 hours of meals.
Beverages other than plain water: may reduce drug absorption. Don't give with drug.

Effects on diagnostic tests
None reported.

Adverse reactions
CNS: anxiety, dizziness, headache, insomnia, involuntary muscle contractions, paresthesia, somnolence, vertigo.
CV: chest pain, edema, hypertension.
EENT: cataracts, conjunctivitis, glaucoma, pharyngitis, rhinitis, sinusitis.
GI: anorexia, constipation, diarrhea, dry mouth, dyspepsia, flatulence, gastritis, nausea, tooth disorder, vomiting.
Metabolic: hyperparathyroidism, vitamin D deficiency.
Musculoskeletal: arthralgia, arthrosis, back pain.
Respiratory: bronchitis, coughing, crackles.
Skin: diaphoresis, pruritus.
Other: *whole body pain.*

Overdose and treatment
No specific information is available. Use standard treatment for hypocalcemia or renal insufficiency, if they occur. Dialysis isn't helpful.

Special considerations
▶ Drug should be given to patients with Paget's disease who have serum alkaline phosphatase level at least twice the upper limit of normal or who are symptomatic or at risk for future complications of disease.
▶ Correct hypocalcemia and other disturbances of mineral metabolism (such as vitamin D deficiency) before therapy starts.
▶ Give drug for 3 months to assess response.

Breast-feeding patients
▶ No data exist to demonstrate whether drug appears in breast milk. Use cautiously in breast-feeding women.

Pediatric patients
▶ Safety and effectiveness in children haven't been established.

Geriatric patients
▶ Plasma levels may be higher in elderly people, but dosage adjustment typically isn't needed.

Patient teaching
▶ Tell patient to take drug with 6 to 8 oz (180 to 240 ml) of water.
▶ Instruct patient not to take drug within 2 hours of eating or taking a calcium supplement, aspirin, or indomethacin.
▶ Advise patient to maintain adequate vitamin D and calcium intake.
▶ If patient takes an aluminum- or a magnesium-containing antacid, caution her to wait 2 hours after taking tiludronate.

▶ timolol maleate
Blocadren, Timoptic, Timoptic-XE

Pharmacologic classification:
beta blocker

Therapeutic classification:
adjunct in MI, antiglaucoma, antihypertensive

Pregnancy risk category C

How supplied
Available by prescription only
Ophthalmic gel: 0.25%, 0.5%
Ophthalmic solution: 0.25%, 0.5%
Tablets: 5 mg, 10 mg, 20 mg

Indications and dosages
Migraine headache
Adults: 10 mg P.O. daily b.i.d., then increased to 20 mg. Or 30 mg/day (10 mg P.O. in the morning and 20 mg P.O. in the evening).
Angina*
Adults: 15 to 45 mg/day P.O. in three divided doses.
◻ DOSAGE ADJUSTMENT. Patients with renal or hepatic impairment may need dosage adjustment.

Pharmacodynamics
Antiglaucoma action: Beta-blocking action of timolol decreases production of aqueous humor, thereby decreasing intraocular pressure.
Antihypertensive action: Exact mechanism is unknown. Timolol may reduce blood pressure by blocking adrenergic receptors (thus decreasing cardiac output), by decreasing sympathetic outflow from the CNS, and by suppressing renin release.
Antimigraine action: Unknown.

Protective action after MI: Exact mechanism by which timolol decreases mortality after MI is unknown. Timolol produces a negative chronotropic and inotropic effects; this decrease in heart rate and myocardial contractility results in reduced myocardial oxygen consumption.

Pharmacokinetics
Absorption: About 90% of an oral dose is absorbed from the GI tract. Plasma levels peak in 1 to 2 hours.
Distribution: After oral administration, drug is distributed throughout the body. Depending on assay method used, 10% to 60% of drug is protein-bound.
Metabolism: About 80% of a dose is metabolized in the liver to inactive metabolites.
Excretion: Drug and its metabolites are excreted primarily in urine; half-life is about 4 hours. After topical application to the eye, effects last up to 24 hours.

Contraindications and precautions
Contraindicated in patients with bronchial asthma, severe COPD, sinus bradycardia and heart block more than first degree, cardiogenic shock, heart failure, or hypersensitivity to drug.

Use cautiously in patients with diabetes, hyperthyroidism, or respiratory disease (especially nonallergic bronchospasm or emphysema). Use oral form cautiously in patients with compensated heart failure and hepatic or renal disease. Use ophthalmic form cautiously in patients with cerebrovascular insufficiency.

◇ Available in Canada only   *Unlabeled use

Interactions
Drug-drug
Antihypertensives: When used as an antihypertensive, timolol may potentiate antihypertensive effects. Monitor blood pressure closely.

Beta-adrenergic blockers, xanthines: Timolol may antagonize the effects of these drugs. Monitor patient closely.

Calcium channel blockers, cardiac glycosides: cardiac arrhythmias may occur. Monitor patient's ECG frequently.

Fentanyl, general anesthetics: Patients receiving ophthalmic or oral timolol may experience excessive hypotension. Monitor blood pressure closely.

NSAIDs: antihypertensive effects may be antagonized. Monitor blood pressure closely.

Phenothiazines: Timolol may increase plasma phenothiazine level. Adjust dosage as needed.

Effects on diagnostic tests
None reported.

Adverse reactions
CNS: confusion, depression, dizziness, fatigue, hallucinations, lethargy, nightmares.
CV: *arrhythmias, bradycardia, cardiac arrest, CVA, heart block, heart failure,* hypotension, peripheral vascular disease, palpitations.
EENT: blepharitis, conjunctivitis, decreased corneal sensitivity with long-term use, diplopia, keratitis, minor eye irritation, ptosis, visual disturbance.
GI: diarrhea, nausea, vomiting.
GU: increased BUN.
Hematologic: decreased hemoglobin levels and hematocrit.
Metabolic: hyperglycemia, hyperkalemia, hyperuricemia.

Respiratory: asthma attacks in patients with history of asthma, **bronchospasm,** dyspnea, increased airway resistance, pulmonary edema.
Skin: pruritus.

Overdose and treatment
Overdose may cause severe hypotension, bradycardia, heart failure, and bronchospasm.

After acute ingestion, induce emesis or perform gastric lavage; give activated charcoal to reduce absorption. Subsequent treatment is usually symptomatic and supportive.

Special considerations
▶ Drug is also used to treat hypertension and glaucoma and to reduce the risk of reinfarction or death after MI.
▶ Although controversial, ophthalmic timolol may need to be discontinued 48 hours before surgery because systemic absorption occurs.
▶ Monitor patient for excessive hypotension.

Breast-feeding patients
▶ Timolol appears in breast milk. Because of the risk of serious adverse reactions in breast-fed infants, an alternative feeding method is recommended during therapy.

Pediatric patients
▶ Safety and efficacy in children haven't been established; use drug only if potential benefit outweighs risk.

Geriatric patients
▶ Elderly patients may require lower oral maintenance doses of timo-

lol because of increased bioavailability or delayed metabolism.
▶ Elderly patients may experience enhanced adverse effects.
▶ Use cautiously because half-life may be prolonged in elderly patients.

Patient teaching
▶ If patient uses ophthalmic form, teach proper administration method.
▶ Instruct patient to invert ophthalmic gel container once before each use.
▶ Instruct patient to administer other ophthalmic drugs at least 10 minutes before the ophthalmic gel.
▶ Warn patient not to touch dropper to eye or surrounding tissue.
▶ Instruct patient to lightly press lacrimal sac with a fingertip after instilling eyedrops to decrease systemic absorption.

▶ tizanidine hydrochloride
Zanaflex

Pharmacologic classification:
alpha₂ agonist

Therapeutic classification:
muscle relaxant

Pregnancy risk category C

How supplied
Tablets: 4 mg

Indications and dosages
Acute and intermittent increase in muscle tone from spasticity
Adults: initially, 4 mg P.O. q 6 to 8 hours, p.r.n. to a maximum of three doses in 24 hours. Dosage can be increased gradually in 2- to 4-mg increments. Maximum, 36 mg/day.

◻ DOSAGE ADJUSTMENT. If patient has renal failure, reduce dosage. If higher dosages are needed, increase individual doses rather than frequency.

Pharmacodynamics
Muscle relaxant action: Unknown. Acts as an alpha₂ agonist. May reduce spasticity by increasing presynaptic inhibition of motor neurons at the level of the spinal cord.

Pharmacokinetics
Absorption: almost completely absorbed after oral administration. Plasma levels peak in 1½ hours.
Distribution: widely distributed throughout the body; 30% bound to plasma proteins.
Metabolism: undergoes extensive first-pass metabolism in the liver. Metabolites are inactive.
Excretion: Half-life is about 2½ hours.

Contraindications and precautions
Contraindicated in patients hypersensitive to drug.
Use cautiously in patients who take antihypertensives, in patients with renal or hepatic impairment, and in elderly patients.

Interactions
Drug-drug
Antihypertensives, other alpha₂ agonists (such as clonidine): may cause hypotension. Monitor patient closely. Don't use with other alpha₂ agonists.
Baclofen, benzodiazepines, other CNS depressants: additive CNS depressant effects. Avoid concomitant use.

Oral contraceptives: decreased tizanidine clearance. Decrease tizanidine dosage as needed.

Drug-lifestyle
Alcohol use: increased CNS depression. Discourage concomitant use.

Effects on diagnostic tests
None reported.

Adverse reactions
CNS: *asthenia, dizziness,* dyskinesia, hallucinations, nervousness, *sedation, somnolence,* speech disorder.
CV: *hypotension.*
EENT: amblyopia, pharyngitis, rhinitis.
GI: constipation, *dry mouth,* vomiting.
GU: urinary frequency, *urinary tract infection.*
Hepatic: elevated liver function test results, hepatic injury.
Other: infection, flulike syndrome.

Overdose and treatment
Overdose may cause severe respiratory depression with Cheyne-Stokes respiration.

Treatment is supportive and symptomatic. Use gastric lavage and forced diuresis as needed.

Special considerations
▶ Obtain baseline liver function test results before treatment; at 1, 3, and 6 months during treatment; and periodically thereafter.
▶ Because of its short duration of effect, give drug at times when relief of spasticity is most important.
▶ Hypotension is common, especially 2 to 3 hours after giving a dose.

▶ Sedation may interfere with everyday activity.
▶ Hallucinations may occur during the first 6 weeks of therapy.
▶ If patient has renal impairment, assess her for increased adverse effects, such as dry mouth, somnolence, asthenia, and dizziness; they may indicate an overdose.

Pregnant patients
▶ Drug should be used in pregnancy only if the benefit to mother justifies the risk to fetus.

Breast-feeding patients
▶ No data exist to demonstrate whether drug appears in breast milk.

Pediatric patients
▶ Safety and effectiveness in children haven't been established.

Geriatric patients
▶ Use cautiously in elderly patients because clearance is decreased.

Patient teaching
▶ Inform patient that orthostatic hypotension can be minimized by rising slowly and avoiding sudden position changes.
▶ Caution patient to avoid hazardous activities until full CNS effects of drug are known; it may cause drowsiness.
▶ Tell patient to avoid alcohol during therapy.

▶ tocainide hydrochloride
Tonocard

Pharmacologic classification:
local anesthetic (amide type)

Therapeutic classification:
ventricular antiarrhythmic

Pregnancy risk category C

How supplied
Available by prescription only
Tablets: 400 mg, 600 mg

Indications and dosages
Trigeminal neuralgia*
Adults: 20 mg/kg/day P.O. t.i.d.
Myotonic dystrophy*
Adults: 800 to 1,200 mg/day P.O.
◩ DOSAGE ADJUSTMENT. Patients with impaired renal or hepatic function may be adequately treated with less than 1,200 mg/day.

Pharmacodynamics
Analgesic action: Unknown.
Antiarrhythmic action: Tocainide is structurally similar to lidocaine and possesses similar electrophysiologic and hemodynamic effects. A class IB antiarrhythmic, it suppresses automaticity and shortens the effective refractory period and action potential duration of His-Purkinje fibers and suppresses spontaneous ventricular depolarization during diastole. Conductive atrial tissue and AV conduction aren't affected significantly at therapeutic levels. Unlike quinidine and procainamide, tocainide doesn't significantly alter hemodynamics when given as usual doses. Tocainide affects the conduction system, inhibiting reentry mechanisms and stopping ventricular ar-rhythmias; these effects may be more pronounced in ischemic tissue. Tocainide doesn't cause a significant negative inotropic effect. Its direct cardiac effects are less potent than those of lidocaine.

Pharmacokinetics
Absorption: Drug is rapidly and completely absorbed from the GI tract; unlike lidocaine, it undergoes negligible first-pass effect in the liver. Serum levels peak 30 minutes to 2 hours after oral administration. Bioavailability is nearly 100%.
Distribution: Tocainide's distribution is only partially known. However, it appears to be distributed widely and apparently crosses the blood-brain barrier and placenta in animals; however, it is less lipophilic than lidocaine. Only about 10% to 20% of the drug is bound to plasma protein.
Metabolism: Drug is apparently metabolized in the liver to inactive metabolites.
Excretion: Drug is excreted in urine as unchanged drug and inactive metabolites. About 30% to 50% of an oral dose is excreted in urine as metabolites. Elimination half-life is about 11 to 23 hours, with an initial biphasic plasma level decline similar to that of lidocaine. Half-life may be prolonged in patients with renal or hepatic insufficiency. Urine alkalinization may substantially decrease the amount of unchanged drug excreted in urine.

Contraindications and precautions
Contraindicated in patients hypersensitive to lidocaine or other amide-type local anesthetics and in

those with second- or third-degree AV block who don't have an artificial pacemaker.

Use cautiously in patients with heart failure, diminished cardiac reserve, bone marrow failure, cytopenia, or impaired renal or hepatic function.

Interactions
Drug-drug
Allopurinol: increased allopurinol effects. Dosage adjustment may be needed.
Antiarrhythmics: tocainide may cause additive, synergistic, or antagonistic effects. Use together cautiously.
Cimetidine, rifampin: may decrease elimination half-life and bioavailability of tocainide. Dosage adjustment may be needed.
Lidocaine: possible CNS toxicity. Use together cautiously.
Metoprolol: may cause additive effects on cardiac index, left ventricular function, and pulmonary wedge pressure. Monitor patient for decreased myocardial contractility and bradycardia.

Effects on diagnostic tests
None reported.

Adverse reactions
CNS: confusion, *dizziness,* drowsiness, fatigue, headache, *lightheadedness,* paresthesia, *tremor, vertigo.*
CV: *bradycardia, heart failure,* hypotension, *new or worsened arrhythmias,* palpitations.
EENT: blurred vision, tinnitus.
GI: anorexia, diarrhea, *nausea, vomiting.*
Hematologic: *blood dyscrasias.*
Hepatic: abnormal liver function test results, *hepatitis.*

Respiratory: pneumonitis, pulmonary edema, pulmonary fibrosis, *respiratory arrest.*
Skin: diaphoresis, rash.

Overdose and treatment
Overdose typically causes extension of common adverse reactions, particularly CNS and GI reactions.

Treatment includes symptomatic and supportive care. In acute overdose, induce emesis or perform gastric lavage. Respiratory depression requires immediate attention and maintenance of a patent airway with ventilatory assistance, if needed. Treat seizures with small incremental doses of a benzodiazepine, such as diazepam, or a short- or an ultrashort-acting barbiturate, such as pentobarbital or thiopental.

Special considerations
▶ Drug is usually used to treat symptomatic ventricular arrhythmias.
▶ Drug is considered an oral lidocaine and may be used to ease transition from I.V. lidocaine to oral antiarrhythmic therapy.
▶ Obtain a chest X-ray if patient has pulmonary symptoms.
▶ Monitor blood drug levels; therapeutic levels range from 4 to 10 mcg/ml.
▶ Monitor periodic blood counts for the first 3 months of therapy and frequently thereafter. Perform CBC promptly if patient develops signs of infection.
▶ Expect adverse effects to be frequent and problematic.
▶ Observe patient for tremors—a possible sign that maximum safe dose has been reached.

Breast-feeding patients
▶ Safety in nursing mothers hasn't been established. An alternative feeding method is recommended during therapy.

Geriatric patients
▶ Use with caution in elderly patients; increased serum drug levels and toxicity are more likely. Monitor patient carefully.
▶ Elderly patients are more likely to become dizzy; provide assistance with walking.

Patient teaching
▶ Tell patient that she may take drug with food to lessen GI upset.
▶ Caution patient to avoid hazardous activities until full effects of drug are known; it may cause drowsiness or dizziness.
▶ Urge patient to notify prescriber about unusual bleeding or bruising, evidence of infection (such as fever, sore throat, stomatitis, chills) or pulmonary symptoms (such as cough, wheezing, or exertional dyspnea).

▶ tolmetin sodium
Tolectin, Tolectin DS

Pharmacologic classification: *NSAID*

Therapeutic classification: *anti-inflammatory, nonnarcotic analgesic*

Pregnancy risk category C

How supplied
Capsules: 400 mg
Tablets: 200 mg, 600 mg

Indications and dosages
Rheumatoid arthritis, osteoarthritis, juvenile rheumatoid arthritis
Adults: initially, 400 mg P.O. t.i.d. Usual dosage ranges from 600 to 1800 mg daily in 3 divided doses. Maximum, 1800 mg/day.
Children age 2 or older: initially, 20 mg/kg/day in three or four divided doses. Usual dosage ranges from 15 to 30 mg/kg/day in three or four divided doses.

Pharmacodynamics
Analgesic and anti-inflammatory actions: Although exact mechanism of action is unknown, inhibited prostaglandin synthesis may be responsible for anti-inflammatory effects. Drug also seems to possess analgesic and antipyretic activity.

Pharmacokinetics
Absorption: Drug is absorbed rapidly from the GI tract; levels peak in 30 to 60 minutes.
Distribution: Drug is highly protein-bound.
Metabolism: Drug is metabolized in the liver.
Excretion: Essentially all of the drug is excreted in urine within 24 hours as an inactive metabolite or conjugates of tolmetin. Elimination is biphasic, with a rapid phase and 1- to 2-hour half-life followed by a slower phase with about a 5-hour half-life.

Contraindications and precautions
Contraindicated in breast-feeding women, in patients hypersensitive to drug, and in patients for whom aspirin or NSAIDs cause acute asthma attack, urticaria, or rhinitis.

 Use cautiously in patients with renal or cardiac disease, GI bleed-

---

ing, history of peptic ulcer, hypertension, and conditions predisposing to fluid retention.

Interactions
Drug-drug
ACE inhibitors: decreased effects of these drugs and an increased risk of renal failure. Use cautiously together, and adjust dosage as needed.

Anticoagulants, thrombolytics: may be potentiated by platelet-inhibiting effect of tolmetin, thus increasing the risk of bleeding. Use cautiously together.

Aspirin: may decrease plasma tolmetin levels. Dosage adjustment may be needed.

Beta blockers: decreased effects of these drugs. Use cautiously together, and adjust dosage as needed.

Drugs that are highly protein-bound (phenytoin, salicylates, sulfonylureas, sulfonamides, warfarin): may cause displacement of either drug and increase adverse effects. Monitor effects of both drugs.

GI-irritating drugs (such as antibiotics, corticosteroids, NSAIDs): may potentiate adverse GI effects of tolmetin. Use together with caution.

Methotrexate: may increase methotrexate toxicity. Avoid concurrent use. If given together, monitor patient closely.

Strontium-89: increased risk of bleeding. Monitor patient closely for evidence of bleeding.

Drug-food
Any food: may delay and decrease tolmetin absorption. Separate administration times.

Effects on diagnostic tests
Tolmetin falsely elevates results of urine protein (pseudoproteinuria) in tests that rely on acid precipitation, such as those using sulfosalicylic acid. Drug doesn't interfere with tests for proteinuria using dye-impregnated reagent strips, such as Albustix and Unistix.

Adverse reactions
CNS: asthenia, depression, dizziness, drowsiness, headache.
CV: chest pain, edema, hypertension.
EENT: tinnitus, visual disturbances.
GI: abdominal pain, anorexia, constipation, diarrhea, dyspepsia, epigastric distress, flatulence, *nausea,* occult blood loss, peptic ulceration, vomiting.
GU: UTI.
Hematologic: decreased hemoglobin and hematocrit, elevated BUN.
Metabolic: weight gain, weight loss.
Skin: irritation.
Other: *anaphylaxis.*

Overdose and treatment
Overdose may cause dizziness, drowsiness, mental confusion, and lethargy.

To treat tolmetin overdose, immediately induce emesis or perform gastric lavage. Then give activated charcoal. Provide symptomatic and supportive measures, including respiratory support and correction of fluid and electrolyte imbalances. Monitor laboratory values and vital signs closely. Alkalinization of urine via sodium bicarbonate ingestion may enhance renal excretion of tolmetin.

Special considerations
▸ Give drug on an empty stomach for maximum absorption. If needed, however, it can be given with meals to lessen GI upset.
▸ Therapeutic effect usually occurs within 1 week of therapy.
▸ Monitor cardiopulmonary status and vital signs closely, especially heart rate and blood pressure.
▸ Assess renal function periodically during therapy; monitor fluid intake, output, and daily weight. Note characteristics of edema.
▸ Evaluate patient's response to drug as evidenced by relief of symptoms.

Breast-feeding patients
▸ Drug appears in breast milk and may adversely affect neonates; avoid use in breast-feeding women.

Pediatric patients
▸ Safety and effectiveness in children under age 2 haven't been established.

Patient teaching
▸ Instruct patient to follow prescribed regimen and recommended schedule of follow-up.
▸ Explain that therapeutic effects may occur in 1 week but could take 2 to 4 weeks.
▸ Caution patient not to take OTC medications (such as NSAIDs) and herbal remedies without consulting prescriber.
▸ Instruct patient to routinely check weight and to report any significant weight gain or loss within 1 week.
▸ Tell patient to report adverse reactions.

▸ **tramadol hydrochloride**
Ultram

Pharmacologic classification: *synthetic derivative*

Therapeutic classification: *analgesic*

Pregnancy risk category C

How supplied
Available by prescription only
Tablets: 50 mg

Indications and dosages
Moderate to moderately severe pain
Adults: 50 to 100 mg P.O. q 4 to 6 hours, p.r.n. Maximum, 400 mg/ day.
▨ DOSAGE ADJUSTMENT. If patient's creatinine clearance is below 30 ml/ minute, increase dosing interval to q 12 hours. Maximum, 200 mg/day. If patient has cirrhosis, recommended dosage is 50 mg q 12 hours.

Pharmacodynamics
Analgesic action: Mechanism of action is unknown. Drug is a central-acting synthetic analgesic not chemically related to opiates; however, it probably binds to opioid receptors and inhibits reuptake of norepinephrine and serotonin.

Pharmacokinetics
Absorption: Tramadol is almost completely absorbed. Mean absolute bioavailability of a 100-mg dose is about 75%. Plasma levels peak at about 2 hours.
Distribution: Drug is about 20% bound to plasma protein; it may cross the blood-brain barrier.

Metabolism: Tramadol is extensively metabolized.
Excretion: About 30% of a dose is excreted unchanged in urine and 60% as metabolites. Half-life of drug is about 6 to 7 hours.

Contraindications and precautions

Contraindicated in patients hypersensitive to drug and patients with acute intoxication from alcohol, hypnotics, central-acting analgesics, opioids, or psychotropic drugs.

Use cautiously in patients at risk for seizures or respiratory depression; in those with increased intracranial pressure or head injury, acute abdominal conditions, and impaired renal or hepatic function; and in patients physically dependent on opioids.

Interactions
Drug-drug

Carbamazepine: increases tramadol metabolism. Patients receiving long-term carbamazepine therapy at doses up to 800 mg daily may require up to twice the recommended tramadol dosage.
CNS depressants: additive effects. Use together with caution, and decrease tramadol dosage as needed.
MAO inhibitors, neuroleptic drugs, selective serotonin reuptake inhibitors: increased risk of seizures. Monitor patient closely.

Effects on diagnostic tests

None reported.

Adverse reactions

CNS: anxiety, *asthenia, CNS stimulation,* confusion, coordination disturbance, *dizziness,* euphoria, *headache,* malaise, nervousness, sleep disorder, ***seizures, somnolence, vertigo.***
CV: vasodilation.
EENT: visual disturbances.
GI: abdominal pain, anorexia, *constipation,* diarrhea, dyspepsia, dry mouth, flatulence, *nausea, vomiting.*
GU: increased creatinine clearance, menopausal symptoms, proteinuria, urine retention, urinary frequency.
Hematologic: decreased hemoglobin levels.
Hepatic: elevated liver enzymes.
Musculoskeletal: hypertonia.
Respiratory: ***respiratory depression.***
Skin: diaphoresis, *pruritus,* rash.

Overdose and treatment

Overdose may cause respiratory depression and seizures. Because naloxone will reverse some, but not all, of the symptoms, supportive therapy is recommended. Hemodialysis removes only a small percentage of drug.

Special considerations

▶ For better analgesic effect, give drug before patient has intense pain.
▶ For chronic pain, higher doses may be used for therapeutic value.
▶ Monitor patient's CV and respiratory status, and stop drug if respirations decrease, rate is below 12 breaths/minute, or patient shows signs of respiratory depression.
▶ Constipation is a common adverse effect and may require laxative therapy.
▶ Prolonged use may lead to physical and psychological dependence

---

and tolerance. However, it may be milder than with opioids.

‣ Drug may reduce seizure threshold; monitor high-risk patients closely.

‣ Because dependence similar to that with codeine or dextropropoxyphene may occur, assess patient for possible abuse.

Breast-feeding patients

‣ Use of drug in breast-feeding women isn't recommended because safety hasn't been established.

Pediatric patients

‣ Safety and effectiveness in children under age 16 haven't been established.

Geriatric patients

‣ Use cautiously in elderly patients because serum levels are slightly elevated and elimination half-life is prolonged.

‣ Don't exceed 300 mg/day in patients over age 75.

Patient teaching

‣ Instruct patient to take drug only as prescribed and not to alter dosage or interval without consulting prescriber.

‣ Caution patient to avoid activities requiring mental alertness and coordination until full CNS effects of drug are known.

‣ Advise patient not to take OTC medications or herbal remedies without consulting prescriber.

‣ trazodone hydrochloride
Desyrel

Pharmacologic classification: *triazolopyridine derivative*

Therapeutic classification: *antidepressant*

Pregnancy risk category C

How supplied
Available by prescription only
Dividose tablets: 150 mg, 300 mg
Tablets: 50 mg, 100 mg
Tablets (film-coated): 50 mg, 100 mg

Indications and dosages
Depression
Adults: initially, 150 mg/day in divided doses. Increase as needed by 50 mg/day q 3 to 4 days. Average dosage is 150 mg to 400 mg/day. Maximum, 400 mg/day in outpatients and 600 mg/day in hospitalized patients.
Aggressive behavior*
Adults: 50 mg P.O. b.i.d.
Panic disorder*
Adults: 300 mg P.O. daily.

Pharmacodynamics
Antidepressant action: Trazodone probably inhibits reuptake of norepinephrine and serotonin in CNS nerve terminals (presynaptic neurons), which increases the level and enhances the activity of these neurotransmitters in the synaptic cleft. Trazodone shares some properties with tricyclic antidepressants: It has antihistaminic, alpha-blocking, analgesic, and sedative effects as well as relaxant effects on skeletal muscle. Unlike tricyclic antidepressants, however, tra-

zodone counteracts the pressor effects of norepinephrine, has limited CV effects and, in particular, has no direct quinidine-like effects on cardiac tissue. It also causes fewer anticholinergic effects.

Pharmacokinetics
Absorption: Drug is well absorbed from the GI tract after oral administration. Effects peak in 1 hour. Taking drug with food delays absorption, extends peak effect to 2 hours, and increases the amount of drug absorbed by 20%.
Distribution: Drug is widely distributed and doesn't concentrate in any particular tissue. Small amounts may appear in breast milk. About 90% is protein-bound. Proposed therapeutic drug levels haven't been established. Steady state plasma levels occur in 3 to 7 days, and therapeutic activity starts in 7 days.
Metabolism: Trazodone is metabolized by the liver. More than 75% of metabolites are excreted within 3 days.
Excretion: Drug is mostly excreted in urine; the rest is excreted in feces via the biliary tract.

Contraindications and precautions
Contraindicated during the initial recovery phase after MI and in patients hypersensitive to drug.

Use cautiously in patients with cardiac disease and in patients at risk for suicide.

Interactions
Drug-drug
Antihypertensives (such as clonidine, guanabenz, guanadrel, guanethidine, methyldopa, reserpine), CNS depressants (such as analgesics, anesthetics, barbiturates, narcotics, tranquilizers): Additive effects likely. Monitor patient closely.
Digoxin, phenytoin: increased serum digoxin and phenytoin levels. Monitor drug levels, and adjust dosages as needed.

Drug-herb
St. John's wort: increased risk of serotonin syndrome. Discourage concurrent use.

Drug-lifestyle
Alcohol use: may worsen CNS depression. Discourage concurrent use.

Effects on diagnostic tests
None reported.

Adverse reactions
CNS: anger, *dizziness, drowsiness,* confusion, fatigue, ***generalized tonic-clonic seizures,*** headache, hostility, insomnia, nervousness, nightmares, tremor, vivid dreams, weakness.
CV: hypertension, orthostatic hypotension, prolonged conduction time on ECG, shortness of breath, syncope, tachycardia.
EENT: blurred vision, nasal congestion, tinnitus.
GI: anorexia, constipation, dry mouth, dysgeusia, nausea, vomiting.
GU: decreased libido, hematuria, priapism that may lead to impotence, urine retention.
Hematologic: anemia, decreased WBC counts.
Hepatic: elevated liver function test results.

Metabolic: altered serum glucose levels.
Skin: diaphoresis, rash, urticaria.

Overdose and treatment

Overdose most often causes drowsiness and vomiting. It also may cause orthostatic hypotension, tachycardia, headache, shortness of breath, dry mouth, and incontinence. Coma may occur as well.

Treatment is symptomatic and supportive and includes maintaining the airway and stabilizing vital signs and fluid and electrolyte balance. Induce emesis if gag reflex is intact; follow with gastric lavage (begin with lavage if emesis isn't feasible) and activated charcoal to prevent further absorption. Forced diuresis may aid elimination. Dialysis is usually ineffective.

Special considerations

▶ Drug has been used to treat painful diabetic neuropathy and other types of chronic pain.
▶ Consider patient to have an inherent risk of suicide until depression improves significantly. Closely monitor high-risk patients during early drug therapy. Provide the smallest quantity of drug consistent with good management.
▶ Giving trazodone with food helps prevent GI upset and increases absorption.
▶ To obtain 50-mg, 75-mg, or 100-mg doses, break 150-mg tablet along the score mark.
▶ Monitor blood pressure because hypotension may occur.
▶ Drug has fewer adverse cardiac and anticholinergic effects than tricyclic antidepressants.
▶ Offer ice or sugarless chewing gum or hard candy to help relieve dry mouth.

▶ To minimize drowsiness, give most of the daily dose at bedtime or reduce the dosage.
▶ Tolerance to adverse effects (especially sedation) usually develops after 1 to 2 weeks of treatment.
▶ Adverse reactions increase with higher doses and are most common when dosage exceeds 300 mg/day.
▶ Drug may cause prolonged painful erections that may need surgical correction. Consider carefully before prescribing for men, especially those who are sexually active.
▶ Don't withdraw drug abruptly, but discontinue it at least 48 hours before surgical procedures.
▶ Trazodone has also been used in alcohol dependence to decrease tremors and relieve anxiety and depression. Dosage ranges from 50 to 75 mg/day.

Pediatric patients

▶ Drug isn't recommended for children under age 18.

Geriatric patients

▶ Elderly patients usually require lower initial doses.
▶ Elderly patients are more likely to develop adverse reactions, but drug may be preferred in these patients because it has fewer adverse cardiac effects.

Patient teaching

▶ Tell patient to take drug exactly as prescribed and not to discontinue drug abruptly or double it after missing a dose.
▶ Tell patient that full effects may take up to 2 weeks to occur.
▶ Suggest taking drug with food or milk if it causes stomach upset.

▶ To minimize dizziness, tell patient to lie down for about 30 minutes after taking drug and to avoid sudden postural changes, especially rising to upright position.
▶ Advise patient to increase fluids to avoid constipation.
▶ Tell patient to avoid alcohol during therapy.
▶ Suggest sugarless chewing gum or hard candy to relieve a dry mouth.
▶ Caution patient to avoid hazardous activities until full effects of drug are known; explain that it may cause drowsiness or dizziness.
▶ Advise patient to immediately notify prescriber about prolonged, painful erections, sexual dysfunction, dizziness, fainting, or a rapid heartbeat. Urge patient to regard an involuntary erection lasting more than 1 hour as a medical emergency.

▶ **triazolam**
Halcion

Pharmacologic classification:
benzodiazepine

Therapeutic classification:
sedative-hypnotic

Controlled substance schedule IV

Pregnancy risk category X

How supplied
Available by prescription only
Tablets: 0.125 mg, 0.25 mg

Indications and dosages
Insomnia
Adults: 0.125 to 0.25 mg P.O. h.s. Maximum, 0.5 mg and only for exceptional patients.

◹ Dosage adjustment. For elderly patients, give 0.125 mg P.O. h.s. Maximum, 0.25 mg.

Pharmacodynamics
Sedative-hypnotic action: Drug depresses the CNS at the limbic and subcortical levels of the brain. It produces a sedative-hypnotic effect by potentiating the effect of the neurotransmitter GABA on its receptor in the ascending reticular activating system, which increases inhibition and blocks both cortical and limbic arousal.

Pharmacokinetics
Absorption: Drug is well absorbed through the GI tract after oral administration. Levels peak in 1 to 2 hours. Onset of action occurs in 15 to 30 minutes.
Distribution: Drug is distributed widely throughout the body and is 90% protein-bound.
Metabolism: Drug is metabolized in the liver, primarily to inactive metabolites.
Excretion: Metabolites of triazolam are excreted in urine. Half-life of triazolam ranges from about 1½ to 5½ hours.

Contraindications and precautions
Contraindicated in pregnant patients and patients hypersensitive to benzodiazepines. Also, contraindicated in patients taking ketoconazole, itraconazole, nefazodone, or any other drug that impairs oxidative metabolism of triazolam by cytochrome P-450 3A.

Use cautiously in patients with impaired renal or hepatic function, chronic pulmonary insufficiency, sleep apnea, depression, suicidal

---

tendencies, or a history of drug abuse.

Interactions
Drug-drug
Cimetidine, disulfiram, isoniazid, oral contraceptives: decreased hepatic triazolam metabolism, which increases plasma levels. Dosage adjustment may be needed.

CNS depressants, such as antidepressants, antihistamines, barbiturates, general anesthetics, MAO inhibitors, opioids, phenothiazines: potentiated CNS depressant effects. Use together cautiously.

Erythromycin: decreased triazolam clearance. Dosage adjustment may be needed.

Haloperidol: decreased serum haloperidol levels. Dosage adjustment may be needed.

Levodopa: benzodiazepines may decrease levodopa effects. Dosage adjustment may be needed.

Drug-food
Grapefruit juice: increases drug levels. Discourage consumption.

Drug-lifestyle
Alcohol use: potentiates CNS depressant effects and enhances amnestic effects. Discourage concurrent use.

Heavy smoking: accelerates triazolam metabolism, thus lowering effectiveness. Discourage concurrent use.

Effects on diagnostic tests
None reported.

Adverse reactions
CNS: amnesia, ataxia, depression, *dizziness, drowsiness, headache,* lack of coordination, lightheadedness, mental confusion,

minor changes in EEG patterns, nervousness, rebound insomnia.
GI: nausea, vomiting.
Hepatic: elevated liver enzymes.
Other: physical or psychological dependence.

Overdose and treatment
Overdose may cause somnolence, confusion, hypoactive reflexes, dyspnea, labored breathing, hypotension, bradycardia, slurred speech, unsteady gait or impaired coordination and, ultimately, coma.

Support blood pressure and respiration until drug effects subside; monitor vital signs. Flumazenil may be useful. Mechanical ventilation via endotracheal tube may be needed. Use I.V. fluids and vasopressors, such as dopamine and phenylephrine, to treat hypotension. If patient is conscious, induce emesis. Perform gastric lavage if ingestion was recent and patient has an endotracheal tube. After emesis or lavage, give activated charcoal with a cathartic. Don't give barbiturates if excitation occurs. Dialysis is of limited value.

Special considerations
▶ Onset of sedation or hypnosis is rapid; keep patient in bed.
▶ Monitor hepatic function studies to detect toxicity.
▶ Store drug in a cool, dry place away from light.

Breast-feeding patients
▶ Triazolam appears in breast milk. Infant may become sedated, have trouble feeding, or lose weight. Avoid use during breast-feeding.

Pediatric patients
▶ Safe use in patients under age 18 hasn't been established.

Geriatric patients
▶ Elderly patients are more susceptible to CNS depressant effects. Use drug with caution.
▶ Assist elderly patients with ambulation and daily activities when therapy starts and dosage increases.

Patient teaching
▶ Tell patient about risk of physical and psychological dependence.
▶ Instruct patient not to alter dosage or take OTC drugs without consulting prescriber.
▶ As needed, teach safety measures to prevent injury.
▶ Suggest other measures to promote sleep, such as warm fluids, quiet music, no alcohol near bedtime, regular exercise, and a regular sleep pattern.
▶ Tell patient that rebound insomnia may occur after stopping drug.
▶ Instruct patient not to take drug when she doesn't have time for a full night's sleep and full drug clearance before activities resume.
▶ Urge women to immediately notify prescriber about planned, suspected, or known pregnancy.

▶ trifluoperazine hydrochloride
Apo-Trifluoperazine◇, Novo-Flurazine◇, Solazine◇, Stelazine, Terfluzine◇

Pharmacologic classification: *phenothiazine (piperazine derivative)*

Therapeutic classification: *antiemetic, antipsychotic*

Pregnancy risk category C

How supplied
Available by prescription only
Injection: 2 mg/ml
Oral concentrate: 10 mg/ml
Tablets (regular and film-coated): 1 mg, 2 mg, 5 mg, 10 mg

Indications and dosages
Nausea and vomiting
Adults: 1 to 2 mg P.O. b.i.d., p.r.n.
◻ DOSAGE ADJUSTMENT. Reduce initial dosage for elderly, debilitated, or emaciated patients, and adjust upward gradually.

Pharmacodynamics
Antiemetic action: Antiemetic effects are attributed to dopamine receptor blockade in the medullary chemoreceptor trigger zone.
Antipsychotic action: Trifluoperazine probably causes postsynaptic blockade of CNS dopamine receptors, thereby inhibiting dopamine-mediated effects.
Other actions: Trifluoperazine has many other central and peripheral effects; it produces alpha and ganglionic blockade and counteracts histamine- and serotonin-mediated activity. It has less sedative and au-

tonomic activity than aliphatic and piperidine phenothiazines.

Pharmacokinetics

Absorption: Rate and extent of absorption vary with route of administration. Oral tablet absorption is erratic and variable, with onset of action ranging from ½ to 1 hour. Oral concentrate absorption is much more predictable. I.M. drug is absorbed rapidly.

Distribution: Drug is distributed widely in the body, including breast milk, and is 91% to 99% protein-bound. Effects peak in 2 to 4 hours, and steady state serum levels occur in 4 to 7 days.

Metabolism: Drug is metabolized extensively by the liver, but no active metabolites are formed. Duration of action is about 4 to 6 hours.

Excretion: Drug is mostly excreted in urine; some is excreted in feces via the biliary tract.

Contraindications and precautions

Contraindicated in comatose patients, patients hypersensitive to phenothiazines, and patients with CNS depression, bone marrow suppression, or liver damage.

Use cautiously in elderly or debilitated patients, patients exposed to extreme heat, and patients with CV disease, seizure disorders, glaucoma, or prostatic hyperplasia.

Interactions
Drug-drug

Antacids that contain aluminum or magnesium, antidiarrheals, phenobarbital: Pharmacokinetic alterations and decreased response to trifluoperazine. Dosage adjustment may be needed.

Antiarrhythmics, such as disopyramide, procainamide, quinidine: increased risk of cardiac arrhythmias and conduction defects. Use together cautiously.

Anticholinergics, such as antidepressants, antihistamines, antiparkinsonians, atropine, MAO inhibitors, meperidine, phenothiazines: increased risk of oversedation, paralytic ileus, visual changes, and severe constipation. Use together cautiously.

Appetite suppressants and sympathomimetics, including ephedrine, epinephrine, phenylephrine, phenylpropanolamine: may decrease stimulatory and pressor effects of these drugs. Using epinephrine for pressor effect in a patient taking trifluoperazine may cause epinephrine reversal or further lowering of blood pressure. Use together with extreme caution, and assess patient's vital signs frequently.

Beta blockers: may inhibit trifluoperazine metabolism, increasing plasma levels and toxicity. Dosage adjustment may be needed.

Bromocriptine: Trifluoperazine may antagonize therapeutic effects of bromocriptine on prolactin secretion. Monitor patient closely.

Central-acting antihypertensives, such as clonidine, guanabenz, guanadrel, guanethidine, methyldopa, reserpine: Trifluoperazine may inhibit blood pressure response. Monitor blood pressure closely.

CNS depressants, including analgesics, barbiturates, epidural anesthetics, general anesthetics, magnesium sulfate (parenteral), opioids, spinal anesthetics, tranquilizers: increased risk of oversedation, respiratory depression, and hypotension. Use together cautiously.

High-dose dopamine: may decrease vasoconstricting effects and effectiveness. Dosage adjustment may be needed.

Levodopa: increased levodopa toxicity by dopamine blockade. Use together with extreme caution.

Lithium: increased risk of severe neurologic toxicity, encephalitis-like syndrome, and decreased response to trifluoperazine. Use together with extreme caution.

Metrizamide: increased risk of seizures. Use together cautiously.

Nitrates: may increase risk of hypotension. Use together cautiously.

Phenytoin: inhibited phenytoin metabolism and increased risk of toxicity. Use together with extreme caution.

Propylthiouracil: increased risk of agranulocytosis. Monitor patient's CBC closely.

Drug-food

Caffeine: increases trifluoperazine metabolism and decreases therapeutic effects. Discourage concurrent use.

Drug-lifestyle

Alcohol use: additive effects. Discourage concurrent use.

Heavy smoking: increases trifluoperazine metabolism and decreases therapeutic effects. Discourage concurrent use.

Sun exposure: increased risk of photosensitivity. Urge precautions.

Effects on diagnostic tests

Drug causes false-positive test results for urine porphyrins, urobilinogen, amylase, and 5-hydroxyindoleacetic acid levels from darkening of urine by metabolites. It also causes false-positive urine pregnancy results in tests using human chorionic gonadotropin as the indicator.

Adverse reactions

CNS: dizziness, drowsiness, *extrapyramidal symptoms,* fatigue, headache, insomnia, pseudoparkinsonism, *tardive dyskinesia.*

CV: ECG changes, *orthostatic hypotension,* tachycardia.

EENT: *blurred vision,* ocular changes.

GI: *constipation, dry mouth,* nausea.

GU: gynecomastia, menstrual irregularities, inhibited lactation, *urine retention.*

Hematologic: *agranulocytosis, transient leukopenia.*

Hepatic: cholestatic jaundice, elevated liver function test results.

Metabolic: weight gain.

Skin: allergic reactions, pain at I.M. injection site, *photosensitivity,* rash, sterile abscess.

Overdose and treatment

Overdose may cause CNS depression characterized by deep, unarousable sleep (possibly coma), hypotension or hypertension, extrapyramidal symptoms, dystonia, abnormal involuntary muscle movements, agitation, seizures, arrhythmias, ECG changes, hypothermia or hyperthermia, and autonomic nervous system dysfunction.

Treatment is symptomatic and supportive and includes maintaining vital signs, airway, stable body temperature, and fluid and electrolyte balance. Don't induce vomiting. Drug inhibits cough reflex, raising the risk of aspiration.

Reactions may be *common*, uncommon, *life-threatening*, or COMMON AND LIFE-THREATENING.

Perform gastric lavage, and then give activated charcoal and sodium chloride cathartics. Dialysis is usually ineffective. Regulate body temperature as needed. Treat hypotension with I.V. fluids. Don't give epinephrine. Give parenteral diazepam or barbiturates for seizures; parenteral phenytoin (1 mg/kg at a rate adjusted to blood pressure) for arrhythmias; and benztropine (1 to 2 mg) or parenteral diphenhydramine (10 to 50 mg) for extrapyramidal symptoms.

Special considerations
▶ Drug is traditionally used for anxiety, schizophrenia, and other psychotic disorders.
▶ Other drugs, such as benzodiazepines, are preferred for treating anxiety. When drug is given for anxiety, don't exceed 6 mg daily for longer than 12 weeks. Some clinicians recommend using drug only for psychosis.
▶ Solution for injection may be slightly discolored. Don't use excessively discolored or precipitated solution.
▶ Give I.M. injection deep into upper outer quadrant of buttock. Massaging the area after injection may prevent abscesses. I.M. injection may cause skin necrosis.
▶ Monitor patient's blood pressure before and after parenteral administration.
▶ Oral forms may cause stomach upset. Give drug with food or fluid.
▶ Protect liquid form from light.
▶ Dilute concentrate in 60 to 120 ml (2 to 4 oz) of liquid, preferably water, carbonated drink, fruit juice, tomato juice, milk, or pudding.

▶ Shake concentrate before giving it.
▶ Drug may cause pink to brown discoloration of urine or blue-gray skin.
▶ Drug commonly causes extrapyramidal symptoms and photosensitivity reactions.
▶ Skin contact with liquid or injectable forms may cause a rash.
▶ Worsening angina has been reported in patients receiving trifluoperazine; however, ECG reactions are less common than with other phenothiazines.
▶ Assess patient at least once every 6 months for abnormal body movements.
▶ Abrupt withdrawal of long-term therapy may cause gastritis, nausea, vomiting, dizziness, tremor, feeling of warmth or cold, diaphoresis, tachycardia, headache, insomnia, anorexia, muscle rigidity, altered mental status, and evidence of autonomic instability.

Breast-feeding patients
▶ Drug may appear in breast milk. Potential benefits to mother should outweigh risk to infant.

Pediatric patients
▶ Not recommended for children under age 6.

Geriatric patients
▶ Elderly patients tend to need lower dosage, adjusted to effect.
▶ Adverse effects, especially extrapyramidal symptoms (particularly tardive dyskinesia) and hypotension, are more likely to develop in elderly patients.

Patient teaching
▶ Explain the risks of dystonic reactions, akathisia, and tardive

dyskinesia, and tell patient to report abnormal body movements.
▶ Caution patient to avoid hazardous activities until full effects of drug are known; it may cause sedation.
▶ Tell patient to minimize sun exposure and to wear sunscreen when going outdoors.
▶ Caution patient to avoid extremely hot or cold baths and exposure to temperature extremes, sunlamps, and tanning beds; drug may cause thermoregulatory changes.
▶ Tell patient to take drug exactly as prescribed and not to discontinue drug abruptly or double the dose to make up for a missed one.
▶ Tell patient to avoid alcohol and other drugs that may cause excessive sedation.
▶ Suggest ice chips, artificial saliva, or sugarless gum or hard candy to help relieve a dry mouth.
▶ Explain that many drug interactions are possible. Tell patient not to take other prescribed drugs, OTC medications, or herbal remedies without consulting prescriber.
▶ Tell patient that adverse reactions may be alleviated by reduced dosage.
▶ Instruct patient to notify prescriber about difficulty urinating, sore throat, dizziness, or fainting. Warn men about possible inhibited ejaculation.

▶ **trimipramine maleate**
Surmontil

Pharmacologic classification:
tricyclic antidepressant

Therapeutic classification:
antianxiety drug, antidepressant

Pregnancy risk category C

How supplied
Available by prescription only
Capsules: 25 mg, 50 mg, 100 mg

Indications and dosages
Peptic ulcer disease
Adults: 25 to 50 mg P.O. daily.
◧ DOSAGE ADJUSTMENT. For elderly and adolescent patients, give 50 to 100 mg/day P.O.

Pharmacodynamics
Antidepressant action: Drug probably equally inhibits reuptake of norepinephrine and serotonin in CNS nerve terminals (presynaptic neurons), which results in increased levels and enhanced activity of these neurotransmitters in the synaptic cleft. Trimipramine also has anxiolytic effects and inhibits gastric acid secretion.
Antiulcer action: Unknown. Drug may inhibit H_2 receptors.

Pharmacokinetics
Absorption: Drug is absorbed rapidly from the GI tract after oral administration.
Distribution: Drug is distributed widely in the body and is 90% protein-bound. Effects peak in 2 hours; steady state occurs within 7 days.
Metabolism: Drug is metabolized by the liver. Significant first-pass effect may explain varying serum

levels in different patients taking the same amount.

Excretion: Drug is mostly excreted in urine; some is excreted in feces via the biliary tract.

Contraindications and precautions

Contraindicated during acute recovery phase of MI, in patients hypersensitive to drug, and in patients who took an MAO inhibitor within 14 days.

Use cautiously in adolescents, in elderly or debilitated patients, in patients taking thyroid hormones, and in patients with CV disease, increased intraocular pressure, hyperthyroidism, impaired hepatic function, a history of seizures, urine retention, or angle-closure glaucoma.

Interactions
Drug-drug

Antiarrhythmics (disopyramide, procainamide, quinidine), thyroid hormones, pimozide: increased risk of cardiac arrhythmias and conduction defects. Monitor patient's ECG frequently.

Anticholinergics, such as antihistamines, antiparkinsonians, atropine, meperidine, phenothiazines: increased risk of oversedation, paralytic ileus, visual changes, and severe constipation. Use together cautiously.

Barbiturates: increased trimipramine metabolism and decreased efficacy. Dosage adjustment may be needed.

Beta blockers, cimetidine, methylphenidate, oral contraceptives, propoxyphene: may inhibit trimipramine metabolism, increasing plasma levels and toxicity. Monitor plasma levels frequently.

Central-acting antihypertensives, such as clonidine, guanabenz, guanadrel, guanethidine, methyldopa, reserpine: decreased hypotensive effects. Monitor blood pressure frequently.

CNS depressants, including analgesics, anesthetics, barbiturates, narcotics, tranquilizers: may cause oversedation. Use cautiously together.

Disulfiram, ethchlorvynol: possible delirium and tachycardia. Use cautiously together.

Haloperidol, phenothiazines: inhibited metabolism and increased blood levels of trimipramine. Dosage adjustment may be needed.

Metrizamide: increased risk of seizures. Use together cautiously.

Selective serotonin reuptake inhibitors, such as fluoxetine, paroxetine, sertraline: increased therapeutic and toxic effects of trimipramine. Monitor patient closely.

Sympathomimetics, including ephedrine, epinephrine, phenylephrine, phenylpropanolamine: may increase blood pressure. Monitor blood pressure frequently.

Warfarin: may increase PT and INR and cause bleeding. Assess patient closely, and monitor PT, PTT, and INR frequently.

Drug-lifestyle

Alcohol use: Additive effects are likely. Discourage concurrent use.

Heavy smoking: induces trimipramine metabolism and decreases efficacy. Discourage concurrent use.

Sun exposure: increased risk of photosensitivity. Urge precautions.

Effects on diagnostic tests
None reported.

Adverse reactions

CNS: agitation, anxiety, ataxia, confusion, delusions, *dizziness, drowsiness,* EEG changes, extrapyramidal symptoms, hallucinations, headache, insomnia, paresthesia, *seizures,* tremor, weakness.
CV: *arrhythmias, CVA, heart block,* hypertension, *MI, orthostatic hypotension,* prolonged conduction time on ECG, tachycardia.
EENT: *blurred vision,* mydriasis, tinnitus.
GI: anorexia, *constipation, dry mouth,* nausea, paralytic ileus, vomiting.
GU: *urine retention.*
Hematologic: altered PT and INR, decreased WBC counts.
Hepatic: elevated liver function test results.
Metabolic: altered serum glucose levels.
Skin: *diaphoresis,* photosensitivity, rash, urticaria.
Other: *hypersensitivity reaction.*

Overdose and treatment

The first 12 hours after acute ingestion are a stimulatory phase characterized by excessive anticholinergic activity (agitation, irritation, confusion, hallucinations, parkinsonian symptoms, seizure, urine retention, dry mucous membranes, pupillary dilation, constipation, and ileus). This is followed by CNS depressant effects, including hypothermia, decreased or absent reflexes, sedation, hypotension, cyanosis, and cardiac irregularities (including tachycardia, conduction disturbances, and quinidine-like effects on the ECG).

Severity of overdose is best indicated by prolongation of QRS interval beyond 100 milliseconds, which usually represents a serum level in excess of 1,000 ng/ml; serum levels are generally not helpful. Metabolic acidosis may follow hypotension, hypoventilation, and seizures.

Treatment is symptomatic and supportive and includes maintaining airway, stable body temperature, and fluid and electrolyte balance. Induce emesis with ipecac if patient is conscious; follow with gastric lavage and activated charcoal to prevent further absorption. Dialysis is of little use. Physostigmine given I.V. slowly has been used to reverse most of the CV and CNS effects of overdose. Treat seizures with parenteral diazepam or phenytoin; arrhythmias with parenteral phenytoin or lidocaine; and acidosis with sodium bicarbonate. Don't give barbiturates because they may enhance CNS and respiratory depression.

Special considerations

▶ Drug is typically used to treat depression. It may also be used to manage some types of chronic, severe, neurogenic pain.
▶ Consider patient to have an inherent risk of suicide until depression improves significantly. Monitor high-risk patients closely during early therapy.
▶ To reduce risk of intentional overdose, provide the smallest quantity of drug consistent with good management.
▶ Tolerance typically develops to sedative effects of drug.
▶ To reduce daytime sedation, give the full dose at bedtime.
▶ Drug may raise the risk of mania or hypomania in patients with cyclic disorders.
▶ Watch for bleeding because drug may alter PT and INR.

▶ Discontinue drug at least 48 hours before surgical procedures.
▶ Abrupt withdrawal of long-term therapy may cause nausea, headache, and malaise (which don't indicate addiction).

Geriatric patients
▶ Elderly patients may be more vulnerable to adverse cardiac effects.

Patient teaching
▶ Tell patient to take drug exactly as prescribed and not to stop taking it suddenly or double the dose after missing a dose.
▶ Explain that full effects of drug may not become apparent for 4 to 6 weeks after therapy begins.
▶ If drug is being taken for neuropathic pain, explain that effects may become apparent in about 1 week.
▶ Suggest taking drug with food or milk if it causes stomach upset.
▶ Advise patient to take full dose at bedtime to minimize daytime sedation.
▶ Caution patient to avoid hazardous activities until full effects of drug are known; explain that it may cause drowsiness or dizziness.
▶ Warn patient not to drink alcohol during therapy.
▶ Suggest ice or sugarless chewing gum or hard candy to relieve a dry mouth.
▶ To minimize dizziness, tell patient to lie down for about 30 minutes after each dose and to avoid abrupt position changes, especially when rising.
▶ Tell patient to promptly notify prescriber about confusion, movement disorders, rapid heartbeat, dizziness, fainting, or difficulty urinating.

▶ tubocurarine chloride
Tubarine ◇

Pharmacologic classification: *nondepolarizing neuromuscular blocker*

Therapeutic classification: *skeletal muscle relaxant*

Pregnancy risk category C

How supplied
Available by prescription only
Injection: 3 mg/ml parenteral

Indications and dosages
Adjunct to general anesthesia to induce skeletal muscle relaxation, facilitate intubation, and reduce fractures and dislocations
Dosage depends on anesthetic used, individual needs, and patient response. Dosages listed are representative and must be adjusted. Calculate at 0.165 mg/kg.
Adults: initially, 6 to 9 mg I.V. or I.M., followed by 3 to 4.5 mg in 3 to 5 minutes if needed. Additional 3-mg doses may be given, if needed, during prolonged anesthesia.
To assist with mechanical ventilation
Adults: initially, 0.0165 mg/kg I.V. or I.M. (average 1 mg), and then adjust subsequent doses to patient's response.
To weaken muscle contractions in pharmacologically or electrically induced seizures
Adults: initially, 0.165 mg/kg I.V. or I.M. slowly. As a precaution, start with 3 mg less than the calculated dose.

◇ Available in Canada only   *Unlabeled use

Pharmacodynamics

Skeletal muscle relaxant action:
Tubocurarine prevents acetylcholine from binding to receptors on motor end plate, thus blocking depolarization. Tubocurarine has histamine-releasing and ganglionic-blocking properties and is usually antagonized by anticholinesterase drugs.

Pharmacokinetics

Absorption: After I.V. injection, onset of muscle relaxation is rapid and peaks within 2 to 5 minutes. Duration is dose-related; effects usually begin to subside in 20 to 30 minutes. Paralysis may persist for 25 to 90 minutes. Subsequent doses have longer durations. After I.M. injection, onset of paralysis is unpredictable (10 to 25 minutes); duration is dose-related.
Distribution: After I.V. injection, drug is distributed in extracellular fluid and rapidly reaches its site of action. After tissue compartment is saturated, drug may persist in tissues for up to 24 hours; 40% to 45% is bound to plasma proteins, mainly globulins.
Metabolism: Tubocurarine undergoes n-demethylation in the liver.
Excretion: About 33% to 75% of a dose is excreted unchanged in urine in 24 hours; up to 11% is excreted in bile.

Contraindications and precautions

Contraindicated in patients hypersensitive to drug and in those for whom histamine release is hazardous (as in asthma).

Use cautiously in elderly or debilitated patients, in patients undergoing cesarean section, in patients with sulfite sensitivity (because some preparations contain sulfite), and in patients with impaired hepatic or pulmonary function, hypothermia, respiratory depression, myasthenia gravis, myasthenic syndrome of lung cancer or bronchiogenic carcinoma, dehydration, thyroid disorders, collagen diseases, porphyria, electrolyte disturbances, fractures, or muscle spasms.

Interactions

Drug-drug

Aminoglycoside antibiotics, beta blockers, calcium salts, clindamycin, depolarizing neuromuscular blockers, furosemide, general anesthetics, lincomycin, local anesthetics, magnesium salts (parenteral), nondepolarizing neuromuscular blockers, polymyxin antibiotics, potassium-depleting drugs, quinidine, quinine, thiazide diuretics, verapamil: may enhance or prolong tubocurarine-induced neuromuscular blockade. Monitor patient closely.
Opioid analgesics, quinidine, quinine: Respiratory depressant effects may be increased. Monitor respiratory status closely.

Effects on diagnostic tests

None reported.

Adverse reactions

CV: *arrhythmias, bradycardia, cardiac arrest,* hypotension.
EENT: increased salivation.
Musculoskeletal: idiosyncrasy, profound and prolonged muscle relaxation, residual muscle weakness.
Respiratory: *apnea, bronchospasm, respiratory depression.*
Other: *hypersensitivity reactions.*

Reactions may be *common*, uncommon, *life-threatening*, or COMMON AND LIFE-THREATENING.

Overdose and treatment

Overdose may cause apnea or prolonged muscle paralysis, which can be treated with controlled ventilation. Use a peripheral nerve stimulator to monitor effects and to determine nature and degree of blockade. Anticholinesterase drugs may antagonize tubocurarine. Atropine given before or with the antagonist counteracts its muscarinic effects.

Special considerations

▶ Drug doesn't affect consciousness or relieve pain; make sure patient receives appropriate analgesic or sedative.
▶ The margin of safety between therapeutic dose and dose that can cause respiratory paralysis is small.
▶ Allow succinylcholine effects to subside before giving tubocurarine.
▶ Decrease dosage if inhalation anesthetics are used.
▶ Assess baseline tests of renal function and serum electrolyte levels before drug administration. Electrolyte imbalance (particularly potassium and magnesium) can potentiate effects of drug.
▶ Tubocurarine is usually given by I.V. injection, which requires direct medical supervision. Give drug slowly over 60 to 90 seconds.
▶ Use only fresh solution. Discard if discolored.
▶ Don't mix with barbiturates or other alkaline solutions in the same syringe.
▶ If patient's veins are inaccessible, drug may be given I.M. in same dose as given I.V. Give drug by deep I.M. injection in deltoid muscle.

▶ Maintain airway, and keep emergency respiratory equipment readily available.
▶ Be prepared for endotracheal intubation, suction, or assisted or controlled respiration with oxygen. Keep atropine and the antagonists neostigmine or edrophonium (cholinesterase inhibitors) readily available. A nerve stimulator may be used to evaluate recovery from neuromuscular blockade.
▶ Muscle paralysis follows drug administration in this sequence: jaw muscles, levator eyelid muscles and other muscles of head and neck, limbs, intercostals and diaphragm, abdomen, trunk. Facial and diaphragm muscles recover first, then legs, arms, shoulder girdle, trunk, larynx, hands, feet, pharynx. Muscle function is usually restored within 90 minutes. Patient may find speech difficult until head and neck muscles recover.
▶ Measure and record intake and output.
▶ Monitor patient's blood pressure, vital signs, and airway until patient recovers from drug effects. Ganglionic blockade (hypotension), histamine liberation (increased salivation, bronchospasm), and neuromuscular blockade (respiratory depression) are known effects of tubocurarine.
▶ After neuromuscular blockade dissipates, watch for residual muscle weakness.
▶ Renal dysfunction prolongs drug action.
▶ Peristaltic action may be suppressed. Check for bowel sounds.
▶ Drug may also be used to diagnose myasthenia gravis. Test is considered positive if drug exaggerates muscle weakness.

Breast-feeding patients
▶ No data exist to demonstrate whether drug appears in breast milk. Use with caution in breast-feeding women.

Pediatric patients
▶ Administer cautiously to children.

Geriatric patients
▶ Administer cautiously to elderly patients.

Patient teaching
▶ Explain all procedures to the patient because she can still hear.

▶ **valproic acid**
Depakene, Epival ◊

▶ **divalproex sodium**
Depakote, Depakote Sprinkle

▶ **valproate sodium**
Depacon

Pharmacologic classification: *carboxylic acid derivative*

Therapeutic classification: *anticonvulsant*

Pregnancy risk category D

How supplied
Available by prescription only
valproic acid
Capsules: 250 mg
Syrup: 250 mg/5 ml
divalproex sodium
Capsules (sprinkle): 125 mg
Tablets (enteric-coated): 125 mg, 250 mg, 500 mg
valproate sodium
Injection: 5 ml single-dose vials

Indications and dosages
Migraine prophylaxis
Adults: 250 mg P.O. b.i.d. Some patients may benefit from up to 1,000 mg/day.

Pharmacodynamics
Anticonvulsant action: Unknown, although effects may result from increased brain levels of GABA, an inhibitory neurotransmitter. Valproic acid may decrease enzymatic catabolism of GABA. Therapeutic effects may require a week or more to begin, so valproic acid may be used with other anticonvulsants.
Antimigraine action: Unknown.

Pharmacokinetics
Absorption: Valproate sodium and divalproex sodium quickly convert to valproic acid after oral administration. Plasma levels peak in 1 to 4 hours for uncoated tablets, 3 to 5 hours for enteric-coated tablets, 15 minutes to 2 hours for syrup, and immediately for I.V. administration. Bioavailability is the same for all drug forms.
Distribution: Valproic acid is distributed rapidly throughout the body and is 80% to 95% protein-bound.
Metabolism: Valproic acid is metabolized by the liver.
Excretion: Valproic acid is excreted mainly in urine; some is excreted in feces and exhaled air. Drug appears in breast milk at 1% to 10% of serum levels.

Contraindications and precautions
Contraindicated in patients hypersensitive to drug. Don't give valproate sodium injection to patients

---

with hepatic disease or significant hepatic dysfunction.

Use cautiously in patients with a history of hepatic dysfunction. Children under age 2 have an increased risk of fatal hepatotoxicity. If benefits outweigh risks, give drug as single therapy.

Interactions
Drug-drug
Aspirin, heparin, NSAIDs, oral anticoagulants, thrombolytics: valproic acid may inhibit platelet aggregation. Monitor bleeding times closely.
Clonazepam: may cause absence seizures. Avoid concurrent use.
CNS depressants, MAO inhibitors: valproic acid may potentiate effects of these drugs. Monitor patient closely.
Felbamate, lamotrigine, salicylates: may increase valproate levels. Dosage adjustment may be needed.
Phenobarbital, phenytoin, primidone: Additive sedative effects because valproic acid increases serum levels. Monitor patient carefully.

Drug-lifestyle
Alcohol use: may decrease valproic acid effectiveness and increase adverse CNS effects. Discourage concurrent use.
Sun exposure: increased risk of photosensitivity reactions. Urge precautions.

Effects on diagnostic tests
Drug may cause false-positive test results for urine ketones.

Adverse reactions
CNS: aggressiveness, ataxia, behavioral deterioration, emotional upset, depression, dizziness, headache, hyperactivity, incoordination, muscle weakness, psychosis, *sedation,* tremor.
EENT: diplopia, nystagmus.
GI: anorexia, abdominal cramps, constipation, diarrhea, increased appetite, *indigestion, nausea, pancreatitis, vomiting.*
Hematologic: *bone marrow suppression,* bruising, eosinophilia, *hemorrhage,* increased bleeding time, *leukopenia,* petechiae, *thrombocytopenia.*
Hepatic: *elevated liver enzymes, toxic hepatitis.*
Metabolic: weight gain.
Skin: alopecia, *erythema multiforme,* photosensitivity, pruritus, rash.

Overdose and treatment
Overdose may cause somnolence and coma. To treat it, provide supportive care. Maintain adequate urinary output, and carefully monitor vital signs and fluid and electrolyte balance. Naloxone reverses CNS and respiratory depression but also may reverse anticonvulsant effects of valproic acid. Hemodialysis and hemoperfusion have been used.

Special considerations
▸ Drug is also administered to treat seizures, mania, and status epilepticus* refractory to I.V. diazepam.
▸ Doses of divalproex sodium are expressed as valproic acid.
▸ Evaluate patient's liver function, platelet count, PT, and INR at baseline and monthly for at least the first 6 months.
▸ Give oral form with food to minimize GI irritation. Enteric-coated form may be better tolerated.
▸ For I.V. use, dilute valproate sodium in at least 50 ml of com-

patible diluent, such as D_5W, normal saline solution, or lactated Ringer's solution.

▶ Use of valproate sodium injection for more than 14 days hasn't been studied. Switch to oral form as soon as possible. When switching from I.V. to oral therapy or vice versa, keep daily dosage and frequency the same.

▶ Therapeutic range of drug is 50 to 100 mcg/ml.

▶ Monitor plasma level and adjust dosage as needed.

▶ Tremors may indicate a need to reduce dosage.

▶ Because drug usually is given with other anticonvulsants, adverse reactions may not be caused by valproic acid alone.

▶ Don't withdraw drug abruptly.

Breast-feeding patients
▶ Valproic acid appears in breast milk at 1% to 10% of serum levels. An alternate feeding method is recommended during therapy.

Pediatric patients
▶ Valproic acid isn't recommended for children under age 2 because this group has the highest risk of adverse effects.

▶ Hyperexcitability and aggressiveness have occurred in a few children.

Geriatric patients
▶ Elderly patients eliminate drug more slowly and typically need a lower dosage.

Patient teaching
▶ Tell patient not to stop drug suddenly, not to alter dosage without consulting prescriber, and not to change brands or use a generic form without consulting prescriber.

▶ Tell patient to swallow tablets or capsules whole to avoid mucosal irritation. Suggest taking them with food if needed.

▶ Caution against taking drug with carbonated beverages because tablet may dissolve before being swallowed, causing irritation and unpleasant taste.

▶ Caution patient to avoid hazardous tasks until full CNS effects of drug are known. It may cause drowsiness and dizziness.

▶ Taking drug at bedtime may minimize CNS depression.

▶ Urge patient to avoid alcohol during therapy because it may decrease drug effectiveness and increase adverse CNS effects.

▶ Review adverse effects and evidence of hypersensitivity; tell patient to notify prescriber about them.

▶ If patient takes drug for a seizure disorder, urge him to wear or carry medical identification that reveals the seizure disorder and the drug therapy being taken for it.

▶ vecuronium bromide
Norcuron

Pharmacologic classification:
nondepolarizing neuromuscular blocker

Therapeutic classification:
skeletal muscle relaxant

Pregnancy risk category C

How supplied
Available by prescription only
Injection: 10 mg (with or without diluent), 20 mg (without diluent)

Indications and dosages
To provide adjunct to anesthesia, to facilitate intubation, to provide skeletal muscle relaxation during surgery or mechanical ventilation
Dosage depends on anesthetic used, individual needs, and response. Dosages are representative and must be individualized.
Adults and children age 10 and over: initially, 0.08 to 0.10 mg/kg as I.V. bolus. Higher initial doses (up to 0.3 mg/kg) may be used for rapid onset. During prolonged surgical procedures, give maintenance doses of 0.010 to 0.015 mg/kg starting 25 to 40 minutes after initial dose. They may be given q 12 to 15 minutes in patients receiving balanced anesthetic. Alternatively, 20 to 40 minutes after the initial dose, start a continuous infusion of 0.001 mg/kg/minute.

Pharmacodynamics
Skeletal muscle relaxant action: Vecuronium prevents acetylcholine from binding to receptors on motor end plates, thus blocking depolarization. Drug has minimum CV effects and doesn't alter heart rate or rhythm, systolic or diastolic blood pressure, cardiac output, systemic vascular resistance, or mean arterial pressure. It has few or no histamine-releasing properties.

Pharmacokinetics
Absorption: After I.V. administration of 0.08 to 0.1 mg/kg, action starts within 1 minute and peaks in 3 to 5 minutes. Duration is about 25 to 40 minutes depending on anesthetic used, dose size given, and number of doses given.
Distribution: After I.V. administration, drug is distributed in extracellular fluid and rapidly reaches its site of action. It's 60% to 90% plasma protein-bound. Volume of distribution is decreased in children under age 1 and may be decreased in elderly patients.
Metabolism: Drug undergoes rapid and extensive hepatic metabolism.
Excretion: Drug and its metabolites appear to be primarily excreted in feces via biliary elimination; it's also excreted in urine.

Contraindications and precautions
Contraindicated in patients hypersensitive to vecuronium and bromides.
    Use cautiously in elderly patients with hepatic disease, severe obesity, bronchogenic carcinoma, electrolyte disturbances, neuromuscular diseases, altered circulation caused by CV disease or edema.

Interactions
Drug-drug
Aminoglycosides, clindamycin, depolarizing neuromuscular blockers, furosemide, lincomycin, magnesium salts (parenteral), nondepolarizing neuromuscular blockers, polymyxin antibiotics, potassium-depleting drugs, quinidine, quinine, thiazide diuretics: may increase vecuronium-induced neuromuscular blockade. Use together with extreme caution.
Anticholinesterase drugs: may antagonize vecuronium effects. Use together with extreme caution.
General anesthetics: may increase neuromuscular blockade. Decrease dosage by 15%, especially with enflurane and isoflurane, and use together with extreme caution.

Opioid analgesics: may increase central respiratory depression. Monitor patient closely.

Effects on diagnostic tests
None reported.

Adverse reactions
Musculoskeletal: skeletal muscle weakness.
Respiratory: *prolonged, dose-related respiratory insufficiency or apnea.*

Overdose and treatment
Overdose may cause prolonged duration of neuromuscular blockade, skeletal muscle weakness, decreased respiratory reserve, low tidal volume, and apnea.

Treatment is supportive and symptomatic. Keep airway clear, and maintain adequate ventilation. Use peripheral nerve stimulator to determine and monitor degree of blockade. Give anticholinesterase drug (edrophonium, neostigmine, pyridostigmine) to reverse neuromuscular blockade and atropine or glycopyrrolate to overcome muscarinic effects.

Special considerations
▶ Drug doesn't relieve pain or affect consciousness and must be accompanied by adequate anesthesia. Assess patient's need for analgesic, anxiolytic, and sedative.
▶ Keep emergency resuscitation equipment immediately available.
▶ Assess serum electrolyte levels, acid-base balance, and renal and hepatic function before drug use.
▶ Reconstitute to 1 or 2 mg/ml using diluent supplied by manufacturer (bacteriostatic water for injection) or a compatible solution, such as normal saline solution,

D_5W, sterile water for injection, 5% dextrose in normal saline solution, or lactated Ringer's solution.
▶ After reconstitution, protect solution from light. Refrigerate or store at room temperature not above 86° F (30° C).
▶ Don't use discolored solution. If reconstituted with supplied bacteriostatic water, solution can be stored for 5 days. Otherwise, discard unused portion after 24 hours.
▶ Use rapid I.V. injection or I.V. infusion. Don't use I.M. route.
▶ Don't mix in same syringe or give through same needle as barbiturates or other alkaline solutions.
▶ After the procedure, monitor patient's vital signs at least every 15 minutes until stable, then every 30 minutes for next 2 hours.
▶ Monitor airway and pattern of respirations until patient recovers from drug effects. Expect ventilation problems in obese patients and those with myasthenia gravis or other neuromuscular disease.
▶ Evaluate recovery from neuromuscular blockade by checking strength of hand grip and ability to breathe naturally, to take deep breaths and cough, to keep eyes open, and to lift head with mouth closed.
▶ Peripheral nerve stimulator may be used to identify residual paralysis during recovery and is especially useful during administration to high-risk patients.

Breast-feeding patients
▶ No data exist to demonstrate whether drug appears in breast milk. Use cautiously in breast-feeding women.

Pediatric patients
▶ Diluent supplied by manufacturer contains benzyl alcohol, which isn't intended for newborns.
▶ Safety and efficacy haven't been established for infants less than 7 weeks old.
▶ Infants 7 weeks to 1 year old are more sensitive to neuromuscular blocking effects; less frequent administration may be needed.
▶ Higher-than-normal doses may be needed by children ages 1 to 9.

Geriatric patients
▶ Administer drugs cautiously to elderly patients.

Patient teaching
▶ Explain all events and procedures to patient because he can still hear.

▶ verapamil hydrochloride
Calan, Calan SR, Covera-HS, Isoptin, Isoptin SR, Verelan

Pharmacologic classification:
calcium channel blocker

Therapeutic classification:
antianginal, antihypertensive, antiarrhythmic

Pregnancy risk category C

How supplied
Available by prescription only
Capsules (sustained-release):
120 mg, 180 mg, 240 mg, 360 mg
Injection: 2.5 mg/ml
Tablets: 40 mg, 80 mg, 120 mg
Tablets (sustained-release):
120 mg, 180 mg, 240 mg

Indications and dosages
Recumbent nocturnal leg cramps*
Adults: 120 mg P.O. h.s. (regular-release tablets).
Migraine prophylaxis*
Adults: 40 to 80 mg P.O. t.i.d. to q.i.d. (regular-release tablets).
Cluster headaches*
Adults: initially, 120 mg P.O. b.i.d. (regular-release tablets).
Prinzmetal's (variant) angina, unstable angina, chronic stable angina
Adults: initially, 80 to 120 mg P.O. t.i.d. May increase at weekly intervals. Some patients need 480 mg/day.

Pharmacodynamics
Antianginal action: Verapamil reduces afterload, both at rest and with exercise, thereby decreasing myocardial oxygen consumption. It also decreases myocardial oxygen demand and cardiac work by exerting a negative inotropic effect, which reduces heart rate, relieves coronary artery spasm (via coronary artery vasodilation), and dilates peripheral vessels. The net result is relief of myocardial ischemia and pain. In patients with Prinzmetal's variant angina, verapamil inhibits coronary artery spasm, which increases myocardial oxygen delivery.
Antiarrhythmic action: Combined effects on the SA and AV nodes helps to manage arrhythmias. Drug's primary effect is on the AV node, where slowed conduction reduces the ventricular rate in atrial tachyarrhythmias and blocks reentry paths in paroxysmal supraventricular arrhythmias.
Antihypertensive action: Verapamil reduces blood pressure mainly by

---

dilating peripheral vessels. Its negative inotropic effect blocks reflex mechanisms that lead to increased blood pressure.

Antimigraine action: Unknown.

Pharmacokinetics

Absorption: Drug is absorbed rapidly and completely from the GI tract after oral administration; however, only about 20% to 35% of drug reaches systemic circulation because of a first-pass effect. Effects peak 1 to 2 hours after regular-release form and 4 to 8 hours after sustained-release form. Effects occur within minutes after I.V. injection and usually persist about 30 to 60 minutes, although they may last up to 6 hours. Therapeutic serum levels are 80 to 300 ng/ml.

Distribution: Steady state distribution volume in healthy adults ranges from about 4.5 to 7 L/kg but may increase to 12 L/kg in patients with hepatic cirrhosis. About 90% of circulating drug is bound to plasma proteins.

Metabolism: Drug is metabolized in the liver.

Excretion: Drug is excreted in urine as unchanged drug and active metabolites. Elimination half-life is normally 6 to 12 hours, although it may reach 16 hours in patients with hepatic cirrhosis. In infants, it may be 5 to 7 hours.

Contraindications and precautions

Contraindicated in patients hypersensitive to drug, in patients receiving beta blockers I.V., and in patients with severe left ventricular dysfunction, cardiogenic shock, second- or third-degree AV block or sick sinus syndrome (unless a functioning pacemaker is in place), atrial flutter or fibrillation with accessory bypass tract syndrome, severe heart failure (unless caused by verapamil), severe hypotension, or ventricular tachycardia.

Use cautiously in elderly patients and those with increased intracranial pressure or impaired renal or hepatic function.

Interactions

Drug-drug

Antihypertensives: increased risk of significant hypotension. Monitor blood pressure closely.

Beta blockers: additive effects may lead to heart failure, conduction disturbances, arrhythmias, and hypotension, especially with high beta-blocker doses, I.V. administration, or moderately severe to severe heart failure, severe cardiomyopathy, or recent MI. Use together with extreme caution.

Carbamazepine, cyclosporine: risk of increased serum levels and toxic effects of these drugs. Dosage adjustment may be needed.

Digoxin: serum digoxin levels may rise 50% to 75% during the first week of oral verapamil therapy. Dosage adjustment may be needed.

Disopyramide: increased negative inotropic effects. Monitor heart rate and blood pressure closely.

Drugs that attenuate alpha-adrenergic response (such as prazosin and methyldopa): may cause excessive blood pressure reduction. Monitor blood pressure closely.

Flecainide: additive negative inotropic effect and prolonged AV conduction. Monitor ECG closely.

Inhalation anesthetics: excessive CV depression. Use together cautiously.

Lithium: increased sensitivity to lithium effects. Use together cautiously.

Neuromuscular blockers: potentiated action of these drugs. Use together cautiously.

Phenobarbital: may increase verapamil clearance. Dose adjustments may be necessary.

Quinidine: may cause excessive hypotension when used to treat hypertrophic cardiomyopathy. Monitor blood pressure closely.

Rifampin: may substantially reduce bioavailability of oral verapamil. Use together cautiously.

Theophylline: inhibited theophylline clearance and increased plasma. Dosage adjustment may be needed.

Drug-herb
Black catechu: possible additive effects. Discourage concurrent use.

Yerba maté: possible decreased clearance of yerba maté methylxanthines and increased risk of toxicity. Urge caution.

Drug-food
Any food: enhances absorption. Give drug with food.

Drug-lifestyle
Alcohol use: prolonged intoxicating effects of alcohol. Discourage concurrent use.

Effects on diagnostic tests
None reported.

Adverse reactions
CNS: asthenia, dizziness, headache.

CV: *AV block, bradycardia, heart failure,* peripheral edema, *transient hypotension, ventricular asystole, ventricular fibrillation.*

GI: *constipation,* nausea.
Hepatic: elevated liver enzymes.
Respiratory: pulmonary edema.
Skin: rash.

Overdose and treatment
Overdose causes primarily extensions of adverse reactions. Heart block, asystole, and hypotension are the most serious reactions and require immediate attention.

Treatment may include administering isoproterenol, norepinephrine, epinephrine, atropine, or calcium gluconate I.V. in usual doses. Ensure adequate hydration. If patient has hypertrophic cardiomyopathy, give alpha-adrenergic drugs (such as methoxamine, phenylephrine, and metaraminol) to maintain blood pressure. Don't use isoproterenol or norepinephrine. If necessary, give inotropic drugs, such as dobutamine or dopamine.

If patient develops severe conduction disturbances (such as heart block and asystole) and hypotension that fails to respond to drug therapy, start cardiac pacing immediately and perform CPR as needed. Patients with Wolff-Parkinson-White or Lown-Ganong-Levine syndrome and a rapid ventricular rate from hemodynamically significant antegrade conduction may need synchronized cardioversion. Lidocaine and procainamide may be used as well.

Special considerations
▶ If patient is receiving carbamazepine when verapamil therapy starts, reduce carbamazepine dosage by 40% to 50% if needed. Do the same if patient is receiving digoxin. Monitor patient closely for signs of toxicity.

▶ Reduce verapamil dosage if patient is receiving beta blockers or has renal impairment, hepatic impairment, or severely compromised cardiac function.

▶ Stop disopyramide 48 hours before starting verapamil, and don't resume it until 24 hours after verapamil has stopped.

▶ Generic sustained-release verapamil tablets may be substituted for Isoptin SR and Calan SR, but not for Verelan capsules. Give capsule form only once daily. When using sustained-release tablets, give amounts over 240 mg/day twice daily.

▶ Give I.V. form by direct infusion into a vein or into the tubing of a free-flowing compatible I.V. solution. Compatible solutions include D_5W, normal saline solution, Ringer's solution, and lactated Ringer's solution.

▶ Give I.V. dose over at least 3 minutes to minimize the risk of adverse reactions.

▶ If patient is receiving I.V. verapamil, monitor ECG and blood pressure continuously.

▶ Obtain periodic liver function tests.

▶ During long-term combination therapy with verapamil and digoxin, assess patient's ECG periodically to detect AV block and bradycardia.

▶ Drug is also used as an antiarrhythmic and antihypertensive.

Breast-feeding patients
▶ Drug appears in breast milk. To avoid possible adverse effects in infants, discontinue breast-feeding during therapy.

Pediatric patients
▶ Currently, only the I.V. form is indicated for children—to treat supraventricular tachyarrhythmias.

Geriatric patients
▶ Elderly patients may need lower dosages.

▶ Give I.V. doses over at least 3 minutes to minimize the risk of adverse effects.

Patient teaching
▶ Instruct patient to notify prescriber about evidence of heart failure, such as shortness of breath or swelling of hands and feet.

▶ If patient is receiving nitrate therapy while verapamil dosage is being adjusted, urge patient to comply carefully with prescribed therapy.

▶ **zolmitriptan**
Zomig

Pharmacologic classification:
selective 5-hydroxytryptamine (5-HT) receptor agonist

Therapeutic classification:
antimigraine

Pregnancy risk category C

How supplied
Available by prescription only
Tablets: 2.5 mg, 5 mg

Indications and dosages
Acute migraine headaches with or without aura
Adults: initially, 2.5 mg P.O. or less. If headache returns after first dose, a second dose may be given after 2 hours. Maximum, 10 mg over 24 hours.

◨ Dosage adjustment. If patient has liver disease, give doses smaller than 2.5 mg.

Pharmacodynamics

Antimigraine action: Zolmitriptan binds with high affinity to human recombinant $5\text{-}HT_{1D}$ and $5\text{-}HT_{1B}$ receptors, aborting migraines by constricting cranial blood vessels and inhibiting release of pro-inflammatory neuropeptides.

Pharmacokinetics

Absorption: Drug is well absorbed after oral administration. Plasma levels peak in 2 hours. Mean absolute bioavailability is about 40%.

Distribution: Apparent volume of distribution is 7 L/kg. Plasma protein-binding is 25%.

Metabolism: Drug is converted to an active N-desmethyl metabolite. Time to maximum concentration for the metabolite is 2 to 3 hours. Mean elimination half-life of zolmitriptan and the active N-desmethyl metabolite is 3 hours.

Excretion: Mean total clearance is 31.5 ml/minute/kg, of which one-sixth is renal clearance. Renal clearance exceeds glomerular filtration rate, suggesting renal tubular secretion. About 65% of the dose is excreted in urine and about 30% in feces.

Contraindications and precautions

Contraindicated in patients hypersensitive to drug or its components and in patients with uncontrolled hypertension, ischemic heart disease (angina, a history of MI, or documented silent ischemia), or other significant heart disease (including Wolff-Parkinson-White syndrome). Avoid use within 24 hours of other $5\text{-}HT_1$ agonists or ergot-containing drugs and within 2 weeks of an MAO inhibitor. Also, avoid use in patients with hemiplegic or basilar migraine.

Use cautiously in patients with liver disease and in pregnant or breast-feeding women.

Interactions

Drug-drug

Cimetidine: doubles zolmitriptan's half-life. Dosage adjustment may be needed.

Ergot-containing drugs: may cause additive vasospastic reactions. Monitor patient closely.

Fluoxetine, fluvoxamine, paroxetine, sertraline: may cause weakness, hyperreflexia, and incoordination. Monitor patient closely.

MAO inhibitors, oral contraceptives: increased plasma zolmitriptan levels. Monitor patient closely, and adjust dosage as needed.

Effects on diagnostic tests

None reported.

Adverse reactions

CNS: asthenia, *dizziness,* hyperesthesia, paresthesia, somnolence, vertigo.

CV: pain or heaviness in chest; *pain, tightness, or pressure in neck, throat, or jaw;* palpitations.

GI: dry mouth, dyspepsia, dysphagia, nausea.

Musculoskeletal: myalgia.

Skin: diaphoresis.

Other: warm or cold sensations.

Overdose and treatment

Overdose may cause sedation. No specific antidote exists. For severe intoxication, provide intensive care that includes establishing and maintaining patient's airway, ensuring adequate oxygenation and

---

ventilation, and monitoring and supporting the CV system. The effect of hemodialysis or peritoneal dialysis on the plasma zolmitriptan levels is unknown.

Special considerations

▶ Drug isn't intended for migraine prophylaxis or for hemiplegic or basilar migraines.

▶ Safety hasn't been established for cluster headaches.

▶ Give drug as soon as symptoms appear.

▶ To obtain a dose below 2.5 mg, break a 2.5-mg tablet in half.

▶ Monitor blood pressure if patient has liver disease.

▶ Although rare and not reported in clinical trials, serious (possible fatal) cardiac events have occurred after use of a $5\text{-}HT_1$ agonist. They include coronary artery vasospasm, transient myocardial ischemia, MI, ventricular tachycardia, and ventricular fibrillation.

Breast-feeding patients

▶ No data exist to demonstrate whether drug appears in breast milk. Use with caution when giving it to breast-feeding women.

Pediatric patients

▶ Safety and effectiveness in children haven't been established.

Patient teaching

▶ Tell patient that drug is intended to relieve migraine symptoms rather than prevent them.

▶ Urge patient to take drug only as prescribed and not to take a second dose unless instructed. If a second dose is allowed, tell patient to take it 2 hours after the first.

▶ Tell patient to immediately notify prescriber about pain or tightness in the chest or throat, heart throbbing, rash, skin lumps, or swelling of the face, lips, or eyelids.

▶ Remind patient not to take drug with other migraine drugs.

▶ Caution women to avoid drug if pregnancy is intended, suspected, or known.

PART 3

Herbs

▶ aloe
aloe barbadensis, aloe vera, Barbados aloe, burn plant, Cape aloe, Curacao aloe, elephant's gall, first-aid plant, hsiang-dan, lily of the desert, lu-hui, medicine plant, miracle plant, plant of immortality, socotrine aloe, Venezuela aloe, Zanzibar aloe

Common trade names
(Various manufacturers; available in combination) All Natural Aloe Vera Gel, Aloe Grande, Aloe Vera Gel, Soft Gel Capsules, Aloe Vera Inner Leaf Capsules, Aloe Vera Jelly, Aloe Vera Juice, Aloe Vera Ointment, Aloe Vesta Perineal, Benzoin Compound Tincture, Dermaide Aloe, Skin Gel Aloe Life, Whole Leaf Aloe Vera Juice

How supplied
Capsules: 75 mg, 100 mg, 200 mg aloe vera extract or powder
Gel: 98%, 99.5%, 99.6% gel
Juice: 99.6%, 99.7% juice
Also available as cream, hair conditioner, jelly, liniment, lotion, ointment, shampoo, skin cream, soap, sunscreen, and impregnated facial tissues

Reported uses
Therapeutic claims center on its use as a topical treatment for minor burns, sunburn, cuts, frostbite, skin irritation, and other dermal wounds and abrasions. Numerous studies have validated these claims by demonstrating that topical application of aloe gel decreases acute inflammation, promotes wound healing, reduces pain, and exerts an antipruritic effect.

Aloe preparations have also been considered for use in treating arthritis, bursitis, hemorrhoids, peptic ulcers, and varicose veins. No well-controlled clinical trials substantiate the use of aloe for any of these disorders.

Dosage
For pruritus, skin irritation, burns, and other wounds (external forms), aloe is applied liberally as needed. Although internal use isn't recommended, some sources suggest 100 to 200 mg aloe or 50 to 100 mg aloe extract P.O., taken in the evening. No dosage information is available for aloe juice.

Actions
When taken internally, aloin is cleaved by intestinal bacteria and produces a metabolite that irritates the large intestine and stimulates colonic motility, propulsion, and transit time. Aloin also causes active secretion of fluids and electrolytes in the lumen and inhibits reabsorption of fluids from the colon. These effects increase peristalsis and cause a feeling of distention. A cathartic effect occurs 8 to 12 hours after ingestion.

Taken externally, aloe reduces inflammation, possibly by blocking production of thromboxane A_2, inactivating bradykinin, inhibiting prostaglandin A_2, and inhibiting oxidation of arachidonic acid. It also moisturizes burns and other wounds,

Aloe's antipruritic effect may result from blockage of the conversion of histidine to histamine via inhibition of histidine decarboxylase. Wound healing is believed to result from increased blood flow to the wounded area.

Some in vitro studies suggest that aloe juice and aloe gel inhibit the growth of bacteria and fungi commonly isolated from wounds and burns, although other studies have found inconsistent activity. Conflicting results may stem from variable aloe content and deterioration of some of active compounds. Because the identity and stability of active components are unknown, the veracity of claims regarding antibacterial and antifungal effects remains unknown as well.

Cautions
Patients hypersensitive to aloe and patients with a history of allergic reactions to plants in the Liliaceae family, such as garlic, onions, and tulips, shouldn't use external preparations. Internal use of aloe should be avoided by pregnant or breast-feeding patients, menstruating patients, children, and patients with kidney or cardiac disease because of the risk of hypokalemia and possible disturbance of cardiac rhythm.

Interactions
Herb-drug
Antiarrhythmics, cardiac glycosides, loop diuretics, other potassium-wasting drugs, corticosteroids, thiazides: increased effects of these drugs with internal aloe use. Avoid internal use of aloe when taking these drugs.

Adverse reactions
GI: damage to intestinal mucosa (may be irreversible), harmless brown discoloration of intestinal mucous membranes, painful intestinal spasms.
GU: accumulation of blood in pelvic region with large doses, red discoloration of urine with frequent use, reflex stimulation of uterine musculature, which may cause spontaneous abortion or premature birth during late pregnancy.
Metabolic: fluid and electrolyte loss from frequent use, loss of potassium from intestine, risk of hypokalemia.
Skin: contact dermatitis.
Other: delayed healing of deep wounds from reduced oxygen permeability through topical forms,

Special considerations
▶ Monitor wounds for delayed healing with topical use.
▶ Severe hemorrhagic diarrhea, kidney damage, and possible death may occur from overdose.
▶ Internal use can cause severe abdominal discomfort and serious hypokalemia and electrolyte imbalance.
▶ Internally, dried latex has been claimed to be useful as a stimulant laxative. Other claims for use of aloe include amenorrhea, asthma, colds, seizures, bleeding, and ulcers. No medical evidence supports the use of aloe for these conditions.
▶ Aloe has also been considered for treating acne, AIDS, asthma, blindness, cancer, colitis, depression, diabetes, glaucoma, and multiple sclerosis. No well-controlled clinical trials substantiate the use of aloe for any of these disorders.
▶ Unapproved use of aloe vera injections for cancer has been linked to deaths. Use of injectable aloe vera or chemical constituents of aloe vera isn't recommended.

Breast-feeding patients
▶ No data exist to demonstrate whether aloe appears in breast milk. Avoid use while breast-feeding.

Pediatric patients
▶ Aloe is contraindicated in children.

Patient teaching
▶ Caution the patient against taking aloe vera gel or juice internally.

▶ arnica
arnica flowers, arnica root, common arnica, leopard's bane, Mexican arnica, mountain arnica, mountain daisy, mountain tobacco, sneezewort, wolf's bane

---

Common trade names
Arnicaid, Arnica Spray, Arniflora (Gel)

How supplied
Available as a spray for topical application and in tablets, teas, gels, tinctures, creams (preferred in Europe), ointments, and S.L. preparations
Creams typically contain 15% arnica oil; salves should contain 20% to 25% arnica oil

Reported uses
Arnica is claimed to be useful for relieving muscle and joint aches and is frequently cited in herbal literature as being able to promote wound healing. In veterinary medicine, it's classified as a counterirritant, an effect most likely related to its isomeric alcohol component.

Analgesic effects failed to be verified in a double-blind study of arnica, metronidazole, and a placebo among postoperative dental patients. Similarly, a homeopathic dose of arnica was tested against a placebo in a population of postoperative abdominal hysterectomy patients. No significant difference was found between the two groups. In a small study of marathon runners, another form of arnica failed to produce statistically significant benefits in muscle stiffness, laboratory measurements of muscle injury, or healing time of muscle injuries.

Dosage
No consensus exists. Homeopathic doses (trace quantities) appear to be most popular.

Actions
Four sesquiterpenoids isolated from *Heterotheca inuloides* in one study demonstrated antibacterial activity in vitro. One compound exhibited gram-positive antibacterial activity and minimal bactericidal concentrations of 12.5 mcg/ml against methicillin-resistant *Staphylococcus aureus*.

An *Arnica montana* extract has been shown to increase phagocytosis in mice.

In a Dutch study, most arnica flavonoids demonstrated moderate to low cytotoxicity in vitro when compared to cisplatin. Helenalin, a sesquiterpene lactone, displayed the strongest cytotoxicity. Another study apparently found a quicker recovery from carbon tetrachloride-induced toxic liver injury in rats when the rats received phenolic compounds of *A. montana.*

An in vitro study found that helenalin and dihydrohelenalin inhibited platelet function in humans. Another study in healthy human volunteers failed to find significant effects on blood clotting immediately after administration of an arnica extract. In vitro studies have documented an anti-inflammatory effect for some components of arnica.

Cautions
Avoid use in pregnant patients because of the risk of oxytocic activity and inadequate knowledge about teratogenic effects.

Interactions
Herb-drug
Antihypertensive drugs: possible reduced antihypertensive effectiveness. Avoid concomitant use.

Adverse reactions
CNS: nervous disorders.
CV: *arrhythmias, cardiac toxicity,* hypertension.
GI: gastroenteritis.
Hepatic: *liver failure.*
Musculoskeletal: muscle weakness.
Skin: allergic dermatitis with topical use.

Special considerations
▶ Arnica shouldn't be applied to abraded skin or open wounds.
▶ Arnica preparations should be kept out of the reach of children.
▶ Arnica has been approved by the German Commission E as a topical remedy with effective anti-inflammatory, analgesic, and anti-bacterial properties. The FDA, however, has classified arnica as an unsafe herb.
▶ Monitor patient for adverse effects.

Pediatric patients
▶ Avoid use in children.
▶ Nausea, vomiting, organ damage, coma, and possible death may occur in children who ingest arnica flowers or roots. Induce emesis and perform gastric lavage to remove undigested contents. Supportive care may be necessary.

Patient teaching
▶ Explain that arnica taken orally or applied to an open wound may cause hypertension, cardiotoxicity, vertigo, and renal dysfunction from activity of sesquiterpene lactones and components of the essential oil.
▶ Advise patient to avoid prolonged topical use because of the risk for allergic hypersensitivity reaction.

▶ birch
birch tar oil, birch wood oil, black birch, cherry birch, sweet birch oil, white birch

Common trade names
None known.

How supplied
Available as essential oil (bark, wood), dried bark, and tea

Reported uses
Claims for this herb include relief of headaches, other analgesic effects, and treatment of kidney stones and GI disorders. Essential oils are claimed to act against rheumatism, gout, and neuralgias.

Dosage
Extract and tea are made by steeping 2 to 3 g of the bark in boiling water for 10 to 15 minutes; the infusion is ingested several times daily.

Actions
Methyl salicylate seems to have antipyretic, anti-inflammatory, and

analgesic properties. Hemostatic function in animals has been shown to be affected by the thromboplastic elements presumably found in *Betula pendula.* The mechanism of action resembles that of human tissue thromboplastin. In other animal studies, birch has been shown to exert diuretic effects.

Cautions
Pregnant and breast-feeding patients shouldn't use birch. Patients with seasonal allergic rhinitis or hypersensitivity to plant allergens should use it cautiously.

Interactions
None reported.

Adverse reactions
EENT: allergic rhinitis from pollen allergens.
Skin: acute contact dermatitis from exposure to birch leaves or sap.

Special considerations
▶ Claims for this herb also include treatment of various acute and chronic skin disorders. Essential oils are claimed to act against tuberculosis, cervical lymphadenitis and bladder infections. In veterinary medicine, essential oil of birch wood has been used to treat various skin diseases.
▶ Cross-sensitization with other plant allergens, such as celery and mugwort pollen, may occur.
▶ Monitor patient for evidence of allergic reaction, particularly if allergic to celery, mugwort, or other plants.

Breast-feeding patients
▶ No data exist to demonstrate whether birch appears in breast milk. Patient should avoid use while breast-feeding.

Pediatric patients
▶ Sweet birch oil is composed of 98% methyl salicylate. Methyl salicylate has been shown to be fatal to children when applied topically to the skin. Poisonings have been reported with as little as 4.7 g of methyl salicylate, applied topically.

Patient teaching
▶ Because of substantial risk of toxicity and death in children, warn patient to store birch preparations safely out of the reach of children.
▶ Tell patient that topical form may irritate the skin and mucous membranes. Encourage patient to report new or unusual skin reactions.
▶ Advise women to avoid use of herb during pregnancy or when breast-feeding.

▶ butterbur
European pestroot, sweet coltsfoot, Western coltsfoot

Common trade names
(Various manufacturers; available in combination) Alzoon, Butterbur Root Extract, Feverfew/Dogwood Supreme, Neurochol, Petaforce, Wild Cherry Supreme

How supplied
Available as 25-mg standardized capsules, *Petasites* extract, and liquid *Petasites* extract (concentration may vary)

Reported uses

Butterbur has been used for thousands of years for GI disorders and GI-related pain as well as for spasms of the urogenital tract. Other therapeutic claims include its use as a sedative and antiarthritic. Butterbur was prescribed in ancient times as an ointment for ulcers and sores. References have also been made to an analgesic effect of *Petasites* extracts, but this effect may be secondary to the herb's spasmolytic properties.

Dosage

No consensus exists. *P. frigidus* is taken as a tea or smoked. It is also used as a poultice by patients residing in areas where the plant is endemic, including the United States.

Actions

Studies with animals have found that *P. hybridus* extracts possess spasmolytic and anti-inflammatory properties. The extracts reduced intestinal ulcerations and blocked gastric damage in rats. The effects were dose-dependent.

Extracts also inhibited peptido-leukotriene biosynthesis in mouse peritoneal macrophages and did not affect prostaglandin synthesis. Proposed mechanisms include inhibition of 5-lipoxygenase or interference with the utilization of calcium ions in leukotriene production.

In 1953, studies found a cytostatic effect of *Petasites* extract on fertilized sea urchin eggs, leading to the herb being used later as an analgesic for cancer patients. This effect isn't substantiated in other available literature.

Cautions

Pregnant and breast-feeding patients should avoid use of *Petasites* extracts; effects are unknown. Also patients with decreased GI or bladder motility should avoid use because symptoms of these disorders may worsen.

Interactions

None reported.

Adverse reactions

EENT: discoloration of the eyes.
GI: abdominal pain or pressure, constipation, discoloration of stool, dysphagia, nausea, vomiting.
GU: dysuria.
Respiratory: dyspnea.
Skin: skin discoloration.

Special considerations

▶ Butterbur has also been used for thousands of years for asthma, cough, and skin diseases. Other therapeutic claims include its use as a diuretic and astringent for cosmetic purposes.
▶ Carcinogenic and hepatotoxic effects are possible resulting from the presence of pyrrolizidine alkaloids in the plant.
▶ Concomitant use with anticholinergic drugs may not be advisable.
▶ Monitor patient for adverse reactions.

Breast-feeding patients

▶ No data exist to demonstrate whether butterbur appears in breast milk. Breast-feeding patient should avoid use.

Patient teaching

▶ Advise women to avoid use of the herb during pregnancy or when breast-feeding.

▶ Discourage the use of butterbur in patients with disorders that might be worsened by any effect on leukotriene synthesis or calcium-modulated smooth-muscle contractility, especially in the GI tract. Also, discourage use in patients with underlying disorders such as asthma that may become dangerous if inadequately treated.

▶ capsicum
bell pepper, capsaicin, cayenne pepper, chili pepper, hot pepper, paprika, pimiento, red pepper, tabasco pepper

Common trade names
Capsin, Cap-Stun, Capzasin, Dolorac, No Pain HP, Pepper Defense, R-Gel, Zostrix (HP)

How supplied
Cream: 0.025%, 0.075%, 0.25%
Gel: 0.025%
Lotion: 0.025%, 0.075%
Self-defense spray: 5%, 10%

Reported uses
Various preparations of capsicum have been applied topically as counterirritants and external analgesics. Topical capsaicin preparations are claimed to be useful for treating pain associated with postherpetic neuralgia, rheumatoid arthritis, osteoarthritis, diabetic neuropathy, postsurgical pain including postmastectomy and postamputation pain, and other neuropathic pain and complex pain syndromes.

Dosage
Because capsaicin is very potent, concentrations of topical preparations range from 0.025% to 0.25%. Preparations are most effective when applied t.i.d. or q.i.d. and have a duration of action of about 4 to 6 hours. Less frequent application typically produces less effective substance P depletion and incomplete analgesia.

Actions
Although topical capsaicin produces an extremely intense irritation at the contact point, vesicle formation usually doesn't occur. The initial dose of capsaicin causes profound pain; however, repeated applications cause desensitization, with analgesic and even anti-inflammatory effects. Heat sensation is caused by stimulation of specific local afferent nerve fibers. Analgesic effects may be explained by capsaicin-induced neuronal depletion of substance P, believed to be a mediator in the transmission of painful stimuli from the periphery to the spinal cord. The analgesic effect may also result from the methoxyphenol portion of the capsaicin molecule that may interfere with the lipoxygenase and cyclooxygenase pathways.

Capsaicin doesn't cause blistering or redness because it doesn't act on the capillaries or other blood vessels. An externally applied 0.1% capsaicin solution inhibits flare formation after I.D. injection of histamine. Areas of skin (control) without pretreatment of capsaicin developed a wheal, flare, and itching. Flare response is believed to be substance P-mediated.

Juices from the fruits have shown antibacterial properties in vitro. I.V. infusion of capsaicin has been reported to stimulate secretion of epinephrine and norepinephrine from the adrenal medulla of rodents.

Cautions
Patients hypersensitive to capsicum or chili pepper products should avoid capiscum. Pregnant patients should avoid it because of possible uterine stimulant effects.

Interactions
Herb-drug
Central-acting adrenergics: may reduce efficacy of antihypertensives such as clonidine or methyldopa. Avoid concomitant use.
MAO inhibitors: may promote toxicity (hypertensive crisis) when used together due to catecholamine release. Avoid concomitant use.

Adverse reactions
EENT: burning pain in nose, serous discharge, sneezing.
GI: GI discomfort.
Respiratory: cough, retrosternal discomfort, transient bronchoconstriction.
Skin: erythema without vesicular eruption, itching, stinging, transient skin irritation.

Special considerations
▶ Traditional claims surrounding use of capsicum include treatment of bowel disorders, chronic laryngitis, and peripheral vascular disease.
▶ Capsaicin has also been suggested for refractory pruritus and pruritus associated with renal failure. A small study has suggested nasal inhalation of capsaicin may be beneficial in nonallergic, noninfectious perennial rhinitis. However, poor tolerability is likely to be of issue with larger clinical trials.

One study has reported capsaicin's use for urinary urgency.
▶ GI discomfort can be minimized if seeds are removed from the product before ingestion.
▶ After topical application, relief occurs as early as 3 days, but may take as long as 14 to 28 days, depending on the condition requiring analgesia.
▶ No evidence exists that topical application causes permanent neurologic injury.
▶ Because of its short-term immobilizing effects, capsaicin is used as a humane self-defense spray. The more popular products contain the capsicum oleoresin, which produces immediate blepharospasm, blindness, and incapacitation for up to 30 minutes.
▶ Monitor patient for adverse effects.
▶ Intensity of adverse reactions are dose- and concentration-dependent.

Patient teaching
▶ Tell the patient to avoid contact with eyes, mucous membranes, or nonintact skin.
▶ Inform the patient to flush the exposed area with cool running water for as long as necessary, if incidental contact occurs.
▶ Caution the patient taking MAO inhibitors or central-acting adrenergics against use of this herb.
▶ Advise women to avoid use of the herb during pregnancy or when breast-feeding.

▌chondroitin
cas, chondroitin sulfate A or chondroitin 4-sulfate, chondroitin C or chondroitin 6-sulfate, css

Common trade names
(Available in combination) 100% CSA, Chondroitin-4 Sulfate, Purified Chondroitin Sulfate

How supplied
Available as 200-mg and 400-mg capsules and as an injection in Europe

Reported uses
Chondroitin is claimed to be useful as a dietary supplement in combination with glucosamine sulfate in osteoarthritis and related disorders.

Chondroitin sulfates were first evaluated using parenteral administration. Other small trials demonstrated improvement in subjective outcomes, such as use of NSAIDs, visual analogue scales for pain, the Lequesne's Index, and patient or physician global assessment.

Dosage
The oral dose is based on the patient's weight; chondroitin is usually given in combination with glucosamine sulfate.
Patients who weigh less than 55 kg (120 lb): 1,000 mg glucosamine sulfate plus 800 mg chondroitin sulfates P.O.
Patients who weigh 55 to 90 kg (120 to 200 lb): 1,500 mg glucosamine sulfate plus 1,200 mg chondroitin sulfates P.O.
Patients who weigh more than 90 kg (200 lb): 2,000 mg glucosamine sulfate plus 1,600 mg chondroitin sulfates P.O.

Total daily amount is usually taken with food in two to four divided doses. Recent studies evaluating chondroitin sulfates alone used doses from 400 mg P.O. b.i.d. or t.i.d., and 1,200 mg P.O. daily as a single dose.

Actions
Because of their large molecular size, it's believed that the oral absorption of chondroitin sulfates is poor. Chondroitin sulfates have been shown to control the formation of new cartilage matrix by stimulating chondrocyte metabolism and synthesis of collagen and proteoglycan.

Chondroitin sulfates are also reported to inhibit the enzymes human leukocyte elastase and hyaluronidase. High concentrations of human leukocyte elastase are found in the blood and synovial fluid of patients with rheumatic disease. Chondroitin sulfates also stimulate the production of highly polymerized hyaluronic acid by synovial cells. Viscosity is subsequently improved and synovial fluid levels return to normal.

Cautions
Pregnant and breast-feeding patients should avoid use of chondroitin; effects are unknown. Patients with bleeding disorders should use it cautiously because of risk of anticoagulation.

Interactions
Herb-drug
Anticoagulants: may potentiate effects. Avoid concomitant use.

Adverse reactions
CNS: euphoria, headache, motor uneasiness.
GI: dyspepsia, nausea.
Other: pain at injection site with parenteral administration.

Special considerations
▶ Risk of internal bleeding exists because of chondroitin's similarity to heparin. Studies in animals found significantly decreased hematocrit, hemoglobin, WBCs, and segmented neutrophils; reduced aggregation in response to adenosine diphosphate and collagen; and significantly decreased platelet count. There's no report of bleeding as a result of chondroitin sulfate use in humans.
▶ Public interest in the combined use of chondroitin sulfates and glucosamine sulfate has risen, especially since the publication of a book, *The Arthritis Cure* (Theodosakis, 1997), which claims that the sulfate combination is "the medical miracle that can halt, reverse, and may even cure osteoarthritis."
▶ The Arthritis Foundation doesn't currently recommend the use of glucosamine sulfate and chondroitin sulfates for osteoarthritis or other types of arthritis.
▶ Offer additional support to the patient with osteoarthritis, such as intermittent moist heat application and exercise.
▶ Chondroitin sulfates have been used in ischemic heart disease and hyperlipidemia, as a preservative of corneas for transplantation, and as an adjunct to eye surgery.
▶ Monitor patient for bleeding.

Breast-feeding patients
▶ No data exist to demonstrate whether chondroitin appears in breast milk. Breast-feeding patients should avoid use.

Patient teaching
▶ Instruct the patient to watch for signs of bleeding, especially if he's taking anticoagulants or has a bleeding disorder.
▶ Advise women to avoid use of the herb during pregnancy or when breast-feeding.

▶ dong quai
Chinese angelica, dry-kuei, FP3340010/FP334015/FT334010, tang-kuei, women's ginseng

Common trade names
Dong Kwai, Dong Quai Capsules, Dong Quai Fluid Extract

How supplied
Dong quai tablet (fluidextract): 0.5 g
Raw root: 4.5 g to 30 g (boil or soak in wine)
Also available as injectable forms in foreign countries

Reported uses
Dong quai has been used for many pain-related disorders, including dysmenorrhea, headache, neuralgia, and toothache.

Dosage
Dosage forms, strengths and extraction forms vary. In the human placebo-controlled study evaluating the estrogenic effects of dong quai on endometrial thickness in postmenopausal woman, 1 g of the

root (equivalent to 0.5 mg/kg of ferulic acid) was used.

Actions

Dong quai alters uterine activity in female rabbits. The volatile oil has an inhibitory action on the uterus whereas the nonvolatile and water- and alcohol-soluble components have stimulatory action. In another study, dong quai alone was found not to produce estrogen-like responses in endometrial thickness or vaginal maturation, and also not to be useful in managing postmenopausal symptoms.

Studies conducted in rats showed increases in metabolism, oxygen use by the liver, and glutamic acid and cysteine oxidation; these actions may be attributed to vitamin B and folinic acid that occur in the herb's root.

Dong quai extracts, especially alcoholic extracts, were also found to exert quinidine-type effects, prolong the refractory period, and correct atrial fibrillation in animals. Other studies in rats showed that the plant may prevent atherosclerosis, expand coronary arteries, and increase coronary blood flow. Some coumarins are known to act as vasodilators. Although studies in animals have shown that the volatile oil exerts vasodilatory action to lower blood pressure, the duration of action is short.

Cautions

Safrole, a component of the volatile oil, is carcinogenic and not recommended for ingestion. Pregnant and breast-feeding patients shouldn't use the herb because its chemical components may cause fetal harm.

Interactions
Herb-drug

Anticoagulants: may potentiate effects. Avoid concomitant use.

Herb-lifestyle

Sun exposure: increased risk of photosensitivity. Urge precautions.

Adverse reactions

GI: diarrhea.
Hematologic: bleeding.
Skin: increased photosensitivity.
Other: fever.

Special considerations

▶ Dong quai is recommended by herbalists for many gynecologic disorders, including irregular menstruation, premenstrual syndrome, excessive fetal movement, and chronic pelvic infection. Most claims are based on data from animal studies or small, uncontrolled human trials. The herb has also anecdotally been reported to treat malaria, constipation, hypertension, herpes zoster, chronic rhinitis, Buerger's disease, Raynaud's disease, hepatitis, hepatocirrhosis, pyogenic infection, ulcerous diseases or abscess, and sepsis.
▶ Question the patient about use of this herb and suggest an appropriate specialist to address these health care concerns.
▶ Monitor patient for potential bleeding.

Breast-feeding

▶ Breast-feeding patients should avoid use because the herb's chemical components may cause fetal harm.

Patient teaching
▶ Warn the patient that some of the herbal components have been shown to increase the risk of some cancers.

▶ Instruct the patient who becomes photosensitive to use sunblock and to wear adequate clothing and sunglasses.

▶ Caution the patient against use of this herb for its yet unproven estrogenic effects.

▶ Advise women to report planned or suspected pregnancy and to avoid use of the herb during pregnancy or when breast-feeding.

▶ elderberry

antelope brush (*Sambucus tridentata*), black elder (*S. nigra*), blue elderberry (*S. caerulea*), boretree, common elder (*S. canadensis*), danewort (*S. ebulus*), dwarf elder, elder, European elder, pipe tree, red elderberry, red-fruited elder (*S. pubens, S. racemosa*), Sambucus, sweet elder

---

Common trade names
(Various manufacturers)
Elderberry Power, Elder Flowers

How supplied
Available as ointments and aqueous solutions of the bark and leaves as well as oils, ointments, and wine; all are derived from the berries.

Reported uses
Reported used for pain include toothache, headache, and neuralgia.

Dosage
No consensus exists.

Actions
The elder and several other herbals have traditionally been used for the treatment of diabetes, although studies in mice indicate that the herb exerts no effects on glucose control. This plant has shown activity against *Salmonella typhi*, *Shigella dysenteriae*, and limited activity against *S. flexneri*. A branch tip extract of the red elder (*Sambucus racemosa*) was found to have strong in vitro antiviral activity against respiratory syncytial virus. No studies in humans or animals have been reported.

A 1997 study indicated that *S. nigra* was somewhat active against the production of inflammatory cytokines in vitro, giving some merit to folklore suggesting that the plant is effective in the treatment of such inflammatory illnesses as rheumatism, fever, infections, and edema. Elderberries have been reported to have antispasmodic and sedative activities, as well as activities as a diaphoretic, diuretic, and laxative. The herb has been used to produce weight loss and to treat colds, "dropsy," kidney disorders, rheumatism, insomnia, and migraines. The cyanogenic glycosides contained in the elder plants release cyanide when hydrolyzed, as when they are chewed; this effect could explain many of the reported actions of this plant.

Cautions
Use elderberry products with caution because of the risk of cyanide toxicity. Berries of the dwarf elder species (*S. ebulus*) shouldn't be

used. All green parts of the elder plant are poisonous. Pregnant and breast-feeding patients should avoid the herb.

Interactions
None reported.

Adverse reactions
GI: diarrhea from berries of the *S. ebulus* and leaves of any species, vomiting with ingestion of excessive amounts of *S. racemosa* berries.
Other: *cyanide poisoning* from bark, roots, leaves, and unripe berries of elder plant.

Special considerations
▶ Ingestion of 60 mg of cyanide has caused death. Emesis and gastric lavage are recommended for known elder plant ingestion. Amyl nitrate, sodium nitrate, and sodium thiosulfate may also be used when cyanide toxicity is suspected.
▶ The dwarf elder (S. ebulus) is regarded as particularly poisonous. Large doses can cause vertigo, vomiting, and diarrhea (signs of cyanide toxicity).
▶ Elder has also been used as an insect repellent, with sprays of the flowers placed in horses' bridles. The powder of the dried elder flowers has been added to water and dabbed on the skin as a mosquito repellent. Clinical support for this use in humans is currently lacking.
▶ Mixed with sage, lemon juice, vinegar and honey, elder has also been used as a gargle. With peppermint and honey in a hot drink, elder is said to be able to treat a cold, inducing diaphoresis to "sweat out" an illness. Elderberry

juice has been used in hair dye and scented ointments. Other reported uses include liver disease, measles, asthma, burns, cancer, chafing, epilepsy, gout, psoriasis, syphilis, reduction of swelling, and wound healing, although there are no scientific data to support such uses.
▶ Monitor fluid intake and output of patients experiencing GI effects from this herb.

Breast-feeding patients
▶ No data exist to demonstrate whether elderberry appears in breast milk. Breast-feeding patients should avoid use.

Pediatric use
▶ Not recommended for use in children because of potentially toxic effects.
▶ Children who make pipes or peashooters from hollowed shafts of the elder can sustain cyanide poisoning.

Patient teaching
▶ Advise the patient that elderberries should never be consumed uncooked because of the risk of cyanide toxicity.
▶ Instruct the patient to keep this plant away from children and pets, and to have the number for the nearest poison control center handy.

▶ feverfew
altamisa, bachelors' button, chamomile grande, featherfew, featherfoil, febrifuge plant, midsummer daisy, mutterkraut, nosebleed, Santa Maria, wild chamomile, wild quinine

Common trade names
(Various manufacturers) Feverfew, Feverfew Glyc, Feverfew Power

How supplied
Available as capsules (pure leaf, 380 mg; leaf extract, 250 mg), liquid, tablets, and leaves, which are commonly used to make infusions or teas

Reported uses
Although initial enthusiasm for feverfew has waned, plant preparations are becoming increasingly popular for use in migraine prophylaxis. Feverfew is also claimed to be useful for the treatment of toothache, rheumatism, stomachache, and menstrual problems.

Dosage
For migraine prophylaxis, 25 mg of freeze-dried leaf extract P.O. daily; 50 mg of leaf P.O. daily with food; or 50 to 200 mg of aerial parts of plant P.O. daily.
For migraine treatment, average dose of 543 mcg P.O. parthenolide daily.

Actions
The main active ingredients are the sesquiterpene lactones, particularly parthenolide, which inhibits serotonin release by human platelets in vitro. This may be the mechanism of action for the herb's purported efficacy in treating migraines.

Parthenolide also inhibits serotonin release. Extracts of feverfew contain chemicals that inhibit activation of polymorphonuclear leukocytes and the synthesis of leukotrienes and prostaglandins.

Cautions
Pregnant or breast-feeding women should avoid use.

Interactions
None reported.

Adverse reactions
GI: *mouth ulcerations* with crude drug.
Other: *hypersensitivity reactions,* post-feverfew syndrome (withdrawal syndrome characterized by moderate to severe pain and joint and muscle stiffness).

Special considerations
▶ Feverfew is also claimed to be useful for the treatment of psoriasis, insect bites, asthma, threatened miscarriage, and as an antipyretic.
▶ Feverfew potency is commonly based on its parthenolide content, which is variable.
▶ The concentration of parthenolide in the leaves and flowering tops is highest during the summer, before the seeds are set, and drops rapidly thereafter. This may explain the difference in parthenolide levels between brands of feverfew capsules and tablets.
▶ The Health Protection Branch of the Canadian government has proposed a standard that formulations contain a minimum of 0.2% parthenolide.
▶ Monitor patient for allergic reaction and for mouth ulcers. Encourage proper oral hygiene.

Breast-feeding patients
▶ No data exist to demonstrate whether feverfew appears in breast milk. Breast-feeding patients should avoid use.

Patient teaching
▶ Instruct the patient not to withdraw the herb abruptly, but to taper it gradually because of risk of post-feverfew syndrome.
▶ Assure the patient that several other strategies for migraine treatment and prophylaxis exist, and that these should be attempted before taking products with unknown benefits and risks.
▶ Remind patient to promptly report unusual symptoms, such as mouth sores or skin ulcerations.

▶ ginger
zingiber

Common trade names
(Various manufacturers; available in combination) Cayenne Ginger, Gingerall, Ginger Peppermint Combo, Ginger Power, Ginger Trips

How supplied
Capsules, liquid, powder: 100 mg, 465 mg
Extract: 250 mg
Root: 530 mg
Tablets (chewable): 67.5 mg
Also available as tea

Reported uses
Claims for ginger include its use as an anti-inflammatory useful for treating arthritis.
　　Ginger was found to provide relief from pain and swelling in patients with rheumatoid arthritis, osteoarthritis, or muscular discomfort. A proposed mechanism is that it inhibits prostaglandin, thromboxane, and leukotriene biosynthesis.

Dosage
Dosage forms and strength vary with each disease state.
To investigate antiemetic action, studies used 500 to 1,000 mg of powdered ginger P.O., or 1,000 mg of fresh ginger root P.O.

Actions
Human studies have shown ginger to inhibit platelet aggregation induced by adenosine diphosphate and epinephrine. Ginger extracts have documented anti-inflammatory effects in rodent models. Specific components of ginger produce varying CV effects. Methanolic extracts of ginger have shown positive inotropic effects in a guinea pig model.
　　Other studies in animals have suggested that components in ginger may be gastroprotective against various chemical insults and stressors. The GI protective action is postulated to be promoted by increased mucosal resistance and potentiation of the defensive mechanism against chemicals or alterations in prostaglandins, providing more protective effects. Additionally, a study of acetone extracts in mice found them to have similar stimulatory effects on GI motility as that seen with metoclopramide and domperidone.

Cautions
The effects in pregnant patients are unknown, so they should avoid use. Patients receiving anticoagulants should use ginger only under

medical supervision because it may affect bleeding time by inhibiting platelet function.

Interactions
Herb-drug
Anticoagulants: may increase bleeding risk. Monitor patient closely.

Adverse reactions
Adverse reactions may occur with overdose
CNS: CNS depression.
CV: *arrhythmias.*

Special considerations
▶ Claims for ginger include, but are not limited to, its use as an antiemetic, GI protectant, a CV stimulant, an antitumor agent, an antioxidant, and also as a therapy for microbial and parasitic infestations. The antiemetic effects of ginger have been extensively studied in humans for morning, motion, or sea sickness, and for postoperative nausea and vomiting; most provide support for this action, although there are some that do not. Doses and duration of therapy varied considerably with each study. The antiemetic properties of ginger are likely to result from local effects on the GI tract rather than on the CNS. Increased gastric peristalsis has been shown in animals, but any mechanism in humans is currently considered speculative.
▶ Monitor patient closely for bleeding, especially those also taking anticoagulants.

Patient teaching
▶ Advise women to avoid use of ginger during pregnancy.

▶ Instruct patient to watch for signs of bleeding when taking ginger.
▶ Explain that no consensus exists with respect to dosing and monitoring.

▶ glucosamine
chitosamine, glucosamine sulfate, gs

Common trade names
(Various manufacturers; available in combination) Arth-X Plus, Enhanced Glucosamine Sulfate, Flexi-Factors, Glucosamine Complex, Glucosamine Mega, Joint Factors, Nutri-Joint, Ultra Maximum Strength Glucosamine Sulfate

How supplied
Various molecular forms of glucosamine are available, including chlorhydrate, D-glucosamine, hydrochloride, *N*-acetyl, sulfate, and with potassium chloride added. The preferred form appears to be glucosamine sulfate.
Capsules: 250 mg, 375 mg, 500 mg, 600 mg, 1,000 mg
Tablets: 63 mg, 87 mg, 375 mg, 500 mg, 600 mg, 750 mg

Reported uses
Glucosamine is thought to be useful as an antiarthritic in patients with osteoarthritis or other joint disorders.

Dosage
The dosage used in several clinical trials was 500 mg P.O. t.i.d. Other dosages used were based on patient weight: if weight was below 120 lb (54 kg), 1,000 mg glucosamine plus 800 mg chondroitin

sulfate; between 120 and 200 lb (91 kg), 1,500 mg glucosamine plus 1,200 mg chondroitin sulfate; and if it is above 200 lb, 2,000 mg glucosamine plus 1,600 mg chondroitin sulfate.

Actions
The administration of glucosamine is believed to stimulate production of cartilage components and allow rebuilding of damaged cartilage. Early in vitro studies have found that culture-derived fibroblast increased mucopolysaccharide and collagen synthesis when glucosamine was added.

In vivo and in vitro studies conducted in rats showed glucosamine can severely impair insulin secretion and beta-cell secretory dysfunction similar to that observed in patients with type 2 diabetes mellitus.

Cautions
Children and pregnant and breast-feeding women should avoid use because the effects in them are unknown.

Interactions
None reported.

Adverse reactions
CNS: drowsiness, headache.
GI: constipation, diarrhea, epigastric pain and discomfort, heartburn, nausea.
Skin: rash.

Special considerations
▶ The Arthritis Foundation doesn't recommend glucosamine for osteoarthritis or for any form of arthritis because of the lack of efficacy data.

▶ The FDA has not reviewed any studies that confirm claims made for this supplement.
▶ Monitor glucose levels in diabetic patients.

Breast-feeding patients
▶ No data exist to demonstrate whether glucosamine appears in breast milk. Breast-feeding patients should avoid use.

Pediatric patients
▶ Children shouldn't take glucosamine; effects are unknown.

Patient teaching
▶ Advise the patient that human clinical trials evaluating glucosamine are lacking.
▶ Suggest other accepted pharmacologic treatment before starting therapy with glucosamine.
▶ Explain that the long-term effect on beta-cell secretory function in humans is unknown and could be potentially harmful, especially to patients with diabetes or impaired glucose tolerance.

▶ hops

Common trade names
(Available in combination) Avena Sativa Compound in Species Sedative Tea, HR 129 Serene, HR 133 Stress, Melatonin with Vitamin B_6, Snuz Plus, Stress Aid
Also available as single-ingredient compounds

How supplied
Available in herbal tea preparations. Both solid and liquid forms are becoming more popular. There

are also anecdotal reports of dried hops being smoked.

Reported uses
Hops have been promoted as an analgesic, hypnotic, antispasmotic, and sedative. Anecdotal reports promote the use of hops as a sedative-hypnotic.

Dosage
No specific dosage is available because hops are often taken either in combination with other herbals or as a tea. However, based upon combination products, the approximate dose of hops may be 2 to 4 mg of the extract.

Actions
The phytoestrogens exert direct estrogenic activity in vitro. Sedative-hypnotic effects have been shown in mice and humans that are attributed to 2-methyl-3-butene-2-ol. Colupulone and avermectin both have antibacterial activity. Humulone has been shown to decrease tumor formation and inflammation in mice. Colupulone has also been shown to induce hepatic microsomal enzymes, whereas xanthohumole inhibits the extramicrosomal hepatic enzyme DGAT in rats, mice, and in vitro.

Cautions
Patients with estrogen-dependent tumors, such as breast, uterine, or cervical cancer, should avoid use. Patients taking CNS depressants or antipsychotics should also avoid use.

Interactions
Herb-drug
CNS depressants (anticholinergics, antidepressants, antihistamines, antipsychotics, anxiolytics): may cause additive effects. Use with caution.
Drugs metabolized by the cytochrome P-450 system: may cause decreased plasma levels of these drugs. Avoid concomitant use.
Phenothiazine-type antipsychotics: may cause additive effects on hyperthermia. Avoid concomitant use.

Herb-lifestyle
Alcohol use: may cause additive effects. Advise caution.

Adverse reactions
CNS: decreased cognitive performance, sedation.
Respiratory: bronchial irritation, bronchitis following inhalation.
Skin: vesicular dermatitis following direct cutaneous contact with raw plants.
Other: allergic reactions (predominantly dermatologic), *anaphylaxis*.

Special considerations
▶ Hops has also been promoted as an anthelmintic and to promote functional activity of the stomach. Anecdotal reports promote the use of hops as an antidepressant and for treatment during menopause.
▶ Herb loses its original activity when stored. Only 15% remains after 9 months.
▶ Monitor patient for adverse effects.

Patient teaching
▶ Warn patient to avoid hazardous activities until CNS effects of the herb are known.

▶ Advise patient to avoid alcohol while using this herb.

▶ kava
ava, awa, kava kava, kawa, kew, sakau, tonga, yagona

Common trade names
Aigin, Antares, Ardeydystin, Cefkava, Kavasedon, Kavasporal, Kavatino, Laitan, Mosaro, Nervonocton N, Potter's Antigian Tablets, Viocava

How supplied
Prepared as a drink from pulverized roots, tablets, capsules, or extract

Reported uses
Medicinal claims of kava include treatment of pain, rheumatism, muscle spasms, and promotion of wound healing.

Dosage
Dosage is usually based on the kavapyrone content, which varies with preparation. Most studies in humans used 70 to 240 mg kavapyrone daily. One study used 90 to 110 mg dried kava extract t.i.d. for the treatment of anxiety. Doses of freshly prepared kava beverages average 400 to 900 g weekly.

Actions
More than one mode of action is involved. There's an unquantified synergism among kava components. Components of the root may cause local anesthetic activity that is similar to cocaine but lasts longer than benzocaine. Kava induced a mephenesin-like muscular relaxation in animals, but was found to lack curare-like activity. The limbic system is inhibited by kavapyrones, an effect associated with suppression of emotional excitability and mood enhancement.

In human studies, kava produced mild euphoria with no effects on thoughts and memory. The neuropharmacologic effects of kava include analgesia, sedation, and hyporeflexia. Kava can impair gait and cause pupil dilation. Some pyrones show fungistatic properties against several fungi, including some that are pathogenic to humans.

Cautions
Pregnant and breast-feeding patients and children under age 12 should avoid use; effects are unknown. Patients with renal disease, thrombocytopenia, or neutropenia should use cautiously.

Interactions
Herb-drug
Alprazolam: may cause coma. Avoid concomitant use.
Benzodiazepines, CNS depressants: additive sedative effects. Avoid concomitant use.
Levodopa: increased Parkinsonian symptoms. Avoid concomitant use.
Pentobarbitol: may cause additive effects. Avoid concomitant use.

Herb-lifestyle
Alcohol use: increased kava toxicity. Discourage concomitant use.

Adverse reactions
CNS: changes in motor reflexes and judgment.
EENT: visual disturbances.

With long-term heavy use:
CNS: Increased patellar reflexes.
EENT: reddened eyes.
Hematologic: *leukopenia, thrombocytopenia.*
Hepatic: decreased bilirubin levels.
Metabolic: reduced plasma proteins and urea levels, weight loss.
Respiratory: pulmonary hypertension, shortness of breath.
Skin: dry, flaking, discolored skin.
Other: dopamine antagonism.

Special considerations
▶ Kava has been shown to be useful in attenuating spinal seizures and also to have antipsychotic properties. Therapeutic trials have shown a degree of seizure control in epileptic patients, suggesting involvement of the GABA receptors. Kava extract has also been studied for anxiety disorders. In a study of patients with anxiety of nonpsychotic origin, kava showed improved scores on the Hamilton Anxiety Scale.
▶ Inform the patient that significant adverse reactions may occur with long term use of kava.
▶ Other medicinal claims of kava include treatment of depression, insomnia, asthma, and venereal disease.
▶ Kava, although a depressant, is nonfermented, nonalcoholic, nonopioid and nonhallucinogenic and doesn't appear to cause physiologic dependence. However, the potential risk for psychological dependence still exists.
▶ Kava is commonly used in the South Pacific as a ceremonial beverage.
▶ Monitor patient for adverse effects, especially with long-term use.

Breast-feeding patients
▶ No data exist to demonstrate whether kava appears in breast milk. Breast-feeding patient should avoid use.

Pediatric patients
▶ Children under age 12 should avoid use because effects are unknown.

Patient teaching
▶ Tell the patient to avoid alcohol and other CNS depressants because they enhance the herb's sedative and toxic effects.
▶ Inform the patient that absorption of kava may be enhanced if taken with food.

▶ lavender
aspic, echter lavendel, English lavender (*Lavandula angustifolia*), esplieg, French lavender, garden lavender, lavanda, lavande commun, lavandin, nardo, Spanish lavender (*L. stoechas*), spigo, spike lavender, true lavender

Common trade names
Lavender, Lavender Flowers

How supplied
Available as oils, flowers, and leaves

Reported uses
Claims include lavender's use in upper abdominal discomfort caused by nervousness, and treatment of migraines and neuralgia. Lavender has also been used for pain caused by strained muscles.

Dosage

Astringent (external): 20 to 100 g of lavender added to 7.7 gallons (20 L) of water to avoid too strong a scent.

Lavender tea: 1 to 2 teaspoons in 150 ml of hot water; steep for approximately 10 minutes.

Oil (internal): 1 to 4 drops of oil on a sugar cube.

Actions

Lavender was found to cause CNS depressant effects, anticonvulsant activity, and potentiation of sedative effects of chloral hydrate in rats. Spike lavender oil has been reported to exert a spasmolytic effect on animal smooth muscle, and *L. stoechas* caused hypoglycemia in normoglycemic rats.

Lavender oil fed to rats was found to cause regression of mammary tumors. The active ingredient has been suggested to be perillyl alcohol. The National Cancer Institute is examining this herb in phase II clinical trials in patients with advanced cancers of the breast, ovaries, and prostate.

In vitro studies report promising results of topical lavender use to eradicate methicillin-resistant *Staphylococcus aureus* and vancomycin-resistant *Enterococcus faecium*. However, no clinical trials are available to confirm these results.

Cautions

Pregnant and breast-feeding patients and those taking sedatives should avoid use.

Interactions

Herb-drug

CNS depressants (benzodiazepines, opioids): may potentiate sedative effects. Avoid concomitant use.

Herb-lifestyle

Alcohol use: may potentiate sedative effects. Discourage concomitant use.

Adverse reactions

With ingestion of large doses (based on opioid-like potential)

CNS: confusion, CNS depression, drowsiness, euphoria, headache, mental dullness.

EENT: miosis.

GI: constipation, nausea, vomiting.

Respiratory: *respiratory depression.*

Skin: contact dermatitis.

Special considerations

▶ Lavender is regarded by herbalists as a sedative to treat insomnia and restlessness. Other claims include its use as an appetite stimulant. Lavender has also been used as an astringent to treat minor cuts, bruises, and burns. It has been used as an indoor scent to induce a calming effect.

▶ Lavender has been used for centuries. Unfortunately, there is inadequate clinical evidence for its efficacy in any disease or condition. Controlled studies are necessary before the use of lavender can be recommended.

▶ Lavender oil should be considered potentially poisonous. No more than 2 drops of the volatile oil should be consumed. Large doses are reported to exert opioid-like effects.

▶ Lavender has been used in small concentrations to flavor food, but it is cultivated mainly for use as a perfume, potpourri, or in decorations.

▶ Monitor the patient using lavender and other sedatives for signs of excessive sedation or opioid-like symptoms.

Breast-feeding patients
▶ No data exist to demonstrate whether lavender appears in breast milk. Breast-feeding patients should avoid use.

Patient teaching
▶ Suggest techniques other than drug therapy (such as behavior modification, light therapy, regular bedtime) to combat insomnia.
▶ Advise women to avoid use of the herb during pregnancy or when breast-feeding.
▶ Inform the patient suffering from insomnia that other sedative or hypnotic drugs with known risks and benefits are available.

▶ meadowsweet
bridewort, dolloff, dropwort, *Filipendula*, fleur d'ulmaire, flores ulmariae, gravel root, meadwort, mede-sweet, queen-of-the-meadow, spierstaude, *Spiraeae flos* (meadowsweet flower), *Spiraeae herba* (meadowsweet herb)

Common trade names
(Available in combination)
Arkocaps, Artival, Neutracalm, Rheuma-Tee, Rheumex, Santane, Spireadosa

How supplied
Available as tablets of dried herb (300 mg), infusion, powder, fluidextract, or tincture

Reported uses
Meadowsweet has been used in folk medicine for gastritis, peptic ulcer, arthritis, indigestion, heartburn, cystitis, rheumatic joints and muscles, sprains, and tendonitis. The French use the herb to treat headache and toothache pain. In Belgium, the herb is used for painful articular conditions.

Dosage
For treatment of diarrhea: 1 cup decoction b.i.d. or t.i.d. P.O.
Dried flowers: 2.5 to 3.5 g P.O. up to t.i.d.
Dried herb: 2 to 6 g P.O. up to t.i.d.
Liquid extract (1:1 in 25% alcohol): 1.5 to 6 ml P.O. up to t.i.d.
Oral infusion: 100 ml every 2 hours.
Powder: ½ teaspoon with a small amount of water t.i.d.
Tincture (1:5 in 25% alcohol): 2 to 4 ml P.O. up to t.i.d.

Actions
Meadowsweet has been used for its anti-inflammatory, antiemetic, antiulcer, astringent, antirheumatic, antiflatulent, diuretic, diaphoretic, laxative, sedative, digestive aid, and mild urinary antiseptic properties. In Russian studies with animals, meadowsweet was reported to lower motor activity and rectal temperature, relax the muscles, and potentiate the action of narcotics; prolong life expectancy of mice; lower vascular permeability and prevent stomach ulcers in mice and rats, in-

crease bronchial tone in cats; potentiate histamine bronchospasm; increase the impact of histamine upon ulcers; increase intestinal tone in guinea pigs; and increase uterine tone in rabbits. Tannins in meadowsweet have an astringent action that may ease stomach complaints.

Cautions
Pregnant and breast-feeding patients should avoid meadowsweet because its effects in them are unknown. Patients with asthma or salicylate sensitivity should also avoid this herb.

Interactions
None reported.

Adverse reactions
Respiratory: *bronchospasm.*

Special considerations
▶ Meadowsweet has also been used in folk medicine for cancer, irritable bowel syndrome (with other herbs), colds and chills, and diarrhea. The French also use the herb as a diuretic and diaphoretic. In Europe, meadowsweet is used as a natural food flavoring.
▶ Although salicylates are present, they appear to cause less GI irritation than acetylsalicylic acid. The FDA lists it as an herb of undefined safety.
▶ Meadowsweet was used as a source of salicylates for aspirin in the late 1800s. Some sources report that aspirin derived its name from this herb (*Spiraea ulmaria*).
▶ The German Commission E reports no known adverse effects or contraindications, except that of salicylate sensitivity, and indicates the use of this herb as supportive therapy for colds. Although its use cannot be recommended currently because of the lack of data, information from the German Commission E suggests that further studies are needed because the herb appears to have potential therapeutic value.

Breast-feeding patients
▶ No data exist to demonstrate whether meadowsweet appears in breast milk. Breast-feeding patients should avoid use.

Pediatric patients
▶ Children shouldn't be given meadowsweet because of salicylate content.

Patient teaching
▶ Advise the patient to avoid taking this herb because there are no clinical data to support its use.
▶ Remind the patient that some contemporary pharmaceuticals have proven antiulcer effects, although efficacy and safety data for meadowsweet are lacking.
▶ Advise women to avoid use of herb during pregnancy or breast-feeding.

▶ **mint**
balm mint, brandy mint, green mint, lamb mint, Our Lady's mint, peppermint, spearmint

Common trade names
(Various manufacturers) Ben-Gay, Rhuli Gel, Robitussin Cough Drops, Vicks VapoRub

How supplied

Peppermint and spearmint are both available as liquid extracts, tea, oil, and inhalants. Peppermint oil is also available as enteric-coated capsules. Menthol is an active component of several topical analgesics, anesthetics, and antipruritics; it's also available as an antitussive ointment, lozenge, and throat spray.

Reported uses

Peppermint is a popular medicinal and commercial mint with several uses. It's considered an anesthetic. Peppermint's antiflatulent and antispasmodic activities have been used for dyspepsia, colic, indigestion, and abdominal pain.

Menthol has been used to relieve the pain of rheumatism, neuralgia, headache, throat infections, and toothache by acting as a local anesthetic, vascular stimulant, disinfectant, antipruritic, antiseptic, and counterirritant. It's used externally in ointments, rubs, and liniments to treat itching, minor pain of sunburn, and musculoskeletal pain of neuralgia, rheumatism, and arthritis.

As a local anesthetic, menthol is used in sprays and lozenges for sore throat, and it's occasionally used to anesthetize gastric nerve endings in motion sickness and nausea.

Dosage

No consensus exists for spearmint preparations. Dosages below are for peppermint:
Capsules (enteric-coated): 1 to 2 capsules (0.2 ml/capsule) P.O. t.i.d. for irritable bowel syndrome.
Spirits (10% oil and 1% leaf extract): 1 ml (20 drops) with water.

Tea: 1 to 1.5 g (1 tablespoon) leaves in 160 ml boiling water, P.O. b.i.d. or t.i.d.
Topicals: apply t.i.d. or q.i.d.; for external use only.
The fatal dose of menthol is estimated to be 1,000 mg/kg body weight.

Actions

Peppermint essential oil is reported to have in vitro antibacterial and antiviral activity. It also relaxes the sphincter of Oddi and stimulates bile flow in animals; this choleretic effect is attributed to flavonoid components.

Most of peppermint's pharmacologic activity is from menthol, which, in concentrations of 0.1% to 1%, depresses sensory cutaneous receptors and alleviates itching and irritation. In higher concentrations, it acts as a counterirritant by stimulating the nerves that perceive cold while depressing the nerves that perceive pain and itching. When applied to the skin, menthol causes an initial feeling of coolness, followed by a sensation of warmth. The cooling effect may result from direct desensitization of warmth receptors, and warming follows vasodilation of small blood vessels under the skin.

Menthol also has a direct spasmolytic effect on smooth muscles of the digestive tract. Its spasmolytic activity is reportedly mediated through a calcium antagonist effect. Azulene (cyclopentacycloheptane) occurs in small amounts in peppermint oil and exerts antiinflammatory and antiulcerogenic effects in animals.

The medicinal action of spearmint is not documented in the literature. Although the herb is reported to have antispasmodic and anti-flatulent properties similar to peppermint, its effects are weaker.

Cautions
Menthol can cause sensitization and allergic reactions in adults and children. Symptoms include urticaria, erythema, and other cutaneous lesions.

Interactions
None reported.

Adverse reactions
GI: hiatal hernia, relaxation of lower esophageal sphincter and GI smooth muscle, worsened symptoms of gastroesophageal reflux disease.
Respiratory: laryngeal or bronchial spasms in infants and small children (with menthol in teas).
Skin: contact dermatitis with external use.
Other: allergic reactions with internal use (flushing, headache, heartburn, irritation of mucous membranes, muscle tremor, rash).

Special considerations
▶ Peppermint is also considered an antiflatulent, diaphoretic, stimulant, digestive aid, antiseptic, antiemetic, aromatic, and flavoring agent. The leaf is also a classic folk remedy for stomach cancer. The enteric-coated capsules are reported to be effective for irritable bowel syndrome; however, efficacy data from European studies are inconclusive.
▶ Menthol is also used in inhalant preparations to alleviate chest complaints, cold, cough, laryngitis, bronchitis, and nasal congestion.

▶ Peppermint oil is widely used in flavoring, pharmaceuticals, cosmetics, toothpastes, and mouth-washes, as well as in local antiseptic, anesthetic, and antipruritic preparations. It's also gaining popularity in aromatherapy and is used to increase concentration and stimulate the mind and body.
▶ Spearmint is mainly used as a flavoring agent, but it's also considered a milder antispasmodic and antiflatulent for colic and other digestive problems, and is claimed to be useful in tumors and stomach cancer. Spearmint is thought to whiten teeth, cure mouth sores, alleviate nausea and vomiting, heal the bites of a rabid dog, relieve pain of wasp stings, and repel rodents. Because its effects are less powerful than those of peppermint, it's considered to cause fewer problems in children.
▶ Menthol is generally recognized as safe and effective when used externally as a local analgesic or anesthetic and as an antipruritic.
▶ The internal use of peppermint and spearmint for purposes other than flavoring isn't recommended.
▶ Peppermint oil has been shown to cause dose-related neurotoxicity and brain lesions in rats fed up to 100 mg/kg/day for 28 days.
▶ Applying a mentholated ointment to an infant's nostrils for cold relief may cause a syncopal event.
▶ Peppermint-flavored toothpaste has been reported to worsen asthma symptoms in a young adult.
▶ Peppermint oil was dropped from nonprescription drug status in 1990 by the FDA Advisory Review Panel on OTC Miscellaneous Internal Drug Products because it lacked safety and efficacy informa-

tion for use internally as a digestive aid.

▶ Monitor patients closely for allergic reactions. Symptoms may include flushing, headache, heartburn, irritation of mucous membranes, muscle tremor, and rash.

Breast-feeding patients
▶ No data exist to demonstrate whether mint appears in breast milk. Breast-feeding patients should avoid use.

Pediatric patients
▶ No safety and efficacy data are available regarding use of these herbs in children.

Patient teaching
▶ Warn the patient not to give peppermint or spearmint products to infants or small children.
▶ Caution the patient against applying topical mentholated products to broken skin.
▶ Instruct the patient not to use topical menthol preparations with a heating pad because skin damage may occur.
▶ Warn the patient to avoid prolonged use of peppermint oil as an inhalant.
▶ Advise the patient with gastroesophageal reflux disease to avoid taking mint products internally.
▶ Advise women to avoid use of the herb during pregnancy or when breast-feeding.

▶ mugwort
ai ye, felon herb, St. John's plant, *Summitates artemisiae*, wild wormwood

Common trade names
None known.

How supplied
Available as dried leaves and roots, fluidextract, infusion, and tincture

Reported uses
Mugwort has been used for dysmenorrhea. It's used in Chinese traditional medicine for *moxa* treatments (moxibustion), in which small cones of dried mugwort leaves are burned in cups on certain points of the body, many of which coincide with acupuncture points. Moxibustion is growing in popularity in the United States.

Mugwort is also used to treat GI conditions such as colic and cramps. It has also been used to treat rheumatism.

Other claimed uses include gout, headache, and muscle spasm.

Dosage
As an appetite stimulant, 150 ml boiling water poured over 1 to 2 teaspoons of the dried herb, allowed to steep for 5 to 10 minutes, and then strained. Two to three cups of the tea is taken before meals.
For heavy menstruation, infusion of 15 g of dried herb added to 500 ml water P.O., or as tincture, up to 2.5 ml P.O. t.i.d.
For stress, 5 ml P.O. root tincture taken 30 minutes before bedtime.
For other complaints, 1 to 4 ml tincture P.O. t.i.d.

Actions

Mugwort is reported to have analgesic, anthelmintic, antibacterial, antiflatulent, antifungal, antirheumatic, antiseptic, aphrodisiac, appetite stimulant, bile stimulant, CNS depressant, counterirritant, diaphoretic, digestive, diuretic, emetic, expectorant, hemostatic, laxative, sedative, uterine stimulant, and uterine vasodilator activities.

Cautions

Pregnant and breast-feeding patients and those with bleeding abnormalities should avoid use. Patients with previous sensitization or hazelnut allergy should also avoid mugwort. Patients with reflux disease should use it cautiously.

Interactions
Herb-drug

Anticoagulants: may potentiate anticoagulant effects. Avoid concomitant use.

Adverse reactions

Skin: contact dermatitis.
Other: *anaphylaxis.*

Special considerations

▶ Mugwort was used similarly to wormwood (*Artemisia absinthium*), namely as an anthelmintic and for amenorrhea.
▶ Mugwort is also used to treat other GI conditions such as diarrhea, constipation, and weak digestion. It has also been used to treat hysteria, epilepsy, persistent vomiting, seizures in children, circulatory problems, menopausal and menstrual complaints, chills, fever, mild depression, and stress.
▶ The roots are claimed to be useful as a tonic and for psychoneu-
roses, neurasthenia, depression, hypochondria, neuroses, general irritability and restlessness, insomnia, and anxiety. Other uses include anorexia, asthma, dermatitis, dysentery, flatulence, hematemesis, hemoptysis, infertility, nosebleed, opium addiction, pinworms, roundworm, snakebite, threadworms, and whitlow. The essential oil is purported to have antibacterial and antifungal properties.
▶ Because there are no clinical data to support mugwort's several therapeutic claims, it cannot be recommended for any use.
▶ Mugwort may have significant uterine stimulant effects.
▶ Mugwort pollen is a known allergen contributing to hay fever in some patients. It has caused IgE cross-reactivity with hazelnut.
▶ Patients hypersensitive to mugwort pollen may be allergic to other foods in the daisy (Compositae) family.

Breast-feeding patients

▶ No data exist to demonstrate whether mugwort appears in breast milk. Breast-feeding patients should avoid use.

Patient teaching

▶ Caution the patient taking anticoagulants against use of this herb.
▶ Warn the pregnant or breast-feeding patient to avoid use of mugwort.
▶ Inform the patient about the lack of clinical safety and efficacy data for mugwort.

⟩ mustard
black mustard, brown mustard, California rape, charlock, Chinese mustard, Indian mustard, white mustard, wild mustard

Common trade names
(Available in combination) Act-On Rub, Musterole

How supplied
Available as a tea, ground mustard seeds (mustard flour), and mustard oil

Reported uses
Mustard has been used in footbaths for rheumatism and arthritis of the feet, and topically to alleviate muscle aches and pains.

Dosage
As a footbath, mix 1 tablespoon of mustard seeds with 1 L of hot water as a soak.
As a topical rubefacient, prepare a paste with 120 g (4 oz) of ground black mustard seeds in warm water. Irritant effect can be eased by applying olive oil after the paste is removed.

Actions
Potent local irritant effects allow mustard to serve as a rubefacient when applied topically. Irritation and copious tearing in the eyes can be attributed to allyl isothiocyanate. Isothiocyanate compounds have produced goiter in animals. The volatile mustard oil has strong antimicrobial properties. Sinigrin, a chemical component of mustard, has been reported to have antilarvicidal properties against some insects.

Mustard oil has been reported to exhibit anticarcinogenic effects in animals with arsenic-induced chromosomal aberrations. This effect was greater than that seen with garlic extract.

Cautions
Pregnant and breast-feeding patients should avoid use. Patients with pulmonary disease should also avoid it because inhalation may aggravate airways.

Interactions
None reported.

Adverse reactions
EENT: severe contact irritation of mucous membranes.
Skin: severe contact irritation.

Special considerations
⟩ The herb has also been used as a stimulant, diuretic, emetic, and antiflatulent, and both orally and topically to the chest to relieve pulmonary congestion.
⟩ Because of its toxic nature, volatile mustard oil should never be tasted or inhaled in undiluted form.
⟩ Mustard flour typically lacks the characteristic pungent aroma when dry, but the aroma is released upon contact with water, which frees allyl isothiocyanate by hydrolysis.
⟩ White mustard doesn't contain the toxic allyl isothiocyanate.
⟩ The highest average maximum level of mustard oil in foods is about 0.02%.
⟩ Topical application of white mustard seed as a poultice is approved in Germany for pulmonary congestion and joint and soft-tissue inflammation.
⟩ The unique pungent properties of mustard entice people to use it as

an herbal remedy. However, if not handled properly, mustard can damage the tissues.
❱ Monitor patient for contact dermatitis and mucous membrane irritation.

Breast-feeding patients
❱ No data exist to demonstrate whether mustard appears in breast milk. Breast-feeding patients should avoid use.

Patient teaching
❱ Caution the patient to use care when preparing mustard herbal products and to wash hands after using products to avoid contact with eyes.
❱ Warn the patient not to apply mustard preparations to mucous membranes.
❱ Advise parents to keep mustard products out of the reach of children and pets.

❱ peyote
anhalonium, big chief, buttons, cactus, mesc, mescal, mescal buttons, mescaline, mexc, moon, pan peyote, peyote button

Controlled substance schedule I

Common trade names
None known.

How supplied
Basic pan peyote: chloroform extract of ground peyote
Button: 45 mg of mescaline
Mescaline hydrochloride or sulfate: 375 mg of hydrochloride salt equals 500 mg of the sulfate salt
Soluble peyote: hydrochloride extract of basic pan peyote used for injection

Tincture: 70% alcohol extract of peyote

Reported uses
Peyote has reportedly been used as a narcotic and sedative. Folk remedies involve use of the herb for angina; as a painkiller for arthritis, backache, burns, and corns; and for headache, rheumatism, and throat irritation.

Dosage
Mescaline doses of 5 mg/kg produce physical effects and hallucinations.

Actions
Mescaline stimulates adenylate cyclase activity at central dopaminergic receptors in the anterior limbic structures. It specifically acts on the pons and pontine raphe nuclei, decreasing neuronal firing and serotonin turnover. It also acts on the catecholamine and indolamine systems. It may inhibit cholinergic neuromuscular transmission by blocking release of acetylcholine and affecting potassium conductance. Mescaline is also thought to have affinity for the $5-HT_{1A}$, $5-HT_{2A}$, and $5-HT_{2C}$ receptors.

Cautions
Pregnant and breast-feeding patients should avoid use. Patients with CNS disorders should use cautiously.

Interactions
Herb-drug
Drugs that act on CNS (opioid analgesics): may potentiate or aggravate effects. Discourage concomitant use.

Herb-lifestyle
Alcohol, marijuana, psychedelics: may potentiate or aggravate effects. Discourage concomitant use.

Adverse reactions
CNS: anxiety, ataxia, *hyperreflexia,* emotional lability, paranoia, tremors.
CV: **bradycardia,** *hypertension,* hypotension, *mild tachycardia,* vasodilation.
EENT: *mydriasis,* nystagmus, photophobia.
GI: nausea, vomiting.
Musculoskeletal: muscle fasciculations.
Respiratory: **respiratory depression.**
Skin: *diaphoresis.*

Special considerations
▶ Peyote has long been used in Native American religious ceremonies. It has also reportedly been used as an antibiotic, cardiotonic, hallucinogenic, intoxicant, poison, psychedelic, and tonic. Folk remedies also involve use of the herb for alcoholism, paralysis, fever, snakebite, and sunstroke.
▶ Peyote that has been mixed with phencyclidine (PCP or "angel dust") or other illicit drugs that may worsen the patient's condition.
▶ Peyote is considered to have no accepted medicinal use and a high abuse potential.
▶ Peyote is used as a sacramental rite in the Native American Church, and its members are, therefore, exempt from prosecution under the Controlled Substances Act.
▶ Peyote is not thought to cause physical dependence, and it isn't known whether it can cause psychological dependence. Tolerance does occur and can cross over to LSD (lysergic acid diethylamide) and DMT (dimethyltryptamine).
▶ Death from high doses is less common than traumatic fatalities resulting from altered perception. Treatment is supportive until the effects have worn off. Place the patient in a semidarkened room and "talk down," if necessary. Diphenhydramine or a mild tranquilizer, such as diazepam, can be given if needed. Avoid antipsychotics because psychosis will resolve spontaneously.
▶ Monitor patient for nausea and vomiting, which commonly occur within 30 to 60 minutes after ingestion.

Breast-feeding patients
▶ No data exist to demonstrate whether peyote appears in breast milk. Breast-feeding patients shouldn't use peyote.

Patient teaching
▶ Inform patient that peyote has no accepted medicinal use and a high risk of abuse.

▶ **primrose, evening**
king's-cure-all

Common trade names
(Various manufacturers; available in combination) Efamol, Epogram, Evening Primrose Oil, Mega Primrose Oil, My Favorite Evening Primrose Oil, Primrose Power

How supplied
Capsules: 50 mg, 500 mg, 1,300 mg
Gelcaps: 500 mg, 1,300 mg

Reported uses

An infusion using the whole primrose plant is reported to have sedative properties. Traditionally, it has been used for breast pain, rheumatoid arthritis, Raynaud's disease, diabetic neuropathy, and as a sedative and analgesic.

Placebo-controlled studies have suggested that gamma linoleic acid (GLA), a component of primrose oil, is superior in the treatment of breast pain and tenderness from premenstrual syndrome and benign breast disease. Animal studies have shown that diabetic neuropathy can be prevented or reversed through GLA supplementation with evening primrose oil.

Evening primrose oil has been studied alone and with fish oils versus placebo in rheumatoid arthritis. These trials showed an improvement in the patient's symptoms, based on the reduced need for pain medication. There was no evidence, however, of evening primrose oil having a disease-modifying action.

Dosage

The following dosages are based on a standardized GLA content of 8%. No consensus exists for other disorders.

For mastalgia, 3 to 4 g P.O. daily.
For eczema, 320 mg to 8 g P.O. daily in adults. In children ages 1 to 12, 160 mg to 4 g P.O. daily; continue for 3 months.

Actions

The claimed therapeutic action of evening primrose oil stems from essential fatty acids that are important as cellular structural elements and as precursors of prostaglandin synthesis. Linoleic acid cannot be manufactured by the body and therefore must be provided through dietary intake. The body relies on the metabolic conversion of linoleic acid (LA) to GLA. Deficient conversion, which has been observed in such disorders as diabetes, CV disease, hypercholesterolemia, viral infections, cancer, and skin conditions, affects prostaglandin-E_1 and E_2 synthesis. It is claimed that LA and GLA supplementation from dietary sources maintains a balance between the inflammatory and noninflammatory prostaglandins that may, in turn, be useful in treating these disorders.

Cautions

Pregnant patients should avoid use because the effects in them are unknown. Schizophrenic patients and those taking epileptogenic drugs should use cautiously.

Interactions
Herb-drug
Phenothiazines: may increase the risk of seizures. Discourage concomitant use.

Adverse reactions
CNS: headache.
GI: nausea.
Skin: rash.

Special considerations
▶ Evening primrose oil has been used as a vegetable with a peppery flavor. An infusion using the whole plant is reported to have astringent properties. Traditionally, it has also been used for asthmatic cough, GI disorders, whooping cough, eczema, premenstrual syndrome, psoriasis, multiple sclerosis, hypercholesterolemia, asthma, and

Sjögren's syndrome. Poultices made with evening primrose oil have been used to speed wound healing.

▶ Hyperactive children are thought to have abnormal levels of essential fatty acids. Supplementation of evening primrose oil has produced controversial results. One trial saw no improvement in the behavioral patterns of children and blood fatty acid levels. However, another study showed a calming effect in two-thirds of children treated with evening primrose oil.

▶ Animal studies have indicated that evening primrose oil produced significant reductions in mammary tumors from baseline size. In vitro experiments found a dose-related inhibition of the growth rate in malignant tumors. High levels of essential fatty acids are toxic to several cancers but not lethal to normal cells. Human studies are currently underway to assess supplementation of essential fatty acids on the growth of cancer cells.

▶ Evening primrose oil is not approved for the treatment of any specific condition.

▶ Monitor patient closely. Temporal lobe epilepsy may occur, especially in schizophrenic patients or those taking epileptogenic drugs such as phenothiazines.

Patient teaching

▶ Instruct the patient with a seizure disorder to reconsider use of this herb.

▶ Caution parents to use this herb for a hyperactive child only under supervision of an experienced practitioner.

▶ rue
herb-of-grace, herbygrass, *Ruta*, rutae herba, Vinruta

Common trade names
(Various manufacturers; available in combination) Joint and Muscle Relief Cream, Rue

How supplied
Available as crude herb, capsules, extracts, and creams

Reported uses
Based on anecdotal data and studies in animals, the herb is currently being promoted for the treatment of sports injuries, arthritis, bruising, sprains and strains, and other joint and muscle disorders. However, there are no human clinical trial data available for these uses. It has also been used for its sedative effects.

Other claims for which there are no supporting data include use in neuralgia, eye strain, earache, dysmenorrhea, and digestive disorders.

Dosage
For earache, place a few drops of infused oil on a cotton plug placed over the ear.
Capsule: 1 capsule P.O. t.i.d. with water and food.
Cream: applied as needed.
Extract: ¼ to 1 teaspoonful P.O. t.i.d. with water and food.

Actions
Rue extracts have shown antimicrobial effects and mutagenic and cytotoxic actions in several cellular models. Studies in mammals have demonstrated an antifertility action, mediated by decreased im-

plantation. An abortifacient action has also been noted. Components of rue nonselectively block potassium and sodium channels in myelinated nerves.

Rue has also demonstrated CV effects in rats. It exhibits positive chronotropic and inotropic effects in isolated rat atria. It acts as a hypotensive in normotensive animals, presumably through a direct vasodilatory mechanism. The alkaloids have demonstrated antispasmodic effects. Rue also exhibits analgesic properties in mice.

Cautions
Pregnant patients should avoid use because of the risk of miscarriage. Patients with a history of heart failure or arrhythmias and those receiving antihypertensive medications should use cautiously.

Interactions
Herb-drug
Antihypertensives: possible increased vasodilatory effects. Use with caution.
Digoxin, dobutamine: enhanced inotropic effects. Use with caution.
Fertility drugs: possible counteraction of therapy. Avoid concomitant use.

Herb-lifestyle
Sun exposure: increased risk of photosensitivity. Urge precautions.

Adverse reactions
CV: hypotension.
GU: increased risk of spontaneous abortion.
Skin: allergic skin reactions (such as erythema, hyperpigmentation, and severe blistering with topical use), photosensitivity.

Special considerations
▶ Rue has traditionally been promoted as a spasmolytic and abortifacient. It has also been used to promote lactation.
▶ Other claims, for which there are no supporting data, include use in edema, amenorrhea, and as an anthelmintic. Rue has also been used by Chinese herbalists for snake and insect bites.
▶ Rue is thought to be a powerful antidote at low doses; larger doses are toxic.
▶ The risks of use outweigh the benefits.
▶ Assess for cumulative effects if patient also takes an antihypertensive.

Patient teaching
▶ Caution patient that insufficient data are available regarding the effects of rue in humans.
▶ Advise women to report planned, suspected, or known pregnancy.
▶ Instruct patient to discontinue use of herb and to notify a health care professional if allergic skin reaction develops.

▶ **turmeric**
Curcuma, **Indian saffron, Indian valerian, jiang huang, radix, red valerian, tumeric**

Common trade names
Turmeric Root

How supplied
Available as capsules, curry spices, dry rhizome, extract, oil, tincture, and turmeric spices

Reported uses

Turmeric has reportedly been used in the treatment of inflammatory conditions such as injuries, osteoarthritis, and rheumatoid arthritis.

Traditional Chinese and Indian (Ayurvedic) philosophies of medicine involve the use of turmeric for toothache, bruises, chest pain, and colic. Poultices of turmeric have been used to relieve local pain and inflammation.

Dosage

The recommended dosage of curcumin is 400 to 600 mg P.O. t.i.d. For turmeric, an equivalent dosage of 8 to 60 g P.O. t.i.d. is necessary. Turmeric should be taken on an empty stomach.

Actions

Turmeric compounds, especially curcumin, have been extensively studied. Curcumin appears to inhibit carcinogenesis at all steps of cancer formation; it promotes detoxification of carcinogens in vitro and in vivo. Antioxidant properties were noted in protein isolated from a liquid extract of turmeric. Rats pretreated with curcumin had fewer and smaller tumors than controls when exposed to chemical carcinogens; this action was partially attributed to the antioxidant properties.

Curcumin shows promise in the treatment of cholelithiasis. Intestinal cholesterol uptake was significantly reduced in rats given curcumin.

Curcumin is as effective as NSAIDs in the treatment of rheumatoid arthritis, osteoarthritis, and postoperative pain. It is thought to stimulate corticosteroid release, sensitize cortisol recep-

tors, or increase the half-life of cortisol through alteration of hepatic degradation processes.

Turmeric extract inhibited gastric secretion and protected gastroduodenal mucosa against ulcer formation induced by stress, pyloric ligation, indomethacin, reserpine, and cysteamine in rats. However, in high doses it may be ulcerogenic.

Curcumin has been used as an antiseptic and antiparasitic internally and externally; it has slowed the growth of most organisms associated with cholecystitis. Curcumin has been found to interfere with the replication of viruses, including viral hepatitis and HIV. Curcumin has increased the CD4 count and inhibited the activity of enzymes that transport the virus into healthy cells.

Cautions

Pregnant and breast-feeding patients should avoid use. The American Herbal Products Association has classified turmeric as a menstrual stimulant; therefore, it may induce miscarriage. Patients with bleeding disorders and bile duct obstruction should also avoid turmeric. Those with a history of ulcers should use it cautiously.

Interactions
Herb-drug

Anticoagulants: possible additive effects on platelets. Avoid concomitant use.

Immunosuppressants: decreased effect. Use cautiously, if at all, in combination.

NSAIDs: may inhibit platelet function and increase the risk for bleeding. Avoid concomitant use.

Adverse reactions
GI: stomach ulcers with high doses or prolonged use.
Skin: allergic contact dermatitis.

Special considerations
▶ Turmeric has also reportedly been used in cancer prevention and as a treatment adjunct. According to the American Institute for Cancer Research, curcumin prevents stomach, colon, oral, esophageal, breast, and skin cancers. It is also used in the treatment of other inflammatory conditions such as irritable bowel syndrome, atherosclerosis, liver disorders, cholelithiasis, GI diseases (ulcerations, gastritis, flatulence), and in infections caused by viruses, GI bacterial overgrowth, and parasitic infestation.
▶ Traditional Chinese and Indian (Ayurvedic) philosophies of medicine also involve the use of turmeric for flatulence, jaundice, menstrual problems, bloody urine, and hemorrhage.
▶ Monitor bleeding studies if medicinal doses are being used.

Breast-feeding patients
▶ No data exist to demonstrate whether turmeric appears in breast milk. Breast-feeding patients should avoid use.

Patient teaching
▶ Tell patient to report evidence of unusual bruising or bleeding.
▶ Advise women to avoid use of the herb during pregnancy or when breast-feeding.
▶ Warn patient to keep turmeric out of reach of children and pets.

▶ vervain
American vervain, blue vervain, enchanter's herb, European vervain, herba veneris, herbe sacrée, herb of the grace, holy herb, pigeon grass, purvain, simpler's joy, wild hyssop

Common trade names
Blue Vervain

How supplied
Capsules: 360 mg

Reported uses
Traditionally, vervain has been claimed to be useful in rheumatism, kidney stones, cramps, dysuria, hemorrhoids, neuralgia, pleurisy, and ulcers. It has also been used as an analgesic and antispasmodic. However, clinical data are lacking.

Dosage
As a purgative and for bowel pain, a decoction of 2 oz to 1 quart P.O. daily has been used.
As a sedative, 360 mg (1 capsule) P.O. h.s.

Actions
In large doses, the glycoside verbenin has been thought to stimulate milk excretion in low doses and inhibit sympathetic nerve endings on the heart, blood vessel, intestine, and salivary glands. Two studies failed to show antidiarrheal, antithyrotropic, or antigonadotropic activity.

Cautions
Patients with multiple allergies and those with asthma or other respiratory disorders should avoid use. Patients with a history of seizure

disorders should use vervain cautiously. In large doses, vervain can induce seizures.

Interactions
Herb-drug
Anticoagulants: possible enhanced effect. Avoid concomitant use.

Adverse reactions
CNS: CNS paralysis followed by stupor and *clonic and tetanic seizures* with large doses.
Skin: contact dermatitis.

Special considerations
▶ Vervain has also been traditionally used in ocular disease, fever, anemia, bronchitis, tumors, colds, eczema, edema, insomnia, malaria, pertussis, tympany, and uterine disorders. It has also been used as an anthelmintic, aphrodisiac, astringent, diaphoretic, diuretic, emetic, and expectorant. However, clinical data are lacking.
▶ The FDA has classified vervain as an herb of undefined safety.
▶ Monitor patient for CNS effects with large doses.
▶ Watch for increased seizure activity in patients with history of seizures.

Patient teaching
▶ Explain that vervain may worsen seizure activity if taken in excessive amounts by patients with seizure disorders.
▶ Tell patient that no clinical data exist to support use of this herb for any medical condition.
▶ Tell patient receiving anticoagulants that, even though vervain has been known in folk medicine to slow blood coagulation, it should be used with caution until more data are available.

▶ wild yam
China root, colic root, devil's bones, Mexican wild yam, rheumatism root, yuma

Common trade names
Mexican Wild Yam Power, Wild Yam Extract, Wild Yam Root, Wild Yam Root & Rhizome Extract

How supplied
Available as a liquid extract, topical oil, and in capsules.

Reported uses
Wild yam is claimed to be useful in the treatment of inflammatory rheumatism, rheumatoid arthritis, dysentary, diverticulosis, stomach and muscle cramps, intermittent claudication, pain in the womb and ovaries, gall or biliary stones, and as an antispasmodic.

Dosage
Average dose is 2 to 4 g or fluid equivalent P.O. t.i.d.
Liquid extract: 2 to 4 ml in water P.O. t.i.d., or 5 to 30 drops P.O. t.i.d.
Oil: external use only.

Actions
This herb was historically the sole source of the raw materials for manufacturing contraceptive hormones, cortisone, and anabolic hormones. It was thought that because wild yam contains dioscin, a precursor for manufacturing progesterone and estrogen, the herb possessed progesterone-like effects.

Wild yam contains large amounts of dioscin, which can be chemically synthesized into progesterone. However, the body doesn't convert this compound into any steroid. Dioscin has anti-inflammatory activity.

Cautions
Pregnant patients should avoid use because of the possibility of fetal masculinization.

Patients with a family history of hormone-induced malignancies, including breast, ovarian, uterine, and prostate cancer should also avoid use.

Interactions
Herb-drug
Estrogen or estrogen-containing drugs: may cause additive effects when coadministered. Discourage concomitant use.
Indomethacin: may increase elimination of indomethacin, reducing plasma levels and anti-inflammatory effects of the drug. Discourage concomitant use.

Adverse reactions
CNS: headache.
GI: diarrhea, nausea, vomiting.
GU: menstrual irregularities, potential for stimulating growth of prostate cancer.
Skin: acne, hair loss, hirsutism, oily skin.

Special considerations
▶ Wild yam is also claimed to be useful in the treatment of adrenal exhaustion, spasmodic asthma, menopausal symptoms, and as a diaphoretic.
▶ Monitor patient for adverse effects.
▶ Closely monitor patient with hormone-induced malignancies.

Patient teaching
▶ Advise patient that wild yam isn't converted into steroids within the body as once believed.
▶ Inform patient that some herbal products have progesterone chemically added, so manufacturers can claim steroidal effects.
▶ Tell women to avoid use of wild yam during pregnancy.
▶ Caution patient that one of the herb's components, dioscorin, may cause CNS stimulation. Poisoning may occur with high doses.

▶ willow
black willow, white willow

Common trade names
(Various manufacturers; available in combination) Aller g Formula 25, White Willow Bark, Willowprin

How supplied
Capsules: 379 mg, 400 mg
Liquid extract: 1 oz

Reported uses
In ancient Egypt, extracts of willow bark were commonly used to treat inflammatory conditions. Willow is claimed to be an effective analgesic and is thought to be useful in the treatment of rheumatism and other systemic inflammatory diseases.

Dosage
Average daily dose of salicin is 60 to 120 mg P.O.
Dried bark: 1 to 3 g as a decoction (cold tea), P.O. t.i.d.
Liquid extract (1:1 in 25% alcohol): 1 to 3 ml P.O. t.i.d.

Actions

The salicylate-like compounds exert anti-inflammatory, analgesic, antipyretic, and uricosuric effects. Tannins exert astringent effects. Flowers of a Russian species (*Salix daphnoides*) have yielded thromboplastin-like effects that trigger procoagulant effects in animals.

Cautions

Patients with salicylate hypersensitivity and pregnant and breast-feeding patients should avoid use.

Patients with asthma, allergic rhinitis, or a history of plant allergy, and those prone to systemic thromboembolism, such as those with prior venous thromboembolic disease or thromboembolic stroke, previous MI, poor ejection fraction, or atrial fibrillation should use cautiously. Patients with renal insufficiency, a history of GI bleeding, or peptic ulcers, and patients with bleeding tendencies should also use willow cautiously.

Interactions
Herb-drug

Anticoagulants: may enhance the risk of bleeding. Avoid concomitant use.
Antihypertensives: may reduce effectiveness. Avoid concomitant use.
Diuretics: enhanced risk for salicylate toxicity; may reduce effectiveness. Avoid concomitant use.
NSAIDs: may increase the risk of stomach ulceration and bleeding. Advise against concomitant use.

Adverse reactions

EENT: allergic rhinitis from aerosolized willow pollen.
GI: GI bleeding.

GU: renal damage.
Hematologic: increased bleeding time.
Hepatic: liver dysfunction.
Respiratory: asthma exacerbations.
Skin: contact dermatitis, local irritation.
Other: *anaphylaxis,* salicylate toxicity (nausea, vomiting, dizziness, tinnitus, CNS confusion, lethargy, metabolic acidosis, diarrhea).

Special considerations

▶ Willow is also claimed to be an effective antipyretic, and is thought to be useful in the treatment of influenza.
▶ Monitor patient for bleeding and for evidence of salicylate toxicity.
▶ If patient has a history of asthma or allergies, watch closely for adverse reactions.

Breast-feeding patients

▶ No data exist to demonstrate whether willow appears in breast milk. Breast-feeding patients should avoid use.

Patient teaching

▶ Counsel the patient with history of allergy or asthma to avoid willow products.
▶ Advise the patient taking anticoagulants to avoid use of willow because of risk of increased bleeding.
▶ Inform patient that insufficient evidence exists to confirm a therapeutic application for willow.
▶ Commercial products containing salicylic acid are readily available. Tell the patient to use standardized products.

❭ yerba maté

armino, Bartholomew's tea, boca juniors, campeche, elacy, el agricultor, flor de lis, gaucho, jaguar, Jesuit's tea, la hoja, la mulata, la tranquera, lonjazo, madrugada, maté, maté bulk loose tea, nobleza gaucha, oro verde, Paraguay tea, payadito, rosamonte, safira, union, yerba-de-maté, yi-yi, zerboni

Common trade names
None known.

How supplied
Available as leaves, tea, and liquid extract

Reported uses
Aside from its popularity as a tea drink in South America, many therapeutic claims have been made for yerba maté; these include use as a antirheumatic and analgesic.

Dosage
Fluidextract (1:1 in 25% alcohol): 2 to 4 ml P.O. t.i.d.
Tea: 2 to 4 g dried leaf P.O. t.i.d.

Actions
The pharmacologic properties of caffeine, theophylline, and theobromine have been evaluated in humans and are well documented. Unlike caffeine and theophylline, theobromine has no stimulant effects on the CNS. Theobromine also has a weaker diuretic effect and is a less powerful stimulant of smooth muscle than theophylline. Large doses of theobromine may result in nausea and vomiting.

Cautions
Patients with hypertension or anxiety should avoid use. Pregnant and breast-feeding patients should also avoid use. Children may be especially susceptible to the toxic effects of yerba maté.

Interactions
Herb-drug
Benzodiazepines, CNS depressants: may counteract effects of these drugs. Discourage concomitant use.
Disulfiram: possible disulfiram reaction if herbal product contains alcohol. Discourage concomitant use.
Diuretics: may have an additive effect. Advise patient not to use together.
Hepatic microsomal enzyme inhibitors (cimetidine, ciprofloxacin, verapamil): may decrease clearance of yerba maté methylxanthines and cause toxicity. Advise patient to use together cautiously.

Herb-food
Caffeine: additive effects. Monitor patient.

Herb-lifestyle
Smoking: additive effects. Monitor patient.

Adverse reactions
CNS: irritability, nervousness, withdrawal headache.
CV: flushing, palpitations.
GI: nausea, vomiting.
Hepatic: *hepatotoxicity*.
Musculoskeletal: muscle twitching.

Special considerations
❭ Many other therapeutic claims have been made for yerba maté, in-

cluding use as a diuretic, antidepressant, cathartic, and CNS stimulant. It has been promoted for the management of diabetes, as well as heart, nerve, and stomach disorders. In Germany, yerba maté is used for the management of physical and mental fatigue because of its purported analeptic properties. In China, yerba maté is reportedly given parenterally for its hypotensive effect and is also used as an appetite suppressant.

▶ Yerba maté is a popular beverage, much like coffee or tea, in parts of South America (primarily Brazil, Paraguay, and Argentina).

▶ Prolonged consumption of yerba maté has been linked to increased cancer risk.

▶ Monitor liver function tests, and observe for evidence of methylxanthine toxicity.

Breast-feeding patients
▶ No data exist to demonstrate whether yerba maté appears in breast milk. Breast-feeding patients should avoid use.

Pediatric patients
▶ Parents shouldn't give this herb to children because they may be especially susceptible to toxic effects.

Patient teaching
▶ Explain that heavy consumption of yerba maté may increase the risk of liver disease, upper digestive tract cancers, and bladder cancer.

▶ If patient takes disulfiram, warn against using an herbal form that contains alcohol.

▶ Advise the patient to avoid caffeine, smoking, and other CNS stimulants while using this herb.

▶ Urge patient to report any unusual signs or symptoms.

PART 4

Appendices and Index

Selected nonnarcotic analgesic combination products

Many common analgesics are combinations of two or more generic drugs. This table reviews common nonnarcotic analgesics.

TRADE NAMES	GENERIC DRUGS	INDICATIONS AND ADULT DOSAGES
Allerest No-Drowsiness Tablets, Coldrine, Ornex No Drowsiness Caplets, Sinus-Relief Tablets, Sinutab Without Drowsiness	▶ acetaminophen 325 mg ▶ pseudoephedrine hydrochloride 30 mg	For common cold, nasal congestion, sinus congestion, sinus pain. Give 2 tablets q 6 hours. Maximum, 8 tablets in 24 hours.
Amaphen, Anoquan, Butace, Endolor, Esgic, Femcet, Fioricet, Fiorpap, Isocet, Medigesic, Repan	▶ acetaminophen 325 mg ▶ caffeine 40 mg ▶ butalbital 50 mg	For headache, mild to moderate pain, migraine. Give 1–2 tablets or capsules q 4 hours. Maximum, 6 tablets or capsules in 24 hours.
Anacin, Gensan	▶ aspirin 400 mg ▶ caffeine 32 mg	For headache, mild pain, myalgia. Give 2 tablets q 6 hours. Maximum, 8 tablets in 24 hours.
Arthritis Foundation Nighttime, Extra Strength Tylenol PM, Midol PM	▶ acetaminophen 500 mg ▶ diphenhydramine 25 mg	For allergic rhinitis, headache, insomnia from pain or pruritus. Give 1 tablet at bedtime.
Ascriptin	▶ aspirin 325 mg ▶ magnesium hydroxide 50 mg ▶ aluminum hydroxide 50 mg ▶ calcium carbonate 50 mg	For fever, mild to moderate pain. Give 1–2 tablets q 4 hours.
Ascriptin A/D	▶ aspirin 325 mg ▶ magnesium hydroxide 75 mg ▶ aluminum hydroxide 75 mg ▶ calcium carbonate 75 mg	For mild to moderate pain. Give 1–2 tablets q 4 hours.

(continued)

◇ Available in Canada only

TRADE NAMES	GENERIC DRUGS	INDICATIONS AND ADULT DOSAGES
Cama, Arthritis Pain Reliever	▶ aspirin 500 mg ▶ magnesium oxide 150 mg ▶ aluminum hydroxide 125 mg	For mild to moderate pain. Give 1–2 tablets q 4 hours. Maximum, 8 tablets in 24 hours.
COPE	▶ aspirin 421 mg ▶ caffeine 32 mg ▶ magnesium hydroxide 50 mg ▶ aluminum hydroxide 25 mg	For mild to moderate pain. Give 1–2 tablets q 4 hours. Maximum, 8 tablets in 24 hours.
Doan's P.M. Extra Strength	▶ magnesium salicylate 500 mg ▶ diphenhydramine 25 mg	For insomnia from mild back pain. Give 2 tablets at bedtime.
Esgic-Plus	▶ acetaminophen 500 mg ▶ caffeine 40 mg ▶ butalbital 50 mg	For headache, migraine, mild to moderate pain. Give 1–2 tablets or capsules q 4 hours. Maximum, 6 tablets or capsules in 24 hours.
Excedrin Extra Strength, Excedrin Migraine	▶ aspirin 250 mg ▶ acetaminophen 250 mg ▶ caffeine 65 mg	For headache, migraine. Give 2 tablets q 4 hours. Maximum, 8 tablets in 24 hours.
Excedrin P.M. Caplets	▶ acetaminophen 500 mg ▶ diphenhydramine citrate 3 mg	For insomnia from pain or pruritus. Give 1 tablet at bedtime.
Fiorinal, Fiortal, Lanorinal	▶ aspirin 325 mg ▶ caffeine 40 mg ▶ butalbital 50 mg	For headache, mild to moderate pain. Give 1–2 tablets or capsules q 4 hours. Maximum, 6 tablets or capsules in 24 hours.
Midrin	▶ isometheptene mucate 65 mg ▶ dichloralphenazone 100 mg ▶ acetaminophen 325 mg	For migraine, tension headache. For migraine, give 2 capsules initially; then 1 capsule q 1 hour to a maximum of 5 capsules in 12 hours. For tension headache, give 1–2 capsules q 4 hours to a maximum of 8 capsules in 24 hours.
Phrenilin	▶ acetaminophen 325 mg ▶ butalbital 50 mg	For headache, mild to moderate pain. Give 1–2 tablets q 4 hours. Maximum, 6 tablets in 24 hours.

◇ Available in Canada only

TRADE NAMES	GENERIC DRUGS	INDICATIONS AND ADULT DOSAGES
Phrenilin Forte, Sedapap	▶ acetaminophen 650 mg ▶ butalbital 50 mg	For headache, mild to moderate pain. Give 1 tablet or capsule q 4 hours. Maximum, 4 tablets or capsules in 24 hours.
Sinus Excedrin Extra Strength	▶ acetaminophen 500 mg ▶ pseudoephedrine hydrochloride 30 mg	For common cold, nasal and sinus congestion, sinus pain. Give 2 tablets q 6 hours. Maximum, 8 tablets in 24 hours.
Sinutab Regular ◇	▶ acetaminophen 325 mg ▶ chlorpheniramine 2 mg ▶ pseudoephedrine hydrochloride 30 mg	For allergic rhinitis, common cold, flu symptoms. Give 2 tablets q 4 hours. Maximum, 8 tablets in 24 hours.
Sinutab Maximum Strength	▶ acetaminophen 500 mg ▶ pseudoephedrine hydrochloride 30 mg ▶ chlorpheniramine maleate 2 mg	For allergic rhinitis, common cold, flu symptoms. Give 2 tablets q 6 hours. Maximum, 8 tablets in 24 hours.
Tecnal ◇	▶ aspirin 330 mg ▶ caffeine 40 mg ▶ butalbital 5 mg	For headache, mild to moderate pain. Give 1–2 tablets or capsules q 4 hours. Maximum, 6 tablets or capsules in 24 hours.
Vanquish	▶ aspirin 227 mg ▶ acetaminophen 194 mg ▶ caffeine 33 mg ▶ aluminum hydroxide 25 mg ▶ magnesium hydroxide 50 mg	For minor aches and pains. Give 2 caplets q 4 hours. Maximum, 12 caplets in 24 hours.

◇ Available in Canada only

Selected narcotic analgesic combination products

Many common analgesics are combinations of two or more generic drugs. This table reviews common narcotic analgesics.

TRADE NAMES AND CONTROLLED SUBSTANCE SCHEDULE (CSS)	GENERIC DRUGS	INDICATIONS AND ADULT DOSAGES
Aceta with Codeine *CSS III*	▶ acetminophen 30 mg ▶ codeine phosphate 30 mg	For fever, mild to moderate pain. Give 1–2 tablets q 4 hours. Maximum, 12 tablets in 24 hours.
Anexsia 7.5/650, Lorcet Plus *CSS III*	▶ acetaminophen 650 mg ▶ hydrocodone bitartrate 7.5 mg	For arthralgia, bone pain, dental pain, headache, migraine, moderate pain. Give 1–2 tablets q 4 hours. Maximum, 6 tablets in 24 hours.
Azolone, Damason-P *CSS III*	▶ acetaminophen 500 mg ▶ hydrocodone bitartrate 5 mg	For moderate to moderately severe pain. Give 1–2 tablets q 4 hours. Maximum, 8 tablets in 24 hours.
Capital with Codeine, Tylenol with Codeine Elixir *CSS V*	▶ acetaminophen 120 mg ▶ codeine phosphate 12 mg/5 ml	For mild to moderate pain. Give 15 ml q 4 hours.
Darvocet-N 50 *CSS IV*	▶ acetaminophen 325 mg ▶ propoxyphene napsylate 50 mg	For mild to moderate pain. Give 1–2 tablets q 4 hours. Maximum, 12 tablets in 24 hours.
Darvocet-N 100, Propacet 100 *CSS IV*	▶ acetaminophen 650 mg ▶ propoxyphene napsykate 100 mg	For mild to moderate pain. Give 1 tablet q 4 hours. Maximum, 6 tablets in 24 hours.
E-Lor, Genagesic, Wygesic *CSS IV*	▶ acetaminophen 650 mg ▶ propoxyphene napsykate 65 mg	For mild to moderate pain. Give 1 tablet q 4 hours. Maximum, 6 tablets in 24 hours.
Empirin with Codeine No. 3 *CSS III*	▶ aspirin 325 mg ▶ codeine phosphate 30 mg	For fever, mild to moderate pain. Give 1–2 tablets q 4 hours. Maximum, 12 tablets in 24 hours.

◇ Available in Canada only

TRADE NAMES AND CONTROLLED SUBSTANCE SCHEDULE (CSS)	GENERIC DRUGS	INDICATIONS AND ADULT DOSAGES
Empirin with Codeine No. 4 *CSS III*	▶ aspirin 325 mg ▶ codeine phosphate 60 mg	For fever, mild to moderate pain. Give 1 tablet q 4 hours. Maximum, 6 tablets in 24 hours.
Fioricet with Codeine *CSS III*	▶ acetaminophen 325 mg ▶ butalbital 50 mg ▶ caffeine 40 mg ▶ codeine phosphate 30 mg	For headache, mild to moderate pain. Give 1–2 capsules q 4 hours. Maximum, 6 capsules in 24 hours.
Fiorinal with Codeine *CSS III*	▶ aspirin 325 mg ▶ butalbital 50 mg ▶ caffeine 40 mg ▶ codeine phosphate 30 mg	For headache, mild to moderate pain. Give 1–2 tablets or capsules q 4 hours. Maximum, 6 tablets or capsules in 24 hours.
Innovar Injection *CSS II*	▶ droperidol 2.5 mg ▶ fentanyl citrate 0.05 mg/ml	For preoperative analgesia, sedation induction. Give 0.09-0.11 mg/kg I.V. (slow infusion, 1 ml over 1–2 minutes) until sleep occurs.
Lorcet 10/650 *CSS III*	▶ acetaminophen 650 mg ▶ hydrocodone bitartrate 10 mg	For moderate to moderately severe pain. Give 1 tablet q 4 hours. Maximum, 6 tablets in 24 hours.
Lortab 2.5/500 *CSS III*	▶ acetaminophen 500 mg ▶ hydrocodone bitartrate 2.5 mg	For moderate to moderately severe pain. Give 1–2 tablets q 4 hours. Maximum, 8 tablets in 24 hours.
Lortab 5/500 *CSS III*	▶ acetaminophen 500 mg ▶ hydrocodone bitartrate 5 mg	For moderate to moderately severe pain. Give 1–2 tablets q 4 hours. Maximum, 8 tablets in 24 hours.
Lortab 7.5/500 *CSS III*	▶ acetaminophen 500 mg ▶ hydrocodone bitartrate 7.5 mg	For moderate to moderately severe pain. Give 1 tablet q 4 hours. Maximum, 8 tablets in 24 hours.
Percocet 2.5/325 *CSS II*	▶ acetaminophen 325 mg ▶ oxycodone hydrochloride 2.5 mg	For moderate to moderately severe pain. Give 1–2 tablets q 4-6 hours. Maximum, 12 tablets in 24 hours.

(continued)

◊ Available in Canada only

TRADE NAMES AND CONTROLLED SUBSTANCE SCHEDULE (CSS)	GENERIC DRUGS	INDICATIONS AND ADULT DOSAGES
Percocet *CSS II*	▶ acetaminophen 325 mg ▶ oxycodone hydro-chloride 5 mg	For moderate to moderately severe pain. Give 1–2 tablets q 4 hours. Maximum, 12 tablets in 24 hours.
Percocet 7.5/500 *CSS II*	▶ acetaminophen 500 mg ▶ oxycodone hydro-chloride 7.5 mg	For moderate to moderately severe pain. Give 1–2 tablets q 4-6 hours. Maximum, 8 tablets in 24 hours.
Percocet 10/650 *CSS II*	▶ acetaminophen 650 mg ▶ oxycodone hydro-chloride 10 mg	For moderate to moderately severe pain. Give 1–2 tablets q 4-6 hours. Maximum, 6 tablets in 24 hours.
Percodan-Demi *CSS II*	▶ aspirin 325 mg ▶ oxycodone hydro-chloride 2.25 mg ▶ oxycodone tereph-thalate 0.19 mg	For moderate to moderately severe pain. Give 1–2 tablets q 6 hours. Maximum, 8 tablets in 24 hours.
Percodan, Roxiprin *CSS II*	▶ aspirin 325 mg ▶ oxycodone hydro-chloride 4.5 mg ▶ oxycodone tereph-thalate 0.38 mg	For moderate to moderately severe pain. Give 1 tablet q 6 hours. Maximum, 4 tablets in 24 hours.
Phenaphen/Codeine No. 3 *CSS III*	▶ acetaminophen 325 mg ▶ codeine phosphate 30 mg	For fever, mild to moderate pain. Give 1–2 tablets q 4 hours. Maximum, 12 tablets in 24 hours.
Phenaphen/Codeine No. 4 *CSS III*	▶ acetaminophen 325 mg ▶ codeine phosphate 60 mg	For fever, mild to moderate pain. Give 1 tablet q 4 hours. Maximum, 6 tablets in 24 hours.
Propoxyphene Napsylate/ Acetaminophen *CSS IV*	▶ acetaminophen 650 mg ▶ propoxyphene napsylate 100 mg	For mild to moderate pain. Give 1 tablet q 4 hours. Maximum, 6 tablets in 24 hours.
Roxicet *CSS II*	▶ acetaminophen 325 mg ▶ oxycodone hydro-chloride 5 mg	For moderate to moderately severe pain. Give 1–2 tablets q 4 hours. Maximum, 12 tablets in 24 hours.
Roxicet 5/500 *CSS II*	▶ acetaminophen 500 mg ▶ oxycodone hydro-chloride 5 mg	For moderate to moderately severe pain. Give 1–2 tablets q 4-6 hours. Maximum, 8 tablets in 24 hours.

◇ Available in Canada only

TRADE NAMES AND CONTROLLED SUBSTANCE SCHEDULE (CSS)	GENERIC DRUGS	INDICATIONS AND ADULT DOSAGES
Roxicet Oral Solution *CSS II*	▶ acetaminophen 325 mg ▶ oxycodone hydro-chloride 5 mg/5 ml	For moderate to moderately severe pain. Give 5–10 ml q 4-6 hours. Maximum, 60 ml in 24 hours.
Talacen *CSS IV*	▶ acetaminophen 650 mg ▶ pentazocine hydro-chloride 25 mg	For mild to moderate pain. Give 1 tablet q 4 hours. Maximum, 6 tablets in 24 hours.
Talwin Compound *CSS IV*	▶ aspirin 325 mg ▶ pentazocine hydro-chloride 12.5 mg	For moderate pain. Give 2 tablets q 6 hours. Maximum, 8 tablets in 24 hours.
Tylenol with Codeine No. 2 *CSS III*	▶ acetaminophen 300 mg ▶ codeine phosphate 15 mg	For fever, mild to moderate pain. Give 1–2 tablets q 4 hours. Maximum, 12 tablets in 24 hours.
Tylenol with Codeine No. 3 *CSS III*	▶ acetaminophen 300 mg ▶ codeine phosphate 30 mg	For fever, mild to moderate pain. Give 1–2 tablets q 4 hours. Maximum, 12 tablets in 24 hours.
Tylenol with Codeine No. 4 *CSS III*	▶ acetaminophen 300 mg ▶ codeine phosphate 60 mg	For fever, mild to moderate pain. Give 1 tablet q 4 hours. Maximum, 6 tablets in 24 hours.
Tylox *CSS II*	▶ acetaminophen 500 mg ▶ oxycodone hydro-chloride 5 mg	For moderate to moderately severe pain. Give 1–2 tablets q 4 hours. Maximum, 12 tablets in 24 hours.
Vicodin, Zydone *CSS III*	▶ acetaminophen 500 mg ▶ hydrocodone bitar-trate 5 mg	For moderate to moderately severe pain. Give 1–2 tablets q 4 hours. Maximum, 8 tablets in 24 hours.
Vicodin ES *CSS III*	▶ acetaminophen 750 mg ▶ hydrocodone bitar-trate 7.5 mg	For moderate to moderately severe pain. Give 1 tablet q 4–6 hours. Maximum, 5 tablets in 24 hours.

◇ Available in Canada only

Resources for pain management

Agency for Healthcare Research and Quality
Department of Health and Human Services
www.ahcpr.gov

American Academy of Hospice and Palliative Medicine
P.O. Box 14228
Gainesville, FL 32604-2288
www.aahpm.org

American Academy of Orofacial Pain
19 Mantua Rd.
Mount Royal, NJ 08061
856-423-3629
www.aaop.org

American Academy of Pain Management
13947 Mono Way #A
Sonora, CA 95370
209-533-9744
www.aapainmanage.org

American Academy of Pain Medicine
4700 W. Lake Ave.
Glenview, IL 60025
847-375-4731
www.painmed.org

American Alliance of Cancer Pain Initiatives
1300 University Ave., Room 4720
Madison, WI 53706
608-265-4013
www.aacpi.org

American Cancer Society
www.cancer.org

American Chronic Pain Association
P.O. Box 850
Rocklin, CA 95677
916-632-0922
www.theacpa.org

American Headache Society
19 Mantua Rd.
Mount Royal, NJ 08061
856-423-0043
www.ahsnet.org

American Pain Society
4700 W. Lake Ave.
Glenview, IL 60025
847-375-4715
www.ampainsoc.org

American Society of Addiction Medicine
4601 N. Park Ave., Arcade Suite 101
Chevy Chase, MD 20815
301-656-3920
www.asam.org

American Society of Pain Management Nurses
7794 Grow Dr.
Pensacola, FL 32514-7072
888-342-7766
www.aspmn.org

American Society of Regional Anesthesia and Pain Medicine
P.O. Box 11086
Richmond, VA 23230-1086
804-282-0010
www.asra.com

Arthritis Foundation
1330 W. Peachtree
Atlanta, GA 30309
800-283-7800
www.arthritis.org

Dannemiller Memorial Educational Foundation
12500 Network Blvd., Suite 101
San Antonio, TX 78249-3302
800-328-2308
www.pain.com

Hospice Foundation of America
2001 S St. NW, Suite 300
Washington, DC 20009
800-854-3402
www.hospicefoundation.org

International Association for the Study of Pain
909 N.E. 43rd St., Suite 306
Seattle, WA 98105-6020
206-547-6409
www.halcyon.com/iasp

Mayday Pain Project
www.painandhealth.org

National Cancer Institute
National Institutes of Health
cancernet.nci.nih.gov

National Center for Complementary and Alternative Medicine
National Institutes of Health
9000 Rockville Pike
Building 31, Room 5B-38
Bethesda, MD 20892
888-644-6226
nccam.nih.gov

National Foundation for the Treatment of Pain
1330 Skyline Dr. #21
Monterey, CA 93940
831-655-8812
www.paincare.org

National Headache Foundation
428 W. St. James Place, 2nd Floor
Chicago, IL 60614-2750
888-643-5552
www.headaches.org

National Hospice and Palliative Care Organization
1700 Diagonal Rd., Suite 300
Alexandria, VA 22314
703-837-1500
www.nho.org

North American Chronic Pain Association of Canada
150 Central Park Dr., Unit 105
Brampton, Ontario L6T 2T9
800-616-7246
www.chronicpaincanada.org

Pain-Aid Information Network
www.geocities.com/~paininfo

Reflex Sympathetic Dystrophy Syndrome Association
116 Haddon Ave., Suite D
Haddonfield, NJ 08033
856-795-8845
www.rsds.org

Sickle Cell Disease Association of America
200 Corporate Pointe, Suite 495
Culver City, CA 90230-7633
800-421-8453
www.sicklecelldisease.org

Society for Pain Practice Management
11111 Nall #202
Leawood, KS 66211
913-491-6451

Trigeminal Neuralgia Association
P.O. Box 340
Barnegat Light, NJ 08006
609-361-1014
www.tna-support.org

Vulvar Pain Foundation
P.O. Drawer 177
Graham, NC 27253
336-226-0704

World Health Organization
www.who.org

Suggested readings

Abram, S. and Haddox, J.D. *The Pain Clinic Manual.* Philadelphia: Lippincott Williams and Wilkins, 1999.

Angelucci, D., et al. "A pain mangement relief plan to improve patient care," *Dimensions in Critical Care Nursing* 18(4):30-34, July-August 1999.

Aronoff, G. *Evaluation and Treatment of Chronic Pain.* Philadelphia: Lippincott Williams and Wilkins, 1998.

Borsook, D., et al. *The Massachusetts General Hospital Handbook of Pain Management.* Philadelphia: Lippincott Williams and Wilkins, 1996.

Cousins, M. and Bridenbaugh. *Neural Blockade in Clinical Anesthesia and the Management of Pain.* Philadelphia: Lippincott Williams and Wilkins, 1997.

Expert Pain Management. Springhouse, Pa.: Springhouse Corp., 1997.

Guru, V. and Dubinsky, I. "The patient vs. caregiver perception of acute pain in the emergency department," *Journal of Emergency Medicine* 18(1):7-12, January 2000.

Kugelmann, R. "Complaining about chronic pain," *Social Science Medicine* 49(12):1663-76, December 1999.

Lefkowitz, M., et al. *A Practical Approach to Pain Management.* Philadelphia: Lippincott Williams and Wilkins, 1996.

Loeser, J., et al. *Bonica's Management of Pain.* Philadelphia: Lippincott Williams and Wilkins, 2000.

Loitman, J. "Pain management: beyond pharmacology to acupuncture and hypnosis," *JAMA* 283(1):118-19, January 2000.

Morton, N. "Prevention and control of pain in children," *Journal of British Anesthesia* 83(1):118-29, July 1999.

Novarro, L. "Pain Management. No-pain gain," *Hospital Health Network* 73(12):17-18, December 1999.

Nursing2001 Drug Handbook. Springhouse, Pa.: Springhouse Corp., 2001.

Otis, J. and McGeeney, B. "Managing Pain in the Elderly," *Clinical Geriatrics* 8(1):48+, 2000.

Pargeon, K. and Hailey, B. "Barriers to effective cancer pain management: a review of the literature," *Journal of Pain Symptom Management* 18(5):358-68, November 1999.

Physician's Drug Handbook, 9th edition. Springhouse, Pa.: Springhouse Corp., 2001.

Portenoy, R and Frager, G. "Pain management: pharmacological approaches," *Cancer Treatment Research* 100:1-29, 1999.

Rhiner, M. and Kedziera, P. "Managing breakthrough cancer pain: a new approach," *Home Healthcare Nurse* 17(6 Suppl):suppl 1-15, June 1999.

Senecal, S. "Pain management in wound care," *Nursing Clinics of North America* 34(4):847-60, December 1999.

Waldman, S. *Atlas of Intervention Pain Management.* Philadelphia: W.B. Saunders Co., 1998.

Index

---

t refers to a table.

---

t refers to a table.

---

t refers to a table.